THERAPEUTIC RADIOLOGY

THERAPEUTIC RADIOLOGY

NEW DIRECTIONS IN THERAPY

Edited by

Carl M. Mansfield, M.D., F.A.C.R.
Professor and Chairman
Department of Radiation Therapy
University of Kansas Medical Center
Kansas City, Kansas
Chairman, Department of Radiation Therapy
Menorah Medical Center
Kansas City, Missouri
Consultant, Veterans Administration Hospital
Kansas City, Missouri

MEDICAL EXAMINATION PUBLISHING CO., INC.
an Excerpta Medica company

Therapeutic radiology.

(New directions in therapy)
Bibliography: p.
Includes index.
1. Radiotherapy. I. Mansfield, Carl M.
II. Series. [DNLM: 1. Neoplasms--Radiotherapy.
QZ 269 M287t]
RM847.T46 1982 616.99'40642 82-12473
ISBN 0-87488-694-5

MEDICAL EXAMINATION PUBLISHING CO., INC.
an Excerpta Medica company
3003 New Hyde Park Road
New Hyde Park, New York

Printed in the United States of America

To our families for their
patience and support

Contents

Contributors

SOLOMON BATNITZKY, M.D., Professor, Department of Diagnostic Radiology, Chief Section of Neuroradiology, Kansas University Medical Center, 39th and Rainbow Boulevard, Kansas City, Kansas

ROGER J. BERRY, M.D., D. Phil., F.R.C.R., Professor, Department of Oncology, Meyerstein Institute of Radiotherapy and Oncology, The Middlesex Hospital Medical School, London, England

FLORENCE C.H. CHU, M.D., F.A.C.R., Chairman, Department of Radiation Therapy, Memorial Sloan-Kettering Cancer Center, 1275 York Avenue; Professor of Radiology, Cornell University Medical Center, New York, New York

BARBARA F. DANOFF, M.D., Associate Professor, Department of Radiation Therapy, Hospital of the University of Pennsylvania, 3400 Spruce Street, Philadelphia, Pennsylvania

STANLEY DISCHE, M.D., F.R.C.R., Marie Curie Research Wing for Oncology, Regional Radiotherapy Center, Mount Vernon Hospital, Northwood, Middlesex, England

SAMUEL J. DWYER, III, Ph.D., Professor, Director, Division of Diagnostic Imaging, Radiological Sciences, Department of Diagnostic Radiology, Kansas University Medical Center, Kansas City, Kansas

JOHN T. FAZEKAS, M.D., Associate Professor, Department of Radiation Therapy, Booth Memorial Medical Center, Flushing, New York

FREDERICK W. GEORGE, III, M.D., F.A.C.R., Professor, Department of Radiation Medicine, University of Southern California School of Medicine, 2025 Zonal Avenue, Los Angeles, California

WALTER G. GUNN, M.D., J.D., Division of Therapeutic Radiology, The Medical College of Wisconsin, 8700 West Wisconsin Avenue, Milwaukee, Wisconsin

GEORGE A. HIGGINS, M.D., F.A.C.S., Chief Surgical Service, Veterans Administration Medical Center; Professor of Surgery, Georgetown University Medical Center, Washington, D.C.

A.M. JELLIFFE, M.D., B.S., F.R.C.P., F.R.C.R., Chairman, Meyerstein Institute of Radiotherapy and Oncology, The Middlesex Hospital; Consultant Radiotherapist and Oncologist, Mount Vernon Hospital; Convener, British National Lymphoma Investigations, London England

MORTON M. KLIGERMAN, M.D., F.A.C.R., Professor, Department of Radiation Therapy, University of Pennsylvania Medical School, Philadelphia, Pennsylvania

EDWARD A. KNAPP, Ph.D., Division Leader, Accelerator Technology Division, Los Alamos National Laboratory, Albuquerque, New Mexico

H.E. LAMBERT, M.B., B.S., M.R.C.O.G., F.R.C.R., Consultant Radiotherapist, Hammersmith Hospital, Ducane Road, London, England

KYO RAK LEE, M.D., Professor, Department of Diagnostic Radiology, Kansas University Medical Center, 39th and Rainbow Boulevard, Kansas City, Kansas

ERROL LEVINE, M.D., Professor, Department of Diagnostic Radiology, Kansas University Medical Center, 39th and Rainbow Boulevard, Kansas City, Kansas

NABIL F. MAKLAD, M.D., Professor, Department of Diagnostic Radiology, University of Texas Health Science Center and Medical School, Houston, Texas

CARL M. MANSFIELD, M.D., F.A.C.R., Professor and Chairman, Department of Radiation Therapy, Kansas University Medical Center, 39th and Rainbow Boulevard, Kansas City, Kansas; Chairman, Department of Radiation Therapy, Menorah Medical Center; Consultant, Kansas City Veterans Administration Hospital, Kansas City, Missouri

EASHWER K. REDDY, M.D., Associate Professor, Department of Radiation Therapy, Kansas University Medical Center, 39th and Rainbow Boulevard, Kansas City, Kansas

BERNARD ROSWIT, M.D., F.A.C.R., Chief, Regional Veterans Administration Radiotherapy Center, Veterans Administration Medical Center, Bronx, New York; Professor, Radiotherapy, Mount Sinai Medical School, New York, New York

MARGARET SNELLING, M.D., M.B., B.S., F.R.C.P., F.R.C.S., F.R.C.R., Department of Radiotherapy, Meyerstein Institute of Radiotherapy and Oncology, The Middlesex Hospital, London, England

RONALD L. STEPHENS, M.D., Professor, Director of Clinical Oncology, Department of Medicine, Kansas University Medical Center, 39th and Rainbow Boulevard, Kansas City, Kansas

C.C. WANG, M.D., F.A.C.R., Professor of Radiation Therapy, Harvard Medical School; Radiation Therapist and Head, Division of Clinical Services, Department of Radiation Medicine, Massachusetts General Hospital, Boston, Massachusetts

BRIGIT VAN DER WERF-MESSING, M.D., Rotterdamsch Radio-Therapeutisch Institute, Groene Hilledijk 301, 3075 EA, Rotterdam, The Netherlands

Preface

In the not too distant past the radiotherapist was the individual who tended to have the broadest understanding of most malignant diseases and their characteristics in terms of their etiology, presentation, methcds of spread, best treatment, and ultimate outcome. At that time, there were few surgical oncologists and essentially no medical oncologists. The radiotherapist did not have to look beyond his specialty when making treatment decisions.

Because of the work of basic and clinical researchers, significant changes in the management of the cancer patient have evolved in recent years. The most notable has been the use of systemic therapy. Thus, the radiotherapist (or radiation oncologist) must have a grasp and understanding of the philosophy and rationale of all the oncologic specialties.

This book is written basically for the practicing radiotherapist. The intent is to reflect the recent advances and some of the currently accepted diagnostic and therapeutic approaches to the treatment of malignancies that are amenable to radiotherapy.

notice

The editor, authors, and the publisher of this book have made every effort to ensure that all therapeutic modalities that are recommended are in accordance with accepted standards at the time of publication.

The drugs specified within this book may not have specific approval by the Food and Drug Administration in regard to the indications and dosages that are recommended by the editor and authors. The manufacturer's package insert is the best source of current prescribing information.

chapter 1

BASIC CONCEPTS IN RADIOBIOLOGY: A REVIEW

R. J. Berry, M.D., D. Phil.

That ionizing radiation had biological effects, capable of application for either good or harm, was recognized very early after the discovery of x-rays by Roentgen. Many early radiation workers received large exposures, both localized and total body, and clinical syndromes such as "radiation dermatitis" and anemia were recognized within the first months of the x-ray era. It was soon found that x-rays and the emanations from radium were capable of curing skin malignancies and in affecting other more unpleasant but superficial malignancies, such as those of the mouth and throat. Within a few years some fundamental radiobiological principles had been established, although not always recognized as such. Schwarz (34), in 1909, had shown by the simple expedient of placing a vacuum cup on the arm of a subject that the response to irradiation was reduced compared to that in skin where the blood flowed freely - now recognized as due to the oxygen effect. Regaud and Blanc (33) showed in the rat testis that mitotic activity was the cellular function most sensitive to interruption by the effect of ionizing radiation. Bergonie and Tribondeau (4), largely from observations, elucidated the "law" that tissues with the most active mitotic future before them were the most sensitive to the effect of ionizing radiation. By the 1920s, studies of relatively simple biological systems such as ascaris eggs were yielding dose-response relationships, and the "dose" portion of the expression was first quantified successfully at the International Congress of Radiology of 1928 with the introduction and specification of the Roentgen as a unit of radiation exposure. In the late 1930s and early 1940s there was a remarkable flowering of biophysical ideas relatively simultaneously around Lea (28) at Cambridge and Timofeev-Ressovsky and Zimmer (39) and Zimmer (45) in Russia and Germany. Dessauer (14) in the 1920s had initiated the suggestion that the form of the radiation dose-effect curve was due to absorption of radiation as quanta following Poisson statistics. Although Dessauer's "point heat" mechanism for radiation damage proved indefensible, the idea that specific biological targets existed within cells and that ionizing radiation inactivated these targets by physical processes opened new vistas in understanding molecular and cellular radiation biology. In the 1940s the detonation of the first nuclear weapons awakened a wider public need to understand the hazards of total-body radiation exposure, and led to animal experimentation in which radiosensitive tissues and their underlying cell renewal systems began to be understood. In the 1950s a momentous step was the development by Puck and Marcus (31) of methodology for the culture of single mammalian cells in vitro and their growth into colonies which could be seen and scored with the naked eye, so that for the first time the survival of cell reproductive capacity could be measured after exposure to radiation. Shortly thereafter, pioneering studies by Hewitt and Wilson (24), Till and McCulloch (38), and Withers and colleagues (42-44), respectively, made it possible to assess cell reproductive capacity in vivo after radiation exposure to tumors, normal hemopoietic cells, and the stem cells of organized epithelia. Since then, mammalian radiobiology has progressed far in understanding the mechanism of the oxygen effect: the protective action of hypoxia against radiation damage, the effects of radiation ionization density, of radiation dose rate, and the effects of radiation on complex cell populations in normal tissues and tumors.

SURVIVAL OF CELL REPRODUCTIVE CAPACITY

The shape of curves for the survival of cell reproductive capacity for all mammalian cells studied so far approximates to a common shape, although there are differences in detail between cells of different origins. As shown in Fig. 1, displayed in a semilog plot, there is a "shoulder" region of relatively minimal cell killing at low radiation doses, followed by a straight line (or a near straight line) portion where reduction in survival of cell reproductive capacity per additional increment of radiation dose is greater than for cells with no prior radiation exposure. Using the biological model of <u>targets</u> or <u>hits</u>, the final slope of the survival curve represents the average radiosensitivity of the vulnerable sites within the cell, and the magnitude of the shoulder in a loose way represents the multiplicity of individual damaging events which need to be accumulated within the cell before one further ionizing event proves lethal. Continuously downbending curves have been analyzed by another model in which cell killing is related to two separate functions of dose, one increasing linearly and the other as a higher (second) power of the dose. This fits the preconceived notion that cell lethality is related to discernible damage to the chromosomes, for which a similar dose-squared response

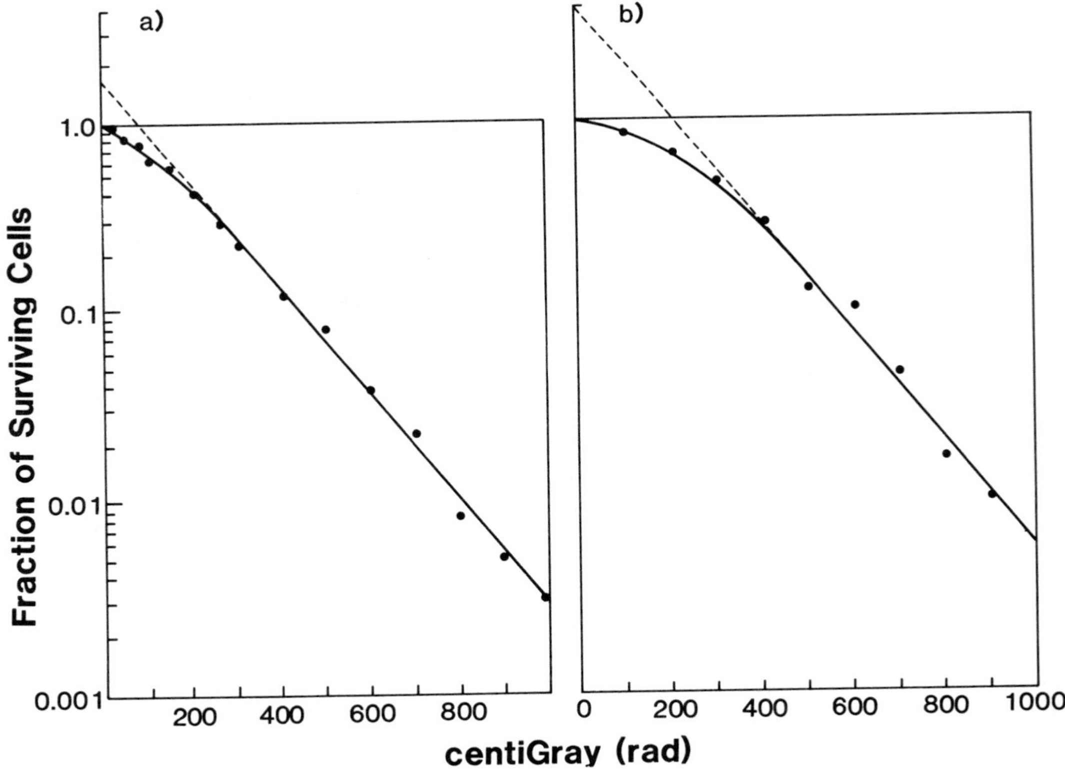

Figure 1. Survival of reproductive capacity of two lines of mammalian cells cultured and irradiated in vitro. A: HeLa S-3_{oxf} of human origin, derived from a carcinoma of the cervix. B: Strain L_{oxf} murine origin, derived from dermal fibroblasts. (Redrawn from Ref. 5.)

is seen, but this seems a rather gross oversimplification of some rather complex biology between the absorption of ionization damage and the expression of cell death (12).

Mammalian cells are not uniformly radiosensitive at all phases of their cell cycle. Terasima and Tolmach (36) in 1963 produced synchronous populations of HeLa cells by harvesting cells in mitosis, replating them in culture, and challenging them with radiation exposure at subsequent times. Sinclair and Morton (35), and others used other and more sophisticated harvesting techniques to produce populations of cells uniformly in one part of the cell cycle, and also studied the change in their response to ionizing radiation as a function of cell cycle phase. Both shoulder and slope alter with position in cell cycle. For mitotic cells the curve appears to be steepest and the shoulder smallest for cells at the end of their DNA synthesis period (late S) the survival curve is least steep and the shoulder is maximally large. Those cells with a long "gap" period between the completion of mitosis and the onset of DNA synthesis (long G1) have a phase of radioresistance with a shallow survival curve and a large shoulder, while at the transition between the end of this gap (G1) and DNA synthesis there is a brief phase of maximal radiosensitivity and minimum shoulder on the survival curve. The post-DNA synthetic gap period until the next mitosis (G2) can be either a sensitive or a resistant phase, depending on the cell type. The sensitivity of tissues to single and fractionated radiation doses will depend on the distribution of cells through the various phases of the cell cycle and the change in this distribution in response to previous treatment.

RECOVERY FROM SUBLETHAL AND POTENTIALLY LETHAL RADIATION DAMAGE

In the 1960s Elkind and Sutton (15) showed that the shoulder on the dose-survival curve for mammalian cells represented not only accumulation of sublethal ionization damage, but that this damage could be rapidly repaired. The results of the series of experiments under which the same total radiation dose was delivered in two fractions at varying intervals showed that even within the first 15-20 min a significant portion of this sublethal damage had been "undone" by the intracellular repair mechanisms. This typical two-dose survival curve often had a "dip" after an initial rise (Fig. 2), and it was suggested that because populations of cells were mixed in their radiosensitivity, depending upon their place in the cell cycle, the initial radiation exposure produced a disproportionately selected population weighted by those cells in the more resistant phases of the cell cycle. As they subsequently progressed around the cell cycle, the second radiation dose could find them parasynchronously in more sensitive phases of the cell cycle. This explanation was confirmed by ourselves, by showing that the presence of this dip depended on the size of the first radiation dose (Fig. 2). Cells subjected to very large first radiation doses, although capable of repair of sublethal damage, were incapable of further progression around the cell cycle and the two-dose survival curve showed no subsequent dip. In vivo experiments showed that at least two other repair mechanisms exist in mammalian cells. First, repair of potentially lethal damage (30) was shown by the difference between survival of tumor cells harvested immediately after irradiation for assay of survival of their reproductive capacity by the Hewitt serial-dilution method with the survival of otherwise identical tumor cells allowed to remain in their irradiated environment for periods of hours before being withdrawn for assay. The stored cells showed marked increases in survival. This finding was analogous to the earlier demonstration in bacteria and later in vitro in mammalian cells that cells held after a single irradiation in relatively non-nutrient

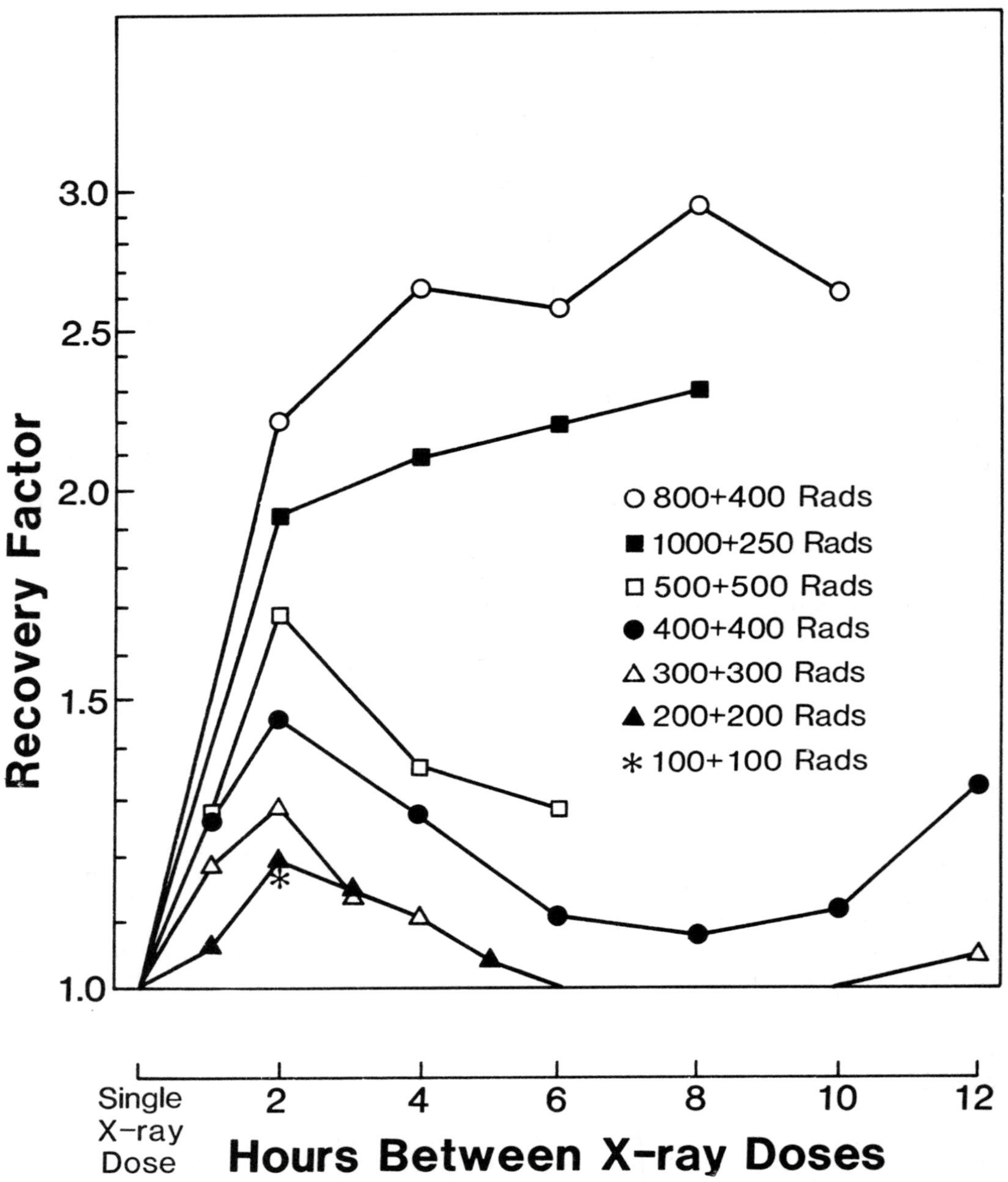

Figure 2. Two-dose recovery curves for well-oxygenated HeLa S-3_{oxf}. cells in vitro after first x-ray doses of 100-1000 CentiGray (rad). Incubation between x-ray doses is at 37°C. (From Ref. 6.)

media for a period of time before plating in an enriched medium which would support colony growth showed higher overall survival after irradiation than did cells plated immediately into full-growth media. A second additional form of repair, termed slow repair, so far has been demonstrated unambiguously only in the rodent lung (17) and has a time scale of weeks or months compared to the rapid time scale of the other two forms of repair. Simply, it is an excess of survival of irradiated cells which cannot be explained by either of the other intracellular repair mechanisms or by cell proliferation. Lajtha and Oliver (26) predicted that intracellular repair would also take place during protracted irradiation, so that radiations delivered at low dose rates would be less effective rad for rad in killing remaining cells. This was first demonstrated in vivo in murine leukemic cells by Berry and Cohen (9) and confirmed in vitro in human tumor cells by Hall (21). As long as the overall length of irradiation was sufficient to allow for repair of sublethal and potentially lethal damage to take place, decreasing radiation dose rates were less and less effective, until a plateau was reached in the region of 1-5 rads/hr.

THE OXYGEN EFFECT

As has already been indicated, it was suspected in the early days of radiation research that in some way the interruption of blood flow protected against radiation damage. Following on earlier studies with lower organisms L. H. Gray (20) and his group began in the 1950s to examine systematically the mechanism of this hypoxic protection called conversely the oxygen effect - the extra effect of radiation delivered in the presence of oxygen compared with its absence. In a variety of mammalian systems, the presence of oxygen proved to be dose modifying. In its absence 2.5-3 times the radiation dose was required to achieve the same amount of cell killing. It was shown that relatively small amounts of oxygen rapidly increased the sensitivity from its minimum level towards full radiosensitivity (Fig. 3). For radiations other than x-rays or gamma rays, the magnitude of hypoxic protection was reduced significantly for those radiations with higher ionization densities (higher LET). This is discussed further in the next section. Thomlinson and Gray (37) showed by histological analysis of human tumors that the distance

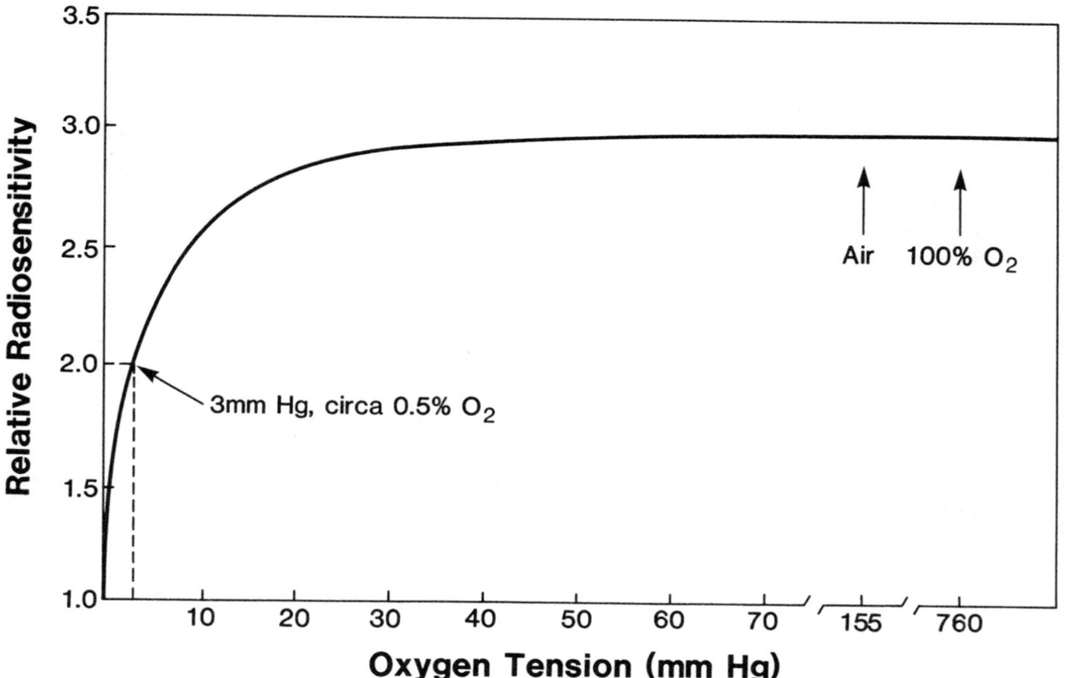

Figure 3. Relative radiosensitivity to x- or gamma radiation as a function of oxygen tension. This curve does not represent any specific experimental data but is a composite of multiple experimental results obtained in microorganisms, eukaryotes, and mammalian cells. (Redrawn from Ref. 22.)

between a blood vessel and the onset of necrosis in rapidly growing human tumors was in close agreement with that predicted by the rate at which oxygen is consumed by respiring tissue. Necrosis began very shortly beyond the maximum diffusion distance of oxygen. This provided an explanation for the apparent radioresistance of some tumors. Fowler and his colleagues (19) showed that at least some rodent tumors were capable of rapid reoxygenation. As the tumor shrank following a first radiation dose, cells previously hypoxic because of their distance from a blood vessel became reoxygenated within 1 to several days as the tumor shrank, and the blood supply once again became sufficient to support the metabolism of the remaining tumor cells. Van Putten (32) showed that some tumors show no such reoxygenation. Adams (1) and his group began a search for chemical compounds which would mimic the radiosensitizing effect of oxygen but which were not actively metabolized by tissue so that they would reach by simple diffusion those tissues which were hypoxic by virtue of their distance from the vessels. They showed that a number of electron-affinic compounds were capable of just this action and that, although nontoxic to aerated cells, they were capable of increasing the cell killing among hypoxic cells to levels approaching those when oxygen was present, as well as having a selective cytotoxicity against hypoxic tumor cells. These compounds are only just reaching the stage of clinical trial and may remain an important growing edge of the interface between clinical radiobiology and radiotherapy.

RADIATION IONIZATION DENSITY (LET)

As early as the 1930s it was realized that radiations of different ionization densities had both quantitatively and qualitatively different biological effects. The use of particle accelerators and the advent of nuclear weapons acted as powerful stimuli to understanding the biological effects on mammalian systems of radiations other than x- or gamma rays. At the cellular level, two groups reported almost simultaneously the effect of radiation ionization density upon the survival of cell reproductive capacity in mammalian cells assessed either in vitro (3) or in vivo (8). We have seen that relatively small doses of x- or gamma rays are inefficient in causing cell reproductive death, in that damage has to be accumulated before one additional ionizing event is lethal. This is reflected in the shoulder on the survival curve. For radiations of high ionization densities, measured as linear energy transfer (LET) in excess of 100 KeV/μm, the dose-response curve for cell reproductive capacity is simply exponential (Fig. 4). In addition, as LET increases from the low values for x- or gamma rays, mean cell killing efficiency increases so that the slope of the survival curve becomes steeper. However, once again above 100-200 KeV/μm (depending on the type of cell being irradiated) the deposition of energy per individual ionizing event exceeds that necessary to cause reproductive death of the cell and ionization is "wasted." For radiations of very high ionization density, although the survival curve remains exponential, the slope of survival curve again becomes shallower (Fig. 4). The effectiveness of different ionizing radiations is usually quoted on the basis of relative biological effectiveness (RBE), the ratio of doses to produce a comparable biological effect. Unlike the oxygen enhancement ratio, RBE is a strong function both of the biological end-point chosen and of the size of the radiation dose used. For all densely ionizing radiations, the change in the shape of the survival curve means that the relative biological effectiveness increases as the radiation dose decreases. In addition, because a smaller shoulder on the survival curve reflects not only less need to accumulate damage before one additional ionizing event proves lethal, but may also reflect decreased repair of sublethal radiation damage after exposure to densely ionizing radiations. The RBE for densely ionizing radiations at low dose rates is considerably higher than that for the same radiation delivered acutely. RBE rises as the dose rate

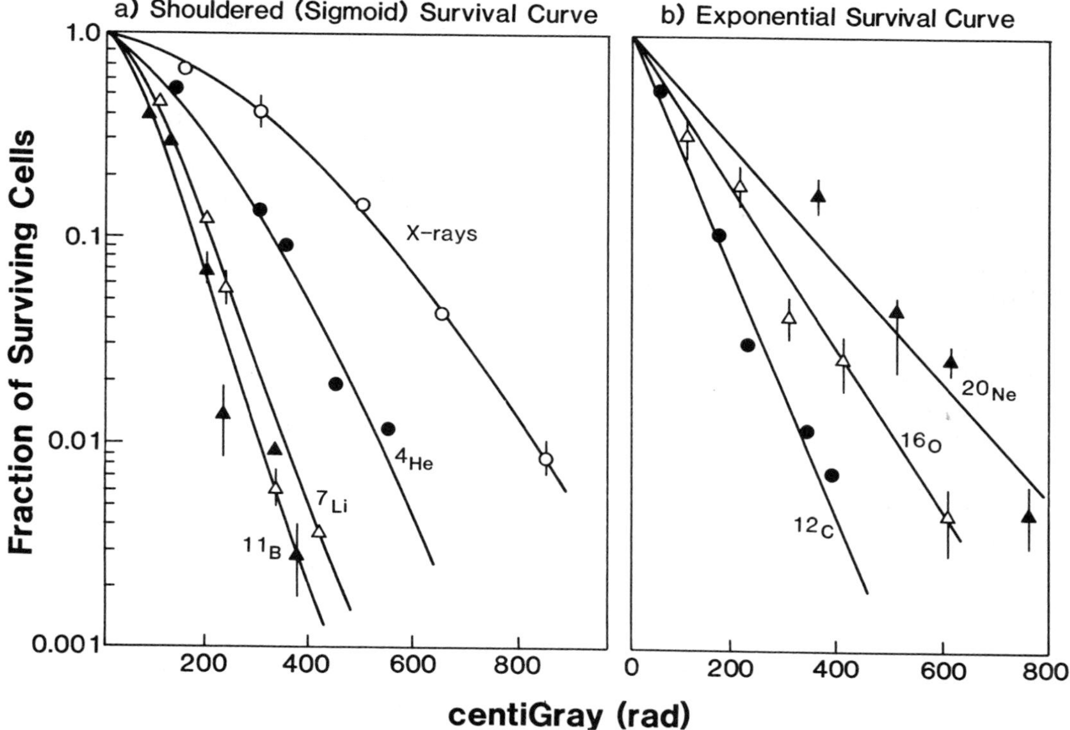

Figure 4. Survival of human kidney-derived T-1 cells irradiated in vitro with x-rays or beams of accelerated charged particles of increasing mass from ^{4}He to ^{20}Ne with correspondingly increasing ionization density. As the ionization density increases, the shoulder on the survival curve becomes smaller and the curve becomes steeper; at very high ionization densities, the survival curve is exponential (no shoulder) and becomes more shallow because of "overkill" from wasted ionization within the sensitive target. (Data redrawn from Ref. 40.)

falls, once again to limiting values of the order of approximately 1 rad/hr. The relative biological effectiveness of densely ionizing radiations also rises as a total acute dose is delivered in multiple fractions. This takes place for the same reason as the increasing RBE with low dose rate; there is repair between fractions of the damage done by sparsely ionizing x- or gamma rays, but little or no repair of the damage done by the more densely ionizing radiations.

High LET radiations are also less susceptible to modification of their lethal effects by the presence or absence of other physiochemical modifiers such as oxygen. Although the oxygen enhancement ratio is a function of radiation ionization density, for all those densely ionizing radiations being considered for use in clinical radiotherapy (e.g., fast neutrons, heavy charged particles, negative pi-mesons), the amount of protection afforded by hypoxia is significantly less than that against sparsely ionizing x- or gamma rays. For the fast neutrons of approximately 8 MeV from the Hammersmith cyclotron on which the greatest volume of clinical experience has been gained, the Oxygen Enhancement Ratio (OER) value of about 1.5 compares favorably with the OER for x- or gamma rays of 2.5-3 when considering treatment of hypoxic tumor cells through well-oxygenated normal tissues.

THE RADIOBIOLOGY OF RADIATION PROTECTION: HAZARDS TO POPULATIONS

As has already been noted, the harmful effects of partial and whole-body exposure to ionizing radiation were tragically demonstrated in many of the earlier radiation workers. The deaths of early radiologists such as Ironside Bruce led to the demand that x-rays should be withdrawn from medical use and to formation of the First International Congress of Radiology in London in 1928, at which a unit of radiation exposure was satisfactorily defined for the first time. The detonation of the first nuclear weapons lent a far greater urgency to understanding both the acute and late effects of radiation exposure. To a first approximation, all total-body exposure can be regarded as life-shortening, the magnitude of the shortening depending on the size of the radiation dose. Natural background radiation, largely from cosmic rays and from the natural radioactivity of soil, rock, and building materials, exposes us all to approximately 100-200 mrem (1-2 mSv) annually, the value being higher in high latitudes. Medical uses of ionizing radiations, particularly diagnostic x-rays, contribute a further approximate 70 mrem (0.7 mSv) per annum in the USA, although somewhat less in the UK, while the contributions from the atmospheric testing of nuclear weapons before 1961 and the current contribution from the nuclear power industry are frankly trivial (approximately 4 and 0.005 mrem/yr, respectively).

The response to acute total-body radiation exposure can be divided into four major syndromes, three of which are acutely lethal (41). Radiation doses in excess of several thousand rads tens of Grays (Gy) results in death within hours from direct interference with the central nervous system function, and a clinical picture of severe intractable vomiting, confusion, coma, and death. Because of the rapidity of these events there are no histopathological changes of significance. Exposures in the range 1000 to 3-4,000 rads (10-40 Gy) damage the gastrointestinal tract and result in death within days. The most rapidly renewing tissue in the body, the epithelium lining the small intestine, requires constant replacement of new cells to maintain the complex villous structure. Cells born in the dividing zone at the base of the crypts migrate up these crypts and on to the villi to be shed from the tip of the villus into the intestinal contents some 4 days later. Even the transient interruption of cell proliferation in the crypts results in a lack of new cells to cover the villi, and the villi respond by shortening. The reduction in effective surface area of the small intestine for fluid absorption results in the symptoms of gastrointestinal damage, diarrhea, and dehydration. If by about day 4 proliferation of crypt cells has not restarted, the villi can shorten no further once they are flat and areas develop where no epithelial cover exists. There is thus no barrier to the passage of body fluid out and of overwhelming infection in, and the animal (or man) dies rapidly of overwhelming dehydration and infection. Only with radiation doses below that at which the gut lining will be preserved is survival possible from total-body radiation exposure. For man these doses are in the region below approximately 1000 rads (10 Gy). The most sensitive limiting tissue system is hemopoiesis. Red blood cells have a peripheral lifetime of about 3 months and are essentially unaffected unless there is gross bleeding, but both white cells and platelets require replenishment in 2-3 weeks, and failure of surviving hemopoietic stem cells to produce sufficient differentiated end-products results in a deficit of white cells and platelets which leads to the clinical syndrome of lack of resistance to infection, bleeding, and death. This latter syndrome can to some extent be protected against by early initiation of cell proliferation (stimulation by bleeding, protein stimuli such as inoculation for typhoid and paratyphoid A/B, TAB , etc.) and by isolation of the patient from the environmental hazard (reverse barrier nursing, sterilization of the gut flora, a padded environment to protect against injury leading to bleeding). The fourth acute radiation syndrome is the rapid interphase cell death in lymphocytes which allows a semiquantitative measure of radiation dose to be made from examination of the blood of accidentally exposed casualties. After surviving these acute radiation hazards, longer-term somatic and genetic hazards are likely to occur. Of the somatic hazards there are the dose-related hazards such as radiation induction of leukemia (lead time 3-10 years) and solid tumors (latent period in excess of 25 years) and the nonstochastic (nondose-related) hazards such as nonspecific life-shortening. This latter has been demonstrated in animals, but never in irradiated populations in man. Irradiation of the fetus can be regarded as somatic damage because the greatest concern is for abnormalities produced in that individual (childhood leukemia, failures of organogenesis, etc.). True genetic hazards tend to be largely self-limiting, because if sufficient radiation damage is accumulative to produce a potentially heritable, unwanted genetic change, the same amount of damage may well have rendered the cell reproductively inert so that the defect cannot be passed on.

A large body of data has been collected from actual exposure of man upon which our best estimates of radiation hazards to populations are based (2). These data have come from many sources, starting with the pioneer radiation workers, the radium dial painters, patients treated for ankylosing spondylitis, children treated with radiation for ringworm or enlarged thymus, uranium miners, women with tuberculosis exposed to repeated fluoroscopies to monitor iatrogenic pneumothorax, and to the survivors of the Hiroshima and Nagasaki nuclear weapons attack. From all these groups dose-risk estimates for late radiation somatic effects on man have been accumulated. For few environmental carcinogens do we have such a large and relevant body of risk data.

IMPLICATIONS FOR RADIOTHERAPY: UNANSWERED QUESTIONS

Does Hypoxia Matter?

We have seen that rodent tumors clearly do contain a significant proportion of hypoxic cells, and all evidence suggests that the human tumors also contain large numbers of radiobiologically hypoxic cells which could well render them resistant to the effects of conventional x- or gamma ray radiotherapy. Positive evidence for this was suggested by Churchill-Davidson et al. (13) and Van den Brenk et al. (10) pioneering studies of the irradiation of human tumors in hyperbaric oxygen, although these studies were criticized in that the former was not randomized, and the latter compared air or oxygen environment for a reduced fractionation schedule which was felt to be less than optimal conventional radiotherapy. Henk et al. (23) confirmed that even when compared against conventionally fractionated radiotherapy delivered in air, irradiation of head and neck tumors in hyperbaric oxygen produced higher tumor local control rates for comparable normal tissue damage. However, other studies of the use of hyperbaric oxygen in tumors of the uterine cervix and bladder failed to show any advantage for hyperbaric oxygen and gave evidence of increased normal tissue damage – all normal tissues are not uniformly oxygenated. The demonstration by Fowler, Thomlinson and Howes (19) of reoxygenation in rodent tumors suggests that success of conventional fractionated radiotherapy might be due in part to overcoming the hypoxic tumor cell problem by this method. The increased tumor local control seen in head and neck tumors irradiated with fast neutrons by Catterall and Bewley (11) may also in part owe success to the reduced hypoxic protection against this densely ionizing radiation. However, the advent of clinically usable selective sensitizers of hypoxic cells may at long last answer this question. If the hypoxic sensitizers, delivered in adequate doses, fail to improve tumor local control at a comparable level of damage to limiting normal tissues, the hypoxic tumor cell can be finally excluded as a major cause of failure in a local control of human tumors by radiotherapy.

Is Repair Important?

From the early misinterpretation of Regaud and Blanc's (33) data on the irradiation of the testis, when ablation of mitoses in the normal testis without subsequent necrosis of the overlying scrotal skin could only be achieved by fractionated dose rather than single radiation doses, fractionated radiotherapy has been the standard mode of treatment. A radiobiological mystique gradually arose, suggesting that tumors had a lower overall repair capacity than did normal tissues, so that the greater the dose fractionation, the greater the net advantage to the normal tissue. Objective testing of this dogma has produced mixed results, however, and many tumors have been shown to have capacity for repair of both sublethal and potentially lethal damage comparable to that of most normal tissues. Certainly there is no all-or-none difference between tumors and normal tissues, and the capacity for repair may well be modified by changes in the distribution of the surviving population through the cell cycle (cf. Survival of Cell Reproductive Capacity, this chapter).

Response of Limiting Normal Tissues: The Therapeutic Ratio

Radiotherapy is usually delivered to the normal tissue tolerance level, determined by individual radiotherapists. The dose to the tumor is largely incidental. As total radiation dose rises, so the chance of rendering the last tumor cell reproductively inert increases (Fig. 5). However, the risk of normal tissue damage also rises with increasing radiation dose, and it is the individual radiotherapist who decides the risk of unacceptable late complications in normal tissues which he will accept as "tolerance." In the days of orthovoltage radiotherapy the tolerance of skin was the limiting normal tissue. With the advent of supervoltage radiotherapy and consequent skin sparing, the most common limiting damage is severe fibrosis in the subcutaneous tissue, unless other and more sensitive organs intrude into the necessary volume of high radiation dose. The mechanism of this late subcutaneous fibrosis, and of much late damage in other tissues is now thought to be vascular injury (25,27). In the acute phase, fluid leakage occurs from the vessels, intravascular proteins leak into surrounding tissues, and while albumin is quickly reabsorbed, fibrinogen is converted to fibrin which remains in the interstitial tissues. Later, when damage to the vessels themselves is recognized and proliferation of surviving endothelial-intimal cells begins, localized vascular obstructions are formed before the mature cells can migrate away down the vessel. This obstruction causes secondary tissue hypoxia and accelerated development of fibrosis.

From clinical observations of normal tissue tolerance and of the doses required for cure of similar tumors, Ellis (16) proposed an empirical formula relating, by a "nominal standard dose," courses of radiotherapy given in different numbers of fractions over different overall times. More recent clinical and animal studies have been directed toward examing in detail the change in normal tissue tolerance with dose fractionation. It has become clear that with reduction in total number of fractions and overall time, there is an increase in the risk of fibrosis following doses of radiation which do not produce acutely limiting early

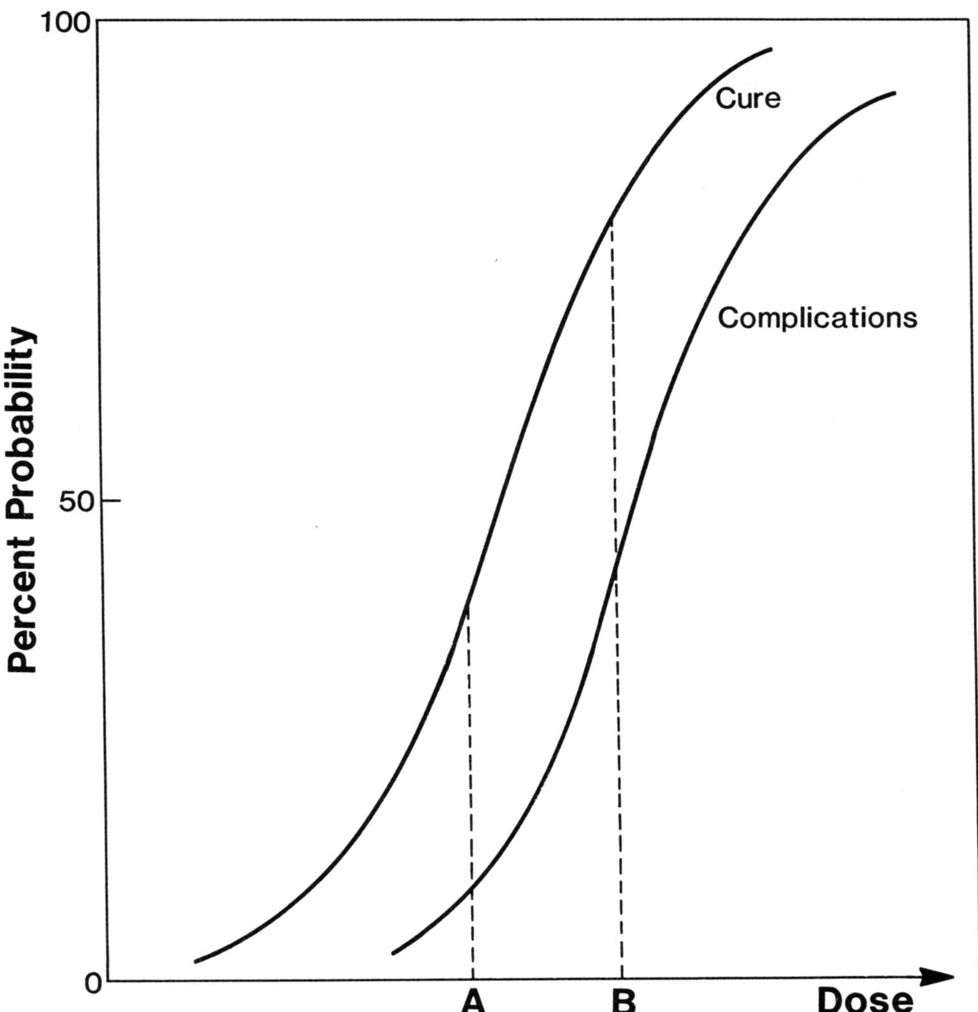

Figure 5. Relationship between radiation dose and probability of tumor cure and late complication. Dose A is associated with a modest probability of cure and a low probability of complication; a small increase in dose (from A to B) might result in a higher cure rate, but only at the expense of a much higher complication rate. Every radiotherapist defines his own maximum acceptable complication rate, which in turn defines the probability that he will achieve tumor cure in a given site.

reactions. These studies provide further justification for the convention of fractionated radiotherapy and need to be extended further into the realms of unorthodox dose fractionation before such techniques are more widely and uncritically used in human cancer radiotherapy.

Possible Combinations of Radiotherapy and Chemotherapy: Have We Gained Anything?

Studies in the early 1960s showed that a number of cytotoxic agents used in cancer chemotherapy also appeared to be effective sensitizers to subsequent killing of tumor cells by x- or gamma rays. On the logical supposition that the cytotoxic agent would deal with any microscopic dissemination of the disease, while at the same time enhancing the local radiation response, a wave of enthusiasm led to the widespread use of combination treatment of this sort in the early 1960s. Unfortunately, the clinical results failed to bear out the optimism shown. Friedman (8) was the first to voice the caveat "combination therapy should save lives not rads." Increased tumor response seen in the combined use of such drugs as methotrexate and radiotherapy was mirrored by increased normal tissue response, which required reduction in the total radiation dose used. Overall tumor control rates remained remarkably similar. The therapeutic ratio, the margin between acceptable damage to normal tissue and tumor local control, had not been widened (7). A variety of cell cycle and phase-specific agents has been used in such combinations: inhibitors of DNA synthesis, mitotic inhibitors, etc. Perhaps the only advantage gained was the clinical experience of being able ethically to exceed conventional normal tissue tolerance in the search for additional tumor control.

Hyperthermia

A further physical modification of tumor environment is the use of hyperthermia. One facet of the poor blood supply of tumors is that they lack the ability to dissipate heat as efficiently as do well-vascularized normal tissues. Tumor cells in vitro have been shown to have an increased sensitivity to temperatures elevated only to as little as from 37-42°C and, in addition, the use of elevated temperatures appears to inhibit intracellular repair of both sublethal and potentially lethal damage (18,29). The major technical problem is the production of suitable temperature increase in the desired volume within the patient, and this has not yet been achieved satisfactorily, although a number of schemes using immersion in warm water or wax or localized heating by microwaves are being attempted. The radiobiological justification is unchallengeable - clinical result is still in doubt; once again, a widened therapeutic ratio between damage to tumor and to limiting normal tissue is the sine qua non for success.

SUMMARY

In summary, radiation biology has taught us that the majority of functions of differentiated cells are highly resistant to the effects of ionizing radiation; cell reproductive capacity is the function most sensitive to inhibition with relatively small radiation doses, and the consequences of loss of cell reproductive capacity are ramified through the kinetics of cell loss and proliferation in tumors and limiting normal tissues. In many cases we have the systems to answer all of the relevant questions of the clinical radiotherapist, but the effort involved is great and the radiotherapy community is unwilling to await the results before attempting new forms of treatment in human cancer. Once again, as at the beginning of our experience of the use of ionizing radiations, man himself is the experimental animal, and we owe it to our patients to be enlightened observers of the biological responses which we produce.

REFERENCES

1. Adams, G.E.: Chemical radiosensitization of hypoxic cells. Br. Med. Bull. 29:48-53, 1973.

2. Advisory Committee on the Biological Effects of Ionizing Radiations (BEIR): The effects on populations of exposure to low levels of ionizing radiation. Washington, National Academy of Science, National Research Council, 1972.

3. Barendsen, G.W.: Impairment of the proliferative capacity of human cells in culture by particles with differing linear energy transfer. Int. J. Radiat. Oncol. Biol. Phys. 8:453-466, 1964.

4. Bergonie, J. and Tribondeau, L.: Interpretation de quelques resultats de la radiotherapie et essai de fixation d'une technique rationelle. Compt. Rend. Acad. Sc. Par. 143:983-985, 1906.

5. Berry, R.J.: A comparison of effects of some chemotherapeutic agents and those of x-rays on the reproductive capacity of mammalian cells. Nature (Lond.) 203:1150-1153, 1964.

6. Berry, R.J.: Effects of small and large first x-ray doses on the two-dose recovery pattern in HeLa S-3 cells in vitro. Radiat. Res. 32:13-20, 1967.

7. Berry, R.J.: Radiotherapy plus chemotherapy - have we gained anything by combining them in the treatment of human cancer? In Frontiers of Radiation Therapy and Oncology, 4, edited by J.M. Vaeth, Basel, Karger, 1979, p. 1.

8. Berry, R.J. and Andrews, J.R.: The effect of radiation ionization density (LET) upon the reproductive capacity of mammalian tumor cells irradiated and assayed in vivo. Br. J. Radiol. 36:49-55, 1963.

9. Berry, R.J. and Cohen, A.B.: Some observations on the reproductive capacity of mammalian tumor cells exposed in vivo to gamma radiation at low dose-rates. Br. J. Radiol. 34:489-491, 1962.

10. van den Brenk, H.A.S., Madigan, J.P., and Kerr, R.C.: Experience with megavoltage irradiation of advanced malignant disease using high pressure oxygen. In Clinical Application of Hyperbaric Oxygen, edited by I. Boerema, W.H. Brunnelkamp, and N.G. Meijne, Amsterdam, Elsevier, 1964, p. 144.

11. Catterall, M. and Bewley, D.K.: Fast Neutrons in the Treatment of Cancer, London, Academic Press, 1979.

12. Chadwick, K.H. and Leenhouts, H.P.: A molecular theory of cell survival. Phys. Med. Biol. 18:78-81, 1973.

13. Churchill-Davidson, I., Sanger, C., and Thomlinson, R.H.: Oxygenation in radiotherapy, II. Clinical application. Br. J. Radiol. 30:406-421, 1957.

14. Dessauer, F.: The cause of the action of x-rays and x-rays of radium upon living cells. J. Radiol. 4:411-415, 1923.

15. Elkind, M.M. and Sutton, H.: Radiation response of mammalian cells grown in culture. I. Repair of x-ray damage in surviving Chinese hamster cells. Radiat. Res. 13:556-593, 1960.

16. Ellis, F.: Dose, time and fractionation: a clinical hypothesis. Clin. Radiol. 20:1-8, 1969.

17. Field, S.B., Hornsey, S. and Kutsutani, Y.: Effects of fractionated irradiation on mouse lung and a phenomenon of slow repair. Br. J. Radiol. 49:700-707, 1976.

18. Field, S.B., Hume, S.P., Law, M.P., and Myers, R.: The response of tissues to combined hyperthermia and x-rays. Br. J. Radiol. 50:129-134, 1977.

19. Fowler, J.F., Thomlinson, R.H., and Howes, A.E.: Time-dose relationships in radiotherapy. Eur. J. Cancer 6:207-221, 1970.

20. Gray, L.H., Conger, A.D., Ebert, M., Hornsey, S., and Scott, O.C.A.: The concentration of oxygen dissolved in tissues at the time of irradiation as a factor in radiotherapy. Br. J. Radiol. 26:638-648, 1953.

21. Hall, E.J.: Radiation dose-rate: a factor of importance in radiobiology and radiotherapy. Br. J. Radiol. 45:81-97, 1972.

22. Hall, E.J.: Radiobiology for the Radiologist, Hagerstown, Md., Harper and Row, 1973.

23. Henk, J.M., Kunkler, P.B., Shah, N.K., Smith, C.W., Sutherland, W.H., and Wassif, S.B.: Hyperbaric oxygen in the radiotherapy of head and neck carcinoma. Clin. Radiol. 21:223-231, 1970.

24. Hewitt, H.G. and Wilson, C.W.: A survival curve for mammalian leukemia cells irradiated in vivo (implications for the treatment of mouse leukemia by whole-body irradiation). Br. J. Cancer 13:69-75, 1959.

25. Hopewell, J.W. and Young, C.M.A.: Changes in the microcirculation of normal tissues after irradiation. Int. J. Radiat. Oncol. Biol. Phys. 4:53-58, 1978.

26. Lajtha, L.G. and Oliver, R.: Some radiobiological considerations in radiotherapy. Br. J. Radiol. 34:252-257, 1961.

27. Law, M.P. and Thomlinson, R.H.: Vascular permeability in the ears of rats after x-irradiation. Br. J. Radiol. 51:895-904, 1978.

28. Lea, D.E.: Actions of Radiations on Living Cells, Cambridge University Press, New York, The Macmillan Co., 1947.

29. Overgaard, J.: Effect of hyperthermia on malignant cells in vivo. A review and a hypothesis. Cancer 39:2637-2646, 1977.

30. Phillips, R.D. and Tolmach, L.J.: Repair of potentially lethal damage in x-irradiated HeLa cells. Radiat. Res. 29:413-432, 1966.

31. Puck, T.T. and Marcus, P.I.: Action of x-rays on mammalian cells. J. Exp. Med. 103:653-666, 1956.

32. van Putten, L.M.: Tumor reoxygenation during fractionated radiotherapy; studies with a transplantable mouse osteosarcoma. Eur. J. Cancer 4:173, 1968.

33. Regaud, C. and Blanc, J.: Actions des rayons x sur les diverses generations de la lignee spermatique; extreme sensibilite des spermatogenies a ces rayons. C.R. Soc. Biol. 61:163-165, 1906.

34. Schwarz, G.: Uber desensibilizierung gegen Rontgen- und Radium-strahlung. Munchen Med. Wchnschr. 56:1217, 1909.

35. Sinclair, W.K. and Morton, R.A.: X-ray sensitivity during the cell generation cycle of cultured Chinese hamster cells. Radiat. Res. 29:450-474, 1966.

36. Terasima, T. and Tolmach, L.J.: Changes in x-ray sensitivity of HeLa cells during the division cycle. Nature (Lond.) 190:1210-1211, 1961.

37. Thomlinson, R.H. and Gray, L.H.: The histological structure of some human lung cancers and possible implications for radiotherapy. Br. J. Cancer 9:539-549, 1955.

38. Till, J.R. and McCulloch, E.A.: Direct measurement of radiation sensitivity of normal mouse bone marrow cells. Radiat. Res. 14:213, 1961.

39. Timofeev-Ressovsky, N.W. and Zimmer, K.G.: Biophysik I. Das Trefferprinzip in der Biologie, Leipzig, Hirzel, 1947.

40. Todd, P.: Heavy ion irradiation of cultured human cells. Radiat. Res. (Supplement) 7:196-207, 1967.

41. Warren, S.: The Pathology of Ionizing Radiation, Springfield, Ill., Charles C Thomas, 1961.

42. Withers, H.R.: The dose-survival relationship for irradiation of epithelial cells of mouse skin. Br. J. Radiol. 40:187-194, 1967.

43. Withers, H.R.: The four Rs of radiotherapy. Adv. Radiat. Biol. 5:241-271, 1975.

44. Withers, H.R. and Elkind, M.M.: Radiosensitivity and fractionation response of crypt cells of mouse jejunum. Radiat. Res. 38:598-613, 1969.

45. Zimmer, K.G.: Studies on Quantitative Radiation Biology. New York, Hafner Publishing Co., 1961.

chapter 2

DIAGNOSIS, LOCALIZATION, AND TREATMENT PLANNING OF MALIGNANCIES

SECTION I. THE HEAD AND NECK

Solomon Batnitzky, M.D.

Tissue biopsy is still the only reliable and definitive method for the diagnosis of malignancies of the head and neck. However, radiological procedures play an integral and indispensable part in the diagnosis, staging, and management of these tumors. Decisions regarding operability and radiation therapy planning require very precise imaging techniques.

In the investigation of tumors of the head and neck, conventional diagnostic radiographic techniques, such as plain film radiography, thin scetion complex motion tomography, radionuclide brain scanning, angiography, and myelography, have been universally practiced and accepted for many years. These procedures permit remarkable accuracy both in the anatomical and pathological diagnosis.

The advent of computed tomography (CT) in the early 1970s has had a profound and dramatic impact on the practice of radiology (4, 6, 79). Computed tomography with its remarkable ability to detect and display minute differences in tissue density has added a new dimension to diagnostic radiology not obtainable by other techniques and has considerably broadened the radiological armamentarium. Computed tomography is a noninvasive, sensitive, accurate, and easily performed technique that produces no appreciable discomfort or morbidity to the patient.

Computed tomography in the transverse, coronal, or sagittal planes provides a third dimension in the spatial localization and definition of known tumors. This information is obviously very important in determining the appropriate treatment modality.

In this section it is the intention to highlight the role of computed tomography as a diagnostic tool and aid to the radiotherapist in the diagnosis, localization, and management of malignancies of the head and neck.

It should be stressed, however, that computed tomography does not rival other conventional radiological techniques. These techniques are complementary to computed tomography and remain an essential part of the investigation of these patients. In many cases more than one study must be performed so as to obtain the maximum amount of information prior to treatment.

INTRACRANIAL AND ORBITAL TUMORS

Computed tomography, especially when utilized in conjunction with the administration of intravenous iodinated contrast material, is probably the most accurate diagnostic tool available for the investigation of intracranial pathology, particularly intracranial tumors. The overall accuracy of computed tomography is of the order of 95-98% in detecting intracranial abnormalities (79).

While many brain tumors are treated with whole-brain radiation, precise localization is therefore not of the utmost importance in these cases. However, in some areas and situations, the precise localization and extent of the tumor as shown on computed tomography permits the radiotherapist to give a larger but more concentrated dose to the tumor while a lower dose is given to the whole brain (Fig. 1).

Computed tomography provides important information in the evaluation of orbital tumors (33). The relationship of the tumor to the globe, optic nerve, and extraocular muscles can be demonstrated, as well as any extension of the tumor into the cranial cavity. In the orbit, CT is the best method of establishing the presence of a mass lesion (46) (Figs. 2 and 3).

In one study assessing the sensitivity of CT in the diagnosis of orbital tumors, CT had an accuracy of 93% compared with 76% for ultrasound (28), another highly sensitive noninvasive technique for the detection of retroorbital masses.

PARANASAL SINUSES

Conventional radiographic techniques such as plain film radiography and multiple thin section complex motion tomography are important and indispensable in the evaluation of these lesions. However, in many instances the radiographic changes that can be seen by these studies are present only when the disease is extensive and advanced. Using conventional x-ray techniques, spread of the tumor outside the sinuses cannot be accurately defined. Complex motion tomography is still the most superior radiographic technique in demonstrating the degree of bone destruction. However, it only delineates the gross extent of tumor and does not demonstrate the precise involvement of the surrounding structures, especially posterior and superior extension.

Computed tomography, because of its ability in delineating soft tissue detail, has established itself as a simple, safe, reliable, and accurate method to assess local tumor spread in paranasal sinus malignancies (25,59). Computed tomography is able to demonstrate posterior and superior extension of the neoplastic process and will reveal intraorbital, intracranial, and infratemporal extension of the tumor. In many instances the CT findings are present before clinical signs of involvement of these areas by the tumor are evident (Figs. 4, 5, and 6). Scans taken in the coronal plane compliment the transverse plane but are especially valuable in demonstrating craniocaudal and nasopharyngeal extension as well as involvement of the skull base (Fig. 7). Follow-up CT scans are especially useful and valuable in monitoring the response to radiation therapy and in the diagnosis of any recurrence.

One of the limitations of computed tomography is that available technology does not allow for differentiation to be made between tissue masses of malignant origin and benign processes. In the management of patients with paranasal sinus malignancy, this may pose both a diagnostic and therapeutic problem in certain situations. Opacification of contiguous paranasal sinuses as seen both on CT and with conventional x-ray studies may be due to tumor spread to the sinuses. However, the opacification may be due to retention of secretions within the sinuses secondary to obstruction of the ostia of the sinuses by the tumor (Fig. 7B). This tends to occur especially when the tumor extends into the apex of the nasal cavity. Differentiation between these two situations may prove difficult at times. In such circumstances repeat CT scans after the completion of radiation therapy may prove helpful to determine the true extent of the tumor. With shrinkage of the tumor mass as a response to the radiation therapy, the ostia may reopen and reestablish drainage indicating that the opacification of the contiguous sinuses was a consequence of obstruction to normal drainage rather than direct tumor extension.

TUMORS OF THE LARYNX, HYPOPHARYNX OROPHARYNX, NASOPHARYNX, AND NASAL CAVITY

In the evaluation of tumors of the larynx, hypopharynx, oropharynx, nasal cavity, and to a lesser extent the nasopharynx, the diagnosis may be obvious clinically in many cases. Conventional radiological studies and other clinical tests provide valuable confirmatory and supplemental information concerning these tumors. The limitations of the clinical and radiographic methods in these areas are their inability to determine the exact size and extent of the tumor and its involvement of adjacent structures. Furthermore, tumors of the nasopharynx, especially those that are small, are difficult to evaluate clinically and radiologically from the standpoint of both diagnosis and management.

CT has established itself as the radiological examination of choice in the workup of these tumors in the above areas (10,47). Computed tomography can delineate anatomical location, size, and extent of the tumor. Invasion of adjacent soft tissue and bony structures as well as any associated intracranial or intraorbital extension can be equally well-appreciated by computed tomography (Figs. 8 and 9).

In a prospective study of 66 patients with laryngeal disorders it was established that computed tomography complimented direct laryngoscopy and biopsy for treatment planning and was superior to both modalities for showing deep infiltration, invasion of cartilage, and extension into the soft tissues of the neck (47). Computed tomography was also useful in demonstrating lymph node extension and was equal or superior to laryngography in approximately 90% of the cases.

NECK MASSES

Computed tomography is an extremely valuable and important diagnostic tool in the evaluation of cervical masses by delineating both the osseous and soft tissue extent of the tumor (52). In addition, the relationship of the tumor to the spinal canal can be demonstrated (Fig. 10). Computed tomography, when used in conjunction with a rapid intravenous drip infusion technique of iodinated contrast material, can demonstrate the relationship of a mass to the major cervical arteries and veins (9) (Fig. 11).

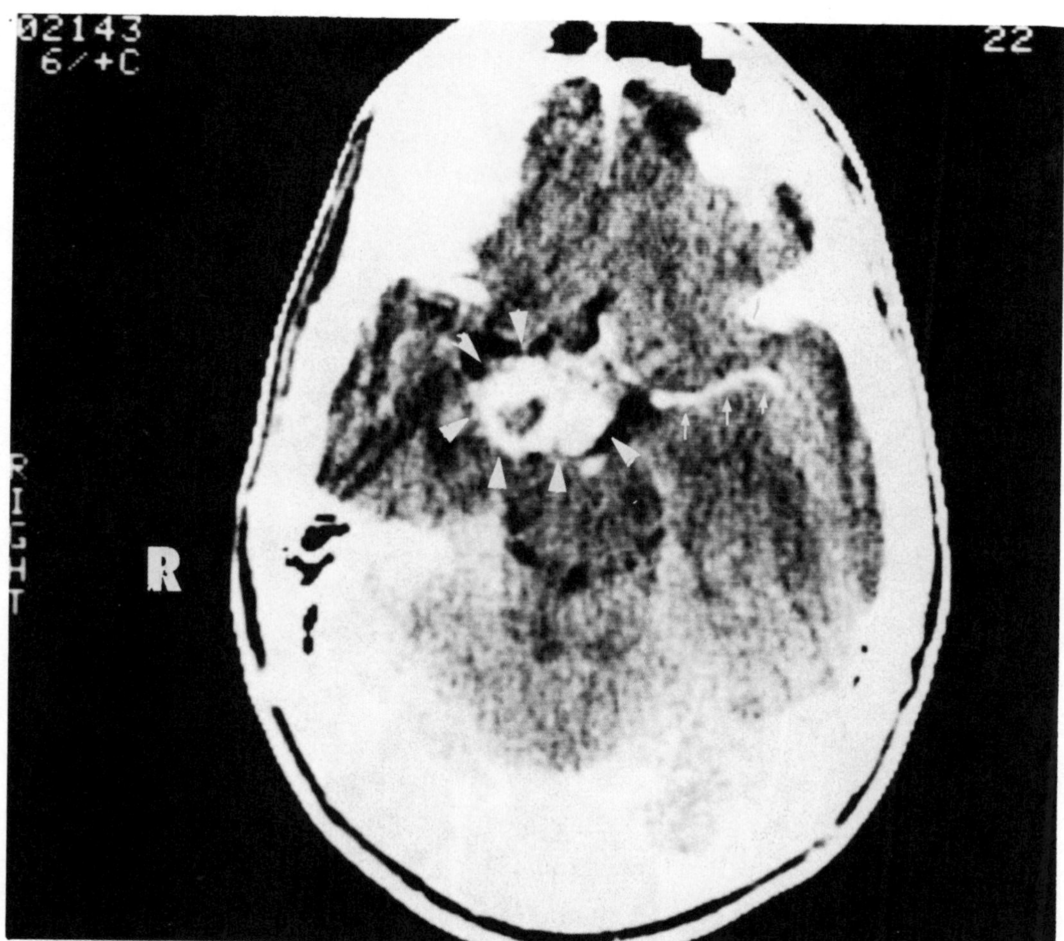

Figure 1. A: Contrast-enhanced transverse CT scan of head of 30-year-old male demonstrates the solid and cystic component of a suprasellar and right parasellar craniopharyngioma (arrowheads). Arrows point to left middle cerebral artery.

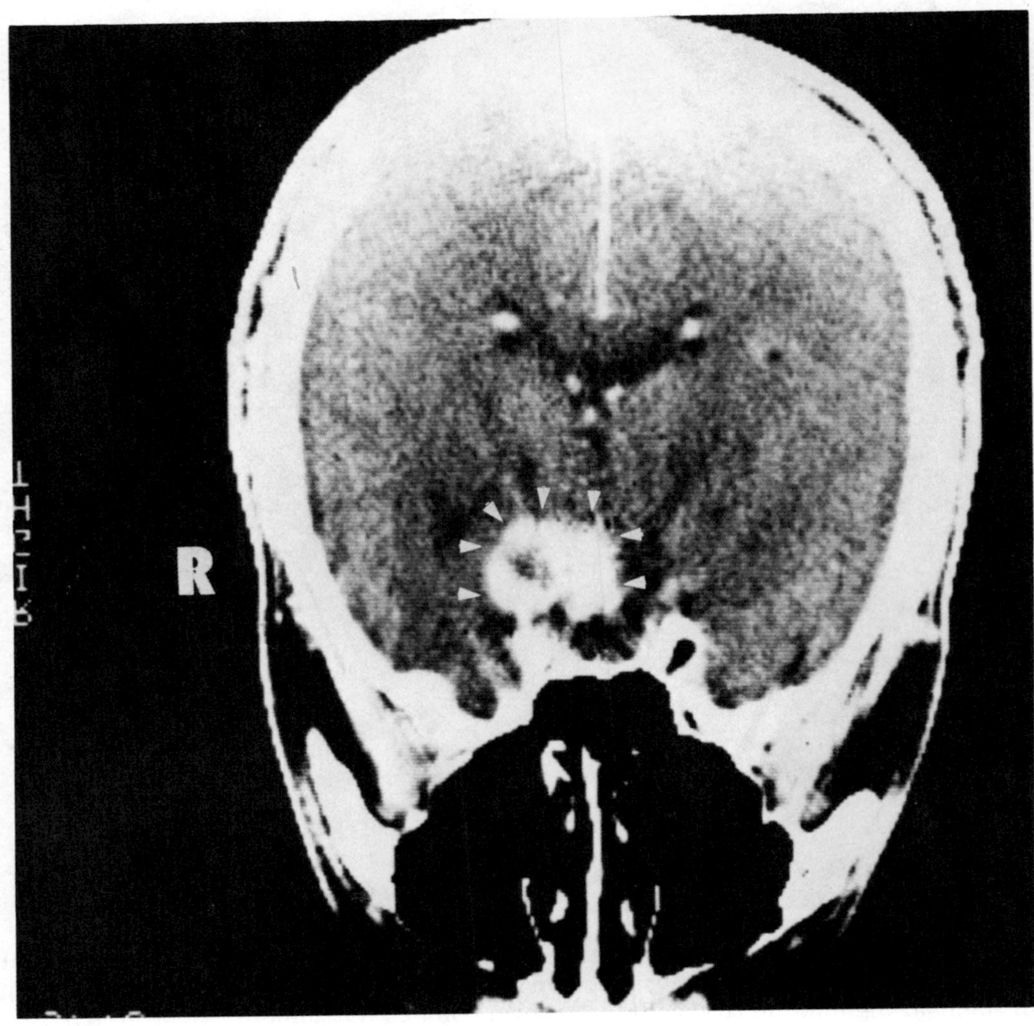

Figure 1. B: Coronal contrast-enhanced CT head scan of same patient shows the superior-inferior extent of the above tumor and its exact relationship to the pituitary fossa. This precise localization allows the radiotherapist to give a higher but more collimated dose of radiation to the tumor.

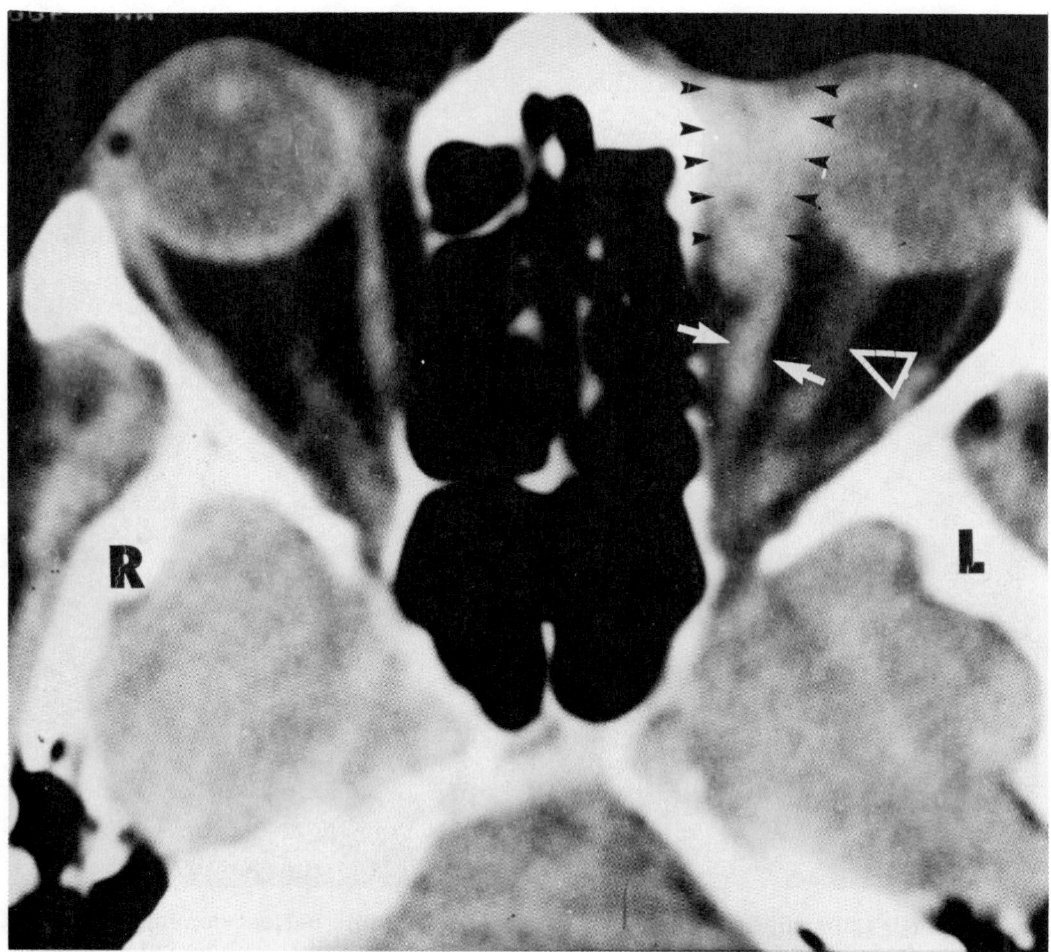

Figure 2. A: CT scan of orbits in transverse plane of a 70-year-old female with left eyelid meibomian gland carcinoma. The left globe is displaced laterally by the tumor (arrowheads) which is extending posteriorly to involve the medial rectus muscle (arrow). No bony destruction is seen. The optic nerve is shown by the open arrowhead.

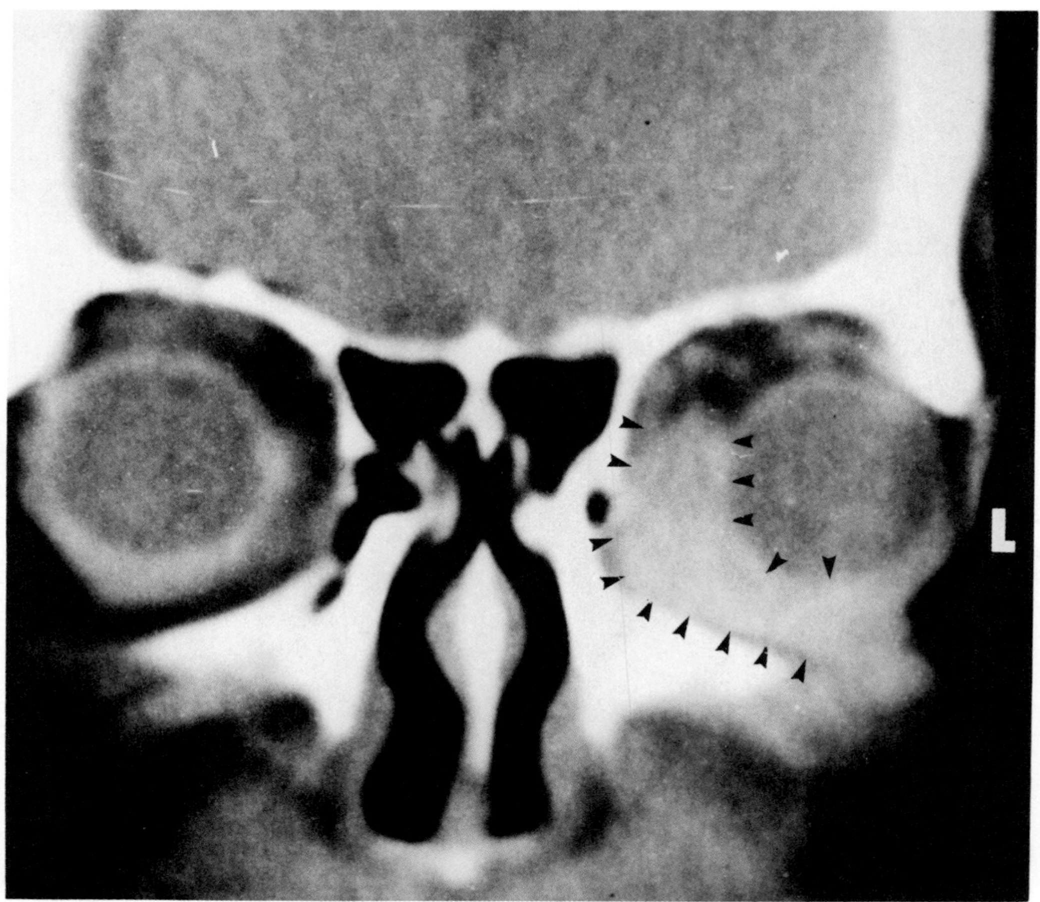

Figure 2.B: CT scan of orbits in coronal plane of same patient demonstrates that the tumor (arrowheads) is not only on the medial aspect of the globe but is also extending inferior to the globe. No extension into the nose or paranasal sinuses is seen.

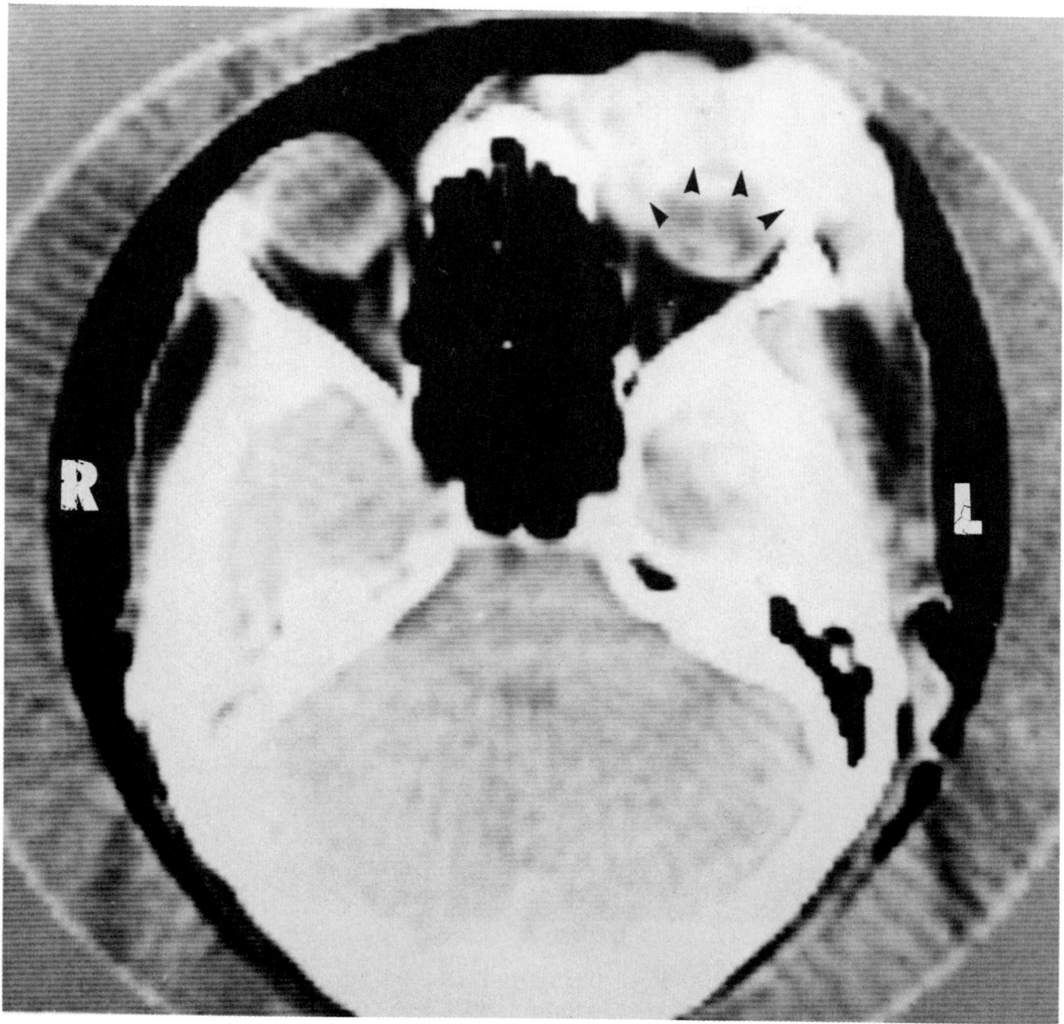

Figure 3. CT scan of orbits in the transverse plane of a 72-year-old female with carcinoma of the meibomian gland of the left eyelid. The large tumor is enveloping the left globe anteriorly but no retroorbital extension of bony destruction is seen. Clinical evaluation of the precise extent of the tumor was difficult due to its large size and position.

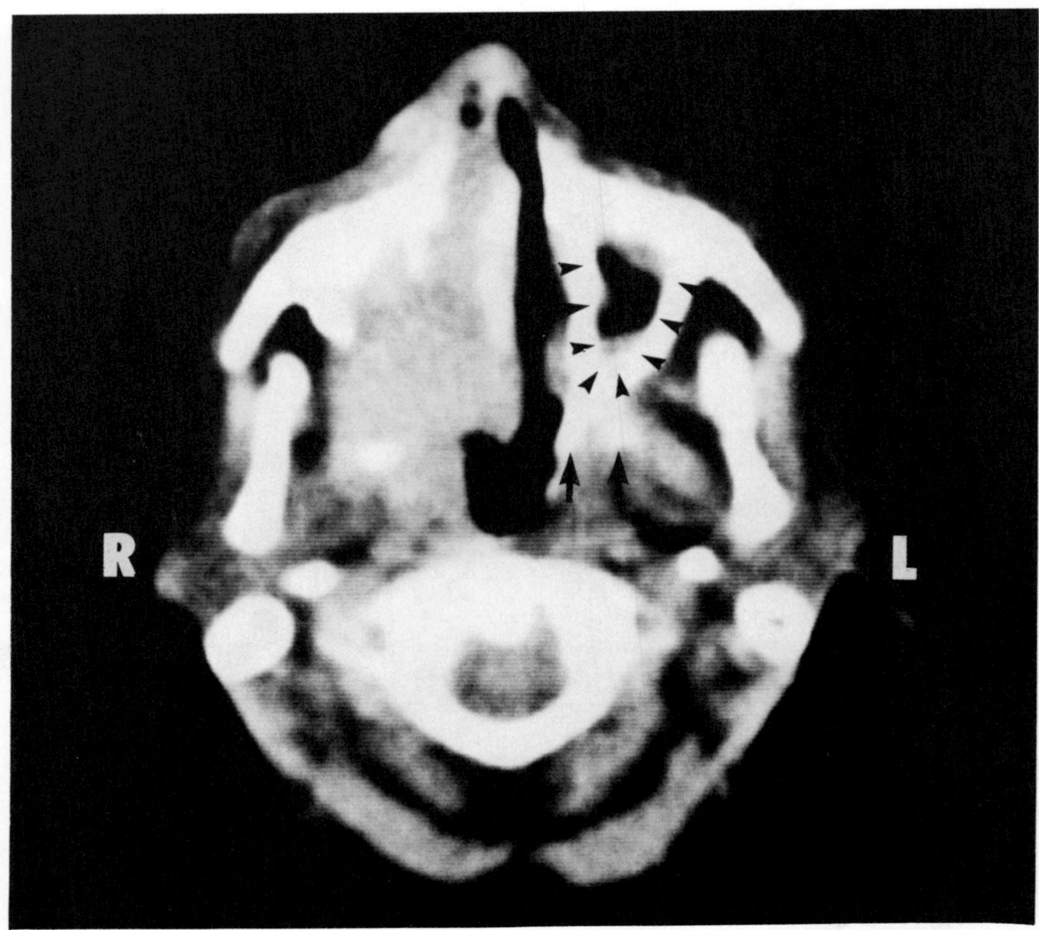

Figure 4. Transverse CT scan of paranasal sinuses of a 63-year-old female demonstrates right maxillary sinus carcinoma with destruction of the medial and posterior lateral walls of the sinus and the medial and lateral pterygoid plates. The tumor extends into the nasal cavity, nasopharynx, and pterygomaxillary fossa. Arrowheads point to the normal bony walls of the left maxillary sinus and arrows point to the normal left pterygoid bone. There is some mucosal thickening of the left maxillary sinus.

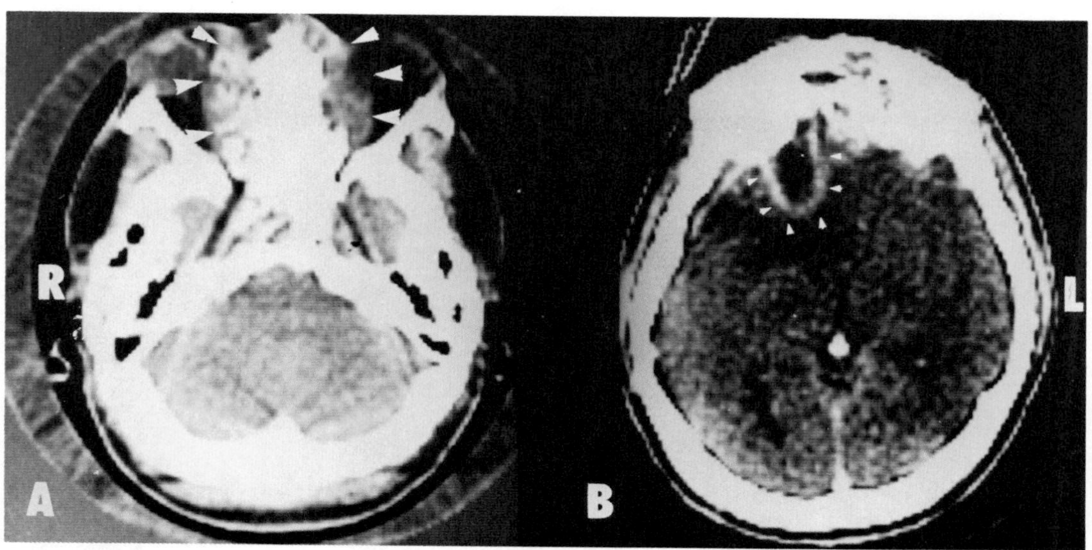

Figure 5. A: CT scan in transverse plane of 27-year-old male demonstrates large chondrosarcoma (arrowheads) involving the nasal cavity, ethmoid, and sphenoid sinuses. The tumor extends into the medial aspect of each orbit displacing each globe laterally. Note the increased density in the central portion of the tumor which represents calcified cartilage. B: Transverse CT scan of same patient at a higher level following the injection of intravenous iodinated contrast material, demonstrated an enhancing peripheral rim (small arrowheads) with a small central lucency in the right frontal lobe. This latter finding indicated intracranial extension of the tumor which was confirmed at surgery.

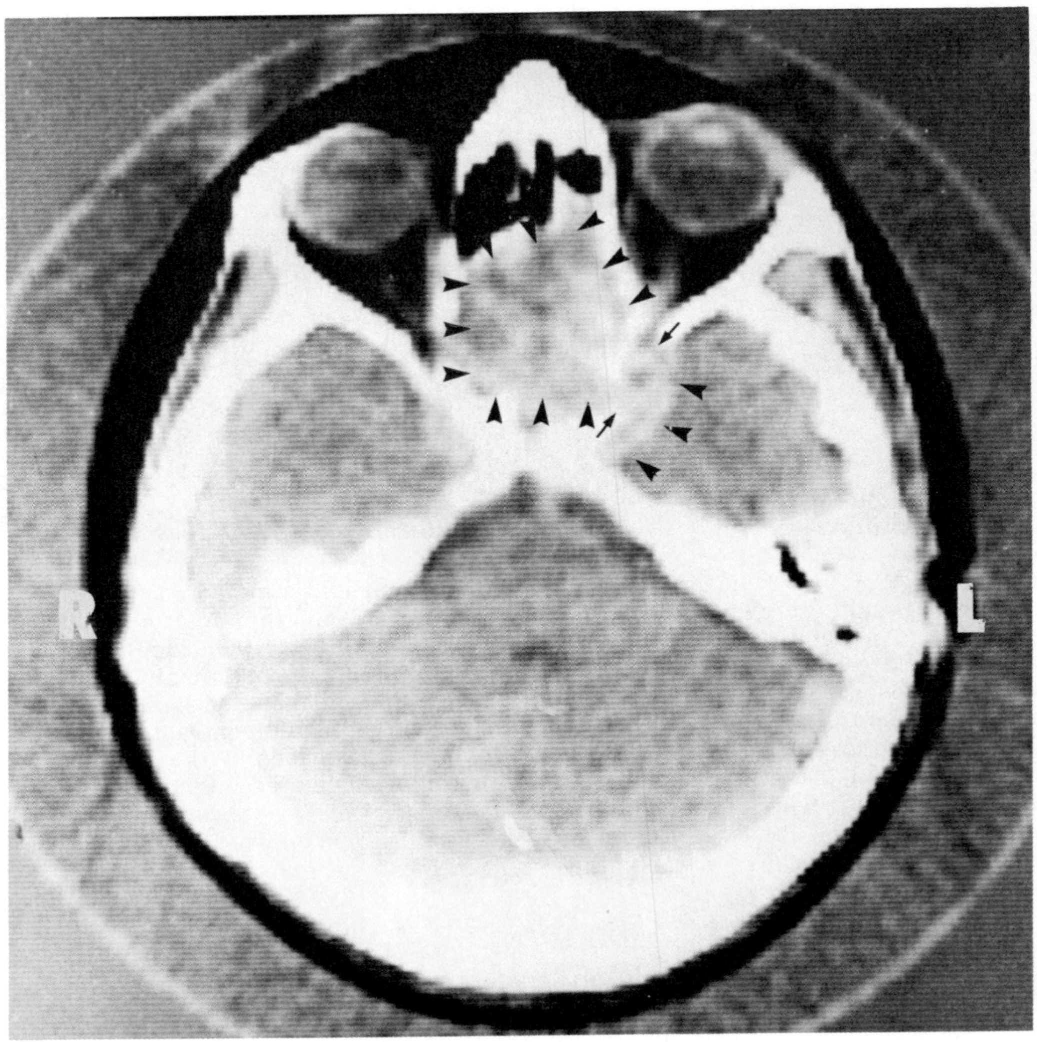

Figure 6. Contrast-enhanced transverse CT scan of head and orbits of a 48-year-old male with metastatic pheochromocytoma. Note that the metastatic tumor (arrowheads) is situated in the ethmoid and sphenoid sinuses. Destruction of the medial aspect of the left sphenoid bone is identified (arrows) with extension of the tumor into the middle cranial fossa.

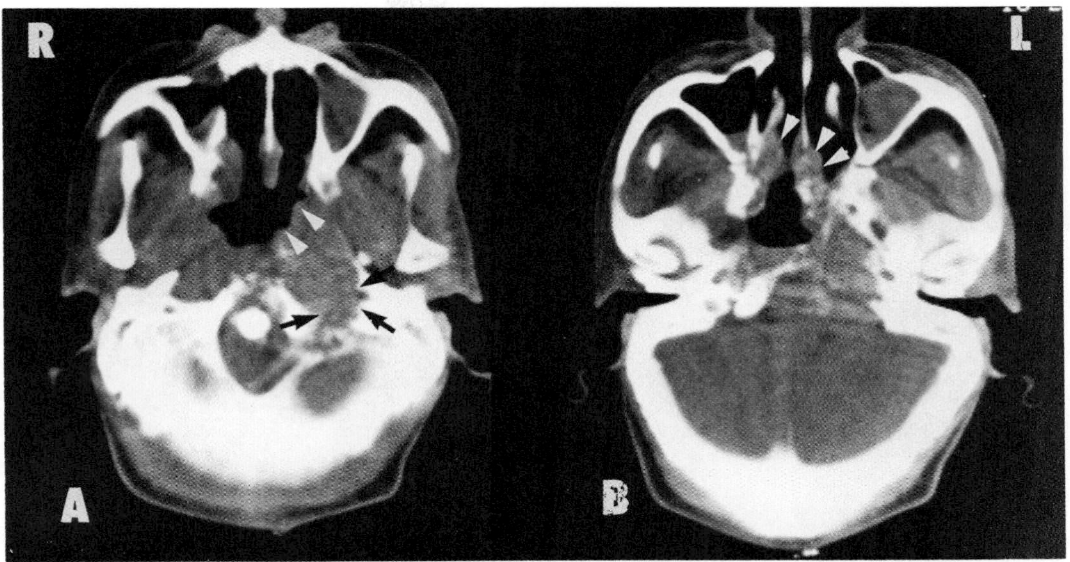

Figure 7. A: Transverse axial CT scan in 48-year-old male with nasopharyngeal carcinoma demonstrates left-sided soft tissue mass distorting the nasopharynx (arrowheads) and extending posteriorly with destruction of base of skull on left (arrows). B: The tumor is seen to be extending into the nasal cavity (arrowheads). Note the air fluid levels in both maxillary sinuses in both Figs. A and B. This is due to retention of secretions within the sinuses secondary to obstruction of the ostia of the sinuses by the tumor.

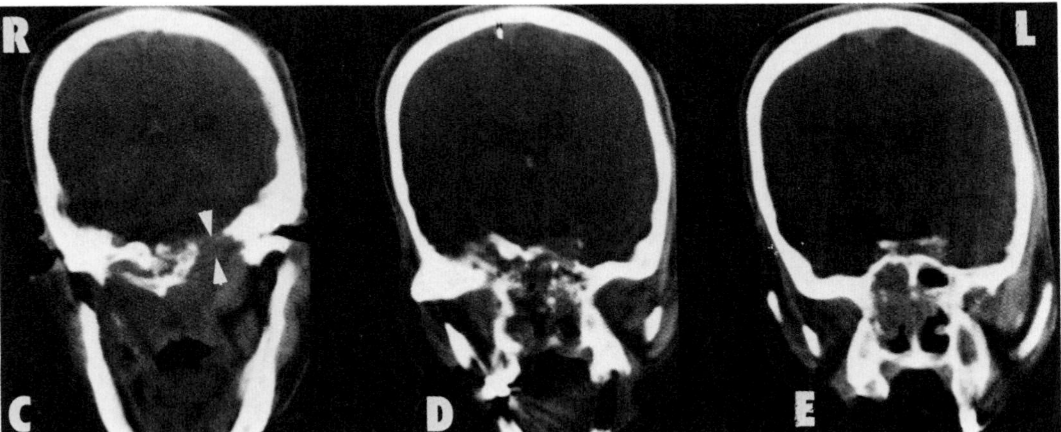

Figure 7. C: Coronal scan of same patient demonstrates the tumor (arrowheads) eroding and destroying the base of the skull in the region of the petrous base on the left side. D and E: Coronal scans showing the tumor mass in the sphenoid sinus and nasal cavity.

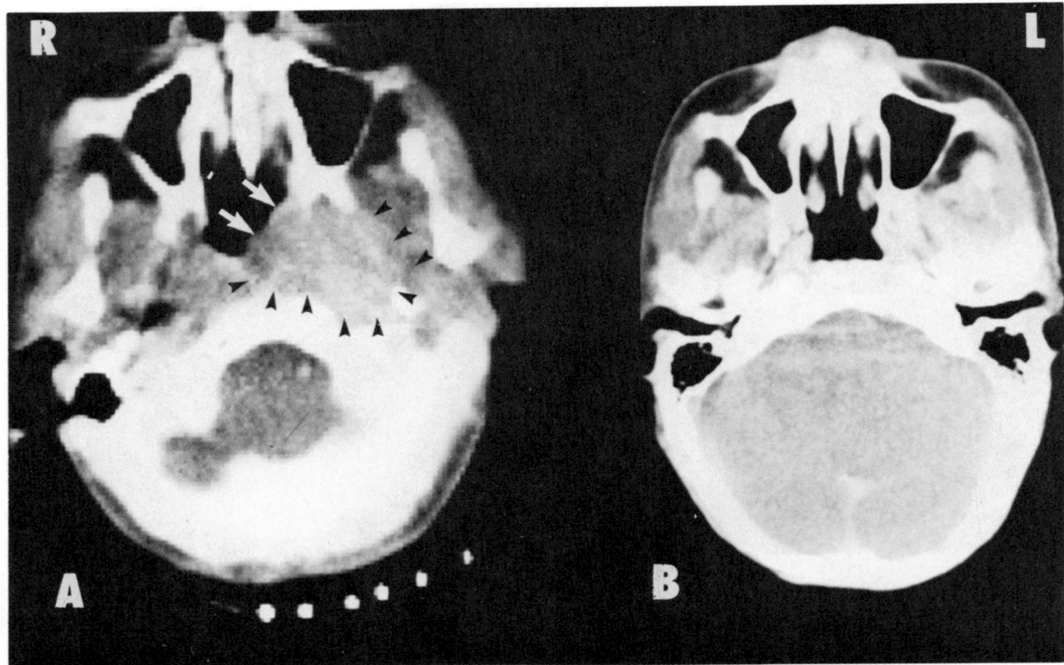

Figure 8. A: Transverse CT scan of 63-year-old female Hodgkin lymphoma demonstrates a left-sided mass (arrowheads) with ill-defined borders impinging on and obliterating the left posteromedial aspect of the nasopharynx (arrows). B: Transverse CT scan same patient taken 9 mo later following a course of radiation therapy and chemotherapy demonstrates complete interval resolution. There is no evidence of the tumor.

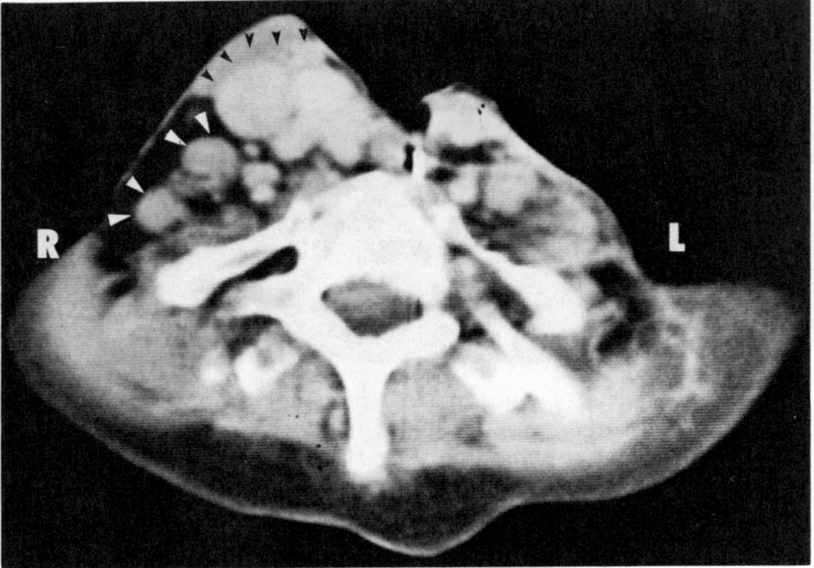

Figure 9. CT scan of neck of 78-year-old male with carcinoma of the pharynx demonstrates multiple enlarged metastatic cervical lymph nodes (arrowheads) mainly on the right side. The arrow points to a tracheostomy tube.

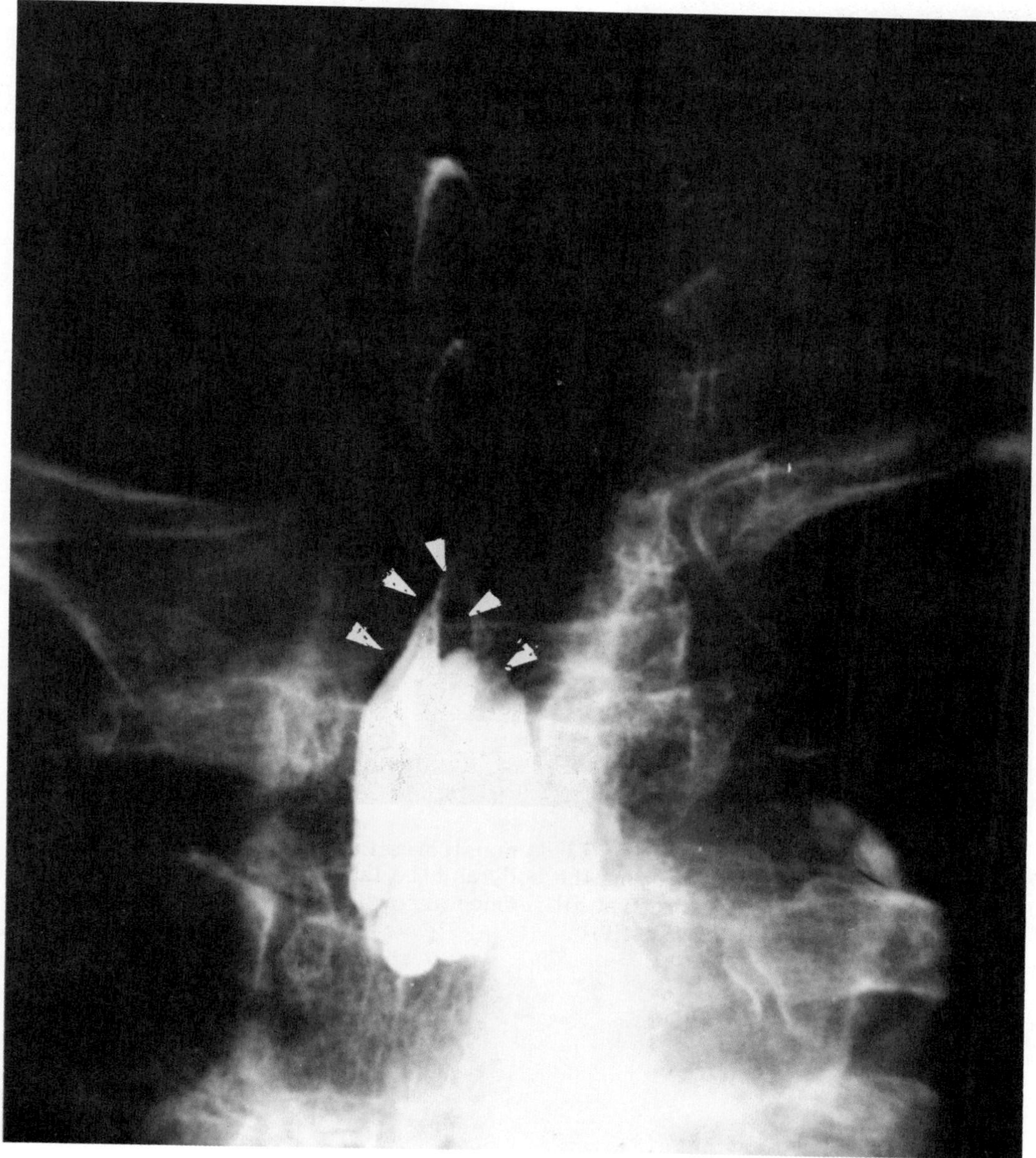

Figure 10. A: Myleography in a 72-year-old male with renal cell carcinoma demonstrates complete block at the level of T1-T2 due to extradural metastases.

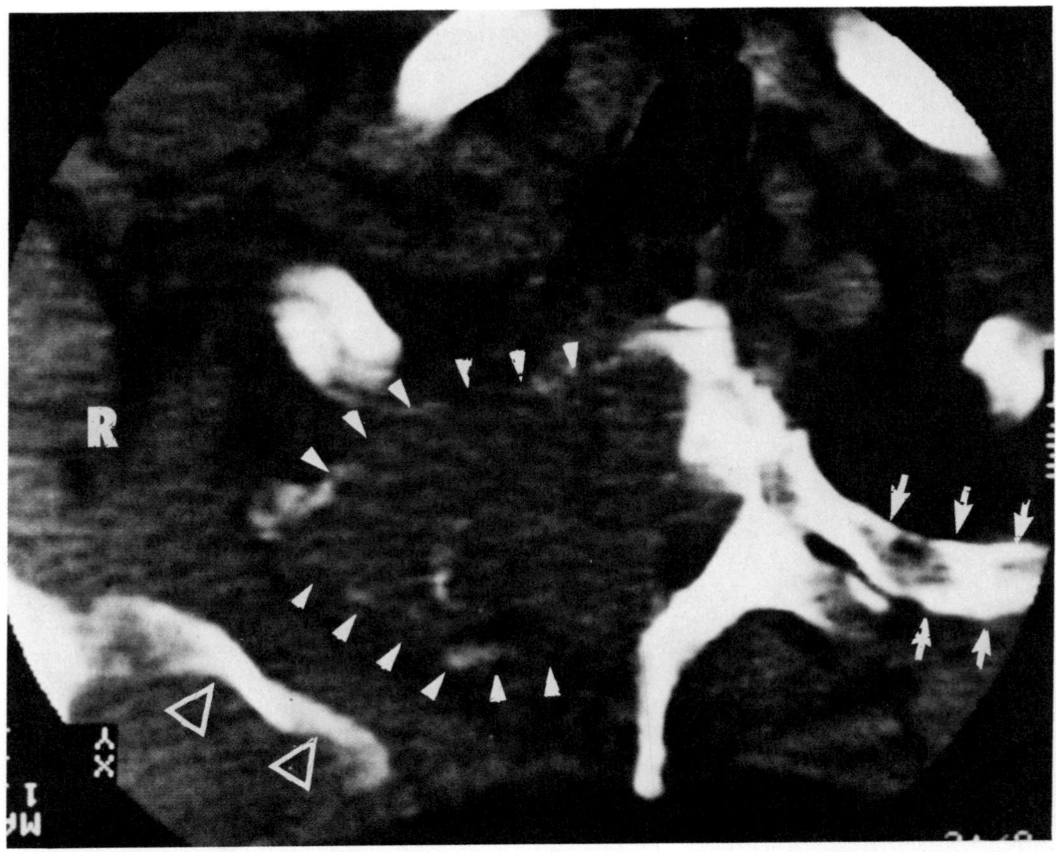

Figure 10. B: CT scan at level of T1 demonstrates large soft tissues mass on the right side (arrowheads) destroying the body and the lateral elements of T1 as well as the proximal portion of the first rib. Open arrowheads point to right scapula. Arrows point to normal left first rib.

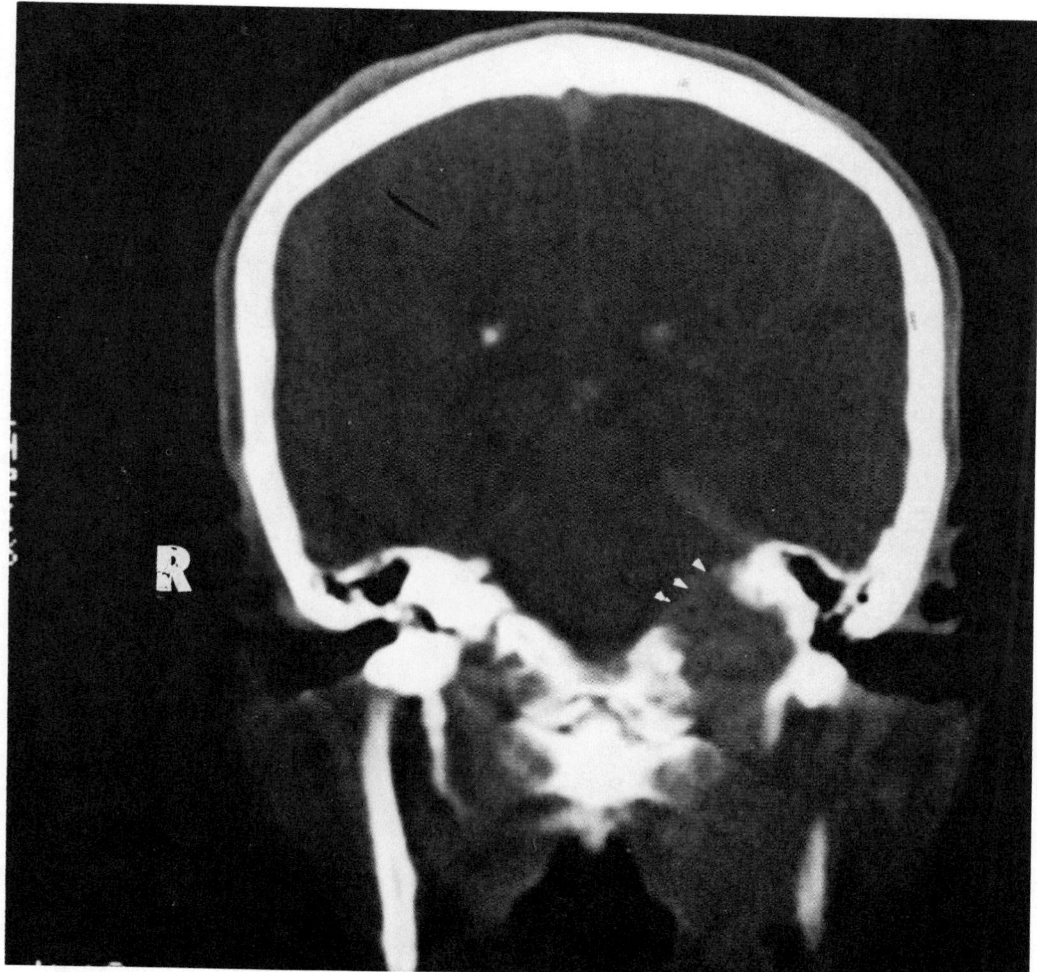

Figure 11. A: Coronal scan of an 84-year-old female with glomus jugulae tumor demonstrates the superior-inferior extension of the tumor in the region of the petrous bone. Note that the tumor is extending into the posterior fossa (arrowheads).

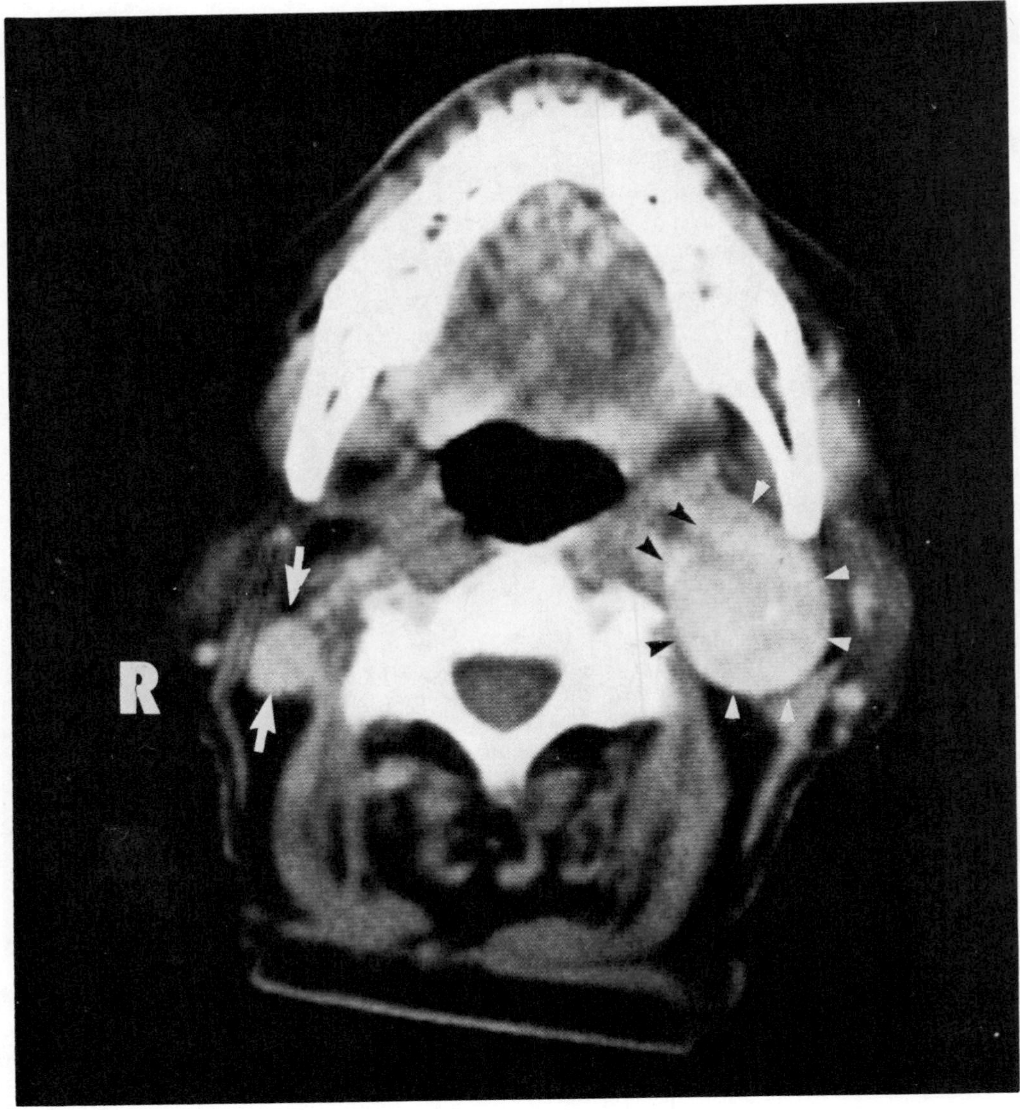

Figure 11. B: Transverse CT scan of neck of same patient at the level of the mandible demonstrates tumor involvement and infiltration of the left jugular vein (arrowheads). The normal jugular vein is seen on the right side (arrows).

SECTION II. PRIMARY BRONCHIAL CARCINOMA, LYMPHOMA, AND COLORECTAL CANCER

Errol Levine, M.D.

The prognosis and management of primary bronchial carcinoma are determined mainly by the cell type and tumor extent at the time of diagnosis. Most authors agree that oat cell carcinoma should be regarded ab initio as a systemic disease and that surgery has little place in its therapy. However, in other types of bronchial carcinoma, staging according to the tumor, node, metastasis (TNM) system is vital for determining the treatment approach. Radiology, along with such other techniques as bronchoscopy, mediastinoscopy, and pleural fluid cytology, plays an important role in staging and treatment planning in patients with bronchial carcinoma.

CT AND CONVENTIONAL RADIOGRAPHY

The Primary Lesion

Peripherally located primary carcinomas may be assessed by either plain films and laminography or by CT. Emami et al. (19) found that CT assessments of tumor size were more accurate than those obtained by conventional radiology and that CT assessments significantly altered radiation fields in over half their patients. However, in most instances pathological proof of CT interpretations was not available. Since lung carcinoma is frequently surrounded by atelectatic or consolidated lung which may be isodense with the tumor, it seems unlikely that either CT or conventional radiology would be capable of providing a precise assessment of tumor size. Further radiology-pathology correlations are necessary in this regard. However, CT does enjoy the advantage that appropriate CT sections can be enlarged to achieve body size and processed directly for radiotherapy planning (29,56). CT is also most useful in evaluation of tumors which are obscured by pleural fluid on conventional radiographs. By virtue of its ability to detect small density differences, CT permits easy distinction between the primary tumor and pleural fluid in most instances (Fig. 12).

Tumor Relationship to the Pleura and Chest Wall

Invasion of the pleura (Figs. 12 and 16), pericardium (Fig. 13), or chest wall generally indicates an inoperable tumor. The unique axial image provided by CT will at times permit recognition of a rim of air containing parenchyma between the pleura and the more centrally located tumor when plain films are equivocal (74). This observation excludes gross pleural tumor extension and thus improves the possibility of successful tumor resection.

Unfortunately, CT demonstration of solid tissue extending from a centrally located cancer to the pleural surface cannot necessarily be interpreted as reflecting direct tumor spread. This results from the inability of CT to distinguish between neoplastic tissue and densely consolidated or atelectatic lung parenchyma intervening between the tumor and chest wall (Fig. 14). While CT demonstration of pleural fluid in such cases will suggest pleural invasion, absence of pleural fluid does not exclude it. Involvement of the spine and chest wall may be shown by conventional radiography or by CT, although in some instances bony erosion is evident on CT study only (Fig. 15).

Evaluation of the Lung Hilum

Endobronchial tumors arising close to the carina are best assessed by bronchoscopy. Hilar lymph node metastasis from peripheral lung carcinoma are most easily detected by oblique hilar tomography (21,53). CT assessment of the hila is difficult as distinction between pulmonary vessels and lymph nodes cannot readily be made.

Mediastinal Tumor Spread

Bronchial carcinoma may involve the mediastinum by direct spread. In many cases it is difficult to determine by plain radiography and laminography whether the mass invades the mediastinum or is merely situated in close proximity to it. The CT scan will often resolve this difficulty (53). Obliteration of fat planes, such as the one contiguous to the aortic arch, will indicate direct mediastinal tumor invasion (Fig. 16).

Metastatic spread to mediastinal lymph nodes is usually assessed by conventional laminography. While this technique has had considerable success, evidence is emerging that contrast-enhanced CT scans of the chest are more sensitive than conventional laminograms in detecting mediastinal masses, including enlarged lymph nodes (19,53,74). All major node groups can be evaluated by CT. However CT is particularly useful in detecting enlargement of subcarinal nodes, periesophageal and paraaortic nodes which often are difficult to identify on conventional laminograms (32). CT is likewise helpful in detecting enlargement of internal mammary, cardiophrenic and tracheobronchial lymph nodes (32). However, mediastinoscopy and biopsy not infrequently reveal microscopic metastatic deposits in normal size lymph nodes which cannot be detected by CT (53). Another limitation of CT is that it cannot distinguish adenopathy due to tumor involvement from that due to reactive hyperplasia. While this is not a common problem, it may cause a patient with a resectable lesion to be denied surgery.

Lung Metastases

The primary tumor may metastasize via the blood stream to the ipsilateral or contralateral lung. Satellite lesions around the primary tumor reflect bloodborne metastases and as such render the lesion inoperable (74). CT has been clearly shown to be more accurate than conventional laminography in the detection of such metastases, particularly if they are subpleural in location (Fig. 17) (53,55). However, the distinction between secondary neoplasm and preexisting granulomas is not always easy and CT-guided biopsy may provide the only method for distinction in such cases.

Radionuclide Scanning in the Staging of Primary Bronchial Carcinoma

In patients with bronchial carcinoma it is well known that regional perfusion to the lung affected by the tumor is often reduced to a degree unsuspected from the size of the lesion on the chest radiograph (65-67,80,81). Regional ventilation may also be impaired in bronchial carcinoma, although ventilation is usually less impaired than perfusion (44,67). The alteration in perfusion is probably related to pulmonary venous obstruction (65). It has been claimed that severe impairment of pulmonary perfusion will usually suggest a nonresectable tumor which has impinged on the pulmonary vasculature and spread to the mediastinum (66). Not all workers agree with this view (48), but there is general agreement that the larger the perfusion defect caused by the tumor, the less likely it is to be resectable. Obviously, tumors associated with a normal lung scan have the best chance of being resectable. Apart from its role in assessing tumor resectability, perfusion-ventilation imaging is useful for assessing the contralateral lung in conjunction with pulmonary function tests in patients in whom pneumonectomy is being considered. Many patients with bronchial carcinoma have coexistent chronic obstructive airway disease.

There is evidence that ventilation-perfusion imaging may prove a most useful method for assessing tumor response to radiotherapy (20). Patients with bronchial carcinoma associated with severe dyspnea often show an immediate amelioration of their breathlessness following radiotherapy, and this is associated with an improvement in regional perfusion and ventilation on the side affected by the tumor. This improvement of regional lung function is probably due to shrinkage of the tumor with partial or total relief of infiltration or compression on airways or blood vessels, particularly pulmonary veins. Subsequent deterioration in regional perfusion and ventilation will often herald the onset of radiation fibrosis (20).

The role of gallium citrate studies in patients with bronchial carcinoma is open to question. Some workers have reported that ^{67}Ga citrate studies yield positive results in 80-90% of patients with bronchial carcinoma, without regard to the cell type of the tumor (16). However, the false positive rate in some series appears rather high (17,74). DeMeester et al. report a 17% false positive rate and a 24% false negative rate in the assessment of lymph nodes as proven by mediastinal biopsy, and a 29% false positive rate as proven by hilar lymph nodes obtained from surgical specimens (17). Despite this, there is evidence that gallium imaging is useful in detection of mediastinal spread of bronchial carcinoma and may help in determining which patients with bronchial carcinoma should have a mediastinoscopy (1). Abnormal ^{67}Ga citrate uptake in the mediastinum is strong, presumptive evidence for mediastinal metastasis. A negative study is a less reliable indicator of the absence of mediastinal spread (1).

Assessment of Distant Metastases

Prominent sites of metastatic spread in bronchial carcinoma include the liver, kidney, brain, adrenals, and bone. The place which radionuclide studies of brain, liver, and bone should occupy in the staging of patients with bronchial carcinoma remains controversial. One prospective study (62) revealed a less than 1% incidence of detection of metastatic disease by scanning in a patient group in which metastatic disease was not suspected after clinical evaluation. This led to the conclusion that the routine use of multiorgan radionuclide scanning was not justified in patients with potentially resectable bronchial carcinoma in whom the history, physical examination, and laboratory studies do not suggest metastatic spread. Another group of workers in a retrospective study using radionuclide scans (58) found evidence of occult metastatic spread in 37% of 59 patients with negative symptoms, signs, and routine laboratory studies. Occult metastases appeared to occur most commonly in bone. Further investigation of the proper role of radionuclide bone, brain, and liver imaging in the staging of bronchial carcinoma is thus warranted.

CONCLUSION

The effectiveness of surgical treatment for primary lung cancer, other than oat cell carcinoma, is dependent on tumor size and extent and the presence or absence of distant metastases. Patients with extensive local disease or distant metastases are candidates for primary treatment by radiotherapy or chemotherapy. However, accurate staging of lung cancer would involve an extensive battery of radiological tests and the efficacy of such an undertaking needs to be questioned. While there is no evidence that extensive radiological workup affects the overall mortality of patients with lung cancer, accurate staging shows evidence of reducing the percentage of patients subjected to unnecessary thoracotomies with the expense, morbidity, and mortality these entail (50,51,74).

MALIGNANT LYMPHOMA

Once the histological diagnosis of malignant lymphoma has been established by biopsy, subsequent management and treatment planning will depend on determination of the extent of the disease. Detection of mediastinal and pulmonary involvement by plain radiography and laminography has been practiced for many years and requires no further discussion. However, assessment of whether or not the abdomen is involved is more difficult and despite the introduction of multiple radiological techniques including lymphangiography, CT scanning, radiogallium scanning, and ultrasound, there is no general agreement as to which of these techniques should be used.

Abdominal Lymph Nodes

With the advent of clinical lymphangiography, an astonishingly high frequency of hitherto unappreciated and thus untreated involvement of paraaortic and pelvic lymph nodes was revealed in patients with malignant lymphoma (40). In patients with newly diagnosed lymphomas, the paraaortic lymph nodes are involved in about one-fourth of patients with Hodgkin disease and in about one-half of those with non-Hodgkin lymphoma (31).

Lymphangiography has been shown to be capable of achieving an overall accuracy of 92% in detecting nodal involvement (11). However, the procedure is time consuming and tedious for radiologist and patient alike. Also, lymphangiography has a moderate false positive rate as a result of confusion caused by reactive lymph node changes (11). Lymphangiography has proved useful in assessing response of disease to therapy and in detecting recurrent disease. Contrast medium will persist in lymph nodes for 6-12 mo after a lymphangiogram permitting recognition of nodal changes. During that time, a single plain film of the abdomen is all that is needed to compare with previous studies. However, some workers have noted that the plain film may remain deceptively normal or unchanged, when in fact, significant abdominal disease can be detected by other techniques such as CT (41).

Computed tomography has provided a dramatic new method for evaluating abdominal lymph nodes. Enlarged paraaortic lymph nodes present as masses which may obliterate the aortic and vena caval contours (Fig. 18). CT enjoys a considerable advantage over lymphangiography inasmuch as it may detect enlarged lymph nodes which will not ordinarily be opacified by lymphangiography. These include nodes above the level of the cisterna chyli, in the root of the mesentery (Fig. 19), and in the hepatic or splenic hila (64). This is important as up to 50% of patients with untreated non-Hodgkin lymphoma may have mesenteric nodal involvement and this may occur in the presence of normal paraaortic lymph nodes (31). Lymph nodes which are completely replaced by lymphomatous tissue will be detected by CT, but not by lymphangiography (Fig. 20) (11).

The overall accuracy of CT in lymphoma has been shown to be approximately 90% (42). However, its main limitation lies in the fact that it cannot correctly detect lymphoma within normal sized or borderline enlarged paraaortic nodes (31).

This is particularly important in Hodgkin disease in which 5-10% of patients show minimal or no enlargement of nodes which are diseased (64,71). Furthermore, CT may yield false positive results when lymph node enlargement results from reactive hyperplasia rather than lymphomatous involvement. Lymphangiography has an edge over CT in this regard inasmuch as it can detect disease in normal sized lymph nodes and is fairly successful in differentiating reactive hyperplasia from lymphoma.

Radionuclide imaging with ^{67}Ga citrate has proven to be useful in detecting involvement of lymph nodes in the neck, mediastinum, and axilla. However, radiogallium scanning of the abdomen has been disappointing inasmuch as it will detect disease in only 50% of surgically proven sites (37). This is in part due to extensive uptake of the radionuclide by the liver and large bowel which tends to obscure the paraaortic lymph nodes and other retroperitoneal structures.

While markedly enlarged paraaortic lymph nodes are detected by ultrasound (Fig. 21), the technique is less successful in detecting moderately enlarged nodes (22). Bowel gas often precludes adequate ultrasonic visualization of the lower retroperitoneum.

It is clear therefore that CT and lymphangiography have a primary role to play in detecting abdominal lymphoma. However, there is no general agreement as to which technique or whether both should be used in any given case. It is our opinion that the CT scan should be the first study for detecting abdominal adenopathy. If the scan is obviously positive then a lymphangiogram need not be carried out. However, if the CT scan is normal or equivocal, lymphangiography should be the next step in the radiological algorithm particularly in patients with Hodgkin disease.

The Spleen

The spleen is frequently involved in both Hodgkin disease and non-Hodgkin lymphoma. Determination as to whether or not the spleen is involved is particularly important in Hodgkin disease as laparotomy studies have shown that it is not infrequently the sole focus of abdominal involvement (38). Unfortunately, most imaging techniques have been disappointing in the detection of splenic involvement. Both CT and 99mTc sulfur colloid liver-spleen scans reveal splenic enlargement. However, enlargement of the spleen in patients with lymphoma, particularly Hodgkin disease, is frequently due to causes other than lymphomatous involvement (38). Furthermore, the spleen may contain tumors while remaining normal in size. Focal intrasplenic lymphoma deposits may be detected by both CT (Fig. 22) (64) and radionuclide scanning (75). Splenic lesions are often less than 1 cm in diameter (45,64), and these usually cannot be detected by either imaging modality. It is possible that with future improvement in the resolution of CT scanners detection of splenic involvement will become more accurate. For the present a normal imaging study cannot be considered to reliably exclude involvement of the spleen.

The Liver

Macroscopic lymphoma deposits within the liver may be readily detected by radionuclide liver scans (2), CT, or ultrasound (Fig. 23). However, in early cases, liver involvement consists of microscopic deposits of lymphoma confined to the portal triad (2,31,64). Normal liver images do not therefore exclude the presence of lymphomatous involvement of the liver.

Other Anatomic Sites

Extranodal involvement occurs frequently in non-Hodgkin lymphoma in such sites as the gastrointestinal tract, pancreas, kidneys (Fig. 24), and adrenals. CT, urography, and barium studies will often document the existence of such disease.

CONCLUSION

Accurate radiological detection of infradiaphragmatic involvement in patients with malignant lymphoma would have a profound effect on patient management. However, all the available imaging techniques have obvious disadvantages and limitations in detecting this involvement. We believe that CT scanning should be the primary method for the assessment of the abdomen. If the scan reveals obvious adenopathy, no further radiological investigation need be undertaken. If, however, the CT scan is normal or equivocal, lymphangiography should be performed, particularly in Hodgkin disease, to detect the small group of patients who have normal sized, but diseased lymph nodes.

There is at present no imaging technique which will reliably detect early involvement of the liver or spleen.

COLORECTAL CANCER

Colorectal carcinoma has an incidence approaching that of lung carcinoma. Despite improvements in technique, radical surgical treatment for colorectal cancer has achieved no significant improvement in overall cure rate (30%) in the last 30 years (54). This has lead to a reexamination of the role of radiotherapy and some centers now use preoperative radiation, particularly in the management of rectosigmoid cancer (63). The advent of newer radiological techniques, including radionuclide scanning, CT, and gray scale ultrasound offers the possibility of more accurate preoperative staging of colorectal cancer and earlier detection of postoperative recurrence.

Staging of Newly Diagnosed Colonic Carcinoma

The Primary Tumor

Primary tumors will usually be diagnosed initially by clinical means, barium enema, or endoscopic examination with biopsy. Preoperative determination of tumor extent and the detection of involvement of adjacent organs is most useful in the case of rectosigmoid cancer. In this area preoperative radiotherapy shows some evidence of improving the overall survival rate (63, 77). CT is helpful inasmuch as it will detect the extent of the primary tumor and appropriate CT sections can be enlarged to actual body size and processed directly for treatment planning (29, 56). CT may show evidence of tumor invasion of the bladder, the uterus and vagina, and the bony sacrum and pelvis (Fig. 25). In the case of carcinoma arising in the cecum, ascending, transverse, and descending portions of the colon, there is no clear role for routine preoperative CT at the present time.

Regional Abdominal Spread and Metastases

Spread of tumor to paraaortic lymph nodes may be detected by CT, ultrasound, or lymphangiography. As detection of such spread does not significantly influence patient management, these techniques are rarely used for this purpose. However, in institutions which use preoperative radiation therapy, demonstration of enlarged paraaortic lymph nodes may lead to their inclusion in the radiation field (63).

Technetium sulfur colloid liver scanning is useful for the exclusion of liver metastasis and is generally used in the preoperative workup of most patients with colon carcinoma. While the technique has a high sensitivity for detection of liver metastasis, its specificity is relatively poor and false positive and equivocal scans are not frequently obtained. In such instances, either CT or ultrasound may be applied in further evaluation of the liver (Fig. 26). Radionuclide scanning of other organs need only be undertaken in patients with symptoms or signs pointing to the presence of metastases. Radiogallium scanning has not proved useful in either the detection or staging of colonic carcinoma. Positive results can be expected in only about 40% of surgically proven cases (60).

Excretory urography is essential in the workup of all cases of rectosigmoid carcinoma for the detection of ureteral obstruction.

Evaluation of Recurrent Colon Cancer

Following surgical resection of the primary tumor and reestablishment of the continuity of the colon, recurrence is detected by serial barium enemas supplemented where necessary by colonoscopy and biopsy. However, the diagnosis of tumor recurrence following abdominoperineal resection for rectal carcinoma is often difficult. Local recurrence is a major factor contributing to death in over 25% of patients (24). CT is of great value for diagnosing suspected recurrence of rectal cancer and in defining tumor extent in those patients with known recurrence (35).

Known Recurrence

CT can define the pelvic mass, its extent and involvement of muscles, organs, bone, and lymph nodes (Figs. 27 and 28). Such information is valuable to the radiotherapist for planning treatment and assessing tumor response to therapy. Ultrasound is not as accurate as CT for detecting precise involvement of adjacent structures. However, it is an inexpensive method for following the response to treatment of patients with known pelvic masses.

Suspected Recurrence

Modern high-resolution CT scans provide information about recurrent rectosigmoid cancers that cannot be obtained by any other techniques (Fig. 29). It is our recommendation that a CT scan should be obtained in the early postoperative period particularly in the high-risk patient with Dukes C carcinoma. Surgery distorts the normal pelvic anatomy and the baseline scan facilitates subsequent distinction between postsurgical changes and tumor recurrence. Because of the high risk of recurrence, a good case can be made for serial scanning in high-risk patients in an attempt to identify local recurrence before symptoms ensue (Fig. 29).

CONCLUSION

Radiology plays a useful role in staging of primary colon carcinoma. The advent of CT has provided an excellent method for postoperative detection of tumor recurrence.

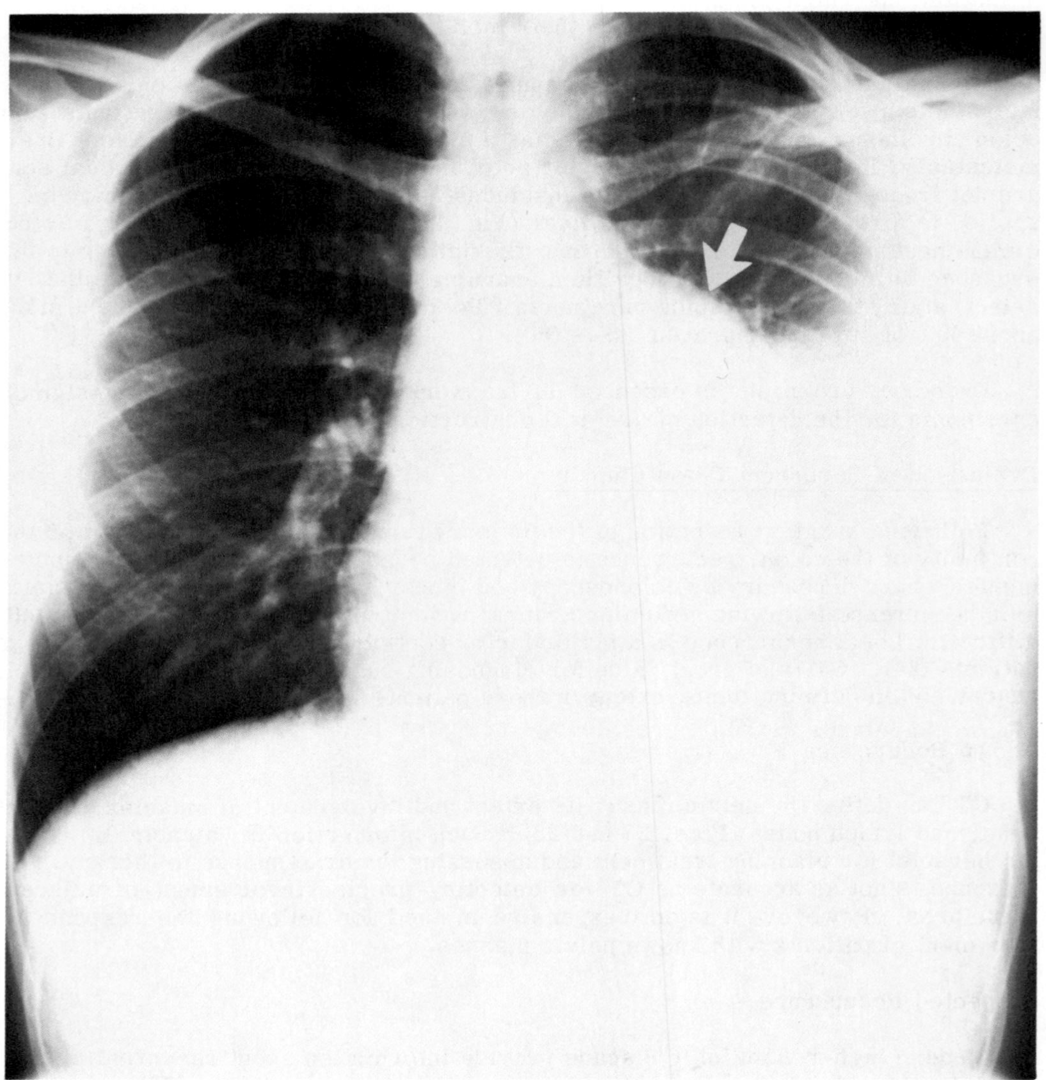

Figure 12. Patient presented with cough and left-sided chest pain. A: Plain film of chest shows a large left pleural effusion. There appears to be a mass (arrow), but its limits cannot be appreciated.

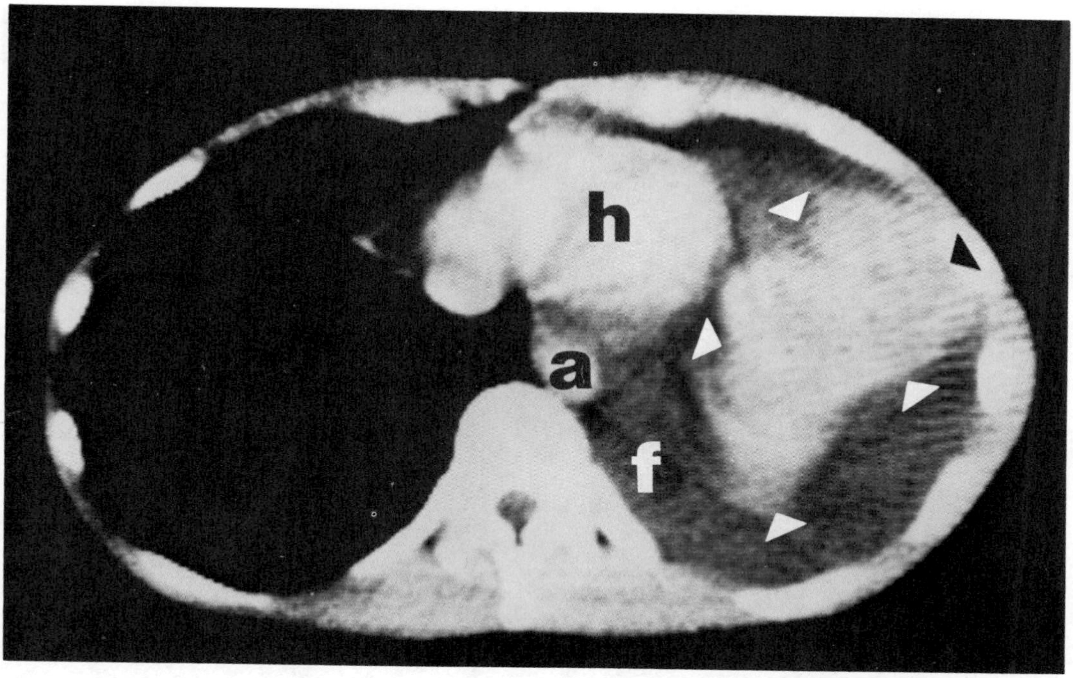

Figure 12. B: CT scan shows mass (arrowheads) surrounded by low-density fluid. The mass extends to the pleural surface laterally (black arrowhead) (f = pleural fluid, a = aorta, h = heart). Percutaneous biopsy showed an epidermoid carcinoma. The patient received radiotherapy.

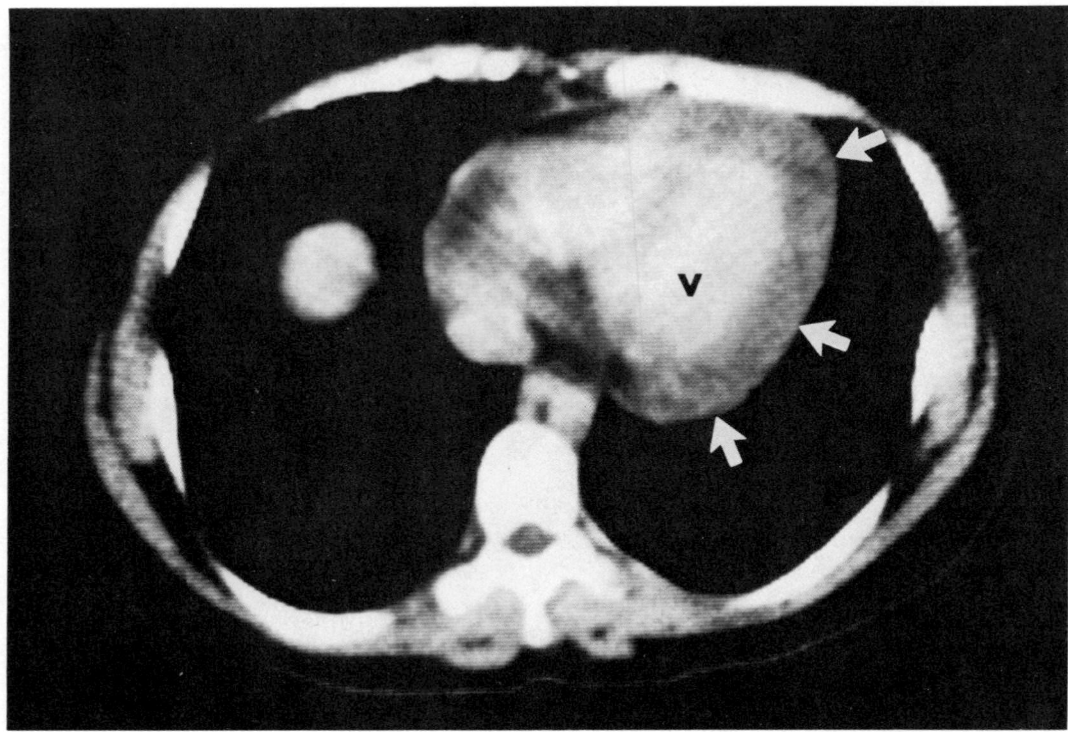

Figure 13. Patient presented with a superior mediastinal mass which at mediastinoscopy and biopsy was shown to be an undifferentiated small cell carcinoma involving lymph nodes. A CT scan below the level of the mass shows an unexpected pericardial effusion presenting as low-density fluid (arrows) surrounding the contrast containing left ventricle (v = left ventricle).

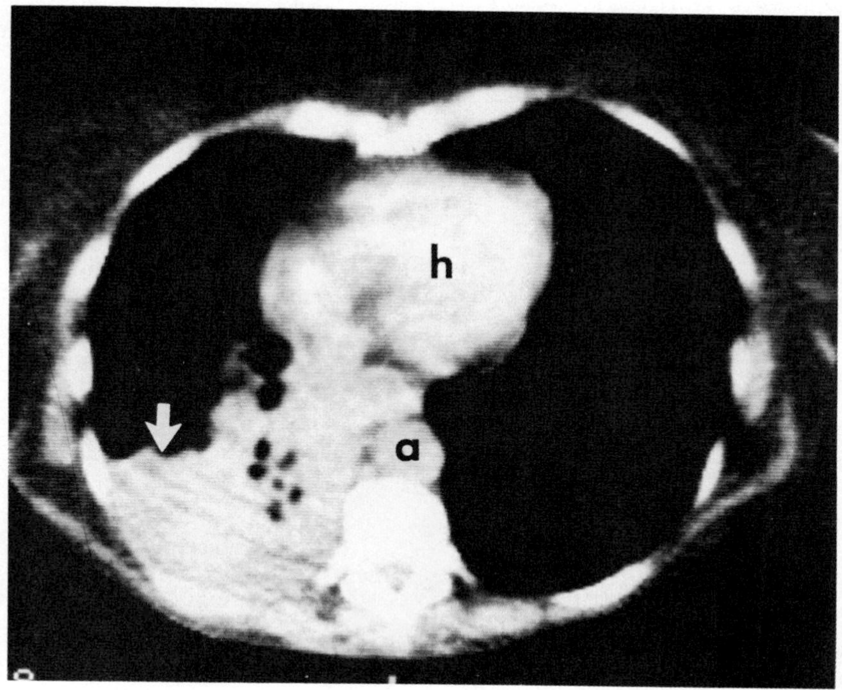

Figure 14. Patient presented with a mass in the inferior part of the right hilum. Bronchoscopy confirmed an epidermoid carcinoma arising in the right lower lobe bronchus. On CT scanning it was not possible to distinguish the tumor from the atelectatic and consolidated lung tissue distal to it (arrow) (h = heart, a = aorta).

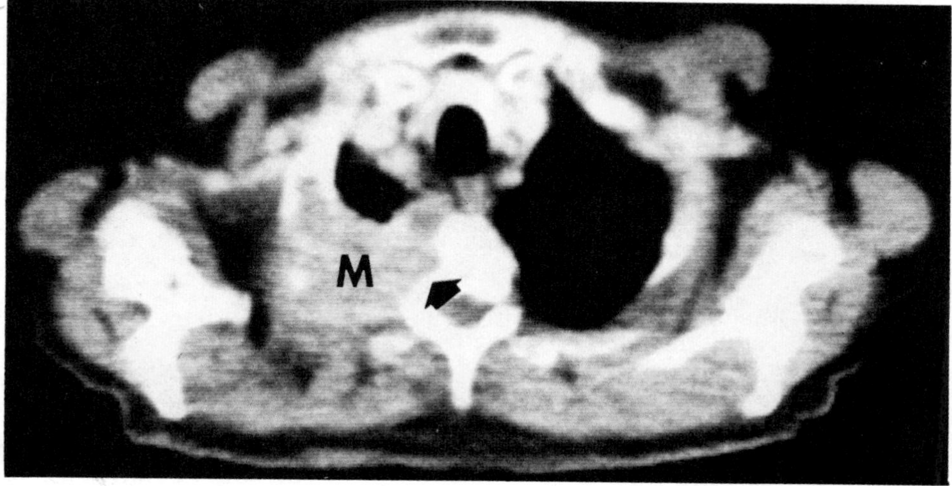

Figure 15. Patient with Pancoast tumor at right apex. The right apical mass and rib destruction were evident on plain films of the chest. However, erosion of the right side of the body of T1 (arrowhead) was shown only on CT (M = mass).

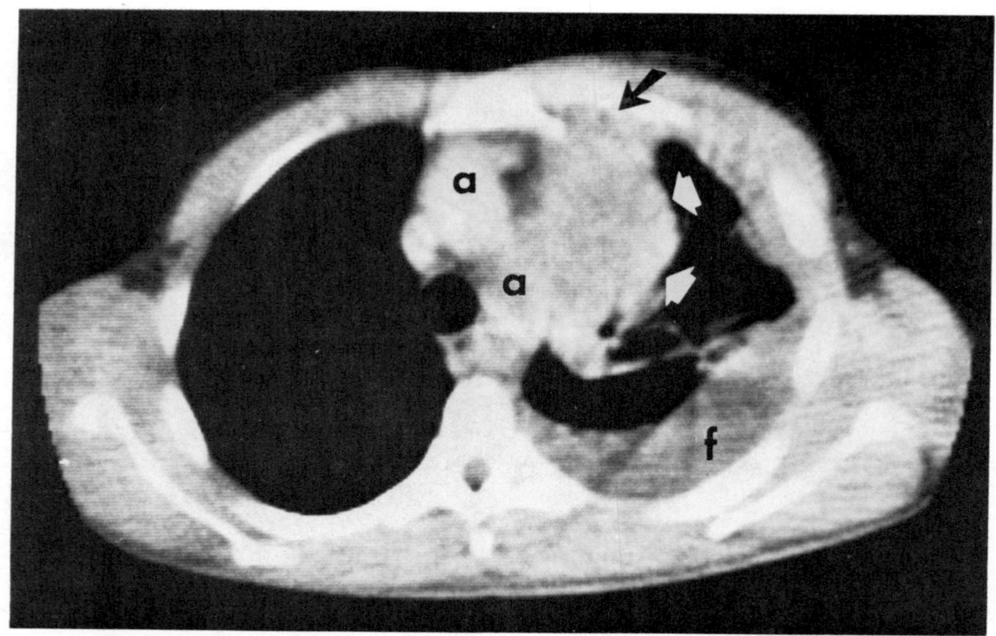

Figure 16. CT scan in patient with left upper lobe carcinoma. The tumor (white arrowheads) is invading the mediastinum as evidenced by obliteration of the fat plane adjacent to the aortic arch. The tumor is also extending anteriorly to the pleural surface (black arrow) and there is an associated pleural effusion (a = aorta, f = pleural effusion).

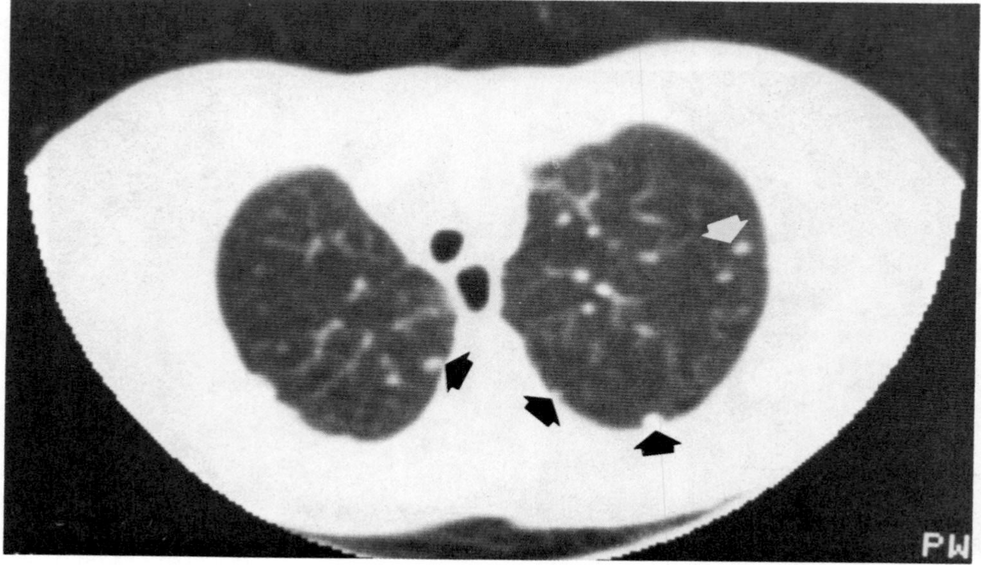

Figure 17. CT scan in patient with bronchial carcinoma right lower lobe (not shown on scan). Scan shows subpleural metastases (arrowheads) which were not evident on conventional laminograms.

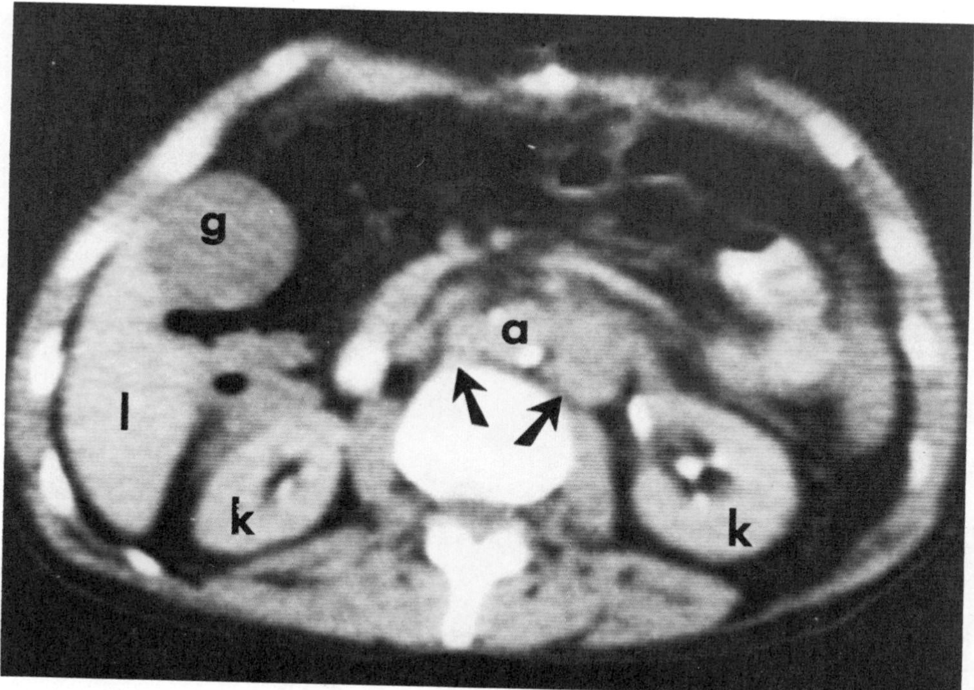

Figure 18. Histiocytic lymphoma. Enlarged paraaortic lymph nodes (arrows) partially obscure the aortic contour (a = aorta, l = liver, g = gallbladder, k = kidney).

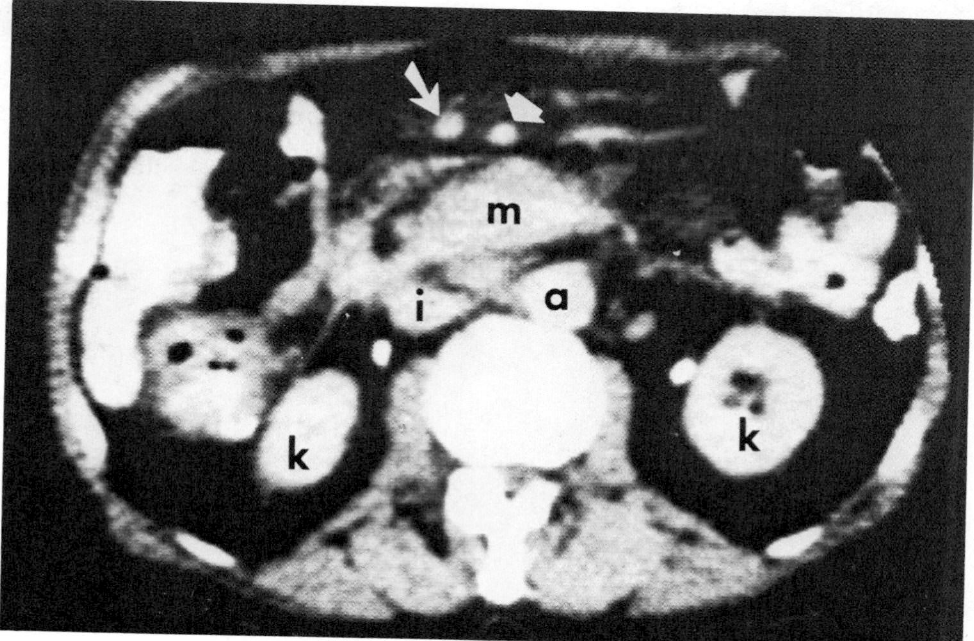

Figure 19. Lymphocytic lymphoma. There is a lymph node mass in the root of the mesentery with anterior displacement of the superior mesenteric vein (long arrow) and superior mesenteric artery (arrowhead) (a = aorta, i = inferior vena cava, k = kidney, m = mesenteric mass).

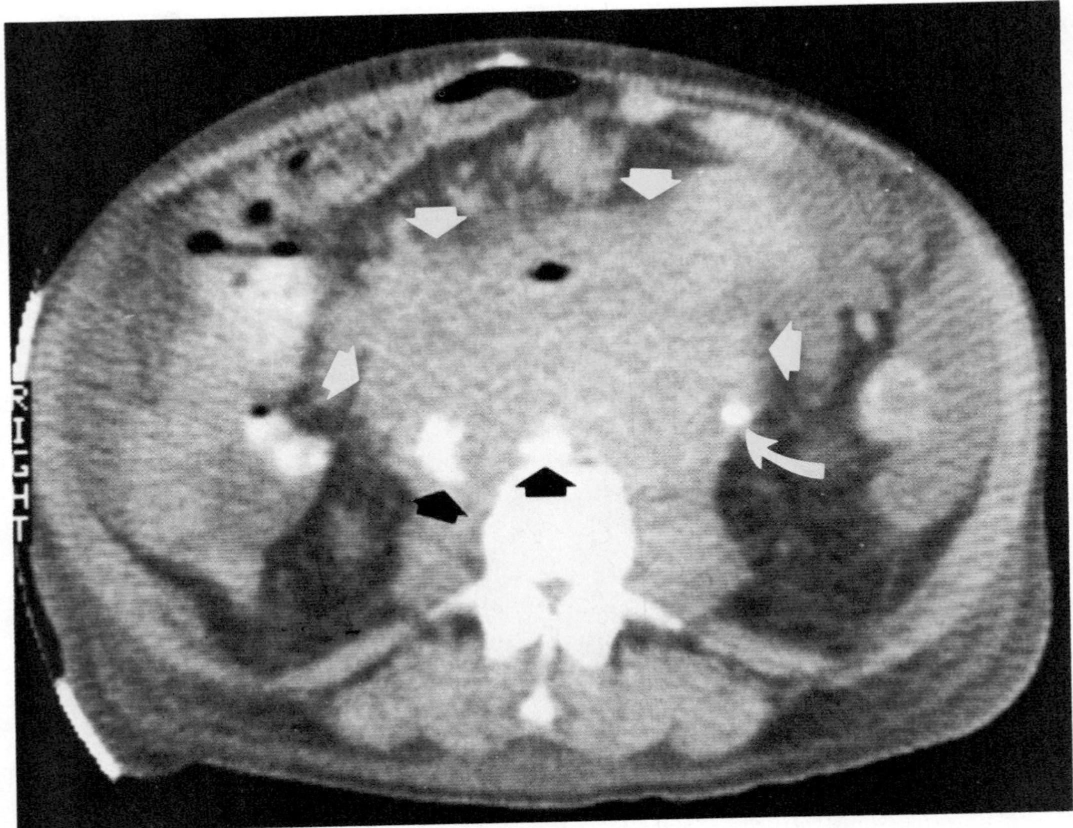

Figure 20. Histiocytic lymphoma. CT scan shows large mass of lymph nodes (white arrowheads) totally obscuring the aortic and inferior vena caval contours. The scan was obtained 3 days after a lymphangiogram. Only partial filling of 2 nodes (black arrowheads) with contrast has occurred. The left ureter (curved arrow) is laterally displaced.

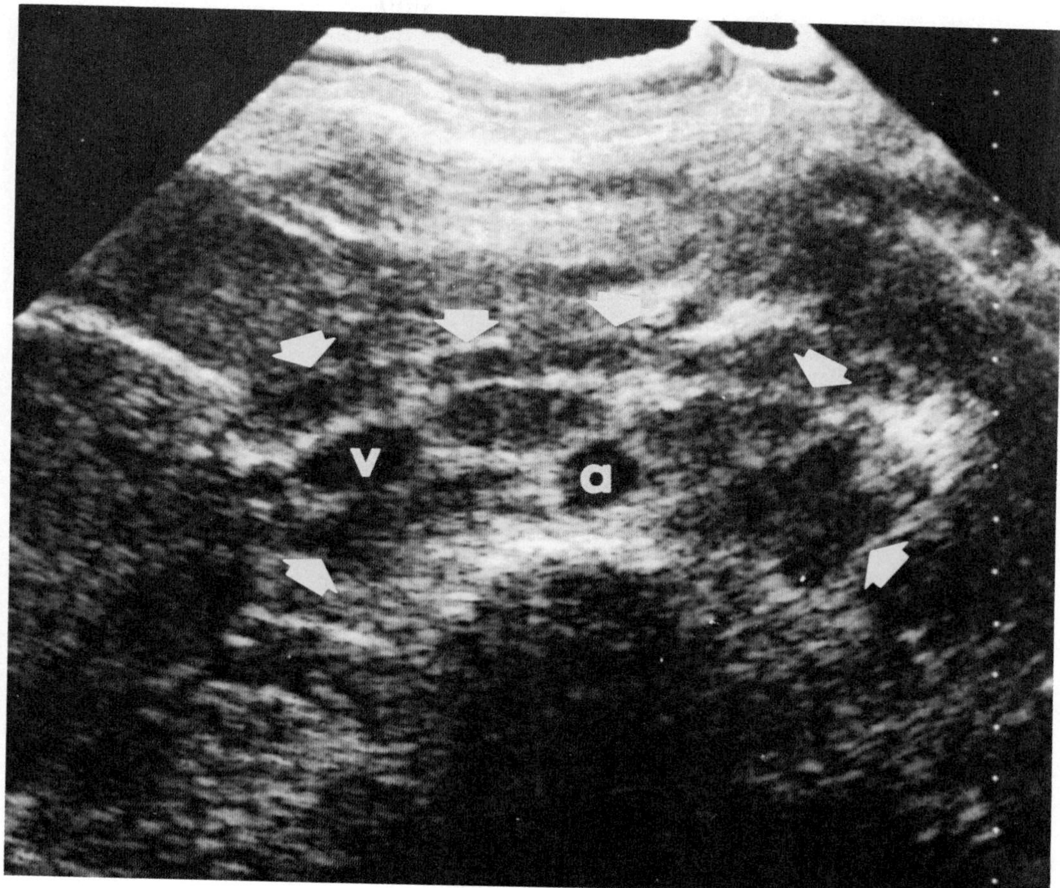

Figure 21. Hodgkin disease. Transverse ultrasonic scan below the level of the pancreas. Enlarged paraaortic and retrocaval lymph nodes (arrowheads) are present (a = aorta, v = inferior vena cava).

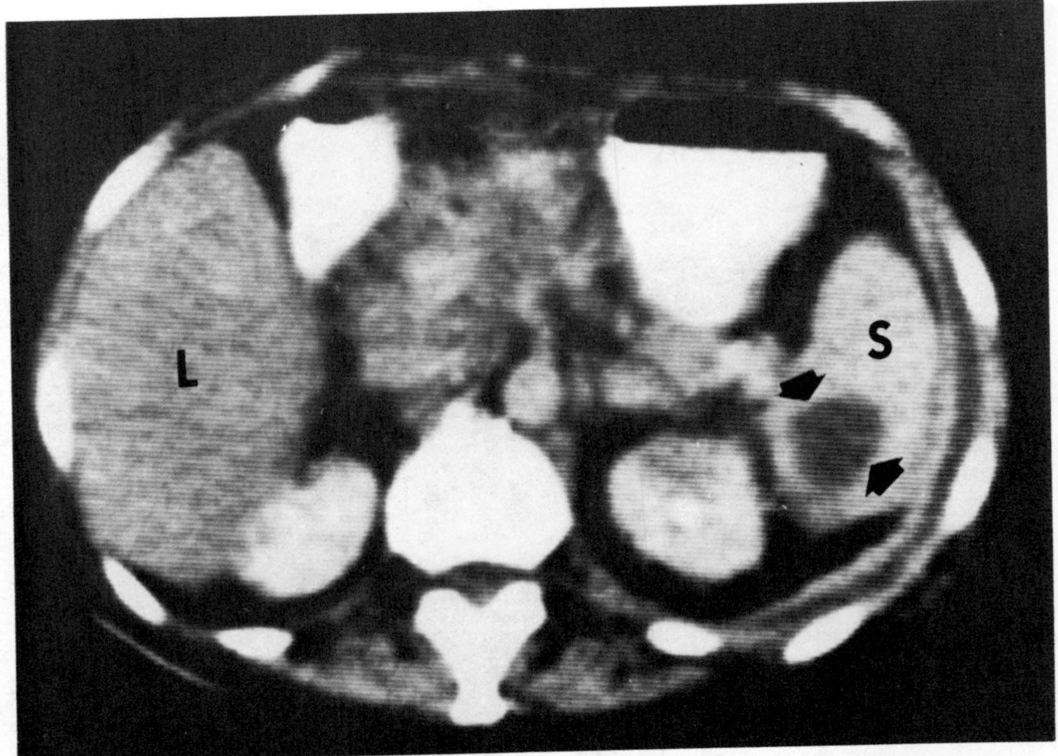

Figure 22. Poorly differentiated lymphocytic lymphoma. The spleen shows a focal deposit of lymphoma (black arrowheads) (L = liver, S = spleen).

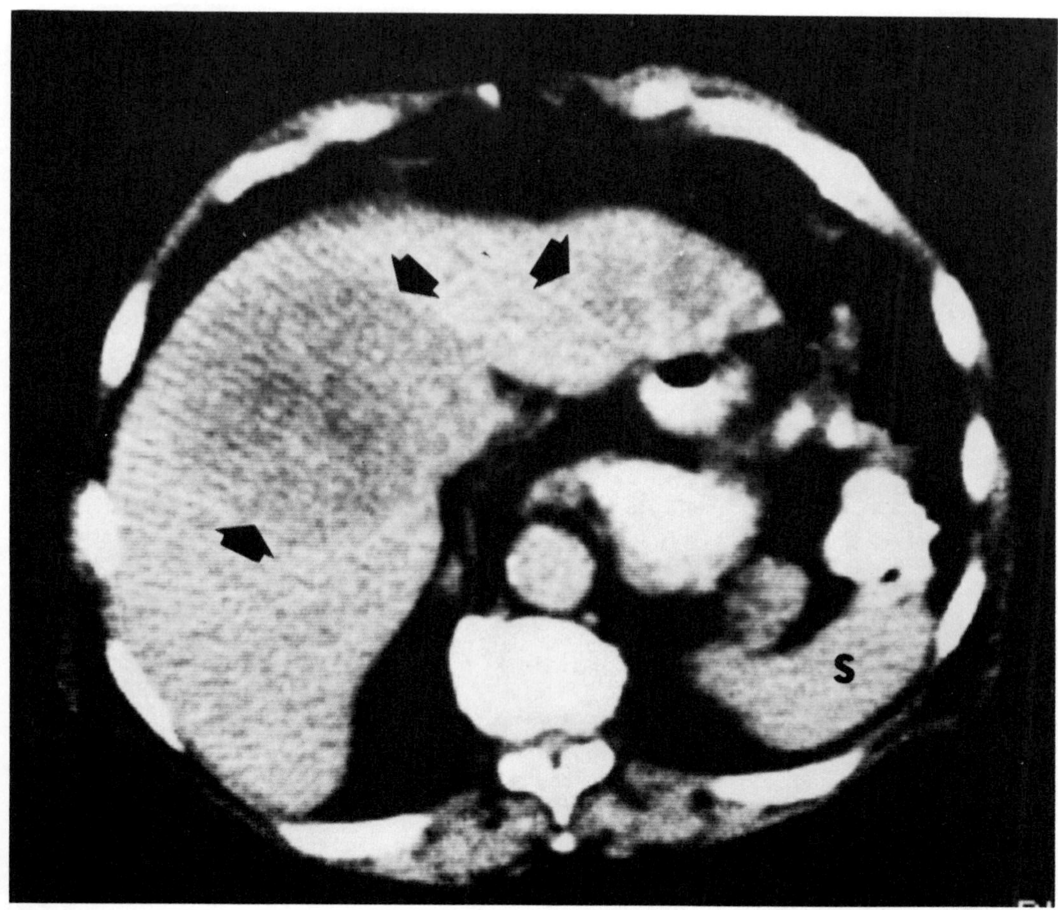

Figure 23. Histiocytic lymphoma. A: CT scan shows biopsy proven lymphomatous masses (black arrowheads) involving the right and left lobes of the liver.

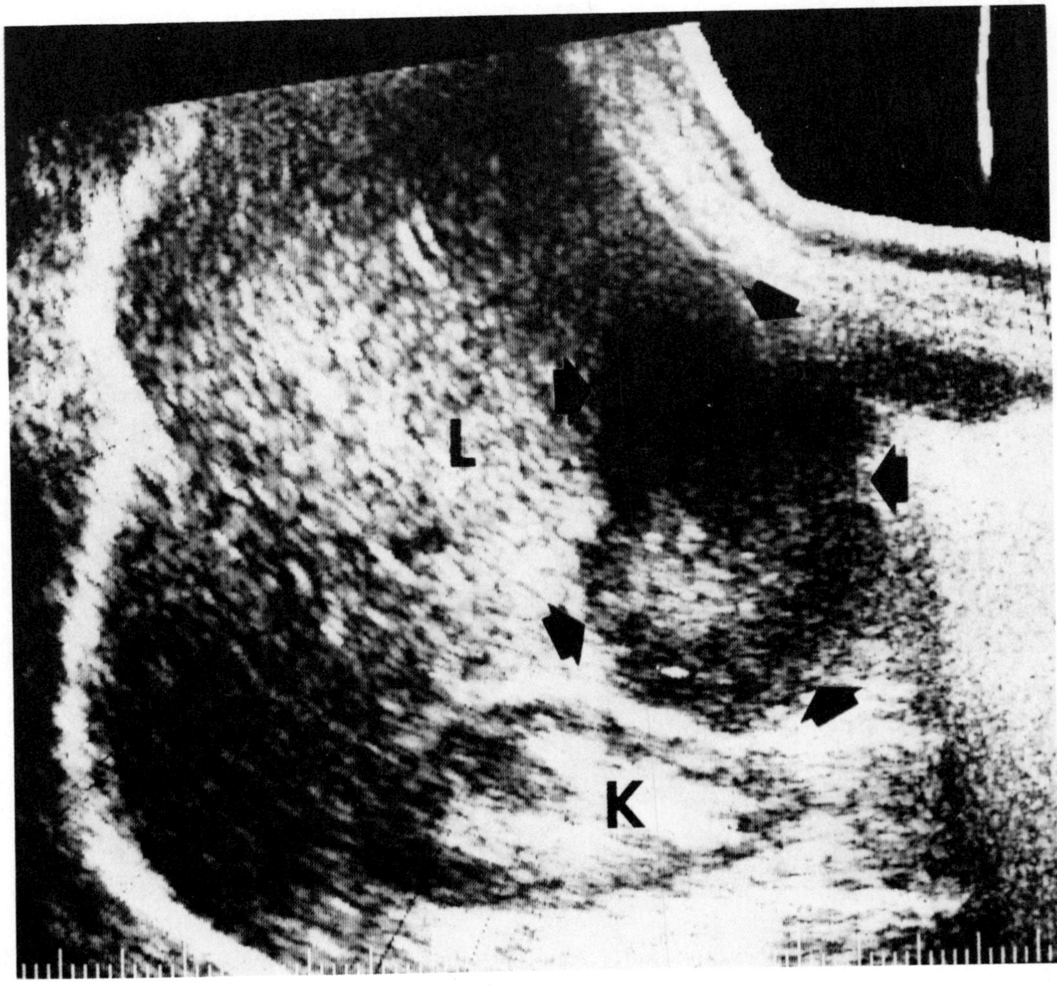

Figure 23. B: Parasagittal ultrasound scan shows the mass in the right lobe of the liver (black arrowheads) (S = spleen, L = liver, K = kidney).

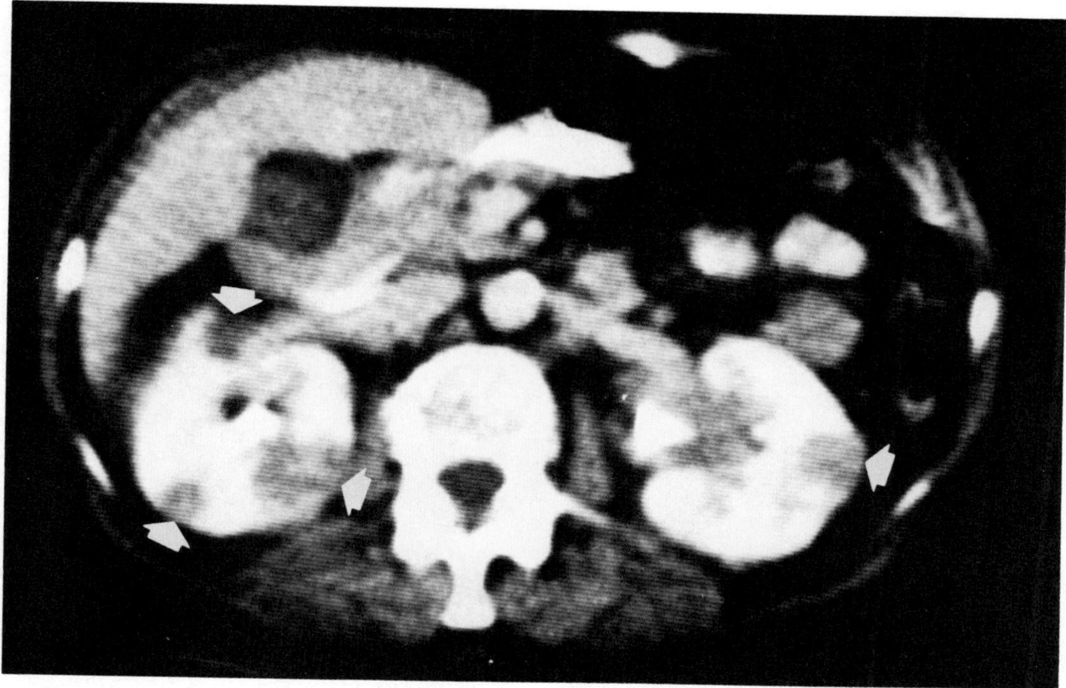

Figure 24. Poorly differentiated lymphocytic lymphoma. Multifocal lymphoma (white arrowheads) involving both kidneys. This patient did not have paraaortic adenopathy.

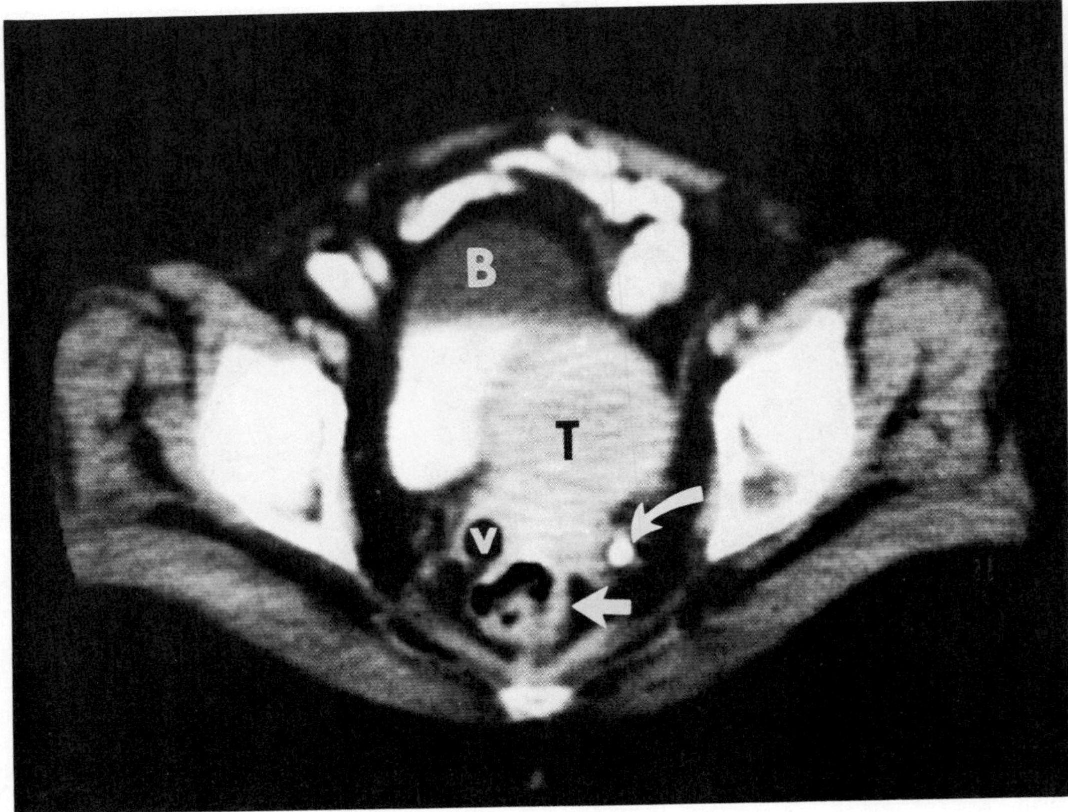

Figure 25. Female patient with rectal carcinoma. The tumor has a large extraluminal component which is displacing the bladder and vagina to the right. The tumor had obstructed the right ureter (not shown) and is close to the left ureter (curved arrow). The vaginal canal is encircled by the tumor mass. Gas is present in the rectal lumen (straight white arrow) (B = bladder, T = tumor, V = vagina).

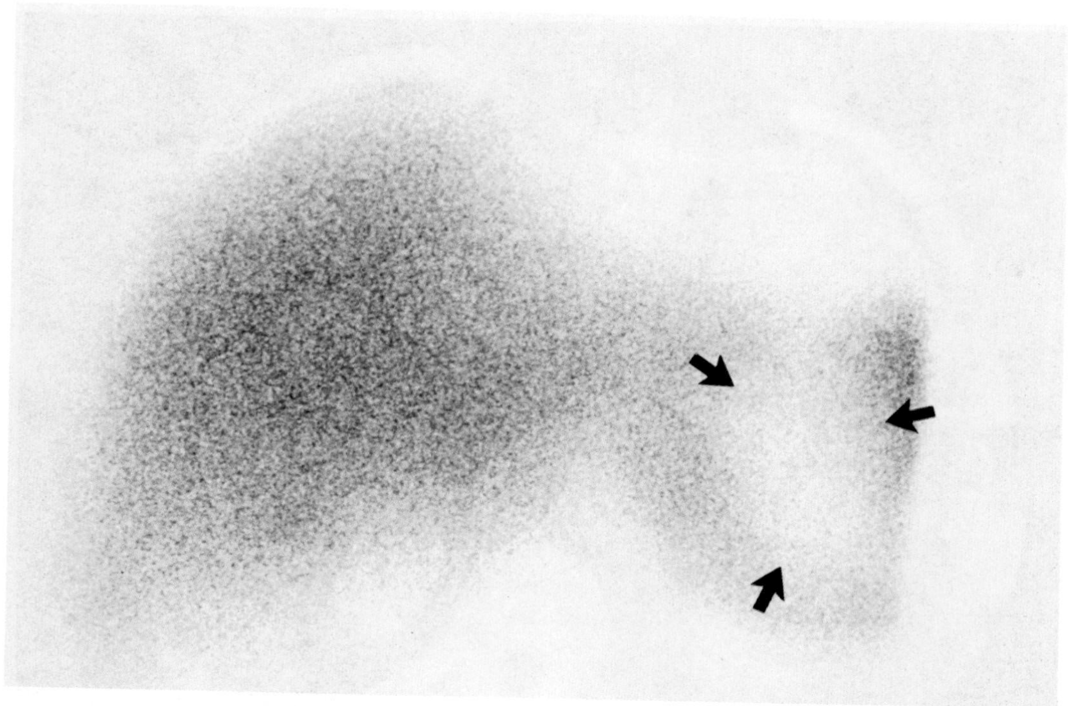

Figure 26. Patient with sigmoid carcinoma. A: Anterior projection of 99mTc = sulfur colloid liver scan. The right lobe of the liver is normal. There is a large area of decreased uptake of radiocolloid in the left lobe of the liver (arrows).

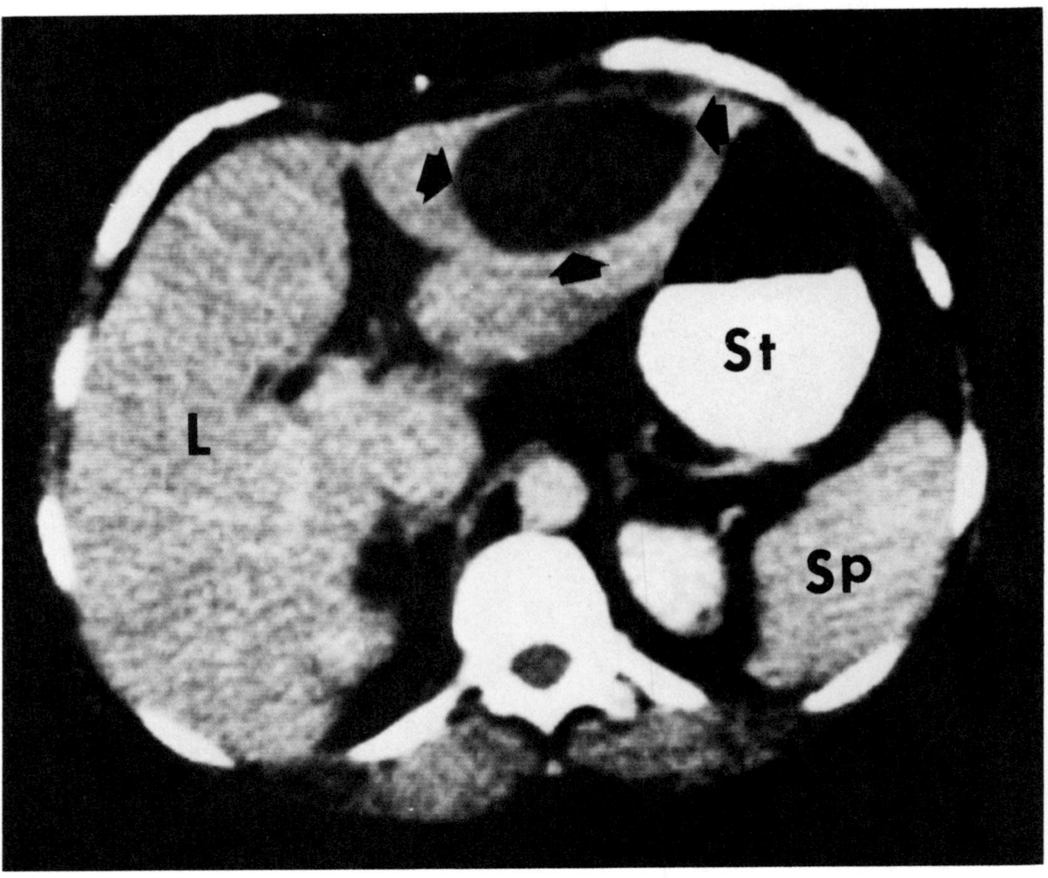

Figure 26. B: CT scan shows well-defined low-density mass in the left lobe of the liver (arrowheads). The CT number was 3 Hounsfield units indicating a fluid containing lesion suggestive of a cyst.

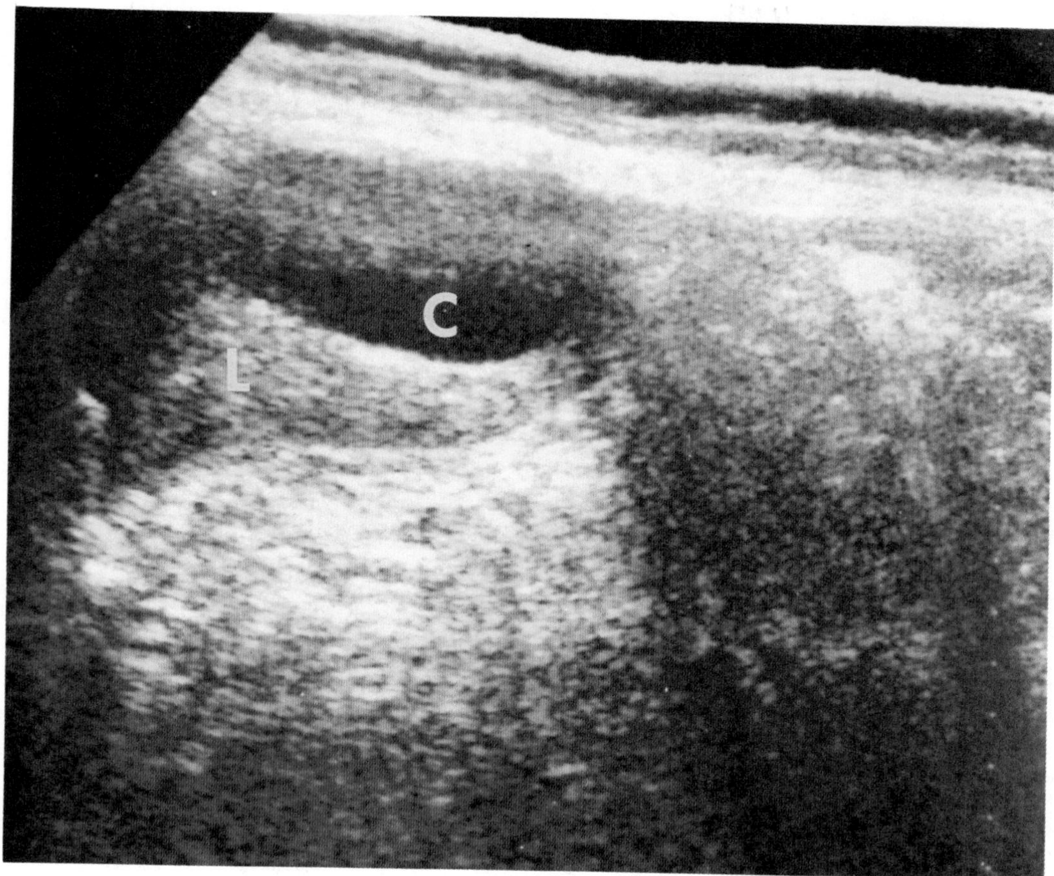

Figure 26. C: Parasagittal ultrasound scan through left lobe of liver. This shows a sonolucent lesion with posterior acoustic enhancement and a smooth posterior wall indicative of a cyst. At surgery for resection of the sigmoid carcinoma, the liver lesion was aspirated and shown to be a simple hepatic cyst (L = liver, St = stomach, Sp = spleen, C = cyst).

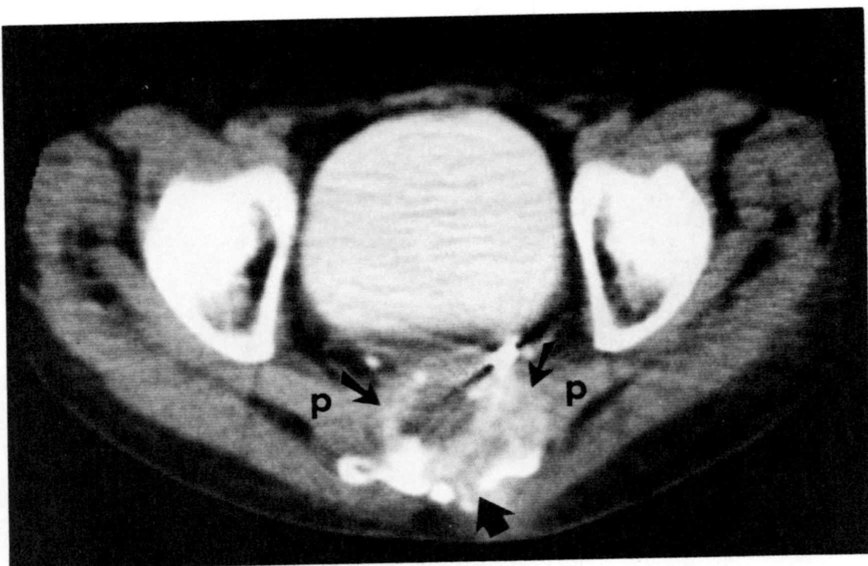

Figure 27. CT scan of pelvis in a patient with lower back and pelvic pain 14 mo following abdominoperineal resection for rectal carcinoma. There is recurrent tumor (small black arrows) posterior to the bladder with invasion of the piriformis muscles and the sacrum (large black arrow) (P = piriformis muscles).

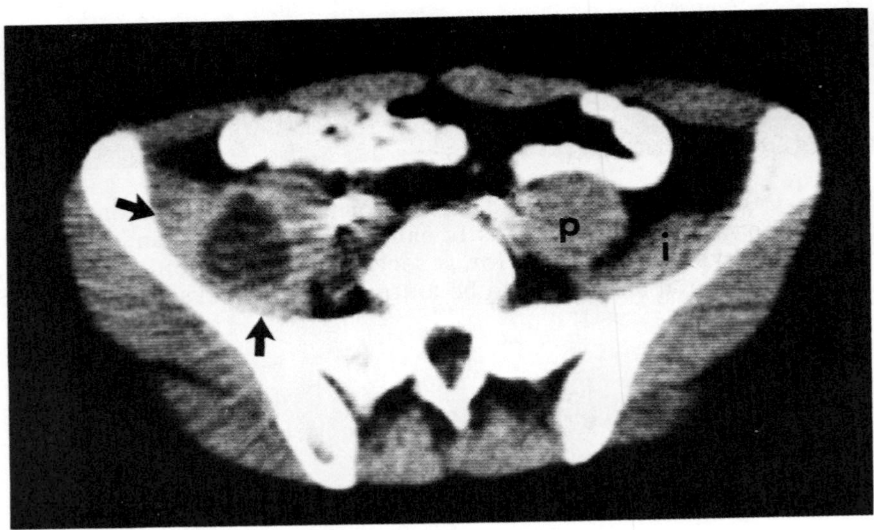

Figure 28. CT scan of pelvis in patient with pain in right thigh 10 mo following abdominoperineal resection for rectal carcinoma. Recurrent tumor (arrows) is invading the right psoas and iliacus muscles in the area of the femoral nerve (P = normal contralateral psoas muscle, i = normal contralateral iliacus muscle).

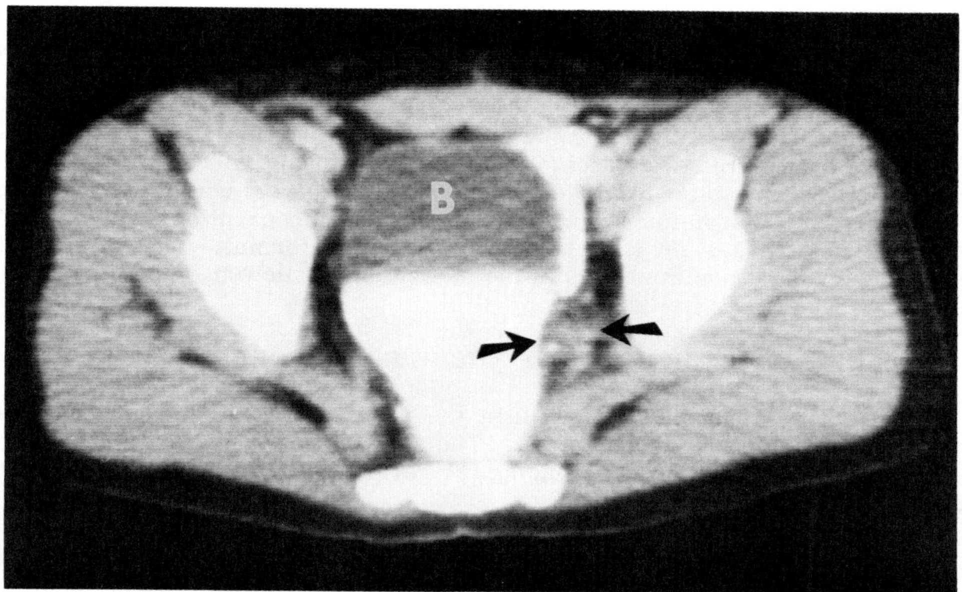

Figure 29. Patient had undergone abdominoperineal resection for rectal carcinoma. A: CT scan 4 mo after surgery, the patient being asymptomatic. There is a small mass (arrows) on the left side of the pelvis adjacent to the bladder.

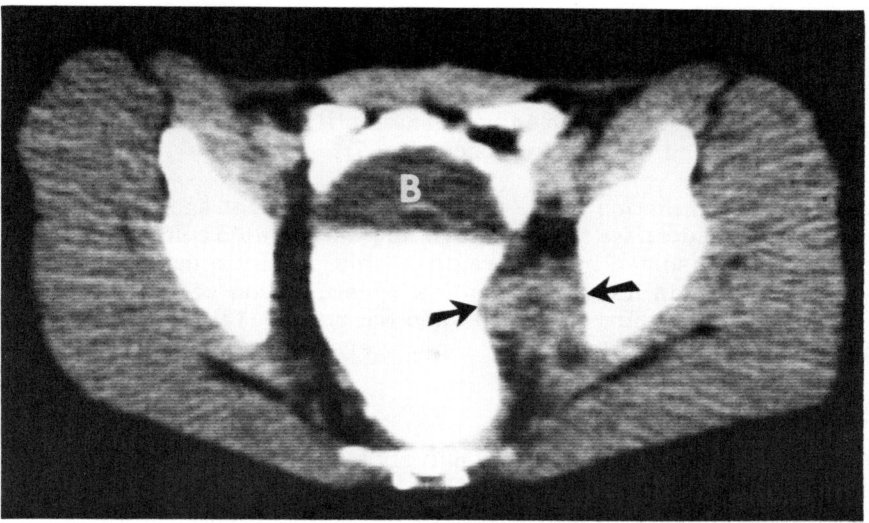

Figure 29. B: CT scan 8 mo after surgery. At this time the patient had pelvic pain. There has been interval enlargement of the pelvic mass (arrows) which now extends to the left lateral pelvic wall. This was interpreted as recurrent tumor and the patient responded satisfactorily to radiation therapy (B = bladder).

SECTION III. PELVIC MALIGNANCIES

Nabil F. Maklad, M.D.

The role of computed tomography and ultrasound in the initial staging of pelvic malignancies and in the evaluation of response to therapy is currently under study in several centers. The advantages of these two relatively noninvasive procedures include minimum discomfort to the patient, no prior preparation, and the display of the size and areas of invasion in a cross-sectional format. The two modalities tend to have complementary roles in the staging and followup of pelvic malignancies.

CARCINOMA OF THE UTERINE CERVIX

Both CT and ultrasound are useful in the pretreatment evaluation of patients with invasive carcinoma of the cervix. The examination should be directed first at the structures immediately surrounding the cervix because this disease spreads mainly by direct extension.

The staging of carcinoma of the cervix has traditionally depended on pelvic examination, including speculum and rectovaginal palpation. The rectovaginal examination is the critical part since it permits the palpation of extension of the disease into the pericervical and parametrial regions. However, Nelson (57) and Averette et al. (5) have shown a significant error in clinical staging. Palpation of induration of the pericervical ligaments is not difficult, but the international classification specifically states that there must be nodular induration in order to consider it extension of the cancer.

Ultrasound examination has been used to determine the size and location of the uterus, and its relationship to other pelvic structures in patients with carcinoma of the cervix. The examination is performed utilizing the full urinary bladder to enable visualization of the pelvic structures (7).

For the CT examination of the pelvis, dilute contrast agent is introduced into the rectum to help identify this structure and the sigmoid colon. In addition, a large vaginal tampon is inserted into the vaginal folds. The vaginal tampon entraps a sufficient amount of air in its fibers to allow identification of the distended vagina. This is helpful in localizing the cervix and the uterus (13). Intravenous contrast agent is usually employed to identify the ureters and opacify the urinary bladder.

Parametrial Invasion

Ultrasound has not been used extensively to detect parametrial invasion in patients with carcinoma of the cervix. This extension manifests itself by thickening of the adnexal structures on ultrasound scans of the pelvis. However, such thickening is nonspecific and is sometimes inaccurate.

CT scanning utilizing a vaginal tampon can provide demonstration of parametrial and paravaginal extension. Tumor extension can be identified by obliteration of normal fat planes and surrounding adipose tissue (Fig. 30).

Extension Onto the Pelvic Wall

Ultrasound examination is not helpful in demonstrating extension onto the pelvic wall because of the intervening bony structures.

CT demonstrates the bony pelvic structures in addition to the musculature of the pelvis. Extension of carcinoma of the cervix onto the pelvic wall can be diagnosed on CT scans of the pelvis (Fig. 31).

Pelvic and Paraaortic Lymphadenopathy

Enlarged lateral pelvic lymph nodes secondary to metastatic carcinoma of the cervix can be outlined by both CT and ultrasound. However, enlargement of the nodes is not absolute proof of metastatic involvement. Lymphangiography is still superior in detecting metastatic disease in the enlarged nodes (82).

Involvement of Bladder and Rectum

Cystoscopic, proctoscopic, and sigmoidoscopic examinations are carried out on all patients with invasive carcinoma of the cervix to rule out direct extension of the disease to the bladder, rectum, and sigmoid colon. It is believed that CT could detect invasion of these organs, but a sufficiently large series is not yet available to estimate the accuracy of this method in detecting such invasion.

Staging of Cervical Carcinoma

Both CT and ultrasound cannot differentiate between stage I and stage IIA. However, stages IIB, III, and IV can be differentiated utilizing CT scans of the pelvis with introduction of a vaginal tampon, contrast agent in the rectum and gas insufflation of the urinary bladder. It is believed that CT evaluation of patients with invasive carcinoma of the cervix will be more accurate for staging then current traditional methods. Both ultrasound and CT can be used to examine the kidneys for diagnosis of obstructive changes.

Response to Therapy and Followup

Serial scans can be done at appropriate intervals during the treatment program and compared to the initial pretherapy scan. Monitoring in this manner allows modification of treatment plans by adjustment of the radiation fields, and the response to therapy can be assessed.

After completion of the initial treatment, a scan should be obtained to serve as a baseline for comparison with future studies. The scans can be done quickly and safely and require little special patient preparation. Incomplete response to therapy or evidence of recurrent disease can be easily diagnosed and appropriate treatment measures can be undertaken.

CARCINOMA OF THE UTERINE CORPUS

Evaluation of the uterus is generally better done by gray scale ultrasound, as the information obtained at CT about the uterus is less specific. The size of the uterus, its location in relation to surrounding structures, and irregularities of the contour and of the internal structure are clearly demonstrated.

The value of ultrasound and CT in this condition is in determining if extrauterine extension of a previously diagnosed endometrial carcinoma has occurred and not in making the primary diagnosis. Extrauterine extension can be detected on CT scans by invasion and replacement of the normal, parametrial, and paravaginal fat. Widespread involvement of the pelvis by extrauterine extension of endometrial carcinoma results in the loss of all fascial plains.

CT and ultrasound can thus be used to differentiate between stage II and stage III uterine carcinoma. Involvement of the mucosa of the bladder or rectum, criteria for stage IV, are still better assessed by cystoscopy and sigmoidoscopy.

Both CT and ultrasound can be used in assessing the response to therapy, in followup after completion of the initial therapy, and in the diagnosis of recurrence.

OVARIAN CARCINOMA

Ultrasound is the primary diagnostic technique used to evaluate the ovaries, distinguish between cystic and solid ovarian masses, and to diagnose pelvic and abdominal ascites. CT scanning can add information about the distant spread of malignant ovarian tumors. The role of ultrasound and CT scanning in staging of ovarian cancer is still evolving.

Recent advances in the staging of ovarian cancer have suggested that many patients with apparently localized disease actually have occult dissemination within the abdomen. Approximately 20% of patients classified as stage I or II at laparotomy have abnormal retroperitoneal lymph nodes by lymphangiography. Half of the stage I or II patients also have advanced disease documented by peritoneoscopy. Ovarian cancer is often discovered to have metastasized to the undersurface of the right diaphragm. This new information about biological behavior of ovarian cancer may help explain the high treatment failure rates in stages I and II disease following surgery and pelvic radiation (23).

Ultrasound is an accurate method of detecting ascites, and thus could aid in differentiating stages IA and IB from stage IC (Fig. 32). Examination of pelvic and retroperitoneal lymph nodes by either CT or ultrasound in patients with ovarian carcinoma could aid in the detection of lymph node involvement and thus correct staging. The under surface of the right diaphragm can be imaged consistently with ultrasound, and metastases in this region could be diagnosed with a high degree of accuracy. If such metastases are found, this indicates a stage IV ovarian carcinoma.

Response to therapy and followup of patients with ovarian carcinoma is best assessed by serial ultrasonic examinations.

CARCINOMA OF THE VAGINA AND VULVA

The role of CT and ultrasound in vaginal and vulval carcinoma is limited to detection of pelvic and abdominal extent of these diseases.

URINARY BLADDER NEOPLASMS

The clinical staging of urinary bladder neoplasms provides the basis for therapeutic recommendations and primarily depends on cystoscopy, biopsy, and bimanual examination under anesthesia. A large number of radiological studies have been used in an adjunctive role to determine the depth of infiltration and/or regional extension of the tumor. These studies include cystography, arteriography, intravesical and perivesical gas insufflation with tomography, triple contrast cystography, and lymphangiography.

The error between the clinically estimated stage and the pathologically determined stage in a group of patients treated by radical cystectomy with pelvic lymph node dissection has been recently reported (84). There was a tendency to understage tumors. Despite varying claims for each of the radiological modalities, the accuracy rate in staging bladder neoplasms has been discouraging (39). In a series of 105 patients 56% were incorrectly staged. Ultrasound has been utilized in the staging of bladder tumors with varying success (49).

Computed tomographic scanning of the pelvis to assist in the clinical staging of bladder neoplasms is fast becoming the diagnostic modality of choice. Several reports (11,68,69) document the accuracy of computed tomography staging of bladder neoplasms. It has been suggested that gas introduced into the bladder provides discrete depiction of the intraluminal projection and nature of the tumor (70). In addition, intravenous iodinated contrast material administered prior to scanning allows visualization of the ureters in the pelvis. In the female patient, a vaginal tampon is introduced prior to scanning to help identify and distend the vaginal canal.

CT in the Staging of Bladder Neoplasms

At the present time, superficial noninvasive lesions limited to the mucosa, stage O; lesions limited to the submucosa, stage A; superficial muscle invasion, stage BI; and deep muscle invasion of the bladder wall, stage BII, cannot be adequately distinguished from each other by CT scanning (Fig. 33). These lesions usually present as intraluminal projections only. In some cases, large superficial tumors may distort the bladder contour by their weight. Stage BII lesions may result in the localized thickening of the wall of the urinary bladder. Lesions located near the ureterovesical junction may result in ureteral obstruction and this can be demonstrated.

The main use of CT is to differentiate stage BII or less lesions from stage C and stage D. Stage C lesions, with extension through the bladder wall and involvement of the perivesical fat, are identified by either loss of definition of the perivesical fat margin compared with the uninvolved portions of the bladder, or obliteration of the normal perivesical fat (Fig. 34). In addition, invasion of the seminal vesicle is seen as obliteration of the angle between this structure and the base of the urinary bladder.

Local extension of the tumor in the pelvis and lymph node involvement, stage D, is usually not difficult to assess. However, involvement of the prostate by a tumor at the base of the bladder is often difficult to detect.

The reported accuracy of CT in staging bladder neoplasms is better than 80%. (As more experience is gained in utilizing CT for staging of bladder neoplasms the accuracy is expected to be greater than what has been achieved.)

PROSTATIC CARCINOMA

Diagnostic Ultrasound

A special instrument utilizing a transrectal ultrasonic probe and a radial scanner attached to a specially designed chair has been developed and extensively used in Japan for imaging of the prostate and surrounding pelvic organs. However, this specialized ultrasonic unit is not widely available in North America. Staging of carcinoma of the prostate utilizing this specialized instrument has been carried out in Japan with some success (30).

Computerized Tomography

The main role of CT with respect to carcinoma of the prostate is to evaluate extension of the tumor, especially stages C and D. Spread of the tumor beyond the prostatic capsule can be diagnosed, especially extension into the seminal vesicles. Metastases to the vesical, sacral external iliac, and lumbar lymph nodes can be detected. Bony metastases, stage D in the pelvis, is also amenable to CT diagnosis.

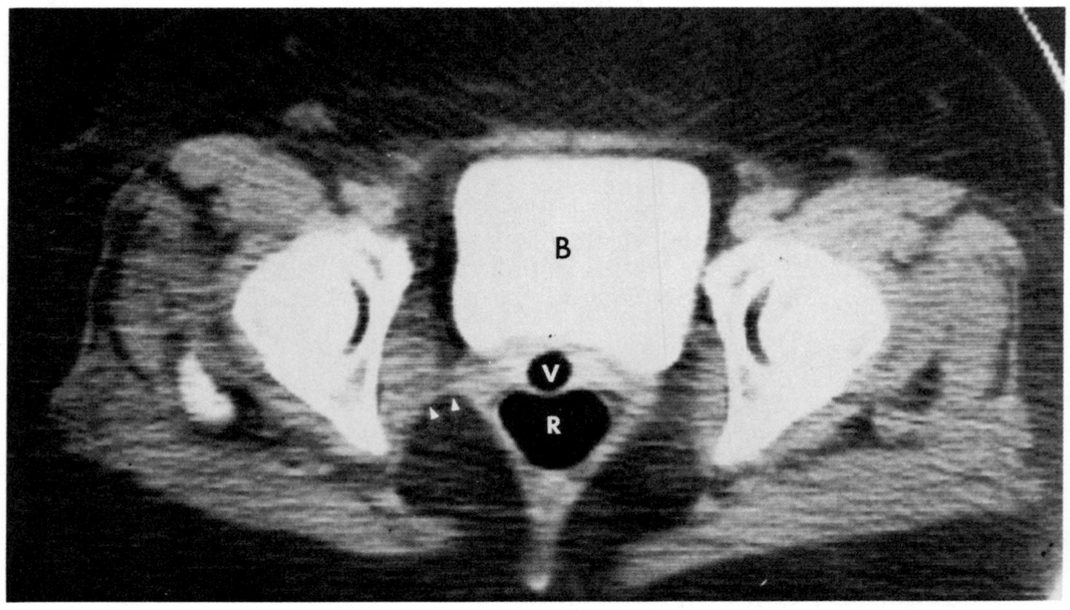

Figure 30. Carcinoma of the cervix with parametrial invasion. CT scan of the lower pelvis shows the urinary bladder (B) distended with contrast. The vaginal tampon (V) identifies the vagina. Paravaginal and parametrial extension of the tumor is seen on the right side (arrowheads) (R = rectum).

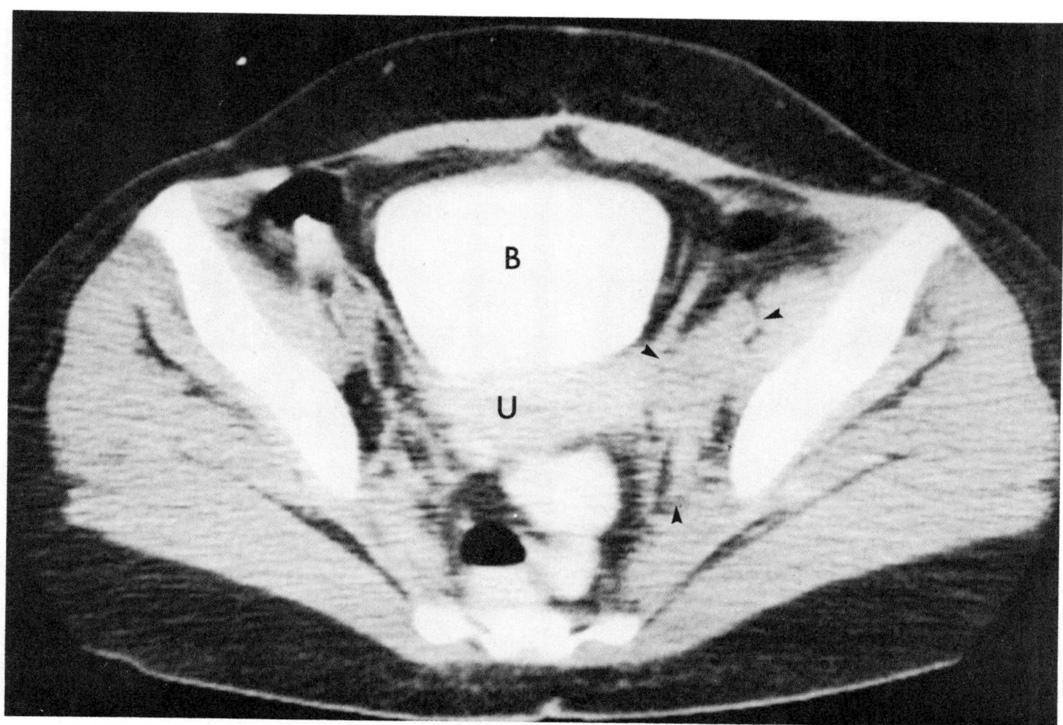

Figure 31. Carcinoma of the cervix with extension onto the pelvic wall. CT scan of the pelvis demonstrates contrast-filled urinary bladder (B). The uterus (U) is seen behind the bladder. There is extension of the tumor onto the left pelvic wall (arrowheads). Note the obliteration of the normal fat planes on the involved left side (compare to the uninvolved right side).

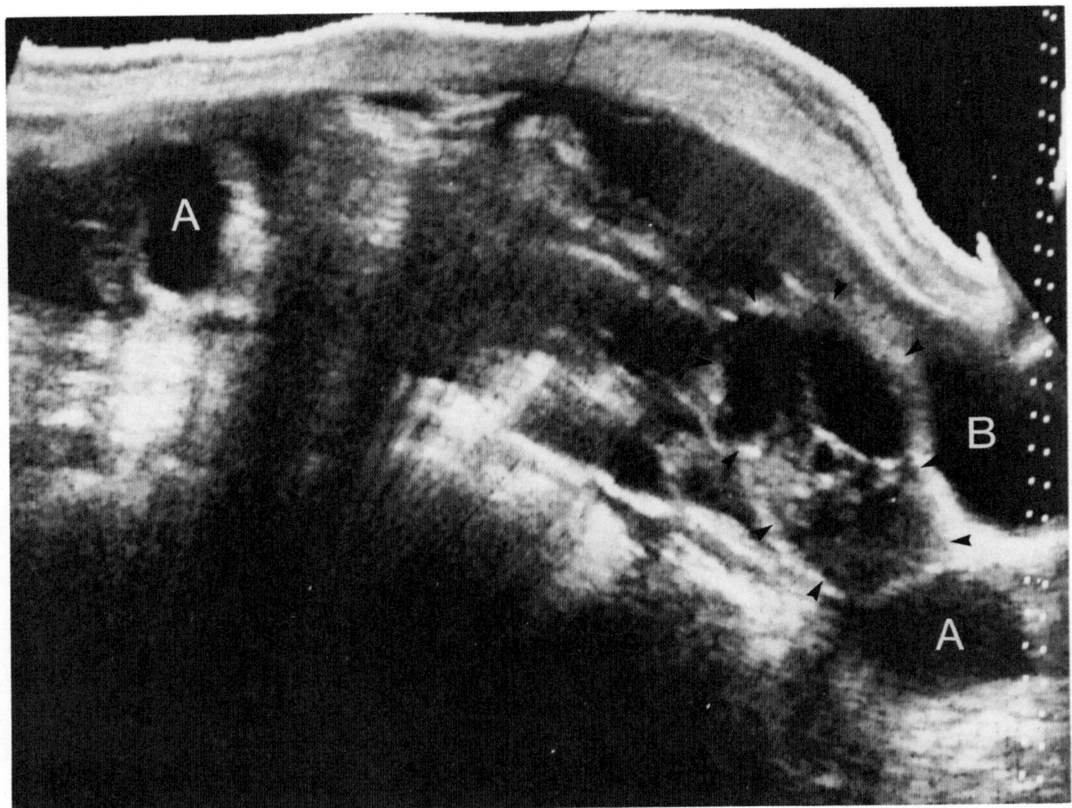

Figure 32. Ovarian carcinoma with ascites. A: Sagittal ultrasound scan shows the ovarian tumor (arrowheads) superior to the urinary bladder (B); ascitic fluid (A) is seen in the pelvis and abdomen.

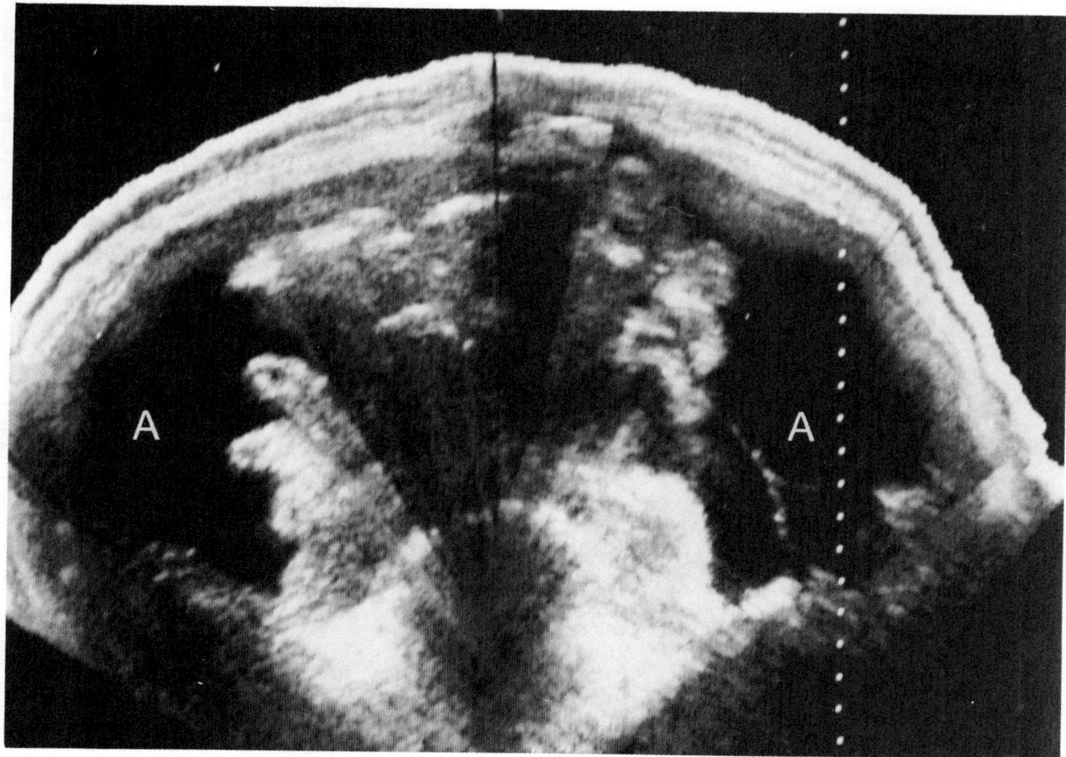

Figure 32. B: Transverse ultrasonic scan in the lower abdomen demonstrates the ascitic fluid (A) on both sides.

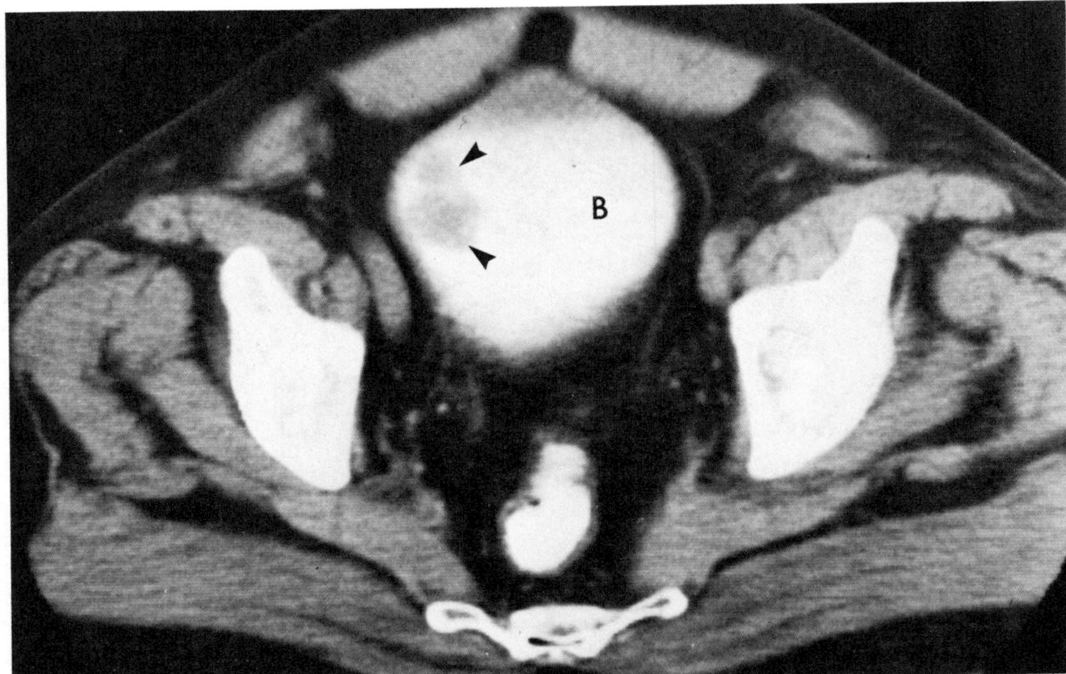

Figure 33. Carcinoma of the urinary bladder, stage B2 or less. CT scan of the pelvis shows an intraluminal filling defect (arrowheads) in the contrast-filled urinary bladder (B). There is no extension of the tumor outside the bladder wall.

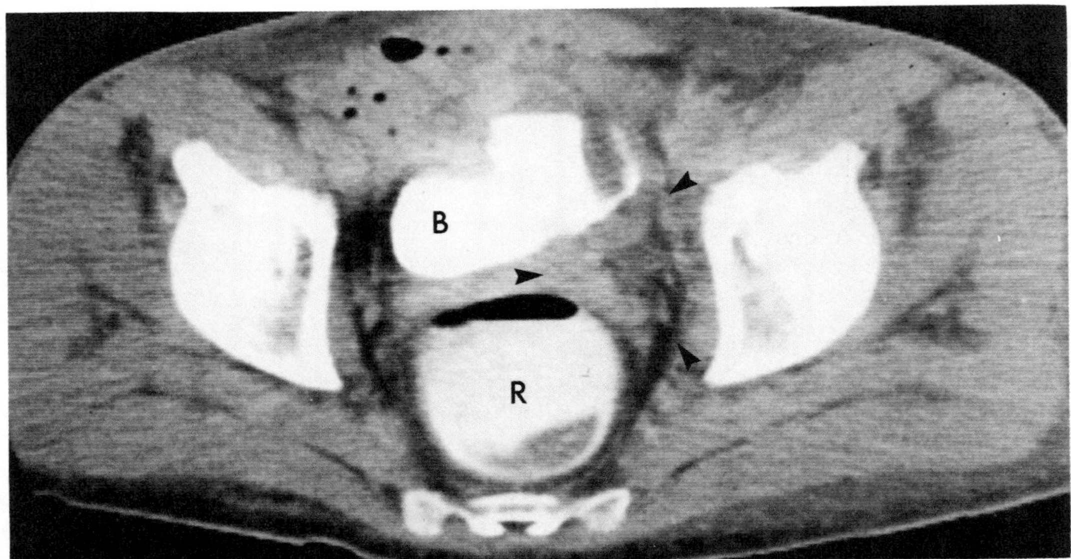

Figure 34. Carcinoma of the urinary bladder stage C. CT scan shows irregular filling of the urinary bladder (B) due to a large intraluminal tumor. There is extension of the tumor through the bladder wall with involvement of the perivesical fat on the left side (arrowheads). Note the obliteration of the perivesical fat margin on the left as compared to the normal uninvolved right side (R = rectum).

SECTION IV. RADIATION THERAPY TREATMENT PLANNING

Kyo Rak Lee, M.D.
Carl M. Mansfield, M.D.
Samuel J. Dwyer, III, Ph.D.

Computed tomography is beginning to play a major role in treatment planning because it is possible to obtain more correct outer contours of the patient and delineate significant tissue inhomogeneities (27,56,76). In brachytherapy, CT has shown potential for depicting three-dimensional anatomic relationships of the implanted radioactive sources, the tumor extent, and surrounding normal structures (43,56). Combining the CT information with computerized radiation therapy treatment planning has improved accuracy and contributed greatly to the solution of complex treatment problems. CT is also useful for evaluating the progress of patients during and following radiation therapy. Therefore, it is anticipated that CT will lead to an improved tumor dose and a decreased dose to surrounding normal tissue. Perhaps these benefits will result in a greater tumor control and less morbidity.

Using all of the clinical information, including the history and physical examination, laboratory and radiological studies, and surgical and pathological findings, a determination is made by the radiotherapist as to the general location of the tumor and the volume to be treated (83). Computerized tomography is now able to provide additional information to the radiotherapist. The capabilities of CT to depict true cross-sectional images of normal and disease tissues within the human body and of providing direct measurement of the density of these tissues has brought a revolutionary impact on diagnostic and therapeutic radiology (3,12,36,56,73,78). CT has made it possible to estimate the tumor volume and to locate normal tissues more accurately for planning a course of radiation therapy (RT).

With this information, an actual treatment technique and setup are simulated using a radiographic machine which is usually referred to as a simulator. This machine may range in complexity from a very simple radiographic device to an elaborate unit especially designed for the purpose.

TREATMENT PLANNING PROCEDURES

Once the treatment volume is established, a computerized tomographic scan can be made through the center of this volume. Additional scans are made through the levels at which dose distributions are desired. The CT scan will depict the cross-sectional images of normal and tumor tissues within the center plane of the volume of interest. This makes it possible to locate these areas and their spatial relationship for treatment planning. It is possible to obtain an outer contour (CT contour) of the patient. With careful refinement of the scanning parameters, this contour can be fairly accurate. Additional efforts in this area should yield a most accurate and reliable method for representing the contour of the patient as it is in the treatment position.

Using the scan that represents the central plane of the treatment volume or the area of interest, appropriate images of this scan can be obtained by changing the window width and level. The widest window width (1000 Hounsfield units) should be used since it provides a more accurate contour of the body and organs, while the narrower window width is used for depicting the tumor and normal structures.

Depending upon the sophistication of the treatment planning facilities, the CT scan can be used in a number of ways:

1. It is possible to trace the image of the CT scan and indicate the tumor volume as well as normal structures, in terms of X and Y coordinates, into a computer using a calibrated rho theta (or theta phi) device (Fig. 35).

2. The image of the CT is superimposed on a contour of the patient, made conventionally at the same level as the scan. This is done by projecting the scan to life size onto the contour using a lantern slide projector. The tumor volume and normal structures are then traced within the contour (56). This anatomical information is entered into the computer as described in example 1.

3. The tumor volume and normal structures can be drawn manually on a contour of the patient using the CT scan to provide the measurements and positions of these areas. This information is entered in the computer as described in example 1.

4. A more elaborate setup using an interactive computer system allows the information to be transferred from the CT scanner into the treatment planning computer. This transfer can be directly or by means of magnetic tapes, discs, or other devices (14,18).

After entering the anatomic information as described above, the physical density for each region representing an internal structure within the treatment volume must be defined and entered into the computer. For convenience, the density may be entered in terms of g/100 cm^3. Average CT numbers for these structures can be used in deriving physical density or one can use values of 100, 150, and 33 g/100 cm^3 for soft tissues, bone, and lung tissue, respectively (27,76). The inhomogeneity corrections using CT numbers require further refinements. When the outline of all internal structures important to the plan and the tumor volume are entered into the computer, the contour configuration is ready for calculating isodense distributions.

The next procedure is to produce a description of the beams tentatively chosen for treatment and to combine them with the contour information to calculate isodose distributions. This beam description is generated by a cartesian or C-Beam program and represents a grid of fan lines and depth lines designed to describe the beam or beams being used in the treatments. The information entered consists of the beam quality chosen (^{60}Co or 4-45 MeV), distance for radiation source, field dimensions, and field shape information, such as wedge or bar characteristics, if appropriate. The final beam description, in the form of a set of fan lines, may be stored in the computer and recalled at any time.

Trial treatment plans are then developed by recalling the contour and beam information, setting up a tentative beam configuration, and calculating the isodose distribution. Further development of the treatment plan is performed by iteration, i.e., the user continues to modify the proposed treatment plan until he feels that an optimal plan has been developed. Beam positions and the relative intensities of the beams may be changed until the final isodose distribution represents the best distribution.

Interactive Graphic Display

Among the primary advantages of CT, important to radiation therapy, is its ability to locate anatomic sites with greater accuracy. Yet this improved location accuracy is underscored by already existing problems consisting of patient registration (position and location), accurate calculation of tumor volume and dose distribution, the use of displays of dose calculations, heterogeneity corrections, and information management systems. Thus, it is necessary to develop an interactive computer system using CT scan data which can be based on the requirements of the radiation therapist. It can be on an off-line medium performance interactive graphics raster display system as shown in Fig. 36. Figure 37 provides a summary of the functions which could be helpful for evaluating the problems associated with developing and evaluating display strategies for efficient and effective radiation treatment planning. The major goal is to make the system as close as possible to a self-sufficient interactive software package which would permit the evaluation of a number of display strategies. The following functions can be incorporated into the interactive computer graphics software.

Acquisition Functions

The acquisition function software permits the user to acquire specific CT scans. It also permits the input of patient contour data using a sonic digitizer, joystick cursor, or TV camera digitizer.

A sonic digitizer is a device which specifies a particular X and Y coordinate using the sound generated by a spark-gap. The digitizer activates a spark-gap at the desired X and Y coordinate. The resultant sound is detected by two sets of sound detectors which use the time of sound progression from the spark-gap to calculate the X and Y coordinate information. The joystick cursor is a device similar to those used in TV games, interfaced to the computer graphics display which enables the user to communicate with the computer to construct lines or curves on the display monitor. A TV camera digitizer acquires the television image information and stores it in the computer as a two-dimensional digital array. These digital arrays are specified by their X, Y coordinates (called a pixel) and the possible value of each X, Y coordinate (called a pixel value). TV camera digitizers are readily available with digital array sizes of 512 x 512 x 8 bits (512 X coordinate values, 512 Y coordinate values, and each pixel with a value of 8 bits). CT data can be acquired by various methods, such as from a magnetic tape transfer (General Electric body scanner), a floppy disc transfer (EMI head scanner) or by CRT entry.

Management Functions

The management function software permits the user to read or write examination images, patient data, or treatment plans into a disc-based data base from a magnetic tape. This software permits the user to transfer data through magnetic tape or other computer systems. The deletion or addition of specific examination images, patient data, or treatment plans into the disc data base is also possible.

Information Processing Functions

The desired information processing functions are selected through the interactive processing module by means of a cursor. The image information processing functions include displaying digital numbers identified by cursor location, histograms, calculated parameters for identified regions of interest, estimated second-order parameters for selected regions of interest, and volume or surface estimation of suspected tumors obtained from contour identification on multiple CT scans.

Image Display Functions

The image display function software permits the user to utilize a number of display algorithms. These formats include display of CT scans, region of interest selection by the user with an interactive device, display of digital numbers, display of an image or region of interest following algorithmic enhancement, the display of information from processing algorithms (such as histograms, maximum digital numbers, parameters from functional imaging, etc.), display of three-dimensional surfaces, display of composite images (such as a three-dimensional display of a resultant treatment planning isodose surface together with a three-dimensional display of the tumor surface obtained from tumor contours as visualized on the CT scans), and display of sagittal, coronal, or planar cuts as selected interactively by the user.

Interactive Processing Functions

The guidelines followed in designing an interactive software include simple interaction sequences focused entirely on the display screen that are adequate for prompting, providing feedback to the user, and providing recovery from user mistakes. The interactive processing functions are controlled by a menu displayed on the raster graphics display and interacting with the user through a positioning cursor. These functions include selection of patient scans through the data-base directory, selection of one of the display formats, modification of the gray-level display ranges for the digital images, and identification of the regions of interest.

External Therapy Treatment Planning

The CT and computer radiotherapy planning can be used in external beam therapy. An external beam treatment planning system can be implemented as previously shown. A spherical sector dose calculation model has also been described (11). The CT image is mapped from a 320 x 320 array into a spherical coordinate image which superimposes all rays emanating from the therapy source into columns representing the digital image array. Attenuation corrections for observed CT values within the body are made by summing along individual columns. Conversion from CT numbers to ^{60}Co attenuation coefficients is accomplished by the use of a simple decision algorithm with the body assumed to be made up of three materials with differing electron density: fat, soft tissue, and bone. An algorithm for computing the scatter contribution to dose is performed by summing pixel-to-pixel scatter contributions on a point-by-point basis. The dose map is displayed on the CT scan either as isodose contours, as intensity or as color modulation of the CT image, or as three-dimensional surfaces viewed in perspective. Figure 38 illustrates the display of an isodose plot of two wedged fields on a CT scan from an interactively designed treatment plan.

Scanners and Scanning Techniques

The requirements of scanners and scanning techniques for radiotherapy are as follows:

1. The patient position information obtained from CT scans must be accurately transferable to a therapy unit. This requires a similar couch top on the scan unit as that on the therapy unit and identical positioning of the patient on both units. The anatomic location of the region scanned must be identified correctly by using a particular method. Several imperfect methods for the purpose have been reported, which include a localization radiograph with a strip of lead markers, triangular metal strips, or angiographic

catheter strips on the skin (8,85). A few scans for localization skin markers which indicate the treatment parts are also used (Fig. 39).

2. The attenuation coefficients of the anatomic structures represented by CT numbers should be constant and reproducible. The following criteria should be met: (a) Hounsfield number of water and air should be reproducible within ± 2%; (b) Hounsfield numbers versus electron density should be linear within ± 2% in the range of water to air; and these should (c) be less than ± 2% variation of Hounsfield numbers across 90% of a 30 cm diameter water flood scan (61).

3. Short scanning time within 5 sec is desirable, but not essential, to eliminate not only poor images but also position change of organs by respiratory motion.

4. Multiple scans reconstructed in transverse, coronal, and a sagittal planes are desirable, but not essential, for better estimation of tumor volume and identification of the three-dimensional relationship of tumor extent and normal structures.

5. A high-contrast spatial resolution of 2 mm with a large number of matrices for improved visualization of low-contrast objects.

6. The attenuation coefficients normalized to water are given at the energies typically used for radiotherapy treatments in a format suitable for the treatment planning computer.

7. An interactive computer system to interface CT data with the treatment planning computer for planning therapy and calculating dose distribution is desirable.

8. A life-size hard copy of the scan image is desirable for correct contouring of the patient and measuring the size and distance of individual organs.

The first two of the above are the absolute requirements for using CT in radiation therapy and can be met with existing diagnostic units without major modification. The remaining are optional and can be achieved with a dedicated scanner for radiation therapy. Dedicated scanners will also provide additional features, including the simulation of a treatment, variable kilovolt peak (KVP) and filter combination, variable scanning time, fast multiplanar reconstruction, and three-dimensional dose calculation and display.

CT TREATMENT PLANNING IN SPECIFIC ANATOMIC SITES

CT scanning can be used in the treatment planning of virtually any anatomical site.

Head and Neck

CT in the head and neck can define the tumor volumes for external or interstitial therapy, provide a correct contour for treatment planning, and localize vital normal structures (36,56,61). Munzenrider et al. (56) and Hobday et al. (34) found that CT showed relatively little effect on total volume treated, tumor coverage, and change in volume of normal tissue irradiated. Danoff et al. (15) recommended that all patients with pituitary tumors should have a CT scan for more accurate radiation therapy treatment planning since a marked discrepancy was noted in tumor extent comparing CT, angiography, and pneumoencephalography.

The following are some examples where CT scanning has been useful: Fig. 40A is a contour and isodose plan of a patient with a squamous cell carcinoma of the maxillary antrum. Figure 40B is a CT scan with the isodose distribution superimposed on the scan. Figures 41A and B are a contour and isodose plan of a patient with a squamous cell carcinoma of the tonsil. Figures 42A and B are a patient with a pituitary tumor and Fig. 43 is a patient with a brain tumor.

Thorax

CT is especially useful in the thorax since it clearly demonstrated the anatomic relationships between the extent of tumor, normal mediastinal structures including heart and spinal cord, and provided accurate localization and quantitative tissue density data of the lungs for inhomogeneity corrections (19,34,56). Figures 44A and B are a patient with an esophageal carcinoma.

Abdomen

The availability of CT information showed significant impact on radiation therapy treatment planning in the abdomen. In the series of Munzenrider et al., 14 of 25 patients (56%) had changes in the tumor and normal tissue volume irradiated, and 15 (60%) had corrections in tumor coverage (56). In the series of Hobday et al. with 19 patients with pancreatic and retroperitoneal tumors, 11 patients showed inadequate tumor coverage and 13 had changes in the total tumor volume (34). Five showed incorrect positioning of the kidneys.

Figures 45A and B are a patient with carcinoma of the pancreas. Figure 46 is a patient with retroperitoneal lymphoma

Pelvis

Although CT is of great value in staging malignant pelvic tumors, its effect on radiation therapy treatment planning in terms of treatment volume and tumor coverage is relatively less pronounced than in the thorax or abdomen. This may be due to relatively uniform treatment techniques which basically consist of total pelvic irradiation with or without brachytherapy. Eighteen of sixty-five patients (28%) with pelvic malignancy had alterations in their treatment plans in the series of Hobday et al. (34). Schlager et al. had 21 patients with bladder carcinoma, in whom 29% of the original treatment plans were changed by the CT information (72).

Figures 47A and B are a patient with a carcinoma of the endometrium. Figures 48A and B are a patient with a carcinoma of the bladder.

BRACHYTHERAPY

The CT scan can be of value in brachytherapy. It has the potential of depicting two- or three-dimensional anatomic relationships of the implanted radioactive sources in many areas, especially in the head and neck, breast, and pelvic regions. For example, Lee et al. has shown that the CT scan clearly identifies the three-dimensional spatial relationships of an intracavitary applicator to the extent of the tumor and to surrounding normal structures (43). This information can be helpful in planning the dosage and loading arrangements of the radioactive sources.

Figure 49A is the isodose plan for a patient with cervical carcinoma. Figure 49B is a scan of this patient with an intracavitary applicator in the uterus and vagina. Figures 50A and B are saggital and coronal reconstructions of the same patient.

Figures 51A and B are transverse scans through the breast of a patient with a stage I carcinoma of the breast that is being treated with an ^{192}Ir interstitial implant. A more accurate isodose distribution is possible. Figures 52A and B are an external radiation therapy plan for the same patient.

THREE-DIMENSIONAL DISPLAY

Three-dimensional display of both the anatomical and dosimetric surfaces can be performed using an algorithm developed by Fuchs et al. (26). This method constructs a three-dimensional model of the surface of an object from serial sections by approximating the surfaces between slices. These surfaces are approximated by using triangular plane segments or <u>tiles</u>, each defined between two consecutive points on an adjacent contour. A tile's boundary consists of a single contour segment and two <u>spans</u>, each connecting one end of the contour segment with a common point on the other contour. There are many sets of triangular tiles which can be defined over all the points on two adjacent contours. Any set chosen to represent the surface must fit together continuously. This requires that each span (line connecting a point on one contour with a point on the other contour) must be the side of exactly two tiles. Within this constraint the surface should also be the one which minimizes the total surface area of the reconstructed object. The algorithm proceeded in three steps: (1) transformation of coordinates of the vertices of the surface elements into a coordinate system with the origin at any arbitrary viewing location; (2) projection of those vertices into a two-dimensional display plane between the surface and the observer; and (3) shading of the surface elements for illumination from an arbitrary point in space (Figs. 53A and B). Solution of the problem of finding this minimal connected surface representation may be considered as a problem in graph theory.

In order to observe the surface of a three-dimensional image from any arbitrary angle and distance, transformation of coordinates into a viewing frame of reference is developed. This transformation of coordinates is made up of sequential, simple transformations such as translation, rotation, and reflection. The image is formed by painting triangles in the order determined by their distances from the observer. The triangle associated with the largest distance is painted first, then struck from the list and the process continued. This information is used to eliminate from view all surfaces hidden by the presence of other surfaces nearer to the viewpoint (Figs. 53B, C, and D). Projection of these vertex coordinates onto a viewing plane then ensures that the object surface is viewed in perspective.

Figure 53C is a patient with a carcinoma of the esophagus. Figures 54A, B, C, and D are a patient with a cervical carcinoma with intracavitary applicator in place.

SUMMARY

It should be apparent from the evidence presented that CT scanning will play a major role in the management of patients being considered for radiation therapy.

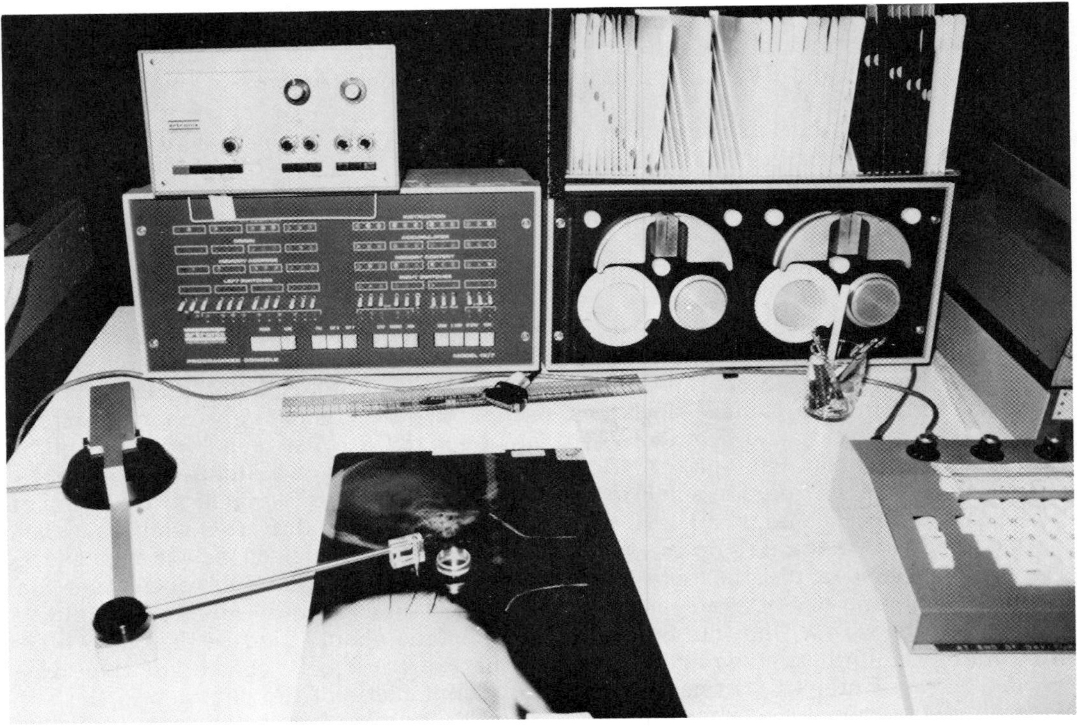

Figure 35. A dedicated treatment planning computer (PC-12) attached with a calibrated rho-theta device.

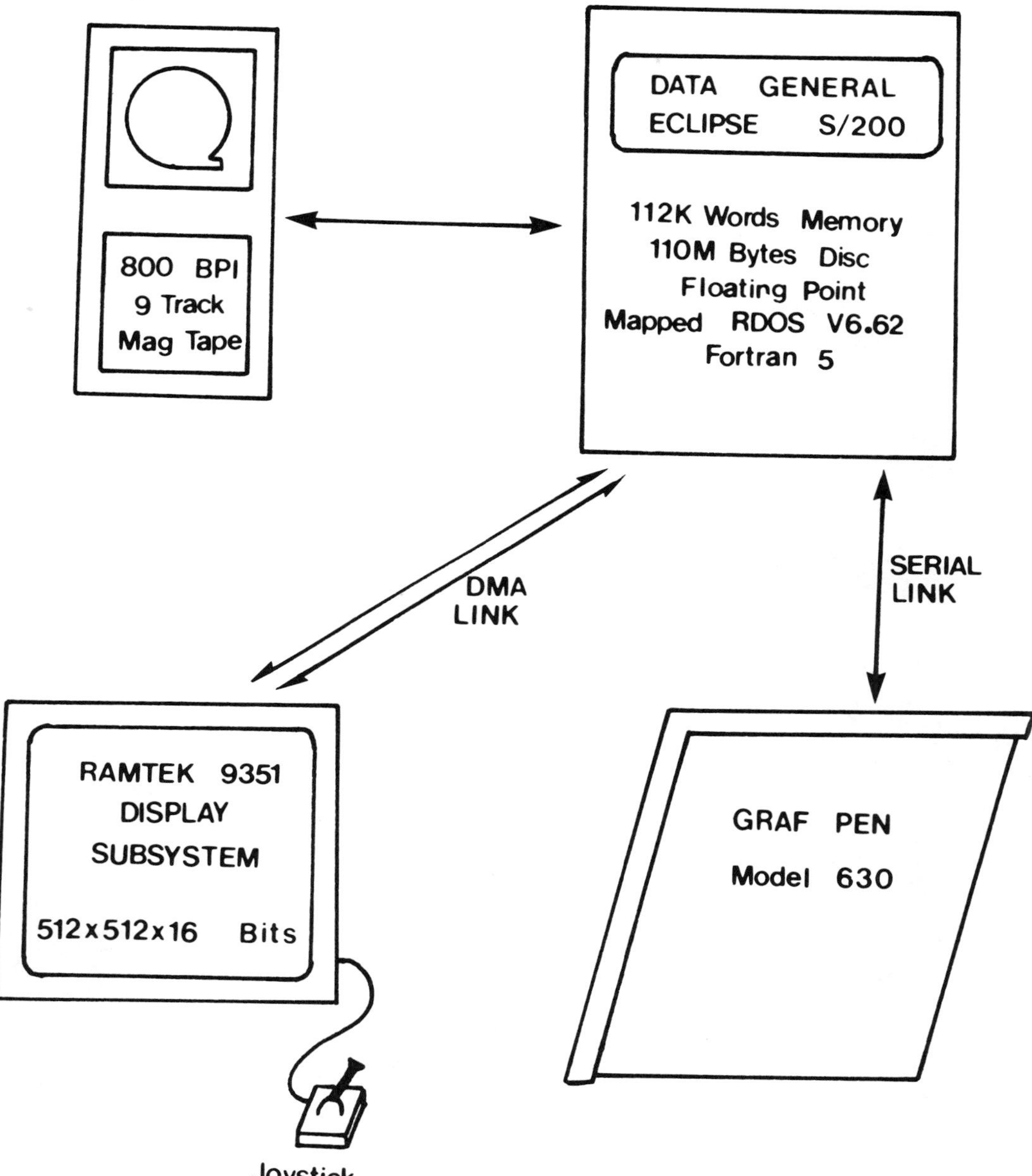

Figure 36. Computer hardware configuration of an off-line medium performance interactive graphics raster display system for treatment planning using CT scan data from a disk or magnetic tape.

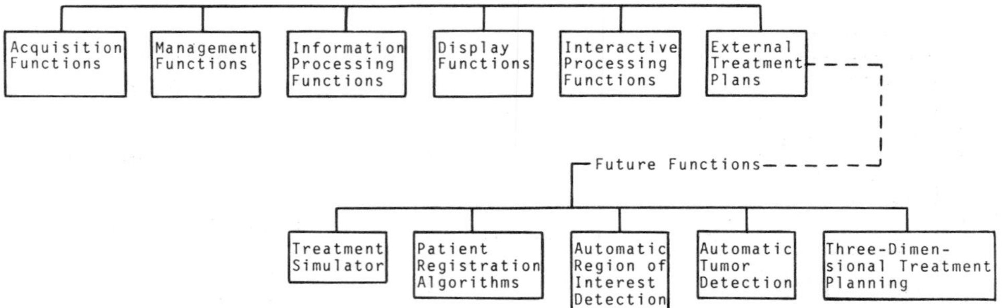

Figure 37. The functions of interactive graphic display system required by a physician.

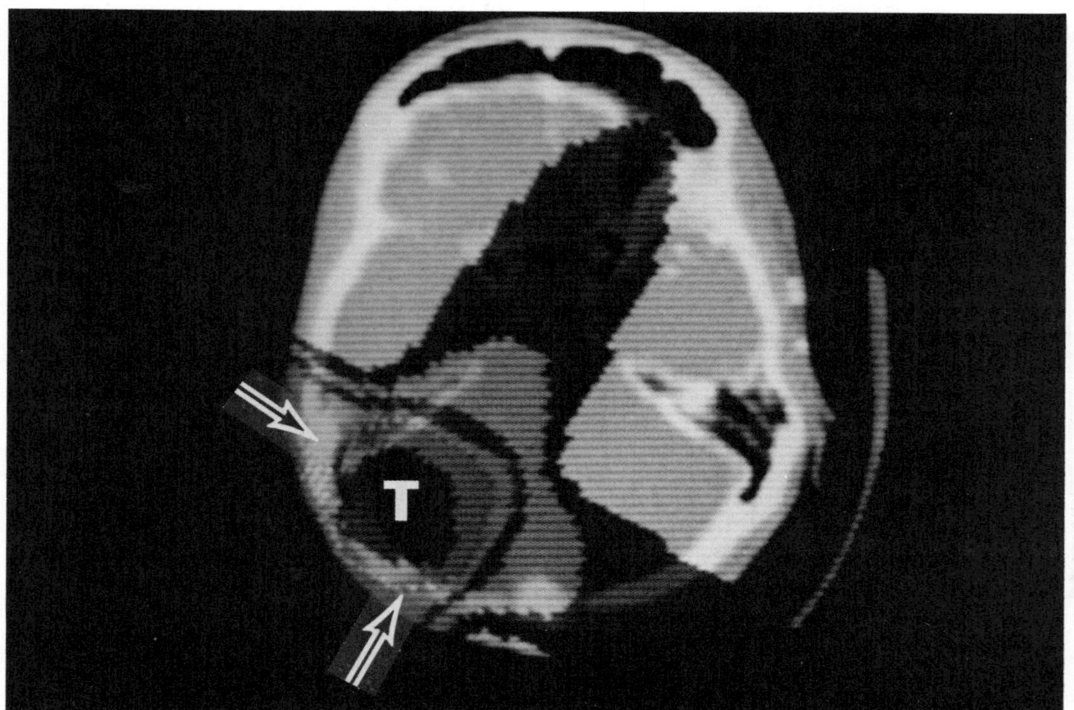

Figure 38. An interactive display of the dose distribution calculated by the spherical sector dose calculation method in a two-wedged fields (arrows), external beam treatment for a brain tumor (T). (Proceedings of MEDINFO '80, by permission.)

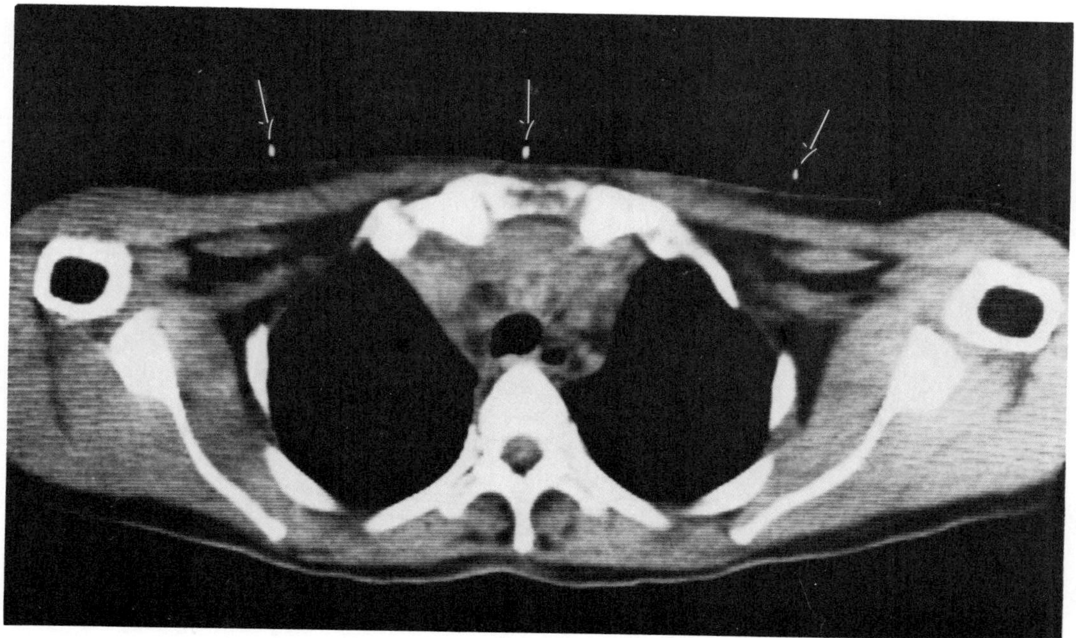

Figure 39. A localization CT scan with skin markers (arrows) which indicate the center and margins of a treatment field.

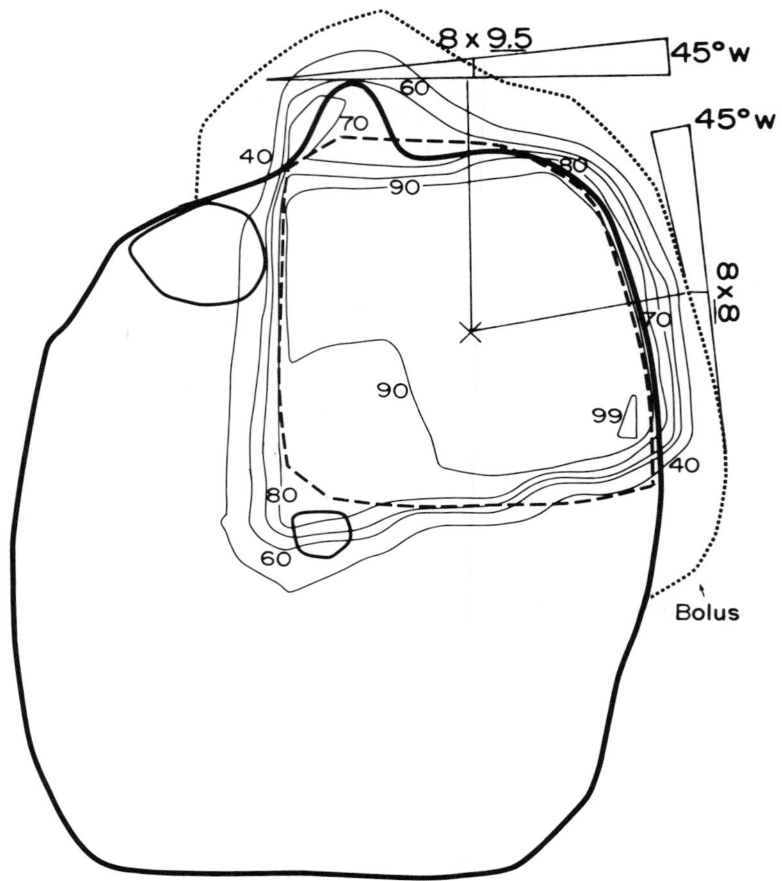

ANTRUM 6MV (with Bolus)

Figure 40. Two treatment plans for the maxillary antrum using the CT scan. A: The outer contour obtained from a T scan showing the isodose distribution for a 6 MV beam. The orbit, spinal cord, and tumor volume are indicated (arrows).

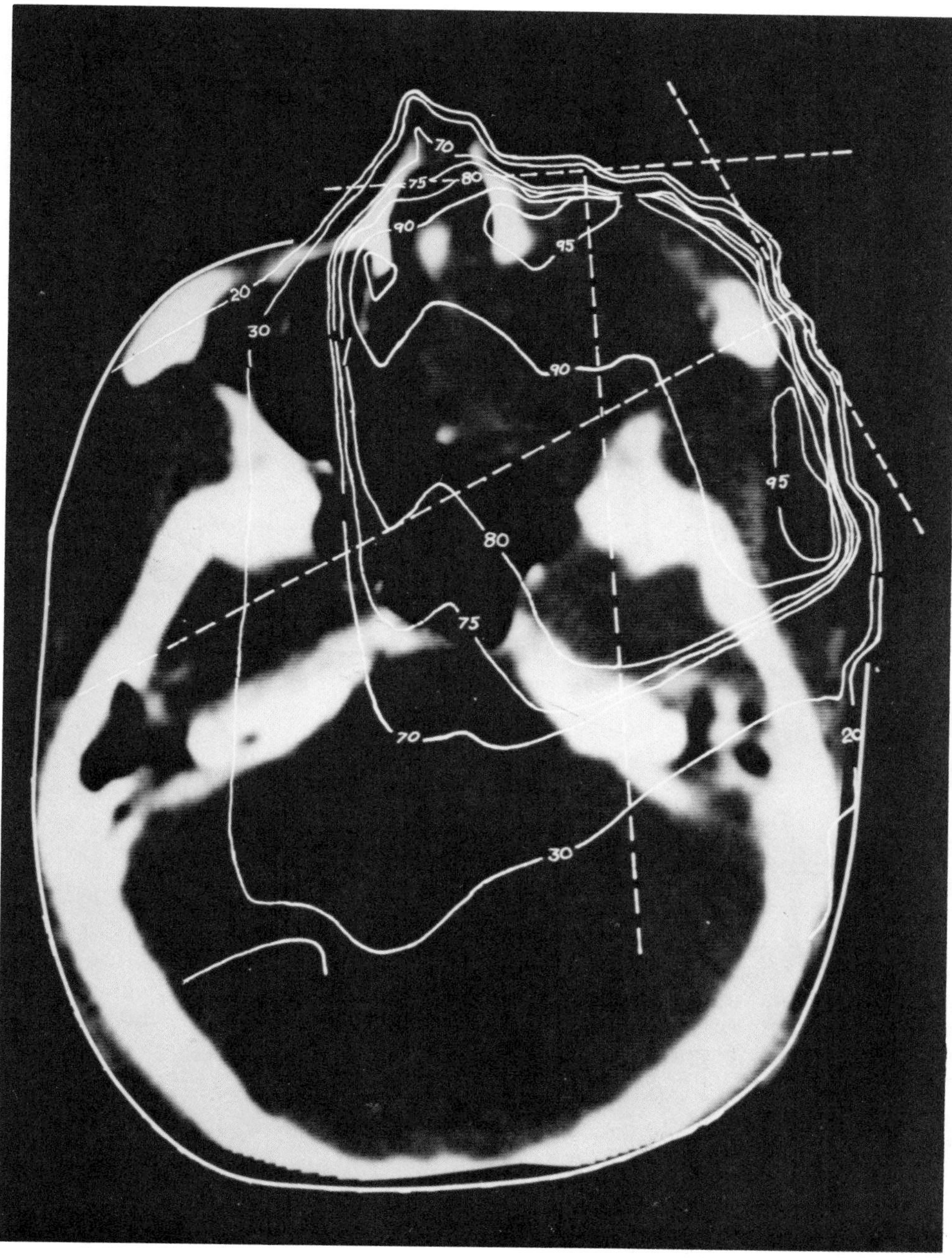

Figure 40. B: The isodose distribution for a 4 MV beam is superimposed on the same CT scan.

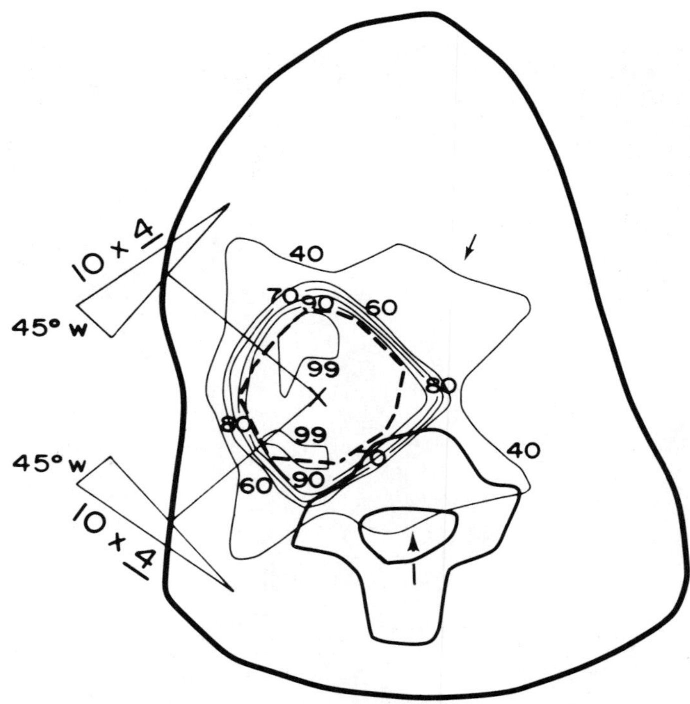

TONSIL 10 MV

Figure 41. A: Two treatment plans for the tonsil using the CT scan. A wedged field, external beam for a squamous cell carcinoma of the right tonsil with 10 MV beam is shown on the CT contour. Notice the 40% isodose line crossing the spinal canal (arrow).

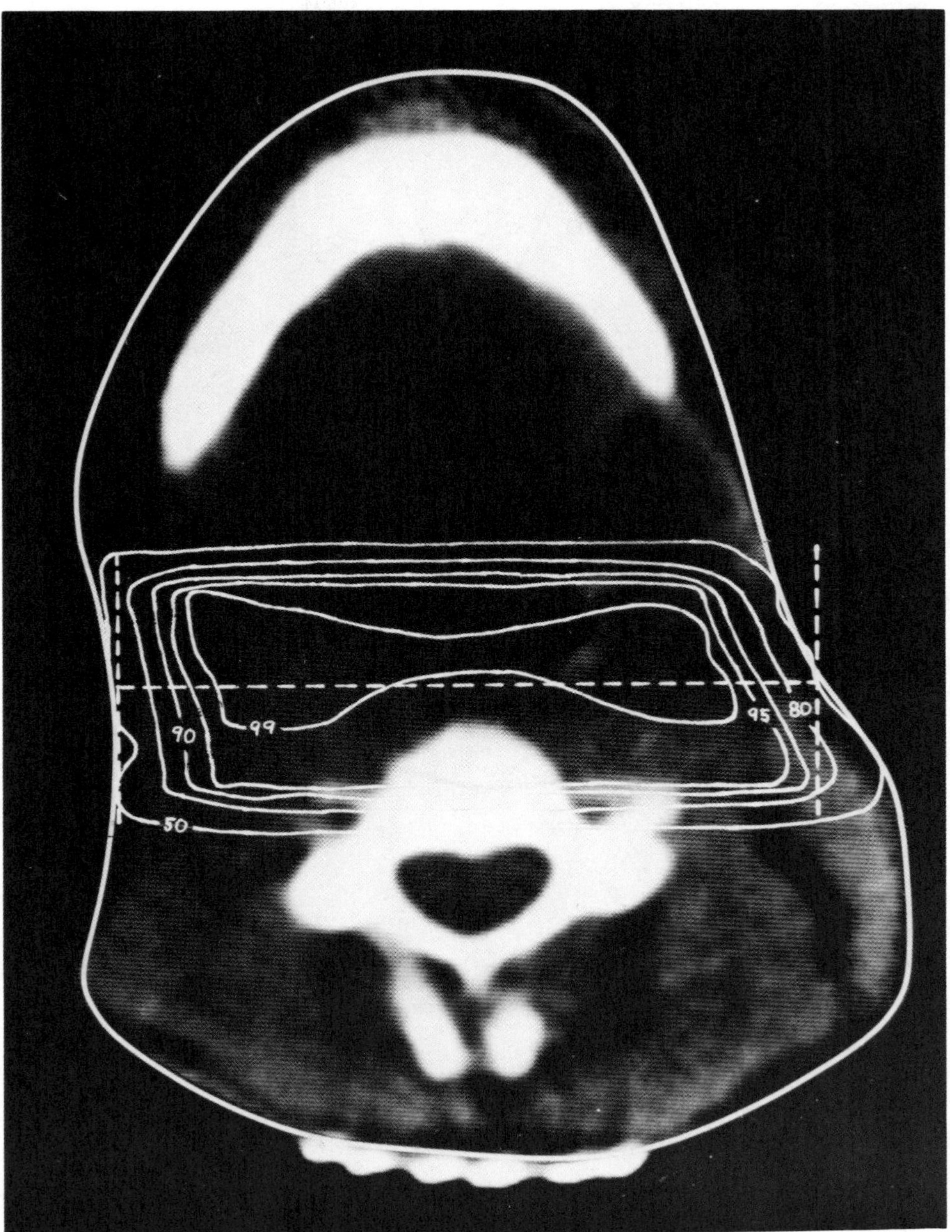

Figure 41. B: The isodose distribution for an opposing 4 MV beam is superimposed on the same CT scan.

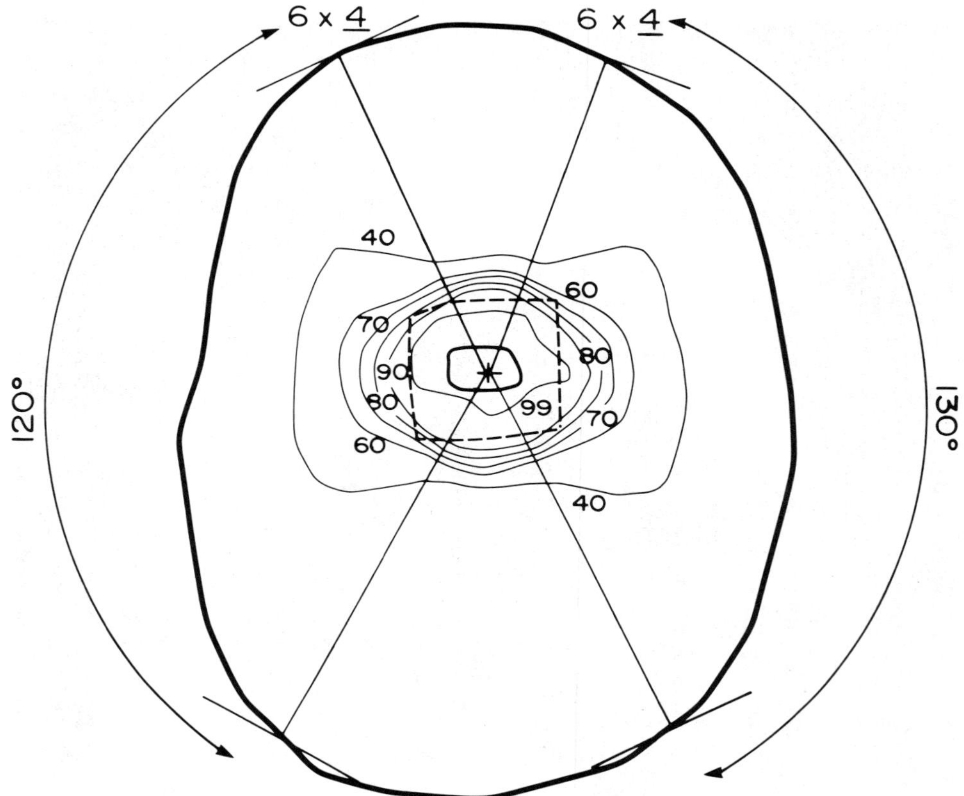

PITUITARY 10MV

Figure 42. A: Opposing arc therapy for a pituitary tumor with 10 MV beam drawn on the CT contour.

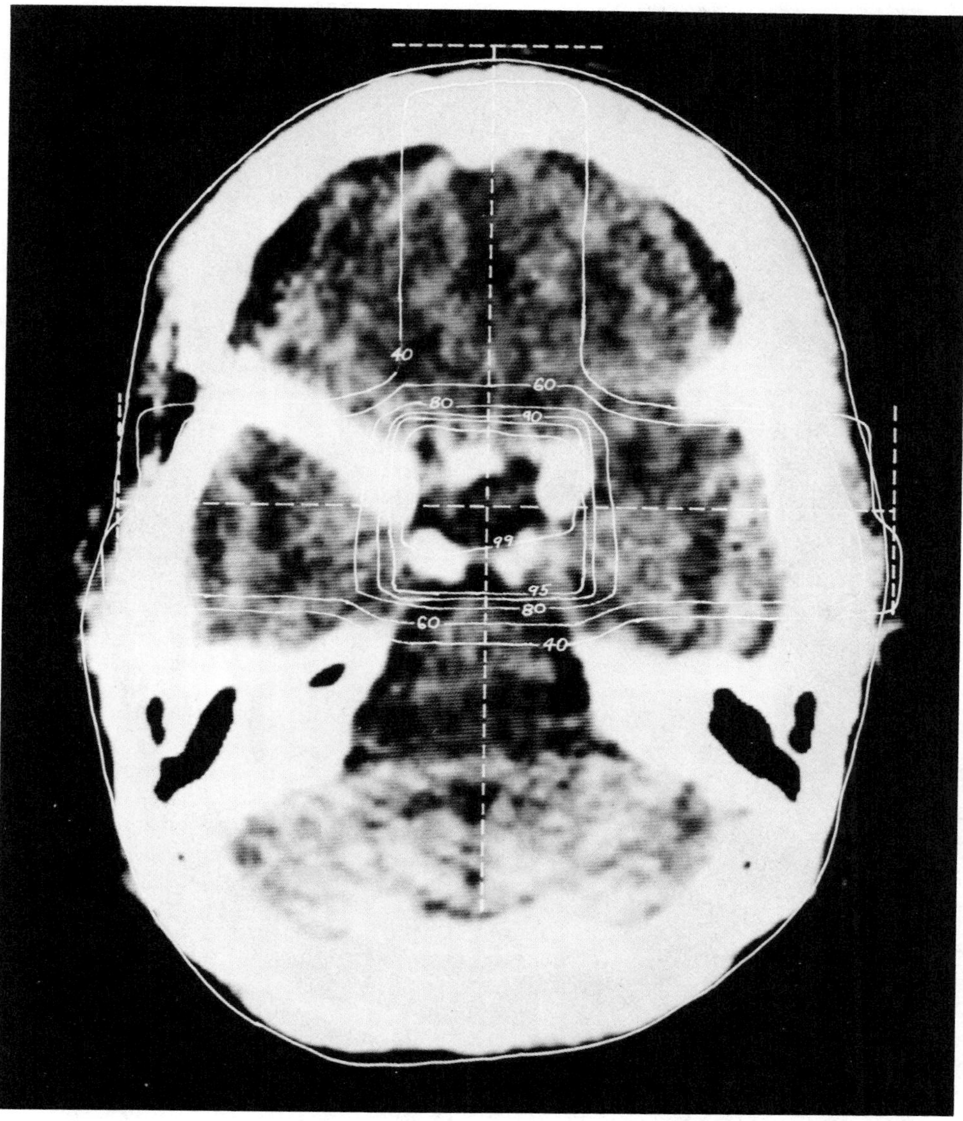

Figure 42. B: The isodose distribution for a 4 MV three-field treatment plan superimposed on the same CT scan.

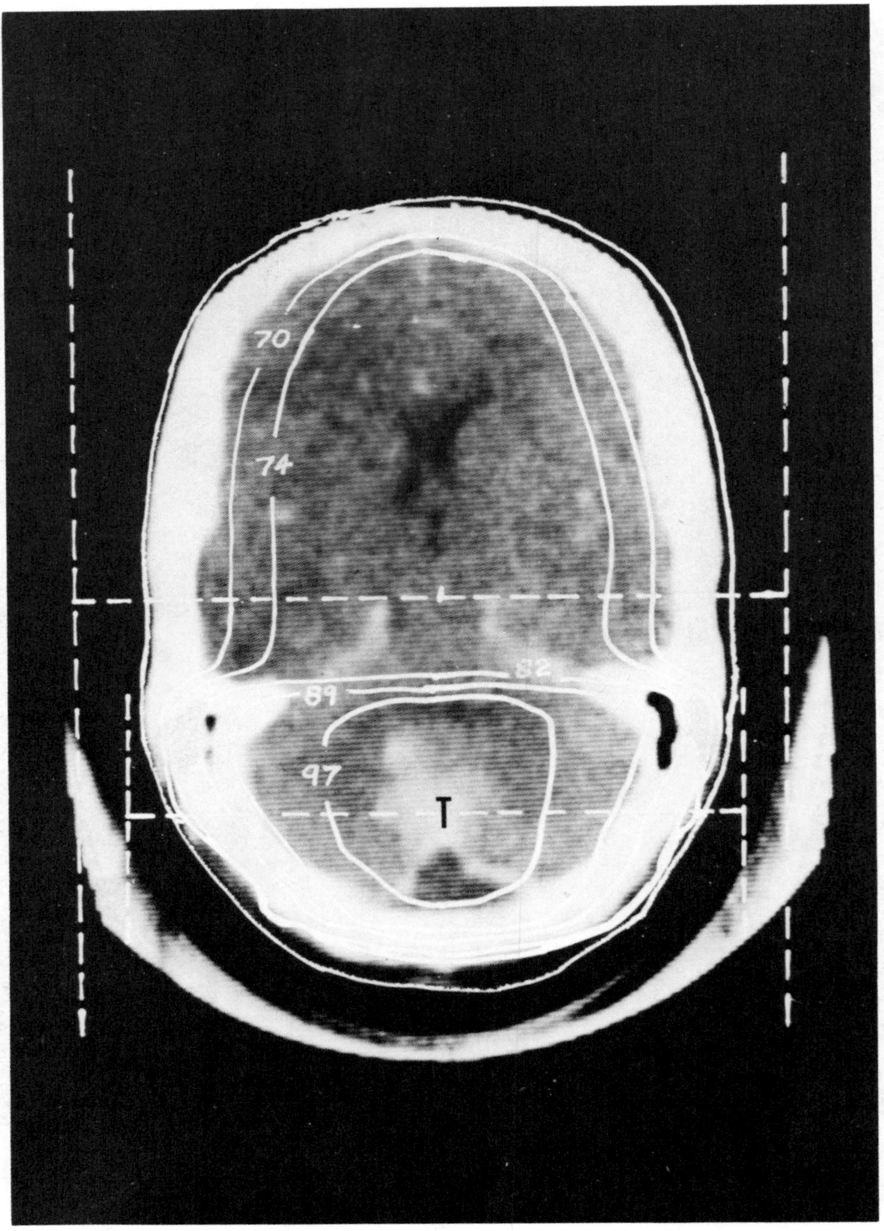

Figure 43. The isodose distribution for opposing 4 MV beams with boost fields for a metastatic tumor in the posterior fossa (T) is superimposed on the CT scan.

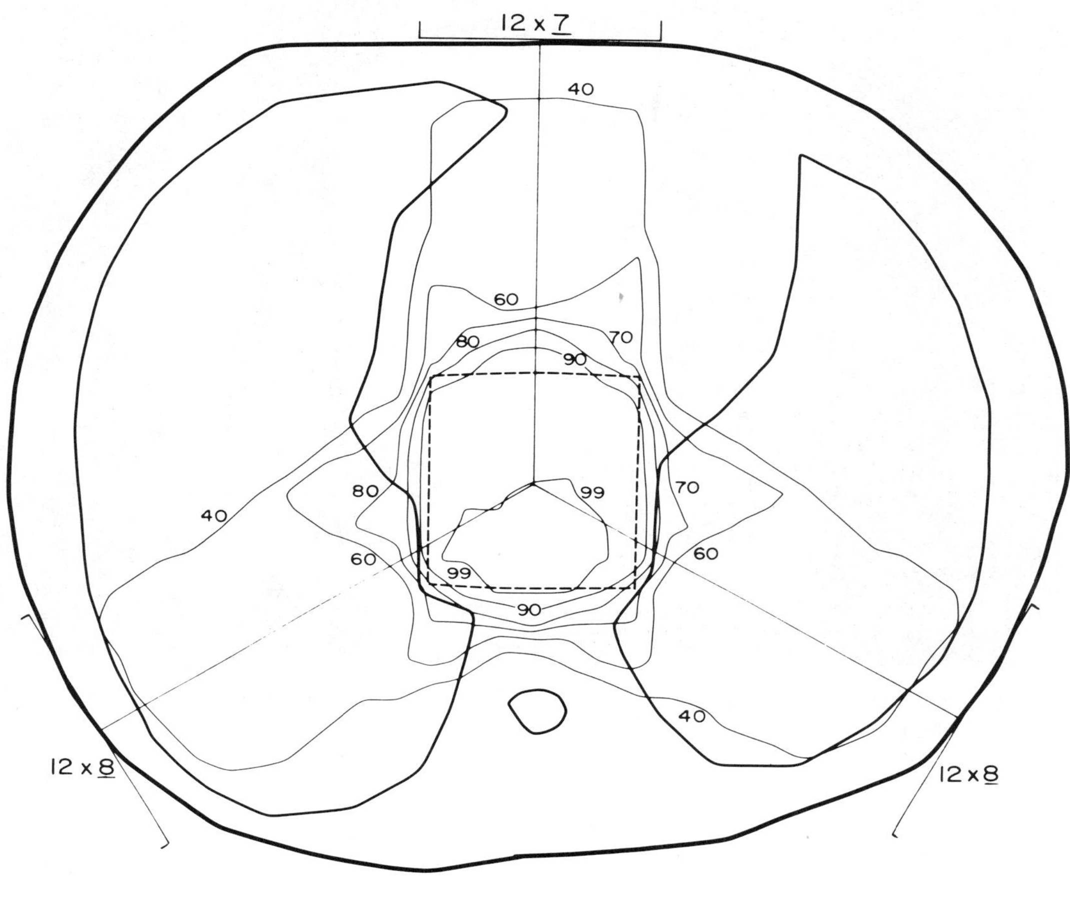

Figure 44. A carcinoma of the midesophagus. A: The CT contour and isodose distribution of a three-field treatment with 10 MV beam. The lungs, spinal canal, and tumor volume are outlined.

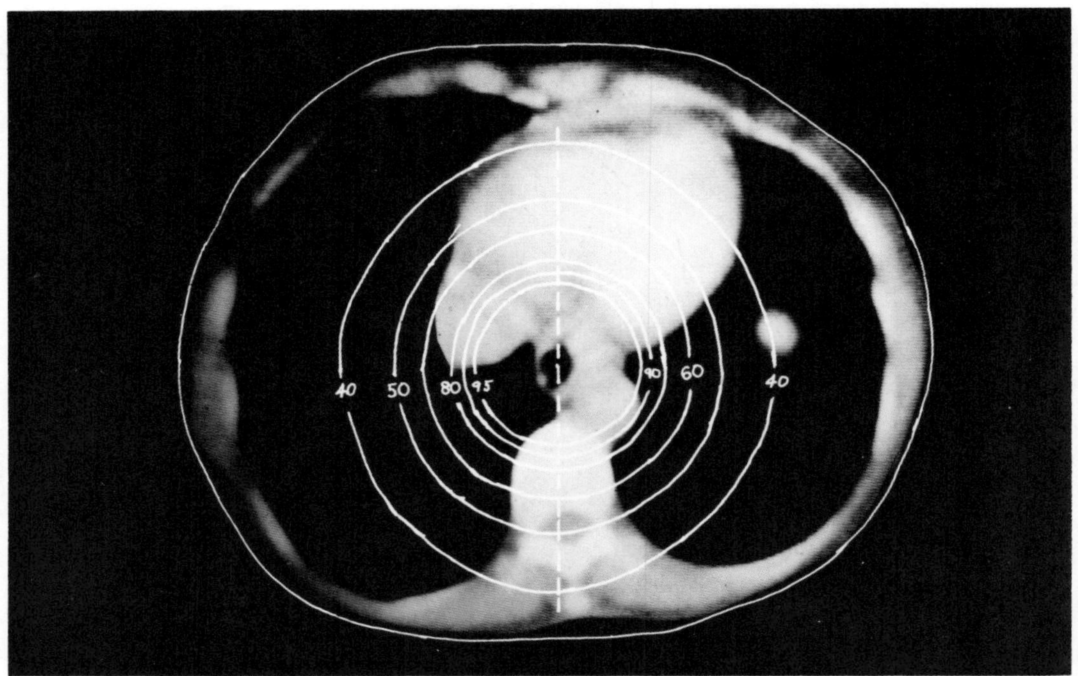

Figure 44. B: The isodose distribution of a rotational treatment with a 4 MV beam is superimposed on the same CT scan.

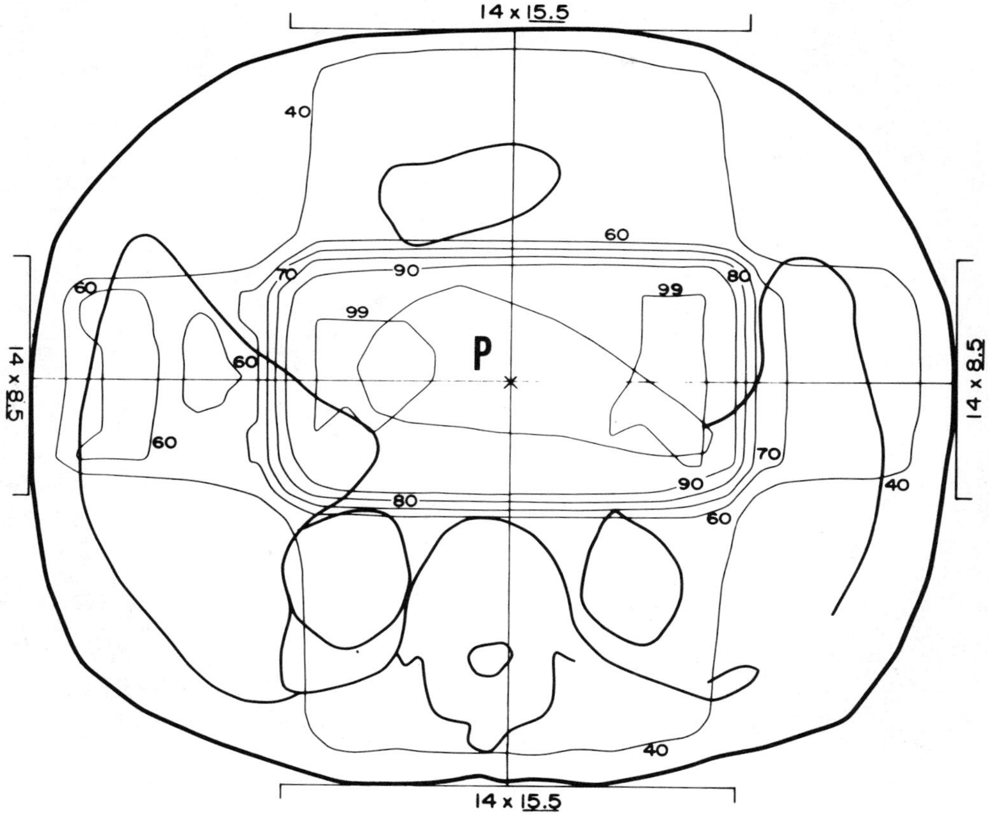

Figure 45. A carcinoma of the pancreas. A: The CT contour and isodose distribution for a four-fields treatment plan with 10 MV beam. The pancreas (P) is outlined by a thin line.

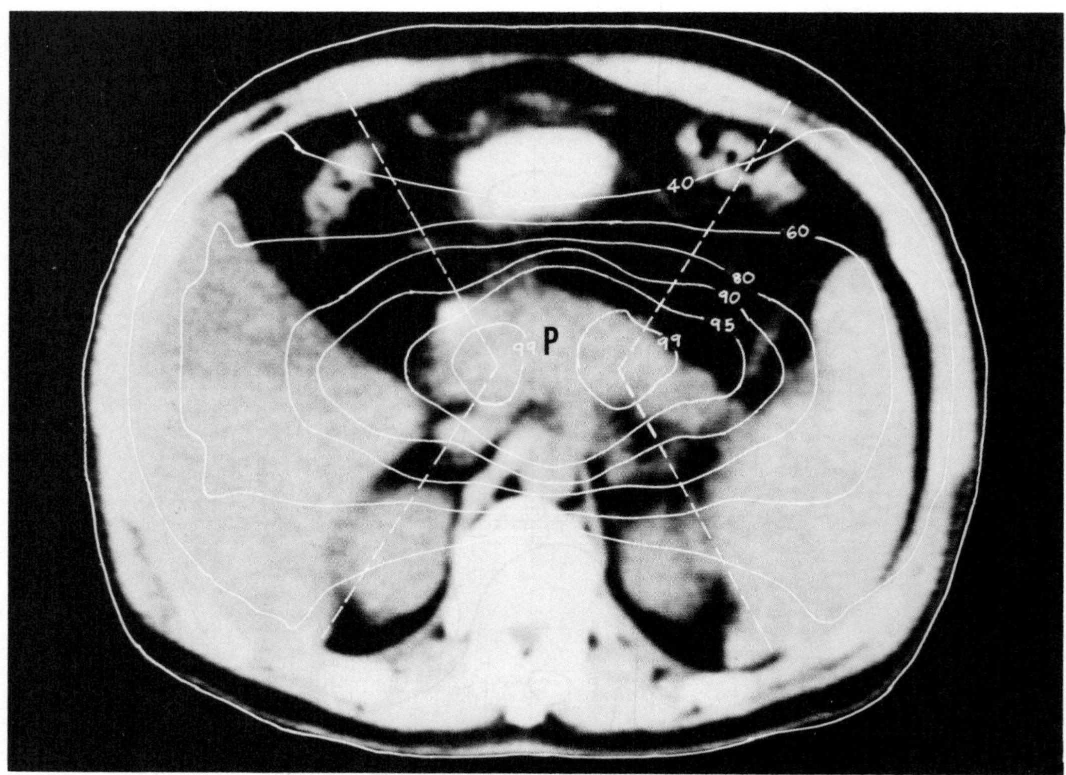

Figure 45. B: The isodose distribution for an opposing arc treatment plan with a 4 MV beam is superimposed on the same CT scan.

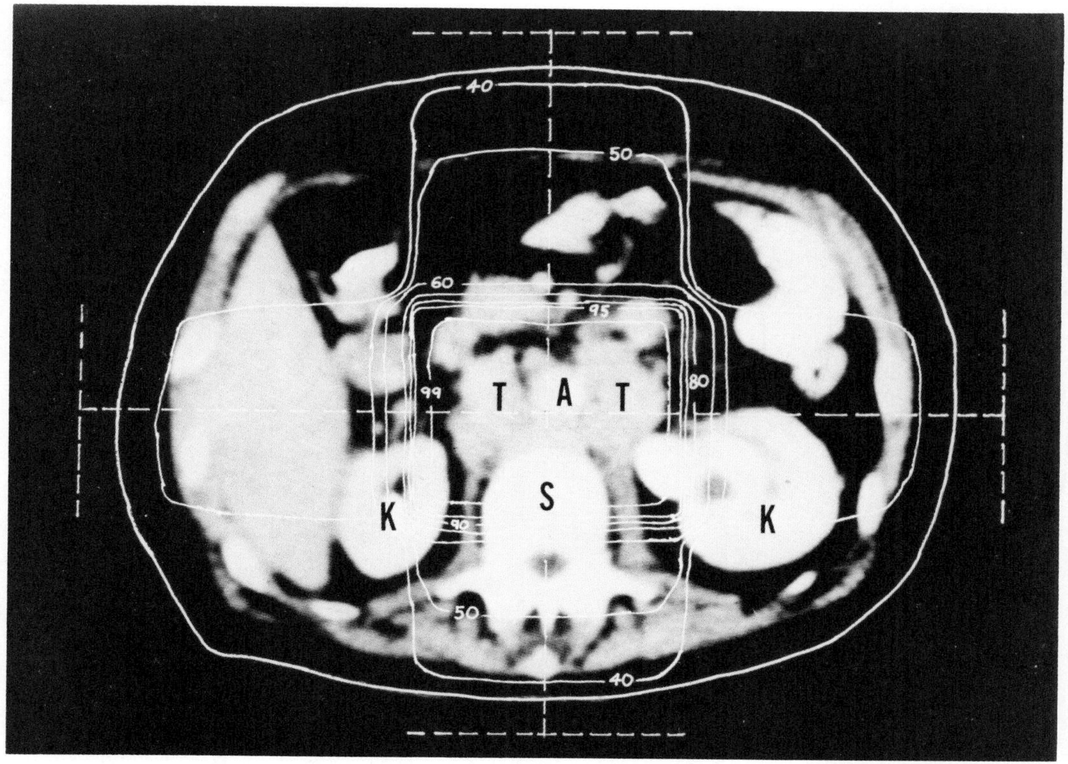

Figure 46. A composite image of the isodose distribution for a 4 MV four-fields treatment superimposed on the CT scan in a patient with retroperitoneal lymphoma (T) (A = aorta, S = spine, K = kidney).

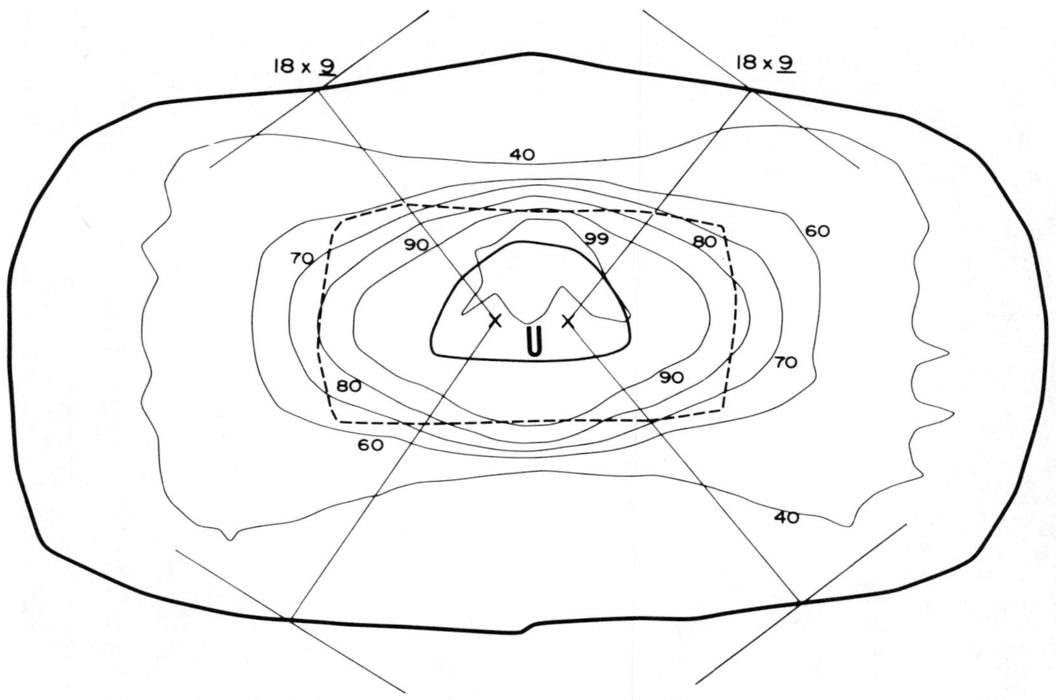

ENDOMETRIUM 6 MV

Figure 47. A carcinoma of the endometrium. A: The CT contour and isodise distribution for opposed arc, treatment with a 6 MV beam. The uterus (U) is outlined with a solid line.

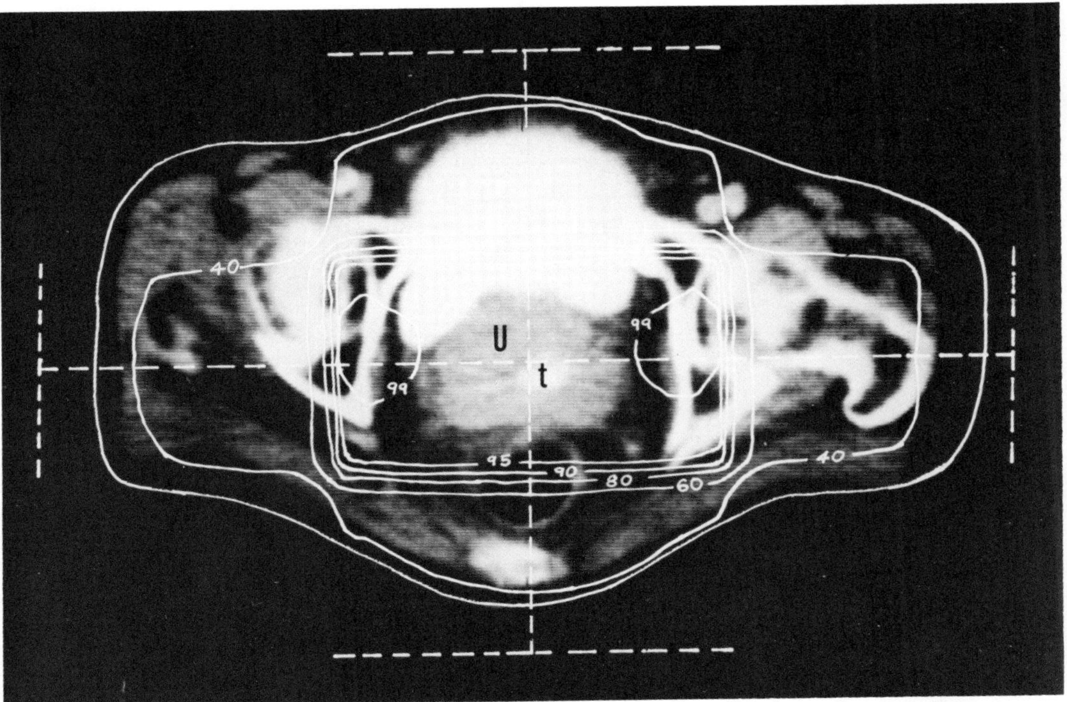

Figure 47. B: A composite image of the 4 MV four-field box isodose distribution on the CT scan. The scan was obtained after insertion of a Fletcher intrauterine tandem (t) into the uterine cavity (U). The bladder is filled with contrast.

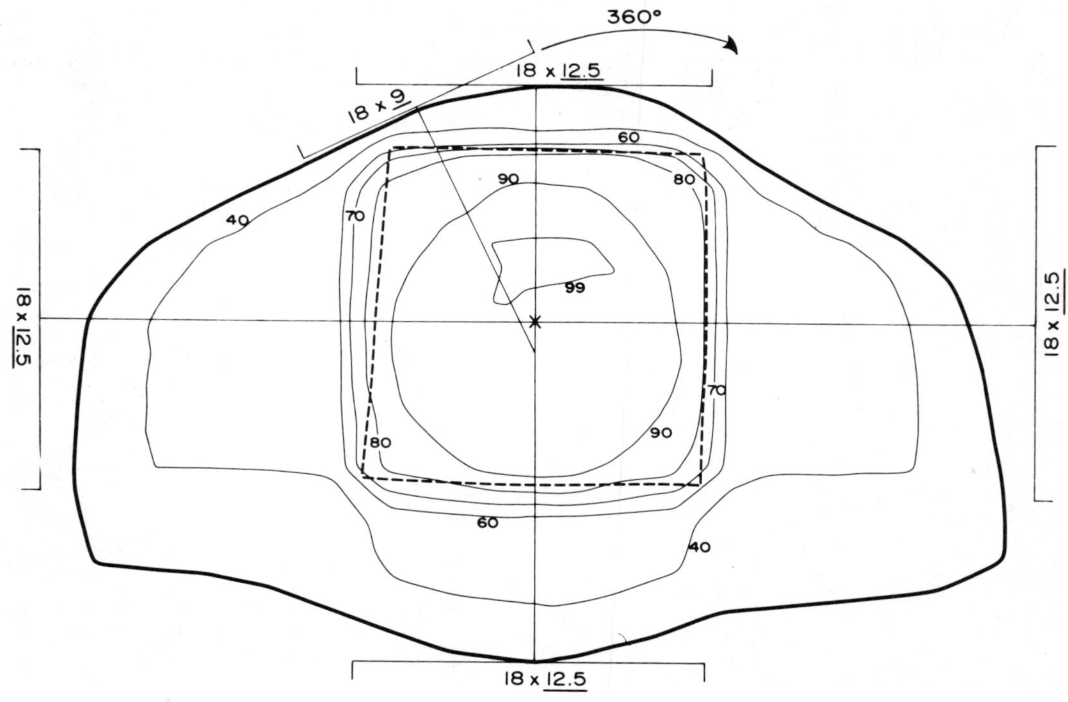

BLADDER 10MV (With 360° rotation to boost volume)

Figure 48. A carcinoma of the bladder. A: The CT contour and isodose distribution of a four-fields therapy with 360° rotation boost with an 18 x 9 cm field. The dash line indicates the tumor volume.

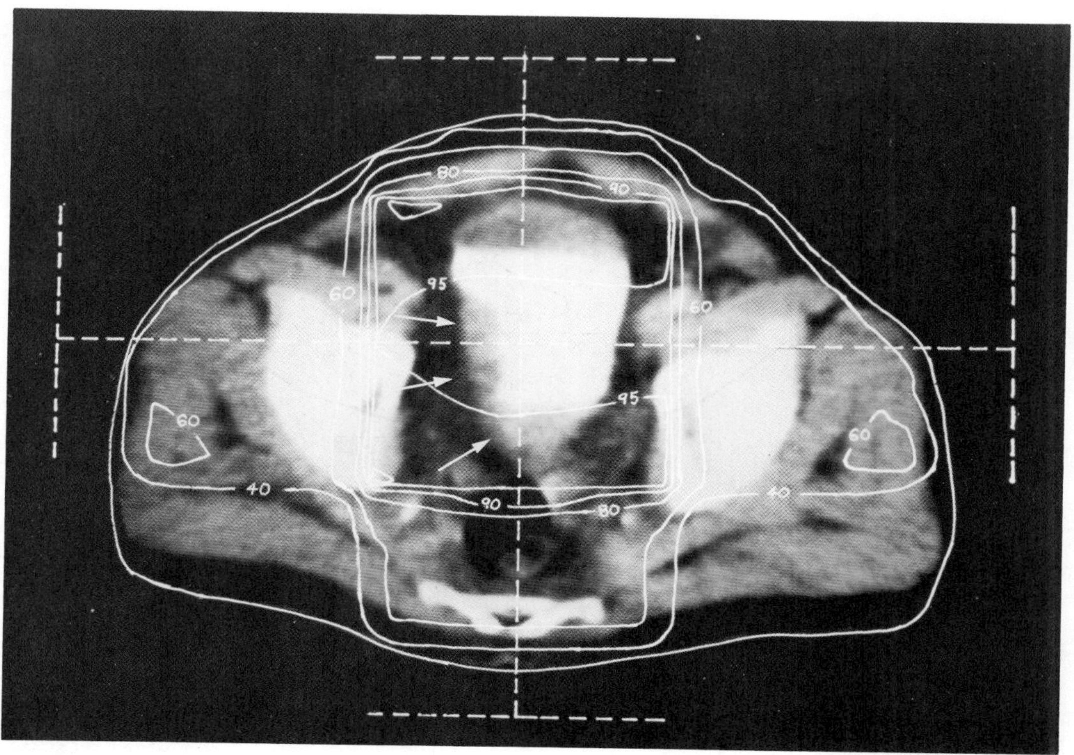

Figure 48. B: A composite image of the isodose distribution for a 4 MV four-field box and CT scan. The tumor involves the right lateral and posterior wall of the bladder (arrows).

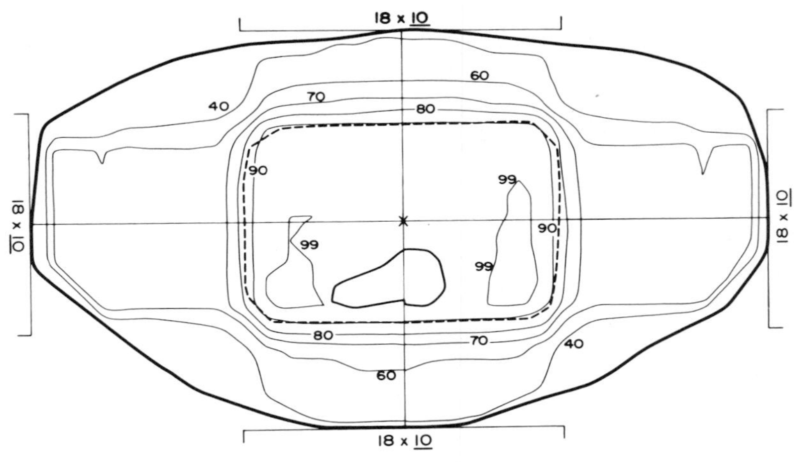

Figure 49. A carcinoma of the cervix. A: The CT contour and isodose distribution of a four-fields box treatment with ^{60}Co. The tumor volume (dash line) is covered by the 80% isodose line. A portion of the sigmoid colon is outlined (arrow).

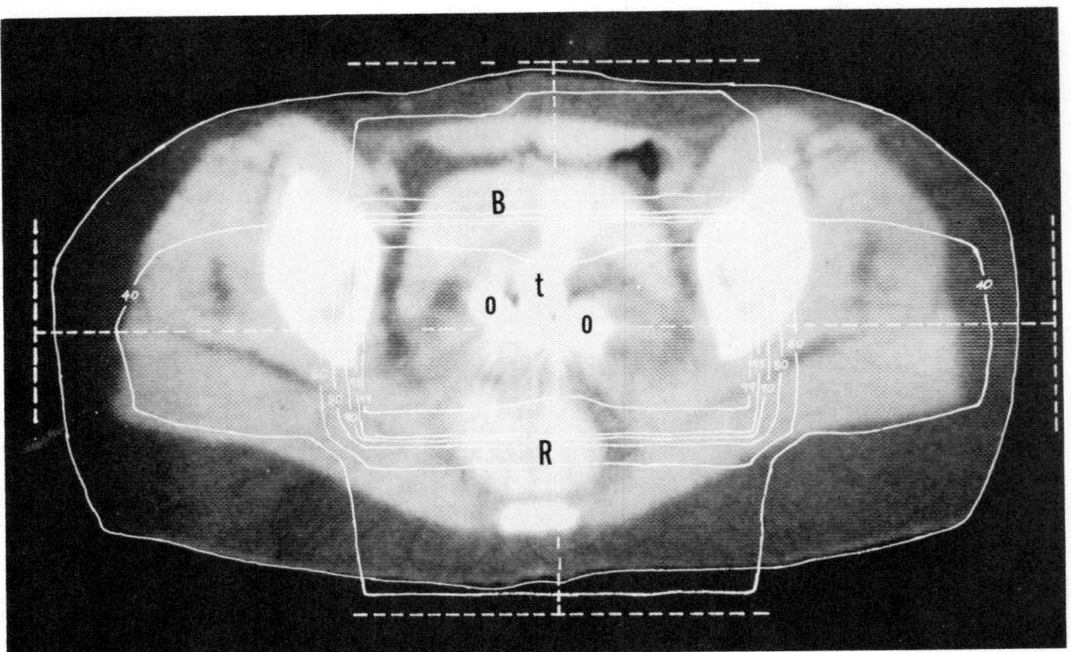

Figure 49. B: A composite image of the isodose distribution for a 4 MV four-field box and CT scan. The scan was obtained after insertion of a Fletcher intracavitary applicator (t = tandem, o = ovoid). The spatial relationships between the applicator and the bladder (B) and rectum (R) are clearly demonstrated.

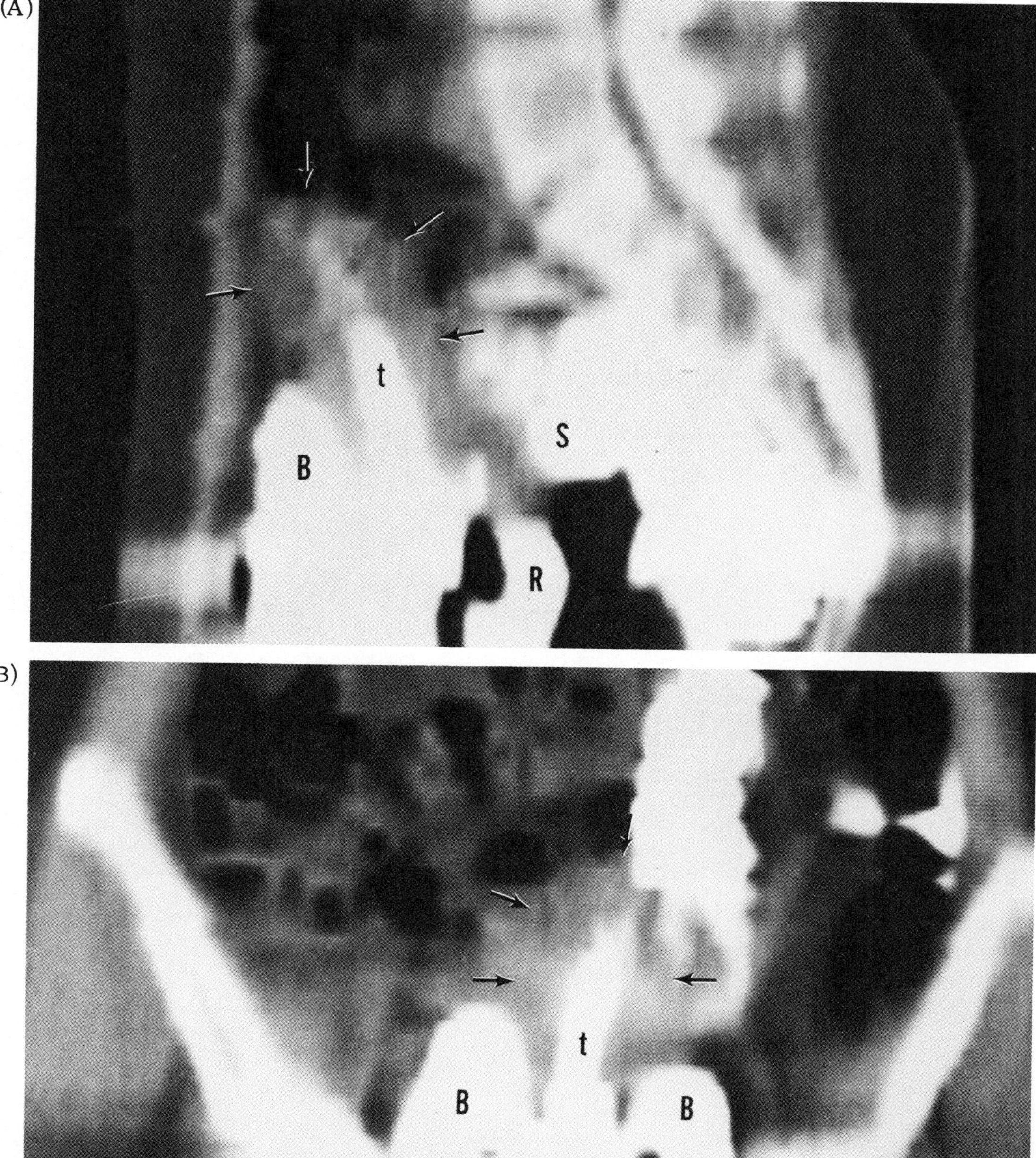

Figure 50. Reconstructed sagittal (A) and coronal (B) scan of the same patient in Fig. 15. The scans demonstrate the entire size and contour of the uterus (arrows) and relation to the intracavitary applicator (t) and the surrounding normal structures including sigmoid (S), bladder (B), and rectum (R).

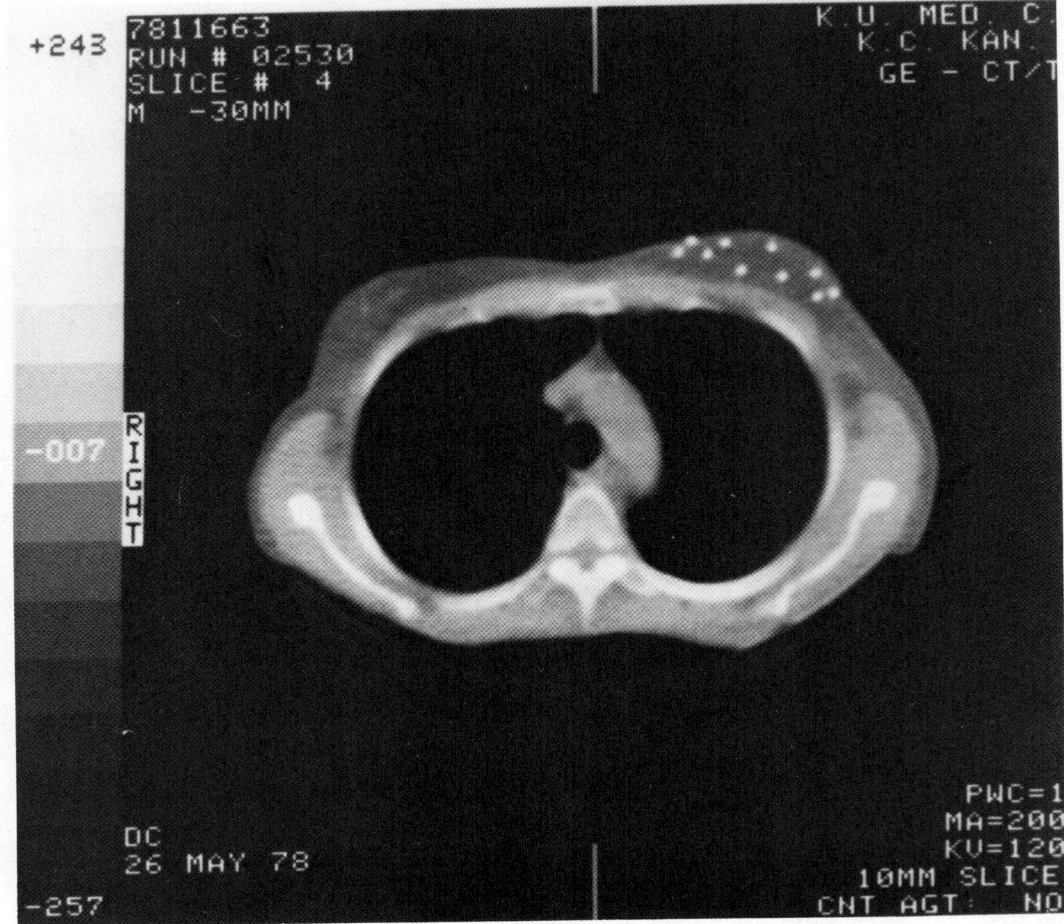

Figure 51. A: An ^{192}Ir interstitial implant for a carcinoma of the breast, stage I. The iridium wires were implanted longitudinally in the breast. The transverse CT scan demonstrates the individual wires.

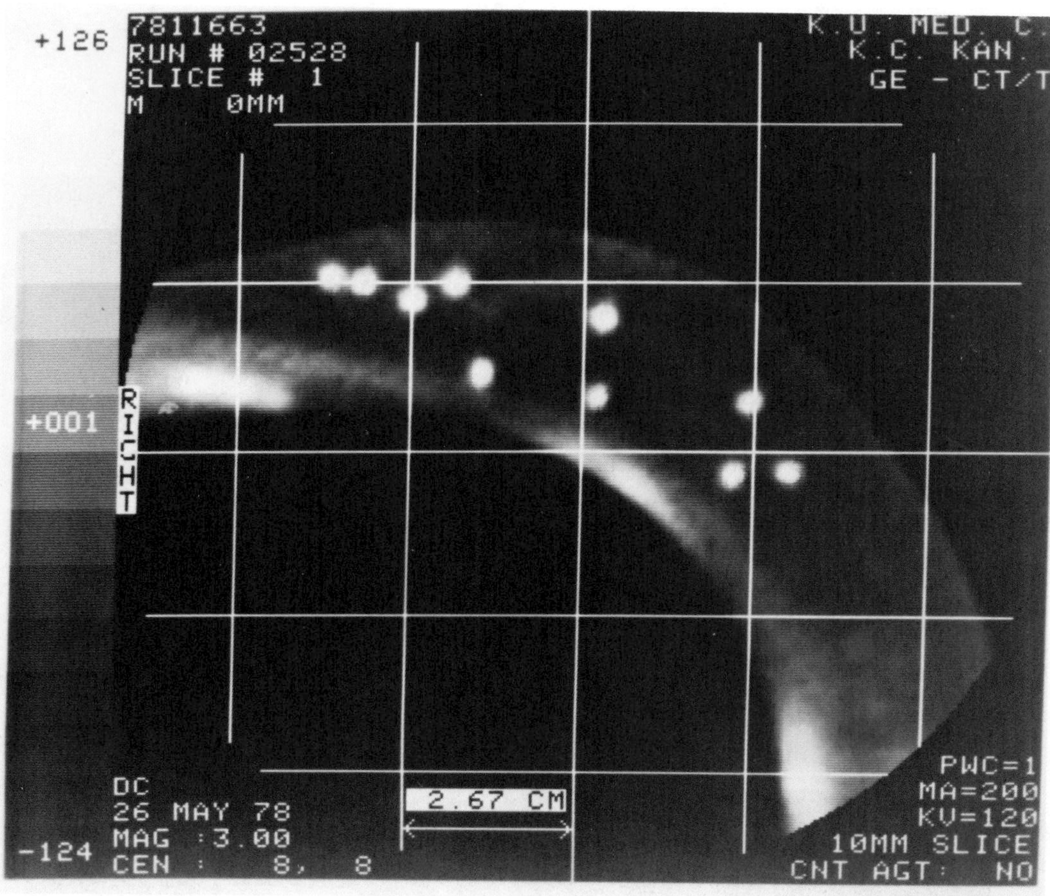

Figure 51. B: The distances between the sources can be accurately measured by a magnified view with a grid.

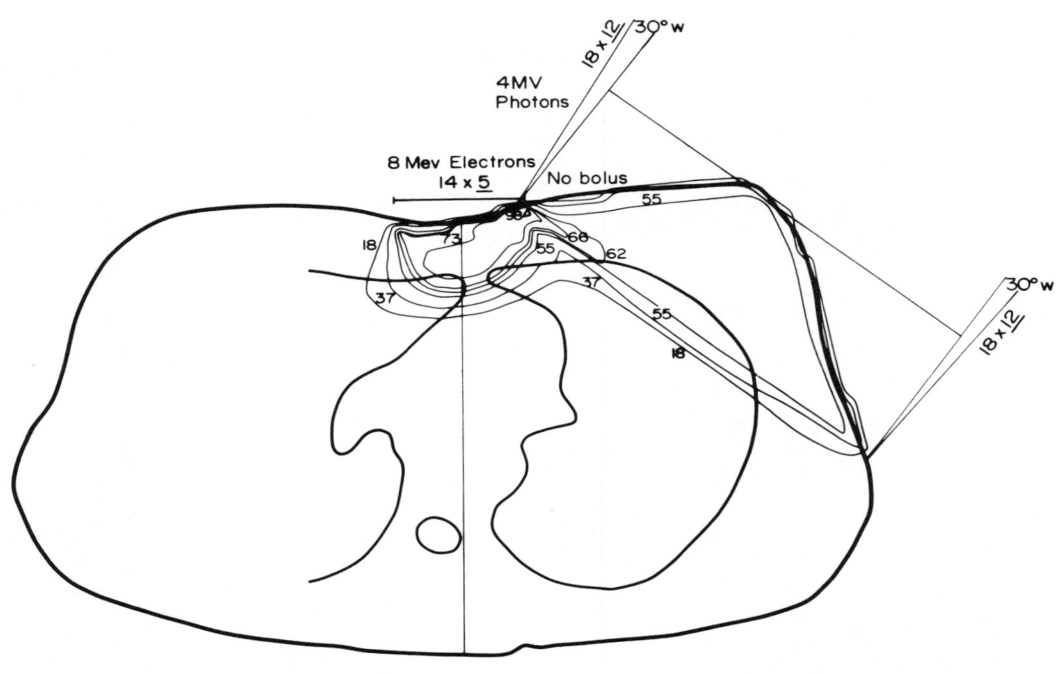

Figure 52. Carcinoma of the breast. A: A CT contour and treatment plan for 8 MeV electrons to the mediastinum and 4 MV beam to the breast.

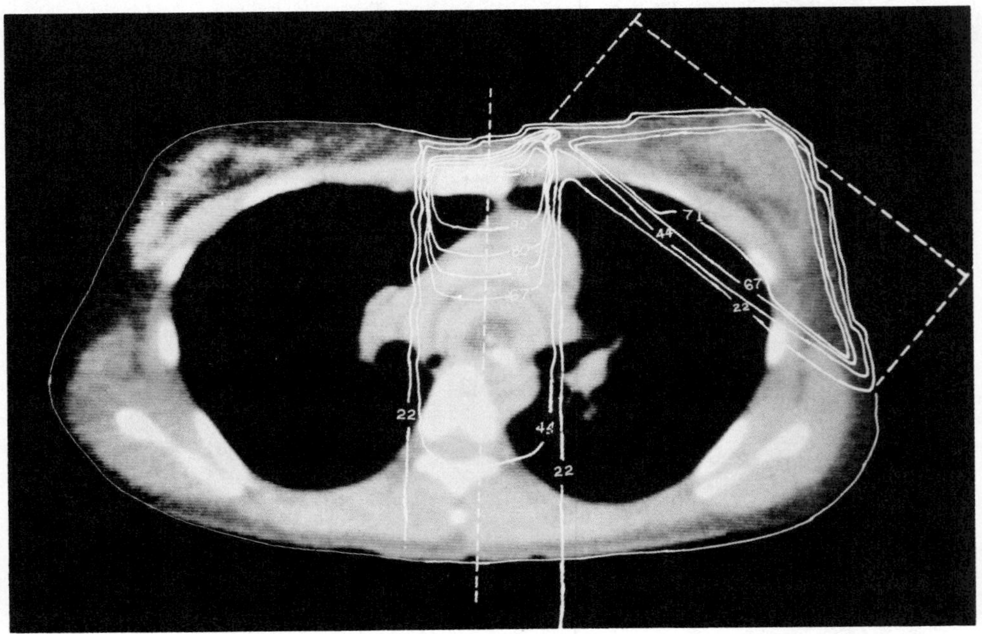

Figure 52. B: The plan with 4 MV beam to the mediastinum and breast superimposed on the same CT scan.

(A)

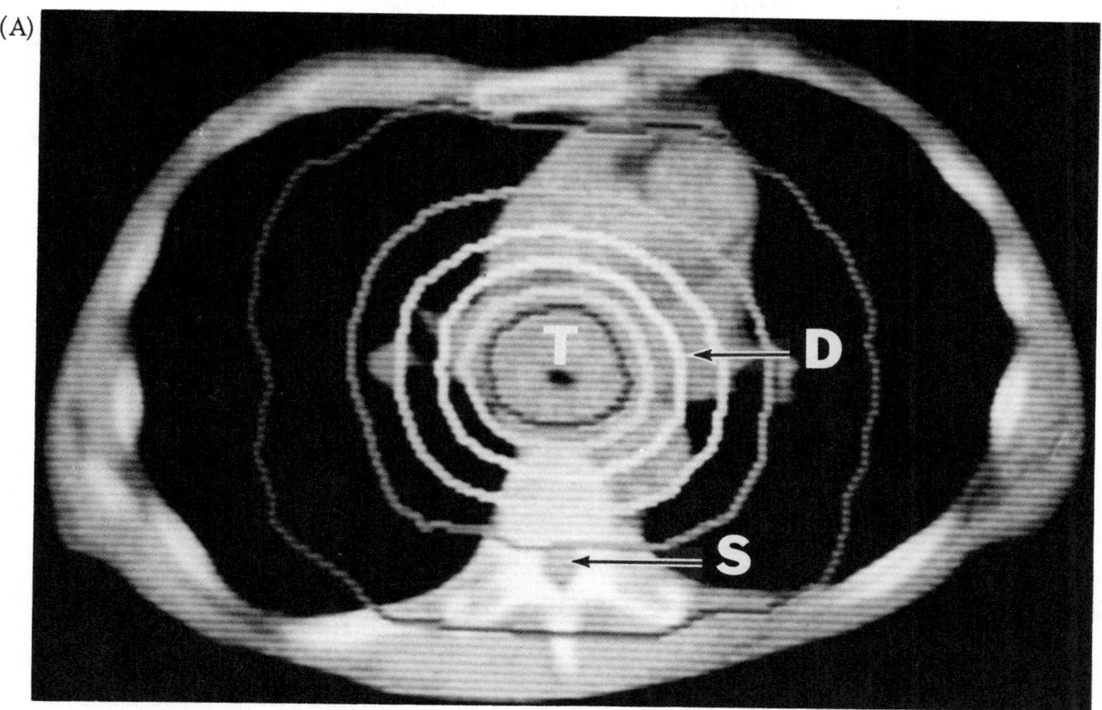

(B)

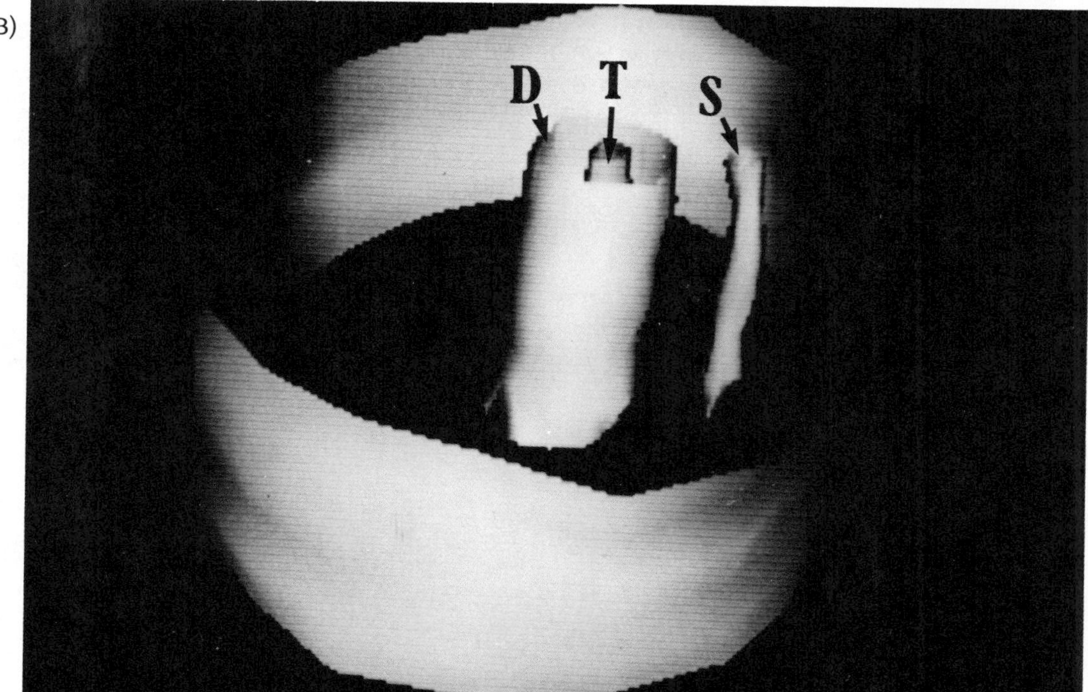

Figure 53. A: A rotational therapy plan for a carcinoma of the midesophagus in transverse and B: perspective displays. Either of these displays might suggest an adequately defined plan.

(C)

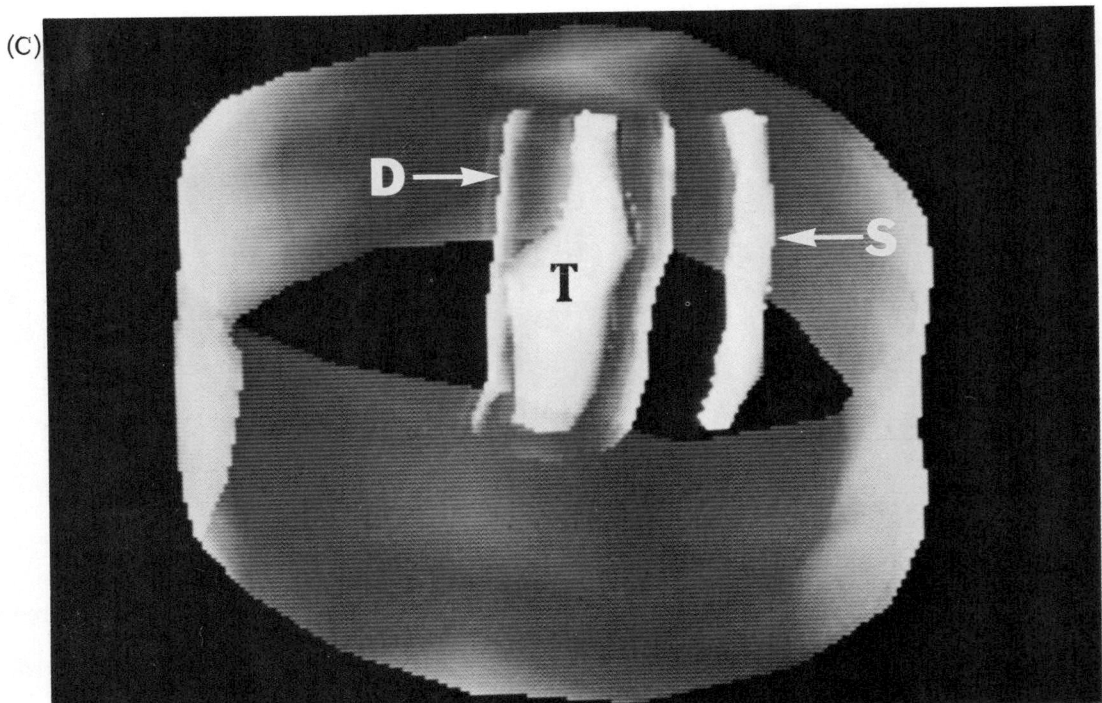

Figure 53. C: But the transparent perspective view shows the relation of esophageal tumor (T), spinal cord (S), and 80% isodose surface (D), and points out that the tumor volume which is irregularly aligned is barely covered by the 80% isodose surface while the spinal cord is spared from the high-dose irradiation. (Proceedings of MEDINFO '80, by permission.)

(A)

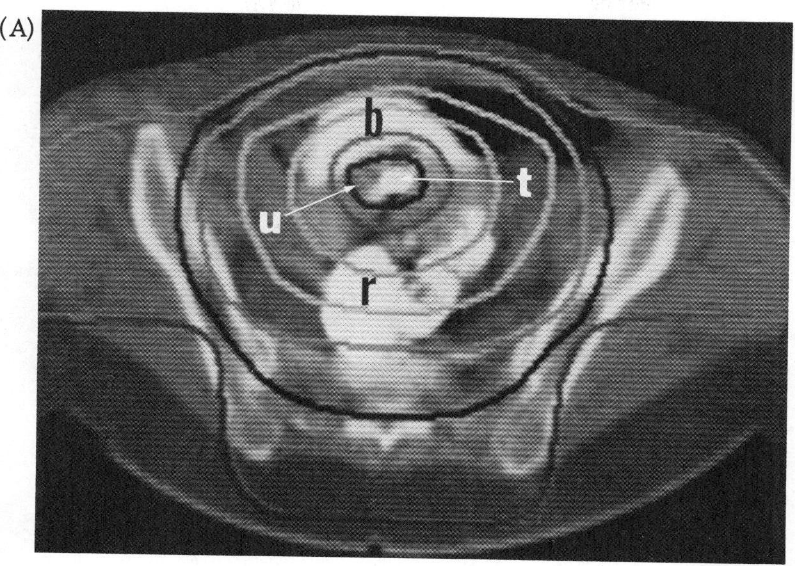

(B)

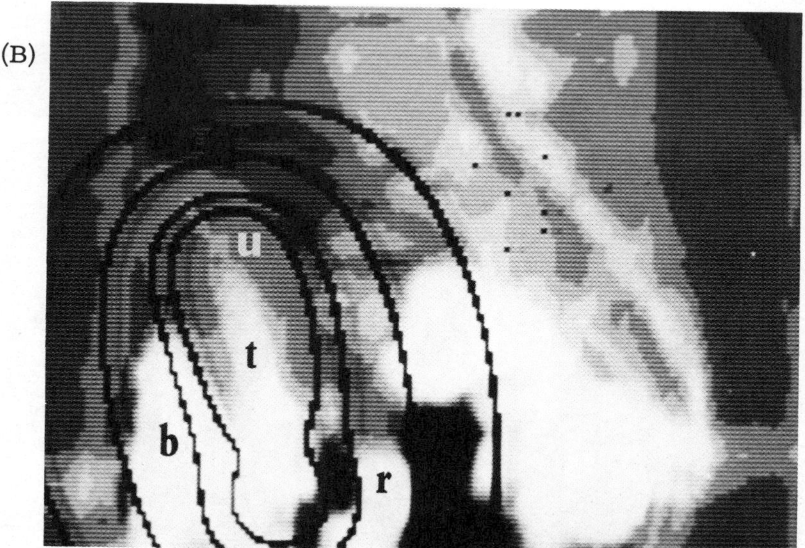

Figure 54. A series of transverse CT scans obtained after insertion of Fletcher afterloading applicator for a carcinoma of the cervix, stage IIA. The isodose distribution of the treatment is superimposed on the transverse (A), sagittal (B), and coronal (C) scans interactively. The transparent perspective view (D) displays the three-dimensional anatomic information regarding the location, size, and shape of the uterus (u), rectum (r), intravaginal ovoids (o), and the 70% dose rate surface (d). (B and C in Proceedings of MEDINFO '80, by permission.)

(C)

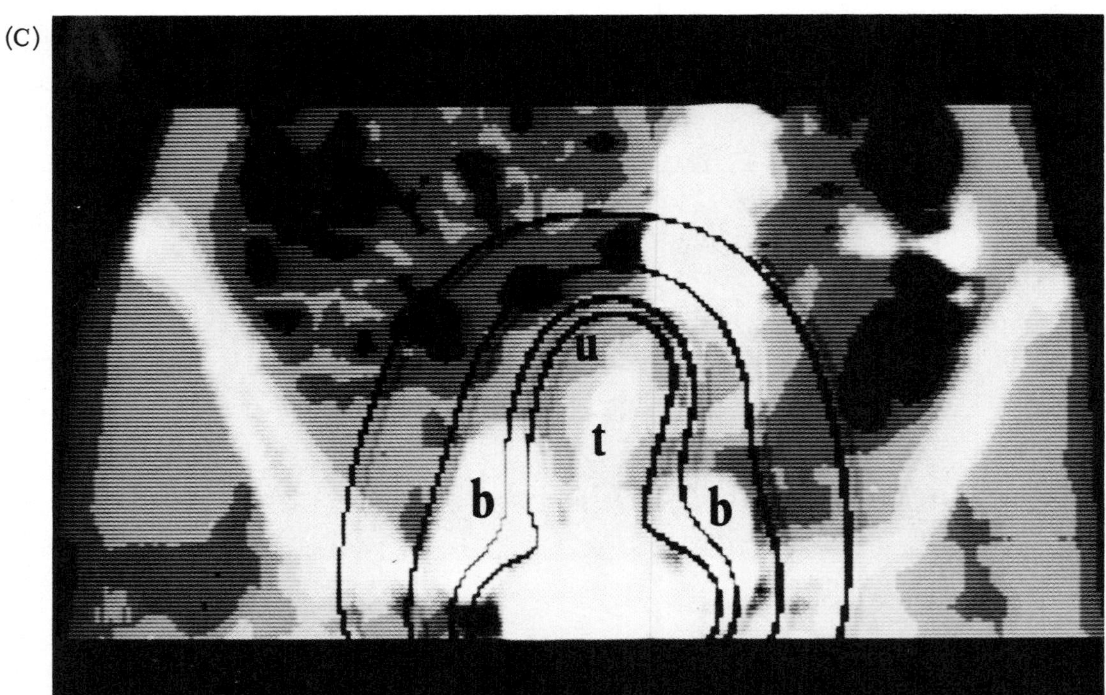

(D)

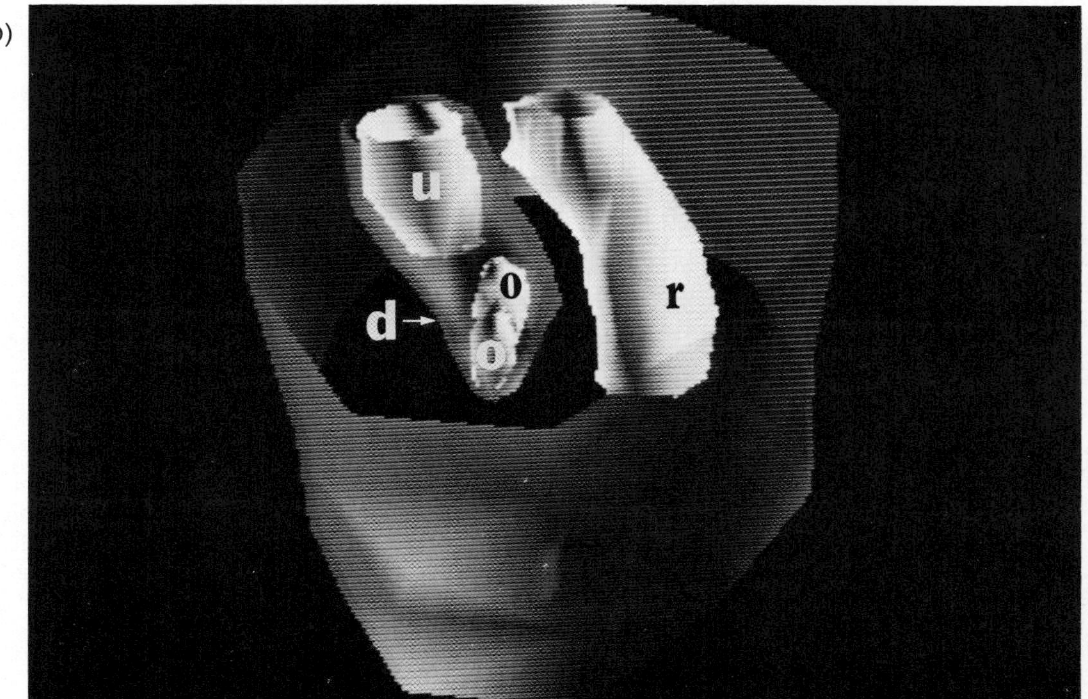

Figure 54. C & D

REFERENCES

1. Alazraki, N.P., Ramsdell, J.W., Taylow, A., Friedman, P.J., Peters, R.M. and Tisi, G.M.: Reliability of gallium scan chest radiography compared to mediastinoscopy for evaluating mediastinal spread of lung cancer. Am. Rev. Respir. Dis. 117:415-420, 1978.

2. Alcron, F.S., Mategrano, V.C., Petansnick, J.P., Clark, J.W.: Contributions of computed tomography in the staging and management of malignant lymphoma. Radiology 125:717-723, 1977.

3. Alfidi, R.J., Haaga, J., Meaney, T.F., MacIntyre, W.J., Gonzalez, L., Tarar, R., Zelch, M.G., Boller, M., Sebastian, C.A. and Jelden, G.: Computed tomography of the thorax and abdomen: A preliminary report. Radiology 117:257-264, 1975.

4. Ambrose, J.: Computerized transverse axial scanning (tomography): Part 2. Clinical application. Brit. J. Radiol. 46:1023-1047, 1973.

5. Averette, H.E., Dudan, R.C., Ford, J.H., Jr.: Exploratory celiotomy for surgical staging of cervical cancer. Am. J. Obstet. Gynecol. 113:1090-1096, 1972.

6. Baker, H.L.: The impact of computed tomography on neuroradiologic practice. Radiology 116:637-640, 1975.

7. Brasho, D.J.: Tumor localization and treatment planning with ultrasound. Cancer 39:697-705, 1977.

8. Burney, B.T. and Klatte, E.: A level marker for whole body computed tomography. Radiology 129:238-239, 1978.

9. Carter, B.L. and Ignatow, S.B.: Neck and mediastinal angiography by computed tomography. Semin. Radiol. 122:515-516, 1977.

10. Carter, B.L. and Karmody, C.S.: Computed tomography of the face and neck. Semin. Roentgenol. 13:257-266, 1978.

11. Castellino, R.A., Billingham, M., and Dorfman, R.F.: Lymphographic accuracy in Hodgkin's disease and malignant lymphoma with a note on the "reactive lymph node" as a cause of most false-positive lymphograms. Invest. Radiol. 9:155-165, 1974.

12. Chernak, E.S., Rodriguez-Antunez, A., Jelden, G.L., Dhaliwal, R.S. and Lavik, P.S.: The use of computed tomography for radiation therapy treatment planning. Radiology 117:613-614, 1975.

13. Cohen, W.N., Siedelman, F.E., and Bryan, P.J.: The use of a tampon to enhance vaginal localization in computed tomography of the female pelvis. Am. J. Roentgenol. 128:1064-1065, 1977.

14. Computed tomography/therapy interfacing. Radiology/Nuclear Medicine Magazine 9:4-13, 1979.

15. Danoff, B.F., Pripstein, S., Croce, N., Kramer, S., and Lee, K.F.: The value of computerized tomography in delineating suprasellar extension of pituitary adenoma for radiotherapeutic management. Cancer 42:1066-1072, 1978.

16. Deland, F.H., Sauerbrunn, J.L., Boyd, C., Wilkinson, R.H., Friedman, B.I., Moinuddin, M., Preston, D.F. and Kniseley, R.M.: 67 Ga-citrate imaging in untreated primary lung cancer: preliminary report of cooperative group. J. Nucl. Med. 15:408-411, 1974.

17. DeMeester, T.R., Bekerman, G., Joseph, J.G., Toscano, M.S., Golomb, H., Bitran, J., Gross, N.J. and Skinner, D.B.: Gallium 67 scanning for carcinoma of the lung. J. Thorac. Cardiovasc. Surg. 72:699-708, 1976.

18. Dwyer, III, S.J., Lee, K.R., Mansfield, C.M., Fritz, S.L., Anderson, W.H., and Cook, P.H.: Display strategies using CT scan data for radiation therapy planning. Proceedings of the 3rd World Conference on Medical Informatics, Tokyo, Sept. 1980, North-Holland Publishing Co., Amsterdam, 1980.

19. Emami, B., Melo, A., Carter, B.L., Muzenrider, J.E. and Piro, A.J.: Value of computed tomography in radiotherapy of lung cancer. Am. J. Roentgenol. 131:63-67, 1978.

20. Fazio, F., Pratt, T.A., McKenzie, C.G., and Steiner, R.E.: Improvement in regional ventilation and perfusion after radiotherapy for unresectable carcinoma of the bronchus. Am. J. Roentgenol. 133:191-200, 1979.

21. Favez, G., Willa, C., and Heinzer, F.: Posterior oblique tomography at an angle of 55° in chest roentgenology. Am. J. Roentgenol. 120:907-915, 1974.

22. Filly, R.A., Marglin, S., and Castellino, R.A.: The ultrasonographic spectrum of abdominal and pelvic Hodgkin's disease and non-Hodgkin's lymphoma. Cancer 38:2143-2148, 1976.

23. Fisher, R.I. and Young, R.C.: Advances in the staging and treatment of ovarian cancer. Cancer 39:967-972, 1977.

24. Floyd, C.E., Corely, R.G., and Cohn, I.J.: Local recurrence of carcinoma of the colon and rectum. Am. J. Surg. 109:153-159, 1965.

25. Forbes, W.S.E.C., Fawcutt, R.A., Isherwoor, I., Webb, R., and Farrington, T.: Computed tomography in the diagnosis of diseases of the paranasal sinuses. Clin. Radiol. 29:501-511, 1978.

26. Fuchs, H., Kedem, Z.M., and Uselton, S.P.: Optimal surface reconstruction from planar contour. Comm. ACM 20:693-702, 1977.

27. Fullerton, G.D., Sewchand, W., Payne, J.T., and Levitt, S.H.: CT determination of parameters for inhomogeneity corrections in radiation therapy of the esophagus. Radiology 126:167-171, 1978.

28. Gawler, J., Sanders, M.D., Bull, J.W.D., DuBaulay, G., and Marshall, J.: Computerized assisted tomography in orbital disease. Brit. J. Ophthalmol. 58:571-587, 1974.

29. Geise, R.A. and McCullough, E.C.: The use of CT scanners in megavoltage photobeam therapy planning. Radiology 124:133-141, 1977.

30. Harada, K., Igari, D., and Tanahashi, Y.: Grey scale transrectal ultrasonography of the prostate. J. Clin. Ultrasound 7:45-49, 1979.

31. Harell, G.S., Beiman, R.S., Glatstein, E.J., Marshall, W.H., and Castellino, R.A.: Computed tomography of the abdomen in the malignant lymphomas. Radiol. Clin. N. Am. 15:391-400, 1977.

32. Heitzman, E.R., Goldwin, R.L., and Proto, A.V.: Radiologic analysis of the mediastinum utilizing computed tomography. Radiol. Clin. N. Am. 15: 309-329, 1977.

33. Hilal, S.K., and Trokel, S.L.: Computerized tomography of the orbit using thin sections. Semin. Roentgenol. 12:137-147, 1977.

34. Hobday, P., Hodson, N.J., Husband, J., Parker, R.P., and Macdonald, J.S.: Computed tomography applied to radiotherapy treatment planning: Techniques and results. Radiology 133:477-482, 1979.

35. Husband, J.E., Hodson, N.J., and Parsons, C.A.: CT in recurrent rectal tumors. J. Comput. Assisted Tomography 3:560, 1979.

36. Jelden, G.L., Chernak, E.S., Rodriguez-Antuniz, A., Haaga, J.R., Lavik, P.S., and Dhaliwal, R.S.: Further progress in CT scanning and computerized radiation therapy treatment planning. Am. J. Roentgenol. 127:179-185, 1976.

37. Johnston, G., Benua, R.S., Teates, C.D., Edwards, C.L., and Kniseley, R.M.: 67 Ga-citrate imaging in untreated Hodgkin's disease: preliminary report of Cooperative Group. J. Nucl. Med. 15:399-403, 1974.

38. Kaplan, H.S.: Hodgkin's disease: multidisciplinary contributions to the conquest of a neoplasm. Radiology 123:551-558, 1977.

39. Kenny, G.M., Hartoner, G.J., Moore, R.M., and Murphy, G.P.: Current results from treatment of stages C and D bladder tumors at Roswell Park Memorial Institute. J. Urol. 107:56-59, 1972.

40. Lee, B.J., Nelson, J.H., and Schwarz, G.: Evaluation of lymphangiography, inferior vena cavography and intravenous pyelography in the clinical staging and management of Hodgkin's disease and lymphosarcoma. N. Engl. J. Med. 271:327-337, 1964.

41. Lee, J.K.T., Stanley, R.J., Sagel, S.S., et al.: Letter to editor. Am. J. Roentgenol. 131:1117, 1978.

42. Lee, J.K.T., Stanley, R.J., Sagel, S.S., et al.: Accuracy of computed tomography in detecting intraabdominal and pelvic adenopathy in lymphoma. Am. J. Roentgenol. 131:311-315, 1978.

43. Lee, K.R., Mansfield, C.M., Dwyer, S.J., III, Cox, H.L., Levine, E., and Templeton, A.W.: CT for intracavitary planning in radiation therapy planning. Am. J. Roentgenol. 135:809-813, 1980.

44. Lipscomb, D. and Pride, N.B.: Ventilation and perfusion scans in the preoperative assessment of bronchial carcinoma. Thorax 32:720-725, 1977.

45. Lipton, M.J., DeNardo, G.L., Silverman, S., et al.: Evaluation of the liver and spleen in Hodgkin's disease. I. The value of hepatic scintigraphy. Am. J. Med. 52:356-364, 1972.

46. Lloyd, G.A.S.: The impact of CT scanning and ultrasonography on orbital diagnosis. Clin. Radiol. 28:583-593, 1977.

47. Mancuso, A.A. and Karafee, W.N.: A comparative elaboration of computed tomography and laryngography. Radiology 133:131-138, 1979.

48. Maynard, C.D. and Cowan, R.J.: Role of the scan in bronchogenic carcinoma. Sem. Nucl. Med. 1:195-205, 1971.

49. McLaughlin, I.S., Morley, P., Deane, R.F., et al.: Ultrasound in the staging of bladder tumours. Brit. J. Urol. 47:51-56, 1975.

50. McNeil, B.J., Collins, J.J., Adelstein, S.J., et al.: Rationale for seeking occult metastases in patients with bronchial carcinoma. Surg. Gynecol. Obstet. 144:389-393, 1977.

51. McNeil, B.J. and Pauker, S.G.: The patient's role in assessing the value of diagnostic tests. Radiology 132:605-610, 1979.

52. Miller, E.M. and Norman, D.: The role of computed tomography in the evaluation of neck masses. Radiology 133:145-149, 1979.

53. Mintzer, R.A., Malave, S.R., Neiman, H.L., et al.: Computed vs. conventional tomography in evaluation of primary and secondary pulmonary neoplasms. Radiology 132:653-659, 1979.

54. Moss, N.H. and Axtell, L.M.: Cancer of the Gastrointestinal Tract - Trends in Method of Treatment and Patient Survival. In Sixth National Cancer Conference Proceedings. Philadelphia, Lippincott, 1970.

55. Muhm, J.R., Brown, L.R., and Crowe, J.K.: Detection of pulmonary nodules by computed tomography. Am. J. Roentgenol. 128:267-270, 1977.

56. Munzenrider, J.E., Pilepich, M., Rene-Ferrero, J.B., et al.: Use of body scanner in radiotherapy treatment planning. Cancer 40:170-179, 1977.

57. Nelson, J.H., Jr.: The incidence and significance of para-aortic lymph node metastases in late invasive carcinoma of the cervix. Am. J. Obstet. Gynecol. 118:749-756, 1974.

58. Operchal, J.A., Bowen, R.D., Grane, R.B.: Efficacy of radionuclide procedures in staging of bronchogenic carcinoma. J. Nucl. Med. 17:531, 1976.

59. Parsons, C. and Hodson, N.: Computed tomography of paranasal sinus tumors. Radiology 132:641-645, 1979.

60. Peterson, A.H.G. and McCready, V.R.: Tumor imaging radiopharmaceuticals. Brit. J. Radiol. 48:520-531, 1975.

61. Pay, N.T., Carella, R.J., Lin, J.P., Kricheff, I.I.: The usefulness of computed tomography during and after radiation therapy in patients with brain tumors. Radiology 121:79-83, 1976.

62. Ramsdell, J.W., Peters, R.M., Taylor, A.T., Jr., et al.: Multiorgan scans for staging lung cancer: Correlation with clinical evaluation. J. Thorac. Cardiovasc. Surg. 73:653-659, 1977.

63. Reddy, E.K., Mansfield, C.M., and Hartman, G.V.: Carcinoma of the rectum and rectosigmoid colon: Role of radiation therapy. J. Natl. Med. Assoc. 70:815-818, 1978.

64. Redman, H.C., Glatstein, E., Castellino, R.A., et al.: Computed tomography as an adjunct in the staging of Hodgkin's disease and non-Hodgkin's lymphomas. Radiology 124:381-385, 1977.

65. Rosen, R.J. and Goodman, L.R.: Occult bronchogenic carcinoma masquerading as recurrent pulmonary embolism. Am. J. Roentgenol. 132:133-135, 1979.

66. Secker-Walker, R.H. and Provan, J.L.: Scintillation scanning of lungs in preoperative assessment of carcinoma of bronchus. Br. Med. J. 3:327-330, 1969.

67. Secker-Walker, R.H., Alderson, P.O., and Wilhelm, J., et al.: Ventilation-perfusion scanning in carcinoma of the bronchus. Chest 65:660-663, 1974.

68. Seidelmann, F.E., Cohen, W.A., and Bryan, P.J.: Computed tomographic staging of bladder neoplasms. Radiol. Clin. North Am. 15:419-440, 1977.

69. Seidelmann, F.E. and Cohen, W.A.: Pelvis in Computed Tomography of Abdominal Abnormalities, edited by J. Haaga and N.E. Reich, St. Louis, C.V. Mosby Company, 1978.

70. Seidelmann, F.E., Temes, S.P., Cohen, W.N., et al.: Computed tomography of gas-filled bladder: Method of staging bladder neoplasms. Urology 9: 337-344, 1977.

71. Schaner, E.G., Head, G.L., Doppman, J.L., et al.: Computed tomography in the diagnosis, staging and management of abdominal lymphoma. J. Comput. Assisted Tomography 1:176-180, 1977.

72. Schlager, B., Asbell, S.O., Baker, A.S., Sklaroff, D.M., Seydel, H.G., and Ostrum, B.J.: The use of computerized tomography scanning in treatment planning for bladder carcinoma. Int. J. Rad. Oncology Biol. Phys. 5:99-103, 1979.

73. Sheedy, II, P.F., Stephens, D.H., Hattery, R.R., Muhm, J.R., and Hartman, G.W.: Computed tomography of the body: Initial clinical trial with the EMI prototype. Am. J. Roentgenol. 127:23-51, 1976.

74. Shevland, J.E., Chiu, L.C., Schapiro, R.L., et al.: The role of conventional tomography and computed tomography in assessing the resectability of primary lung cancer: A preliminary report. J. Comput. Tomography 2:1-19, 1978.

75. Silverman, S., DeNardo, G.L., Glatstein, E., et al.: Evaluation of the liver and spleen in Hodgkin's disease. II. The value of splenic scintigraphy. Am. J. Med. 52:362, 1972.

76. Sontag, M.R., Battista, J.J., Bronskill, M.J., and Cunningham, J.R.: Implications of computed tomography for inhomogeneity corrections in photon beam dose calculations. Radiology 124:143-149, 1977.

77. Stearns, M.W., Jr., Deddish, M.R., and Quan, S.H.O.: Preoperative roentgen therapy in cancer of the rectum. Surg. Gynecol. Obstet. 109:225-229, 1959.

78. Stewart, J.R., Boone, M.L.M., Hicks, J.A., and Simpson, L.D.: Computed tomography in radiation therapy: Report of the Committee on Radiation Oncology Studies, NIH, 1977.

79. Taveras, J.M. and Wood, E.M.: Diagnostic neuroradiology, Baltimore, Williams and Wilkin, 1976, pp. 997-1020.

80. Vassullo, C.L., Gee, J.B.L., Wholey, M.H., et al.: Lung scanning in hilar bronchogenic carcinoma. Am. Rev. Resp. Dis. 97:851-858, 1968.

81. Wagner, H.N., Lopez-Majano, V., Tow, D.E., et al.: Radioisotope scanning of lungs in early diagnosis of bronchogenic carcinoma. Lancet 1:344, 1965.

82. Wallace, S., Jing, B., and Zornosa, J.: Lymphangiography in the determination of the extent of metastatic carcinoma. Cancer 39:706-718, 1977.

83. Wharam, M.D. and Order, S.E.: Treatment planning in radiation therapy: Maximization by CT. Appl. Radiology 6:50-56, 1980.

84. Whitmoe, W.F., Jr.: Assessment and management of deeply invasive and metastatic lesions. Cancer Res. 37:2756-2758, 1977.

85. Zimmerman, R.A., Bilaniuk, L.T., Grundy, G., and Littman, P.: Computed tomographic localization for radiotherapy of cerebral tumors. Radiology 119:230-231, 1976.

chapter 3

BRAIN TUMORS

SECTION I. BRAIN TUMORS IN CHILDREN

Barbara F. Danoff, M.D.

Intracranial tumors represent the second most common neoplasm in children exceeded only by leukemia. Approximately 1000 new cases are diagnosed annually in the United States accounting for 20% of all childhood malignant disease (32). The peak incidence occurs in the latter half of the first decade of life. Overall, males and females are equally affected (80). However, a definite male predominance is evident in medulloblastoma.

Sixty percent of intracranial neoplasms in patients below age 15 are infratentorial and 40% are supratentorial (80). The principal infratentorial tumors are cerebellar astrocytomas, medulloblastomas, brain stem gliomas, and fourth ventricle ependymomas, with the frequency of occurrence in that order. Cerebral astrocytomas, ependymomas of the lateral ventricles, craniopharyngiomas and pinealomas are the most common supratentorial tumors. Meningiomas and pituitary tumors are rare in children (Table 1).

Gliomas comprise 70% of verified brain tumors in children compared to 45% in adults (15). Low-grade astrocytomas and medulloblastomas constitute 70% of gliomas in children, whereas glioblastoma multiform is the most common glioma in adults (15).

The etiology of intracranial neoplasms is unknown. A higher incidence of central nervous system tumors has been noted with neurofibromatosis (34), von Hippel Lindau disease (43), and tuberous sclerosis (55). Teratomas, dermoid and epidermoid cysts, craniopharyngiomas, and chordomas are of congenital origin (59).

Brain tumors in children tend to occur along the central neural axis, i.e., within the third and fourth ventricles, the midline of the cerebellum, the brainstem, hypothalamus, or optic pathways. This location accounts for the frequent absence of localizing neurological signs. Early obstruction of cerebrospinal fluid (CSF) flow results in signs and symptoms of increased intracranial pressure. Focal signs and symptoms result from invasion or compression of adjacent structures.

BRAIN TUMORS IN CHILDREN

The clinical diagnosis of a brain tumor is often prompted by an accurate history and neurological examination. Radiological investigations delineate the anatomic location of the tumor and the presence or absence of hydrocephalus. Surgical treatment includes biopsy to establish a diagnosis, insertion of a shunt to relieve increased intracranial pressure, and complete or partial tumor removal when

Table 1. Intracranial Neoplasms in Childhood (%)

Cerebellar astrocytoma	25
Medulloblastoma	20
Cerebral astrocytoma	15
Brainstem glioma	15
Ependymoma	10
Craniopharyngioma	10
Optic nerve glioma	4
Pinealoma	2
Miscellaneous	8

possible. For certain tumors (thalamic, brainstem) biopsy is too hazardous and a presumptive diagnosis is based on clinical and radiographic findings.

With few exceptions, radiotherapy is universally employed with or without surgery in the treatment of brain tumors in children. An overall 5-year survival of 47% and a 10-year survival of 40% have been achieved (12). Prognosis is related to histology, anatomic site, age of presentation, and degree of surgical resection.

Chemotherapy has been of benefit in the treatment of recurrent tumors (118) and is under investigation as adjuvant therapy for medulloblastomas, ependymomas, brain stem gliomas, and grade III and IV astrocytomas. The use of radiosensitizers has been proposed and is currently under study.

With the achievement of improved survival, attention has now been directed towards the assessment of treatment-induced sequelae. Diminished bone and soft tissue growth, secondary neoplasms including thyroid carcinoma and intracranial sarcomas, and altered intellectual and social behavior have been reported. Other potential late effects require longer periods of observation for documentation. It is often difficult, however, to determine whether these changes are related to the effect of the tumor, hydrocephalus and/or treatment, genetic predisposition, or a combination of factors.

Medulloblastoma

Medulloblastomas comprise 4% of all intracranial neoplasms (14) and 20% of all brain tumors in children (14,118). Eighty percent occur in patients less than 15 years of age (14) and males predominate with a male/female ratio of 2-4:1 (12, 14,83). The tumor first described by Bailey and Cushing in 1925 (8) is an embryonic tumor composed of largely primitive or poorly differentiated cells which arise from the cerebellum. The desmoplastic variant occurs more commonly in adults, is often extracerebellar and, therefore, more amenable to surgical resection, and associated with a better prognosis (23,106).

Patients with medulloblastoma commonly present with symptoms of increased intracranial pressure, i.e., early morning headaches, nausea, and vomiting. Other symptoms include a clumsy, ataxic gait and personality changes. The most common signs on admission include papilledema, truncal and/or limb ataxia, nystagmus, and cranial nerve defects.

Medulloblastomas may spread via direct extension, CSF seeding, or hematogenous dissemination and may extend inferiorly between the cerebellar tonsils towards the foramen magnum and into the upper cervical subarachnoid space. A striking feature is the dissemination of malignant cells through the cerebrospinal fluid to the leptomeninges, the walls of the ventricular system, the spinal cord, and the cauda equina. These deposits may be diffuse or nodular. McFarland et al. (83) in a review of 430 cases of medulloblastoma found 33% with evidence of CNS metastases; 94% of these were along the spinal canal and 6% were intracranial. Sheline (125) postulated that the overall incidence of CSF metastases was higher since many of McFarland's patients had received prior radiotherapy. Hematogenous dissemination occurs in approximately 5% of cases. Osteolytic and osteoblastic bone metastases are the most common extra CNS metastases. Lung and lymph node metastases also occur. Extraneural metastases are primarily associated with surgical manipulation and the placement of CSF shunts (56).

Surgery alone has not produced a single documented cure in patients with medulloblastoma (145). Its primary objectives are to confirm the diagnosis, create a rapid decompression, and restore the flow of cerebrospinal fluid. Wilson (145), Bloom and Walsh (15), Jenkin (53), and Sheline (125) advocate resection of as much tumor bulk as possible without compromising neurological function. The results following gross subtotal and total tumor removal appear to be superior to those of biopsy or minimal tumor resection (13, 41, 96, 145). Operative mortality is now in the range of 10% (13, 58). Routine prophylactic permanent shunts are to be avoided since tumor cells may seed through the shunt (56). A surgical staging system was proposed by Chang et al. in 1969 (21) (Table 2) and more recently has been shown to correlate well with survival (41). A wider application of the staging system by other investigators is needed to confirm the prognostic value.

The survival of patients with medulloblastoma has increased since the introduction of postoperative radiotherapy in the 1920s (13). Substantially improved survivals have been achieved with the use of craniospinal irradiation. Five- and ten-year survival rates of 35 and 25% respectively, have been reported (11). Because of the propensity for medulloblastomas to spread along the subarachnoid space and into the cerebrospinal fluid, the whole neural axis must be irradiated.

The preradiotherapy evaluation of the patient with medulloblastoma should include cerebrospinal fluid cytology for tumor cells to detect possible microscopic spinal seeding. A myelogram should be performed to detect clinically unsuspected asymptomatic gross spinal deposits (30). Known areas of spinal involvement would then receive additional radiotherapy above the prophylactic level.

Several techniques have been utilized to irradiate the entire craniospinal axis. These include the simultaneous irradiation of the whole brain and spinal cord (25, 92), irradiation of the whole brain followed by irradiation of the spinal cord (14, 41), and timed sequential overlapping irradiation of the intracranial contents and spinal cord (62). The advantage of simultaneous irradiation is that malignant cells cannot be harbored in any area of the CNS which is not being irradiated at a particular time.

Current policy is to irradiate the whole brain and spinal canal simultaneously. Megavoltage equipment is employed. The whole brain and cervical spine to C-5 or C-6 are treated with parallel opposed lateral fields. The spinal cord and dural sac (S-2) are treated by direct posterior field(s). The posterior fossa is irradiated using lateral parallel opposed fields. Postoperative radiotherapy is initially begun to the posterior fossa alone. A tumor dose (central axis at the

Table 2. Operative Staging System for Medulloblastoma (Chang)

T1	Tumor less than 3 cm in diameter and limited to the classic midline position in the vermis, the roof of the fourth ventricle and less frequently to the cerebellar hemispheres.
T2	Tumor more than 3 cm in diameter, invading one adjacent structure or partially filling the fourth ventricle.
T3a	Tumor invading two adjacent structures or completely filling the fourth ventricle with extension into the aqueduct of Sylvius, foramen of Magendie, or foramen of Luschka, thus producing marked internal hydrocephalus.
T3b	Tumor arising from the floor of the fourth ventricle or brain stem and filling the fourth ventricle.
T4	Tumor spreading through the aqueduct of Sylvius to involve the third ventricle or midbrain or tumor extending to the upper cervical cord.
MO	No evidence of gross subarachnoid or hematogenous metastases.
M1	Microscopic tumor cells found in the cerebrospinal fluid.
M2	Gross nodular seedings demonstrated in the cerebellar, cerebral subarachnoid space, or in the third or lateral ventricles.
M3	Gross nodular seeding in the spinal subarachnoid space.
M4	Extraneuroaxial metastases.

midplane of the opposed fields) of 1000 rads is delivered in five fractions (200 rads/ fraction) over 5-7 days. During this period an anterior half-body cast is made in the supine position from the patient's forehead to the upper thighs for immobilization. The cast is then mounted on supports to allow sufficient elevation so that the nose and face are not in direct contact with the treatment table. The lateral whole-brain and cervical spine fields are then stimulated with the patient in the cast in the prone position. Alloys are made to shield the globes, facial structures, and anterior portion of the neck. The retroorbital space is included in the treatment field and a generous margin is left around the anterior portion of the middle cranial fossa. Posterior and lateral films are taken of the entire length of the spine with lead markers placed on the posterior skin surface. These films are used to determine the depth of the anterior surface of the spinal cord (posterior surface of the vertebral body) and the straightness of the spine. In an older child or adult more than one posterior field may be required in order to cover the entire cord. A gap is left on the skin surface at the junction of the upper posterior field and the lateral head fields and between each of the posterior fields. The length of this gap is determined by the length of each field and the depth at which they are to be matched (anterior surface of the spinal cord). The gaps are moved 1 cm every 1000 rads cord dose. In general we have chosen to have a gap between the lateral whole-brain fields and the upper posterior field rather than rotate the head fields such that the inferior border of these fields follows the line of divergence of the upper posterior field. In cases where the spine is located at an unusually large depth, a combination of photons and electrons (mixed beam) may be used for one or more of the posterior field(s). Craniospinal irradiation begins once the posterior fossa boost fields are completed. A tumor dose of 4500 rads is delivered to the whole brain in 5 weeks. Four thousand rads is delivered prophylactically to the spinal cord in 5 weeks. The lateral head fields receive 180 rads/fraction and the posterior spinal field 150-160 rads/fraction. If gross disease exists in the spinal cord the dose is increased to that local area of involvement to 5000 rads/6 weeks. The total dose to the posterior fossa is therefore 5500 rads/6 weeks. Using this technique and ^{60}Co radiation, Van Dyk et al. (140) have estimated that the overall dosage variation to the brain and spinal cord is within $\pm$ 10% for the average adult and $\pm$ 5% for the average child. For children under the age of 2-3 years Bloom (13) recommends a posterior fossa dose of 4000-4500 rads/6-7 weeks and 3000 rads to the spinal cord in 6 weeks.

Craniospinal irradiation includes 20-40% of the bone marrow depending on the age of the patient (110). Leukopenia and thrombocytopenia develop during treatment and occasionally may be severe enough to warrant interruption. Treatment can usually be resumed within a week. Rapid recovery of the total leukocyte count occurs following completion of treatment (25). Cumberlin et al. (25) noted that the peripheral lymphocyte count decreased markedly during treatment and recovery was slow. Not only were the total number of T cells decreased but their function was also impaired. Other acute problems related to craniospinal irradiation include dysphagia and gastrointestinal distress secondary to the exit dose from the spinal field. Most patients, however, experience improvement in their presenting signs and symptoms during treatment.

Recently attention has been drawn to the late sequelae of craniospinal irradiation. Probert and Parker (97) found 28 out of 44 patients who received spinal irradiation to have a sitting height more than two standard deviations below the mean for the normal control group. This reduction occurred in 12 out of 15 patients receiving less than 2500 rads of megavoltage irradiation as well as in 16 out of 29 patients receiving more than 4200 rads/25 days. There was a greater reduction in sitting height than standing. Children appeared most sensitive to radiation when their vertebral column was irradiated at puberty or at less than 6 years of age. Kyphoscoliotic deformities are avoided by including both pedicles in the irradiated field (107). Growth deficiency secondary to decreased growth hormone production has been documented in children who have received craniospinal irradiation (25, 119,142). Mental retardation and learning disabilities have been noted in children treated for medulloblastoma. Bloom et al. (14) reported 2 demented patients out of 22 long-term survivors of craniospinal irradiation for medulloblastoma. Jenkin (54) found 1 mentally retarded patient and 3 with learning disabilities in a group of 30 patients completing such treatment. Harisiadis and Chang (41) reported 4 patients with learning disabilities in a group of 11 patients surviving 5 or more years with no evidence of disease. It appears that children under the age of 2-3 years at the time of diagnosis and treatment are particularly vulnerable to the subsequent occurrence of disability (14,58). Five cases of thyroid carcinoma (5,100,105) and two cases of intracranial sarcoma (83) have been reported following craniospinal irradiation for medulloblastoma. It has been estimated that approximately 80% of surviving medulloblastoma patients lead active, productive lives (14,54).

Five-year survival rates ranging from 20-63% (Table 3) have been reported for patients with medulloblastoma treated with craniospinal irradiation. With adequate doses, 35-50% (13,41,125) of the children can be expected to survive 5 years.

Table 3. Medulloblastoma

	5-Year Survival %	5-Year Survival No. of Patients	10-Year Survival (%)
Bloom et al. (14)	38	(22/58)	28
McFarland et al. (83)	38	(7/23)	30
Harisiadis and Chang (41)	40	(17/43)	30
Smith et al. (127)	32	(7/32)	
Sheline (125)	63	(5/8)	
Marsa et al. (77)*	47	(28)	
Onoyama et al. (88)	20	(20)	
Hope-Stone (46)*	58	(11/19)	
Jenkin (54)	27	(8/30)	17
Aron (7)*	31	(4/13)	26
Bouchard (17)	27	(10/37)	17
Bamford et al. (9)	37	(31/84)	
Kramer (62)	50	(6/12)	

*Adults and children.

Prognostic factors include the local extent of the tumor, the type of surgery, histology, sex, age, and the radiation dose to the posterior fossa. Harisiadis and Chang (41) have correlated survival with local tumor extent by the use of an operative staging system. Tumor spread to the third ventricle, midbrain, or upper cervical spine was associated with a 0% 5-year survival. Brain stem involvement significantly decreased the 10-year survival (39% vs. 17%) but did not alter the 5-year survival. Gross subtotal or total tumor removal is associated with improved survival rates as compared to those having biopsy only (13,41,96,145). Histological grading does not influence prognosis (23,106). Females appear to do better than males (13). Adults have higher survival rates for the first 5 years following treatment. After 5 years the younger patients do better (14,41). The disease in young children appears to run a faster course (13). Improved survival rates and decreased recurrence rates are obtained by increasing the radiation dose to the posterior fossa. With doses of 4700-5000 rads or less, overall recurrence rates of 76% (41) and 83% (25) have been reported. In comparison, recurrence rates of 14% (25) and 46% (41) are noted with doses greater than 5200 rads to the posterior fossa. Harisiadis and Chang (41) reported 48% 5-year survival with 5400 rads to the posterior fossa and 35% with a dose of 4000-4700 rads.

Treatment failure in medulloblastoma is due to local recurrence in the posterior fossa with or without cerebral or spinal involvement in 75% of the cases (115). The average time for recurrence is 17.5 months (115) with more than 90% occurring within 5 years (113). Bloom et al. (14) and Harisiadis and Chang (41) found that recurrences from medulloblastoma obey Collin's law, i.e., they occur within a period of risk equal to the patient's age at diagnosis plus 9 months for gestation. However, late recurrences from medulloblastoma have been reported (58). Spinal metastases tend to occur earlier than cerebral metastases (58).

The treatment of recurrent disease may consist of radiotherapy, radiotherapy and/or chemotherapy, or supportive measures alone. Harisiadis and Chang (41) advocate retreatment with craniospinal irradiation to tolerance dose. They found that within the first year after diagnosis of recurrence those treated with radiotherapy and chemotherapy or chemotherapy alone did better than those treated with radiotherapy alone. This finding has been confirmed by Mealey and Hall (81). The Children's Cancer Study Group (CCSG)-Radiation Therapy Oncology Group (RTOG) phase III study of medulloblastoma (99) proposes the use of chemotherapy alone for those recurrences manifesting within 1 year of initial diagnosis and chemotherapy and radiotherapy for those occurring after 1 year. Radiotherapy is limited to the area of recurrence with the doses of 3000-4000 rads/3. 5-5. 5 weeks being employed. Bloom et al. (14) recommend retreatment with radiotherapy to the affected area with doses not exceeding 2000 rads. Vincristine, CCNU, and intrathecal methotrexate have shown to be effective in the treatment of recurrent medulloblastoma (120,145). The CCSG-RTOG protocol employs procarbazine, CCNU, and vincristine for recurrent disease.

Despite the advances of modern surgery and megavoltage radiotherapy, local recurrence in the posterior fossa accounts for the majority of treatment failures. In an attempt to increase survival and decrease local recurrence as well as distant metastases, chemotherapy has been added on an adjuvant basis. Bloom in 1970 initiated a pilot study at the Royal Marsden Hospital using intrathecal vincristine, oral CCNU, and intrathecal methotrexate following surgery and craniospinal irradiation. Chemotherapy was begun upon completion of the radiotherapy. The survival of 21 consecutive patients treated in this manner as of 1977 was better than that of a historical series receiving conventional radiotherapy alone (13). A prospective randomized cooperative trial was then established through the International Society of Pediatric Oncology. Patients are randomized to receive or not receive adjuvant chemotherapy. The chemotherapy arm consists of vincristine administered weekly during radiotherapy followed by a maintenance program of CCNU and vincristine for 1 year. The RTOG and the CCSG in 1975 initiated a phase III study of adjuvant chemotherapy for medulloblastoma. The protocol includes a no chemotherapy control arm in which patients receive craniospinal irradiation and an adjuvant chemotherapy arm consisting of weekly vincristine during radiotherapy followed by maintenance CCNU, vincristine, and prednisone for 1 year.

Future efforts to eradicate the primary tumor may include the use of radiosensitizers (particularly nitroimidiazole compounds) and particle beam irradiation.

Ependymomas

Intracranial ependymomas account for 10% (31) of all brain tumors in children. Fifty to sixty percent (15,31,66) occur under the age of 15. Approximately 70% of intracranial ependymomas (35,66) are infratentorial. The majority arise from the floor of the fourth ventricle. There is no striking male predominance as seen with medulloblastoma.

Ependymomas arise from the cells lining the cerebral ventricular system and the central canal of the spinal cord. They are characterized by ependymal rosettes and perivascular pseudorosettes (106).

Low-grade ependymomas should be distinguished from high-grade ependymomas (ependymoblastomas). The former exhibit a relatively benign behavior while the latter are extremely aggressive. The majority of ependymomas are low grade (106,112).

Ependymomas may extend locally into adjacent structures, seed the CSF pathway, invade adjacent dura, bone, or scalp, and produce extracranial metastases. Approximately one-third of infratentorial ependymomas project extraventricularly into the cisterna magna and cervical subarachnoid space (10,66,112). Local extension into the cerebellopontine angle, central canal of the spinal cord, or cerebellum is less common. Extracranial metastases are rare. They occur more frequently in males and with supratentorial ependymomas (36). The most common metastatic sites are lung, bone, and cervical lymph nodes.

The actual incidence of CSF seeding by intracranial ependymomas remains controversial. Autopsy studies have documented a 30% incidence (112) of spinal subarachnoid seeding. However, a significant proportion of these cases had uncontrolled primary tumors or had received inadequate therapy. Therefore, this figure does not reflect the natural history of optimally treated ependymomas and does not correlate with clinical experience. The incidence of clinically symptomatic seeding is less than 5% (Table 4). It appears greatest for high-grade infratentorial ependymomas (Table 5).

The role of surgery in the treatment of intracranial ependymomas is to establish the diagnosis and remove as much tumor as possible without producing significant morbidity and mortality. Complete surgical resection cannot be achieved in the majority of cases especially when the tumor extends out of the fourth ventricle through one or both lateral recesses (146). Five-year survival rates of 20 (27), 25 (31), and 27% (104) have been reported with surgery alone.

Ependymomas are among the most radiosensitive gliomas. The addition of postoperative radiotherapy has been responsible for increased survival rates (10, 31,126) (Table 6). Supratentorial ependymomas are treated with whole-brain radiotherapy to 4500 rads followed by a 1000 rads boost to the primary. High-grade infratentorial ependymomas receive craniospinal irradiation using a technique similar to that described for medulloblastoma. Low-grade infratentorial ependymomas

Table 4. Intracranial Ependymomas: Clinical Incidence of Spinal Seeding

	Cases	Cases with Symptomatic Seeding
Tarlov and Davidoff (134)	8	3
Svien et al. (133)	126	0
Dricheff et al. (66)	70	1
Phillips et al. (94)	42	2
Marsa et al. (77)	6	0
Bouchard and Pierce (17)	12	0
Barone and Elvidge (10)	47	0
Bloom and Freeman (15)	31	5
Salazar et al. (112)	28	1
Shuman et al. (126)	60	3
Shuman et al. (126)	32	7
Total	462	22 (4.8%)

Table 5. Ependymoma: Symptomatic Spinal Subarachnoid Seeding by Tumor Site and Grade

<table>
<tr><th></th><th colspan="2">Supratentorial</th><th colspan="2">Infratentorial</th></tr>
<tr><th></th><th>High Grade</th><th>Low Grade</th><th>High Grade</th><th>Low Grade</th></tr>
<tr><td>Bloom and Walsh (15)</td><td colspan="2">0/11</td><td>4/7</td><td>1/13</td></tr>
<tr><td>Svien et al. (133)</td><td>0/12</td><td>0/9</td><td>0/12</td><td>0/21</td></tr>
<tr><td>Sheline (122)</td><td>0/3</td><td>0/2</td><td>0/2</td><td>0/7</td></tr>
<tr><td>Kim and Fayos (57)</td><td>1/8</td><td>0/3</td><td>5/13</td><td>1/8</td></tr>
<tr><td>Salazar et al. (112)</td><td colspan="2">0/11</td><td colspan="2">0/17</td></tr>
</table>

Table 6. Intracranial Ependymoma

	5-Year Survival		
	Low Grade (%)		High Grade (%)
Sheline (122)	78		20
Onoyama (88)		44	
Bouchard (17)		58	
Bloom (15)	83	39	14
Salazar (112)*	63	33	13
Kricheff (66)*		41	
Phillips (94)*		56	
Shuman (126)	18		
Barone (10)	34	33	30
Kim and Fayos (57)*	68		21
Dohrmann (31)	21		15

*Adults and children.

are treated with whole-brain fields that encompass the first five cervical vertebrae to 4500 rads with an additional 1000 rads boost to the primary tumor. The cervical spine extension of the field allows for the frequent projection of the infratentorial lesions beyond the cisterna magna. Any ependymoma with a positive CSF cytology for malignant cells or with gross spinal subarachnoid implants should receive craniospinal irradiation.

Overall 5-year survival rates of 33-58% have been reported with addition of postoperative radiotherapy (Table 6). Prognostic factors include tumor location and local extent, age, histologic grade, and radiation dose to the primary. Certain authors have found improved survival associated with an infratentorial location while others have noted just the reverse (Table 7). Gross invasion of the brain stem or cerebellum is associated with a 7.6% 3-year survival (66). Extension to the cervical subarachnoid space adversely affects survival (Table 8). Younger patients tend to do worse (53,66,126). High-grade ependymomas have a worse prognosis (Table 6). Patients who receive less than 4500 rads to the primary site have a decreased survival rate (Table 9).

Table 7. Intracranial Ependymoma

	5-Year Survival	
	Supratentorial (%)	Infratentorial (%)
Kricheff (66)*	33	45
Phillips (94)*	31	47
Bloom (15)	20	46
Dohrmann (31)	21	10
Jenkin (53)	42	28

*Adults and children.

Table 8. Infratentorial Ependymomas: Local Extension

	5-Year Survival	
	(-) Cervical Subarachnoid	(+) Cervical Subarachnoid
Kricheff (66)	90%	33%
Jenkin (53)	43%	23%

Table 9. Survival Intracranial Ependymoma: Radiation Dose to Primary

	Survival	
	4500 rads	4500 rads
Salazar (112)	10 %	56 %
Kim and Fayos (57)	20 %	46 %
Phillips (94)	10 %	87 %
Jenkin (53)	8 %	43 %
Shuman (126)	0 %	47 %

The majority of treatment failures are due to local recurrence. In an attempt to increase survival and decrease the incidence of local recurrence, adjuvant chemotherapy has been instituted in various protocol studies for high-grade lesions. The period of observation remains too short for definite conclusions. CCNU and BCNU have produced beneficial responses in recurrent disease (120).

Pinealoma

Pinealomas are rare tumors and comprise only 2% of intracranial lesions in children. They occur primarily in older children, adolescents, and young adults. Young males are predominantly effected. The peak incidence occurs in the second decade. Pinealomas can be divided into two groups based on location: those occurring in the midline in the region of the pineal gland and those occurring in the suprasellar region (ectopic pinealoma, atypical teratoma). Pineal tumors include tumors of germ cell origin (germinoma, teratoma, choriocarcinoma, embryonal carcinoma), tumors of pineal parenchymal cell origin (pineocytoma, pineoblastoma), and a miscellaneous group (astrocytomas, ependymomas, ganglioneuroma, and ganglioglioma). Germinomas constitute greater than 50% of tumors in the pineal region and ectopic pinealomas (106).

Signs and symptoms of midline pineal tumors include headache, nausea, vomiting, diplopia, somnolence, ataxia, loss of upward gaze (Parinaud's syndrome), abnormal pupillary reflexes, diabetes insipidus, delayed gonadal function, or sexual precocity. Suprasellar germinomas are characterized by a triad of diabetes insipidus, bitemporal hemianopsia, and hypopituitarism.

The diagnosis of midline pineal tumors is usually based on clinical findings and the roentgenographic appearance of a tumor mass in the area of the pineal gland indenting the posterior third ventricle with bilateral obstructive hydrocephalus. Because of the high operative morbidity and mortality associated with a direct surgical approach to tumors of the pineal, patients are often referred for radiotherapy without histological verification. The primary role of surgery in midline pineal tumors is the placement of a shunt for decompression and biopsy of the tumor mass if feasible. Radical extirpation is rarely indicated (89,131) or possible.

Suprasellar germinomas present as a noncalcified suprasellar mass. This location lends itself more readily to a surgical approach. Exploratory craniotomy is indicated for biopsy, decompression of the optic chiasm, and subtotal removal (131). Total tumor removal is rarely achieved.

Pineal tumors may extend locally into adjacent structures, seed the cerebrospinal fluid pathways, or disseminate rarely via the bloodstream. The overall incidence of spinal cord seeding is less than 10% (Table 10). Germinomas and pineoblastomas tend to metastasize to the spinal subarachnoid space more often than

Table 10. Incidence of Spinal Seeding in Cases of Intracranial Pinealoma

	Cases	Cases with Seeding
Wara et al. (143)	19	0
Mincer et al. (84)	12	1
Maier and Dejong (75)	10	0
AFIP (106)	100	8
Rubin and Kramer (109)	36	3
Bradfield and Perez (18)	16	4
Cummins et al. (26)	32	2
Dayan et al. (28)	114	11
Sugn et al. (131)	72	9
Onoyama et al. (89)	58	4
Smith et al. (128)	14	1
Salazar et al. (116)	22	2
Total	505	45 (8.9%)

other tumors in this region. Sung et al. (131) found that 6 of 14 (43%) of histologically verified germinomas produced spinal subarachnoid seeding. The majority of ectopic pinealomas are dysgerminomas and this accounts for the increased incidence of spinal seeding seen with tumors in the suprasellar region. Sung et al. (131) found that 9% of midline pineal tumors produced spinal seeding compared to 27% of ectopic pinealomas.

Conservative surgery followed by radiotherapy is the treatment of choice for tumors of the pineal region (131). Dysgerminomas of the pineal and suprasellar region have a radiosensitivity similar to seminomas. Whole-brain irradiation is given to 4500 rads/4.5-5 weeks followed by an additional 1000 rads boost/1-1.5 weeks to the primary. Most authors recommend irradiation initially to the entire ventricular system and not whole brain (18, 89, 109, 131). Doses below 5000 rad to the primary have been associated with decreased survival rates (Table 11). Sung et al. (131) found a 47% incidence of intracranial relapse with doses less than 4500 rads compared to 10% with 5000-5500 rads to the primary. Craniospinal irradiation is recommended for all biopsy-confirmed germinomas and pineoblastomas, extensive tumors, and those with a positive CSF cytology for malignant cells. A technique similar to that for medulloblastoma is employed.

Overall 5-year-survival rates of 44-73% have been achieved with radiotherapy in the treatment of pinealomas (Table 12). Patients with ectopic pinealomas tend to have a higher survival rate than those with midline pineal tumors (Table 13). This observation is probably due to a more varied nature of tumors (gliomas, teratomas, etc.) occurring in the midline location. Onoyama et al. (89) noted that 85%

Table 11. Survival of Pinealoma Related to Radiation Dose

	Dose to Primary	
	5000 rads	5000 rads
Salazar et al. (116)	50%	65%
Bradfield and Perez (18)	57%	75%
Onoyama et al. (89)	47%	90%

Table 12. Five-Year Survival Pinealomas and Suprasellar Germinomas Treated by Radiation

	%	No. of Patients
Mincer et al. (84)	73	(8/11)
Bradfield and Perez (18)	44	(4/9)
Cummins et al. (26)	61	(20/33)
Wara et al. (143)	69	(9/13)
Onoyama et al. (89)	61	(58)
Salazar et al. (116)	63	(22)

Table 13. Five-Year Survival Pinealoma and Suprasellar Germinoma

	Suprasellar Germinoma		Midline Pineal Tumor	
	%	No. of Patients	%	No. of Patients
Onoyama et al. (89)	82	(17)	55	(41)
Mincer et al. (84)	100	(2/2)	67	(6/9)
Sung et al. (131)	77	(16)	79	(61)
Maier and Dejong (75)			62	(5/8)
Bradfield and Perez (18)	50	(1/2)	38	(3/8)
Rubin and Kramer (109)	50	(2/4)		
Cummins et al. (26)	100	(2/2)	46	(6/13)
Smith et al. (128)			50	(7/14)
Salazar et al. (116)	33	(1/3)	54	(7/13)

of the patients with histologically verified dysgerminomas survived 5 years whereas none of the patients with gliomas or teratomas survived this period. The majority of treatment failures are due to recurrent or persistent tumors (89,131).

Cerebral Astrocytomas

Approximately 15% of childhood astrocytomas are located in the cerebral hemispheres. The most common location is the frontal lobe. The majority of these tumors are low grade although glioblastomas are not uncommon. Signs and symptoms include nausea and vomiting, headaches, papilledema, seizures, lethargy, behavioral and personality changes, and hemiparesis.

Treatment policies are similar to those for adult supratentorial astrocytomas. The surgical objective is the removal of as much tumor as possible allowing for preservation of neurological function. Total gross removal is rarely accomplished due to the diffusely infiltrative nature of the tumors. The addition of postoperative radiotherapy for incompletely resected tumors has resulted in improved survival rates. Leibel et al. (70) noted a 50% 5-year survival for incompletely excised childhood astrocytomas compared to 80% for those receiving postoperative radiotherapy. In general, the whole brain is treated to 4500 rads/5 weeks (180/day) followed by a 1000-1500 rads boost to the primary in 1.5-2 weeks.

Prognosis is related to sex, histological grade, and the degree of surgical resection. Five-year survival rates for various series are listed in Table 14. Males tend to do better than females (53). Increasing histological grade is associated with decreasing survival. In a series of 52 childhood cerebral astrocytomas, Jenkin (53) found that in those who underwent complete resection recurrence at the primary site was the major cause of treatment failure.

Cerebellar Astrocytoma

The cerebellar astrocytoma is the most common childhood brain tumor (15,45, 80,106). The peak incidence occurs during the first decade of life. The majority of the tumors are slow growing, well-circumscribed, cystic low-grade astrocytomas. They preferentially involve the cerebellar hemispheres producing signs and symptoms of headache, nausea, vomiting, papilledema, and ataxia. In cystic lesions, the actual tumor is often localized to a small area of the cyst wall making

Table 14. Cerebral Hemisphere Astrocytomas: 5-Year Survival for Surgery and Radiation

	5 Year	
	%	No. of Patients
Marsa et al. (76)	33	(2/6)
Onoyama et al. (88)	49	(26)
Sheline (122)	50	(6/12)
Bamford et al. (9)	13	(4/31)
Jenkin (53)	37	(52)
Bloom (15)	33	(39)

total gross surgical resection feasible. Approximately 40% of these tumors are entirely solid and are characterized by diffuse infiltration. Complete resection in this instance is often not possible.

The primary mode of treatment is surgical removal. For those completely resected, 5-year survivals greater than 90% have been reported (115). For those incompletely resected, the addition of postoperative radiotherapy has resulted in 5-year survival rates of 50-80% (Table 15). The posterior fossa is treated to a tumor dose of 5500 rads/6 weeks at the rate of 180 rads/fraction. Craniospinal irradiation should be considered in high-grade (grade III and IV) astrocytomas arising in the posterior fossa (115).

Brain Stem Glioma

Brain stem gliomas account for approximately 15% of all brain tumors in children. The peak incidence occurs at 4-8 years of age and 80% occur in individuals less than 20 years of age. The brain stem includes the medulla and pons which are infratentorial in location and the midbrain which is supratentorial. Brain stem tumors are often divided into two groups: those occurring in the medulla and pons and those occurring in the midbrain-thalamic region.

At the time of autopsy or biopsy 95% of brain stem tumors are gliomas (115). Almost 50% are high-grade astrocytomas. These observations justify the treatment of unbiopsied brain stem lesions as presumptive gliomas.

Table 15. Cerebellar Astrocytoma: 5-Year Survival for Surgery and Postoperative Radiation

	5-Year Survival (%)
Marsa et al. (76)	66
Onoyama et al. (88)	50
Sheline (122)	80
Bamford et al. (9)	62
Bloom (15)	50

The diagnosis of brain stem tumors is frequently based on clinical and neuroradiological findings. Intrinsic tumors of the brain stem are not resectable and biopsy is hazardous (146). Histological confirmation is not feasible in most cases. Characteristic signs and symptoms include multiple cranial nerve palsies, ataxia, and hemiparesis without evidence of raised intracranial pressure. Posterior displacement of the fourth ventricle is found on the pneumoencephalogram. Approximately 20% of these tumors are cystic and this finding is best demonstrated by computerized tomography.

The role of surgery in the treatment of brain stem tumors is primarily that of shunt placement for relief of raised intraventricular pressure. Indications for surgical exploration include: (1) enlargement of the brain stem out of proportion to the neurological deficit which suggests the presence of a cyst that can be surgically drained; (2) a mass that occupies or distorts the fourth ventricle; (3) an extraaxial mass occupying the cerebellopontine angle cistern; (4) herniation of the cerebellar tonsils; (5) atypical clinical and neuroradiological findings that raise the doubt of a primary intrinsic brain stem tumor (146).

Radiotherapy is the primary mode of treatment for brain stem gliomas and has been responsible for increased survival rates (Table 16). Treatment is initiated often without a histological diagnosis. Controversy exists as to whether treatment should be directed to the primary plus a margin or the whole brain initially followed by a boost to the primary. Autopsy studies have shown that less than 10% of brain stem tumors are confined to the primary site at the time of death (115). The majority of tumors extend to adjacent structures infratentorially and/or supratentorially. Approximately 40-50% of brain stem tumors, biopsied pretreatment or at autopsy, are glioblastomas (69,111,115). Based on these observations some authors (69,115,138) recommend initial large fields followed by a cone down to the primary. Others (38,111,125) maintain that comparable survival rates are achieved with local fields. In general, fields that encompass the primary plus an adequate margin are used. The superior border should include the midbrain and posterior third ventricle. The inferior border should include the upper cervical cord. Tumor doses greater than or equal to 5000 rads have produced improved survival rates (Table 17). Fifty-five hundred rads is delivered to the primary in 6 weeks at the rate of 180 rads/fraction, five fractions/week. Seventy (38,111,125) to ninety percent of patients receiving radiotherapy will experience significant symptomatic improvement.

Table 16. Survival Brain Stem Gliomas Related to Treatment with Radiotherapy

	5-Year Survival (%)	
	No Radiation	Radiation
Panitch et al. (90)	0	30
Redmond (101)	0	13

Table 17. Brain Stem and Midbrain Tumors: Survival Related to Radiation Dose

	3000-4999 rad (%)	5000 rad (%)
Lee (69)	17	45
Salazar (115)	15	55

Prognosis is related to tumor grade, location, and response to radiotherapy. Glioblastomas of the brain stem are uniformly fatal. Variations in reported 5-year survival rates result from the varying proportions of high-grade lesions. Tumors in the midbrain-thalamic area have a better 5-year survival than those of the brain stem (Tables 18 and 19). Patients who respond to radiotherapy have an increased survival (Table 20). Children appear to do worse than adults (144).

Table 18. Brain Stem Gliomas Treated with Radiation

	5-Year Survival	
	(%)	No. of Patients
Marsa et al. (76)	20	(2/14)
Onoyama et al. (88)	13	(4/32)
Sheline (122)	41	(10/24)
Bouchard (16)	25	(5/20)
Urtasun (138)	16	(2/12)
Lee (69)	14	(2/14)
Whyte et al. (144)	38	(23/61)
Lassman et al. (68)	0	(0/15)
Greenberger et al. (38)	28	(26)
Ryoo et al. (111)	30	(6/20)
Salazar (115)	23	(3/13)
Bloom (15)	17	(5/29)

Table 19. Midbrain, Thalamic Gliomas Treated with Radiotherapy

	5-Year Survival	
	(%)	No. of Patients
Marsa et al. (76)	72	(9)
Onoyama et al. (88)	32	(15)
Sheline (122)	63	(5/8)
Bouchard (16)	57	(8/14)
Lee (68)	42	(5/12)
Greenberger et al. (38)	57	(14)
Ryoo et al. (111)	40	(8/20)

Table 20. Survival Brain Stem Gliomas Related to Response to Radiation

	Average Survival Month	
	No Response	Response
Panitch et al. (90)	5.6	60.8
Bray et al. (19)	4.8	11.2

Optic Nerve Gliomas

Optic nerve gliomas comprise 1-5% of all intracranial tumors in children. Seventy-five percent occur during the first decade of life (137). Histologically, the majority of these tumors are benign pilocytic astrocytomas. Approximately one-third of patients will have von Recklinghausen neurofibromatosis. For prognostic and therapeutic considerations, gliomas confined to the optic nerve should be distinguished from those involving the chiasm and/or hypothalamus.

Signs and symptoms of intraborbital lesions include exophthalmos, decreased visual acuity, central scotoma, and papilledema. Optic nerve gliomas which arise or extend intracranially may produce decreased vision, visual field defects, and increased intracranial pressure. Posterior extension to the hypothalamus may result in diabetes insipidus, obesity, lethargy, and sexual precocity.

Considerable controversy exists regarding the natural history and optimum treatment of optic nerve gliomas. The tumors are characterized by a slow but often unpredictable growth pattern. Long-term survival following incomplete excision or observation only has been reported with stabilization or improvement of signs and symptoms (49,50,95). As a result, certain authors (37,49,148) recommend conservative management after initial diagnosis. Others have recognized the potentially aggressive nature of these tumors especially with chiasmatic or hypothalamic involvement and have advocated surgical resection (48,73,74) when feasible and/or radiotherapy (22,42,73,74,85,135,136). In general total surgical resection is accomplished only with lesions confined to the optic nerve. For those extending intracranially, surgery is limited to transcranial exploration and inspection of the tumor, biopsy for histological confirmation, and the insertion of shunt for hydrocephalus.

Indications for radiotherapy in the management of optic nerve gliomas include patients with progressive visual loss, tumor involvement of the chiasm and/or hypothalamus, and presence of hydrocephalus. Stabilization or improvement of vision, decrease in proptosis, and reduction in radiological and gross tumor mass as well as long-term survival have been reported in patients treated with radiotherapy for optic nerve gliomas (22,42,85,135,136). In general the primary tumor plus an adequate margin is treated. Parallel opposed fields, a three-field technique (two lateral fields and a vertex field), or a rotational technique may be used depending upon the extent of tumor. A tumor dose of 5500 rads is delivered in 6 weeks at a rate of 180 rads/day. In children under the age of 2 years the dose should not exceed 4500 rads/6 weeks.

Table 21. Optic Nerve Glioma: Results with Radiotherapy

	5-Year Survival	
	%	No. of Patients
Marsa et al. (76)	66	(2/3)
Taveras et al. (135)	79	(15/19)
Chang and Wood (22)	73	(88)
Throuvalas et al. (136)	80	(15)
Montgomery et al. (85)	75	(16)
Lloyd (73)	83	(23)

For patients with lesions confined to the optic nerve who undergo surgical resection, the 5-year survival approaches 100% (49,73,148). Table 21 lists the 5-year survival rates reported by various authors for patients with intracranial lesions receiving radiotherapy. These range from 66-83%.

Prognostic factors include tumor extent, the presence or absence of hydrocephalus, and histological grade. Lesions with posterior extension to the hypothalamus or third ventricle tend to exhibit a more aggressive course (22,49). Hydrocephalus is associated with a grave prognosis (49). High-grade lesions are rare in children, but as in adults, have a decreased survival.

SECTION II. BRAIN TUMORS IN ADULTS

John T. Fazekas, M.D.

Although primary brain tumors are relatively rare (11,600 new cases in USA, 1979) (3) in comparison to malignancies occurring within other parenchymal organs, their overall impact is devastating. Overall, only 18% of its victims will survive therapy and the prognosis for the worst histological type of malignant brain tumor, glioblastoma multiforme, is a discouraging 1-4% at 5 years. Yet, these tumors represent a spectrum of disease with prognosis ranging from the benign, radiosensitive, and curable pinealoma (80% survival free of disease) to the highly malignant and radioresistant astrocytoma, grade IV (0-1% survival).

One unique property of all tumors occurring within the cranial cavity is their ability to prove lethal to the patient regardless of the benign appearance under microscopic scrutiny. Even histologically malignant brain tumors rarely metastasize. Death is virtually always related to the phenomenon of locally persistent or recurrent disease. Long periods of physical disability may precede the terminal events, although many patients return to fully productive lives. More importantly, the overall prospects for effective treatment have improved significantly with the advent of new microsurgical techniques, the addition of chemotherapy, and the synthesis of effective sensitizer drugs.

CLINICAL PRESENTATIONS

When should a primary brain tumor be considered as a likely clinical diagnosis? The specific neurological clue(s) are primarily functions of the exact tumor localization (within the dominant or nondominant hemisphere) and whether intracranial pressure has become elevated. The specific tumor histopathology frequently determines the degree of peritumor edema, often accounting for the majority of the clinical complaints and symptoms. The presence of one or more of these five clinical signs/symptoms may herald an underlying cerebral tumor:

1. Headache, although not particularly suspicious when it is the sole clinical symptom, may accompany other nonspecific signs or findings.

2. Personality changes, most prominent with tumor infiltration and/or edema involving the anterior frontal region (a favorite site for glioblastoma), may be subtle and insidious.

3. Frequently memory loss will not be noted or admitted by the patient. Close relatives will usually be more reliable sources for history in these recall skills.

4. Confusion, also a nonspecific finding, frequently accompanies an increase in CSF pressure, and may be associated with deterioration of other higher cognitive functions, such as the ability to abstract.

5. Nausea and/or vomiting, the direct result of elevated intracranial pressure, usually secondary to blockade of CSF flow or peritumor edema, may result in moderate weight loss incorrectly attributed to medical causes.

Specific findings often accompany one or more of these five nonspecific complaints. Although patients may ignore a subtle change in personality, they will rarely minimize the significance of a grand mal seizure, tolerate the presence of diplopia, or ignore a progressive muscle weakness.

IS BIOPSY ALWAYS NECESSARY?

The majority of patients will be referred to the radiation oncologist after a tissue diagnosis has been obtained. Yet, the radiation oncologist may be consulted prior to biopsy, perhaps during the early "suspect brain tumor" stage of evaluation. Primary brain tumor-suspect patients are frequently found to have metastatic cancer. The occult primary (usually breast or lung carcinoma) will be discovered prior to craniotomy only if an appropriate search is undertaken. Remember that metastatic cancer to brain is more common than primary brain tumors. Solitary metastatic lesions may mimic glioblastoma multiforme on CT imaging.

Surgical removal of accessible primary brain tumors continues to be the mainstay of accepted management. However, computerized tomography (CT) equipment and techniques have advanced sufficiently to allow prediction of the location, size, and histology of almost all brain tumors with a 90% accuracy (39). The angiogram, isotopic brain scan, and pneumoencephalogram have been rendered nearly extinct by the rapid proliferation of CT units. The radiation oncologist can now, with greater confidence, administer therapy without a tissue diagnosis when the primary tumor is located deep within the dominant hemisphere (e.g., the hypothalamus or motor strip), near or within the corpus callosum, or within the brain stem itself. Even a small biopsy performed within these critical areas can frequently result in severe and permanent disability. Conversely, the value of complete tumor resection, when clinically and surgically feasible, cannot be overstressed. Total or gross removal of astrocytomas, regardless of histopathological grade, improves prognosis and prolongs survival. Radiation therapy cannot compensate for the lack of tumor excision. The single exception to this basic premise may be glioblastoma multiforme, in which Marshall and Langfitt (78) have shown that median survival with biopsy plus generous steroids (5.5 months) is identical to that obtained with radical tumor excision (6 months).

COMPUTERIZED TOMOGRAPH IN ADULT BRAIN TUMORS

The value of the CT scanner in diagnosis, upon radiotherapy treatment planning, and in following results (regression-recurrence) cannot be overstressed. Pay et al. (93), Ambrose and colleagues (2), Norman et al. (87), and Steinhoff et al. (130) have reported the specific CT findings as a function of histological type in over 500 cases. Essentially all grade III-IV astrocytomas enhance with intravenously administered contrast, while virtually no grade I astrocytomas display that phenomenon. Surprisingly, most grade II astrocytomas do enhance (16 of 18). Only 4 oligodendrogliomas enhanced among Steinhoff's series of 14 cases. Perifocal edema also correlates well with histological type, exhibiting a progressive increase in frequency from 11% in grade I astrocytomas to 74% in grade II and 88% in glioblastoma multiforme (III-IV). Only half of the oligodendrogliomas exhibited peritumor edema. McCollough et al. (82) correlated estimates of tumor size on CT with actual autopsy size in two cases, reporting generally good agreement (in one instance 417 cm^3 on CT compared to 437 cm^3 on autopsy).

Kretzschmar et al. (65) demonstrated that the CT is also valuable in follow-up assessment of radiotherapy results. In his series of 73 patients, 35 showed definite improvement with 24 of these 35 having no clinical signs of persistent tumor. Twenty-two showed no tumor effect, and CT evidence of tumor growth was demonstrated in another 16. Although persistent defects do not necessarily equate to residual tumor, the CT is of great value in assessing the effect of irradiation.

ROLE OF STEROIDS

Although the classic work by Rubin (109) showed no enhancement of normal CNS edema by the therapeutic administration of radiation, peritumor edema frequently accounts for a major portion of the clinical symptoms accompanying brain tumors. Steroids usually dexamethasone (Decadron) is chosen for its maximum antiedema properties and minimal systemic side effects exert their effects upon peritumor edema by these three mechanisms (40):

1. Inhibition of growth among human glioblastoma cells

2. Reversal of the blood flow impairment present surrounding brain tumors

3. Decrease of sodium and water content within peritumor brain tissues, while exerting no effect upon more distant normal brain

The amount of dexamethasone required to eliminate or minimize the edema surrounding primary brain tumors displays a dose-effect relationship up to 96 mg/day in divided doses (40). Whether dexamethasone should be routinely given prior to radiotherapy remains a matter of debate, although the authors advised its administration routinely during the first week of radiotherapy in dosages of 16-32 mg/day to prevent increased brain edema.

TOLERANCE OF BRAIN TO RADIATIONS

In deciding the optimal (i.e., maximum benefit/risk ratio) dose of radiation to administer in each clinical situation, the tolerance of normal brain structures must always be kept in mind. Microscopic radiation damage in a critical area (e.g., brainstem or precentral gyrus or temporal lobe) may be manifested by major neurological deficits, while macroscopic necrosis of the anterior frontal lobe may be relatively asymptomatic. Frequently, the radiation oncologist must set upon a time-dosage based not upon known tumoricidal dosage but instead upon the potential consequences inherent in a radiation-induced necrosis of normal brain. Early clinical reports of "safe" CNS dosage by Lindgren (72), Rider (103), Lampert and Davis (67), and Kramer and colleagues (61, 63) have formed the guidelines for whole-brain radiotherapy which remain clinically valid. Arnold et al. (6) established similar standards for brain stem radiotherapy reporting damage at a dose as low as 4500 rads/30 days. Two syndromes of radiation effect (damage) upon normal brain have been described. Specifically these consist of an early response primarily upon myelin observed at 3 months or beyond, which can mimic multiple sclerosis and included formation of MS-like plaques and a late effect, seen at 1 year or beyond, characterized by white matter degeneration and vascular damage.

Not until the fractionated radiotherapy studies upon intact monkey brains by Nakagaki et al. (86), Caveness (20), and others did the specific pathology become clear within time-dose parameters used in human radiotherapy. These authors discovered that 4000 rads (20 fractions/4 weeks) produced no demonstrable histopathological lesions at 6 months or at 1 year. A fractionated dose of 8000 rads/8 weeks (1000 rads/5 fractions/week), however, resulted in profound histopathological damage at 6 months. These changes consist of micronecrotic (less than 1 mm each) foci within white matter accompanied by brain swelling resultant from breaks in the blood-brain barrier. Similar results were noted following a fractionated dose of 6000 rads/6 weeks after a latent period of 12 months. Telangectasia is characteristic of the late effect (1 year), consistent with the pathology underlying virtually all delayed radiation complications. These observations should not be interpreted to mean 6000 rads/6 weeks is ultimately as damaging as 8000 rads/8 weeks, or that either dosage is safe for clinical radiation therapy. Yet, these histopathological studies upon monkey brains may be predictive in that 6000 rads to the entire human brain is not without sequelae. Dexamethasone, even in large doses, does not seem to alter or reverse the radiation-induced damage, at least under experimental conditions (79), however, the steroid may reduce edema and indirectly the severity of symptoms (149).

COMMON TYPES OF BRAIN TUMORS

Low Grade (Benign) Astrocytomas

This class of brain tumor may be described by various morphological or descriptive terms of little prognostic significance apart from categorizing into the low-grade (I-II) group. The value of radiation therapy following surgical excision (complete or incomplete tumor removal) has been reviewed by Sheline (123). Although eight series generally show improved survival at 3 or 5 years when radiotherapy was administered following craniotomy, the 5-year survival results (with radiotherapy) vary from a low of 32% (129) to a high of 85% (124). A review of 63 cases by Fazekas (33) revealed a direct correlation between postoperative radiotherapy and the presence or absence of total gross tumor removal. If tumor excision was complete, as judged by the neurosurgeon at time of craniotomy, postoperative radiotherapy added nothing to survival at 5 years (90%) and 10 years (25%).

Recurrence were frequent beyond 5 years, in contrast to the high-grade gliomas, in which recurrences usually become manifest within the first 18 months. However, when excision has been judged incomplete, the addition of radiotherapy improved survival substantially, increasing from 13% at 5 years without radiotherapy to 41% (5 years) when irradiation was delivered. Survival at 10 years among 23 nonirradiated cases and 22 grossly excised patients was a similar 30 and 25%.

Whether the entire cranial contents need be included in the radiation portal remains controversial; however, the authors recommend that the entire brain be given a dose of about 5000 rads/5-6 weeks (adults) even in histological grade I astrocytic tumors. The rationale for this philosophy is threefold. First, these tumors are frequently poorly defined and may extend beyond their obvious borders, as judged by CT or at direct craniotomy. Second, the gliomas may occasionally occur in a multifocal fashion (117). Finally, an area of high-grade glioma may lie deep to the biopsy excision site from which the tissue diagnosis was obtained. A boost or cone-down field is suggested to a total dose of 6000-6500 rads/5-7 weeks depending upon field size and region of brain included within the high-dose portal.

Meningiomas

Although these intracranial tumors are generally benign, slow growing, and usually resectable, recurrence is a frequent occurrence. Even when the growth is well encapsulated and totally excised, regrowth occurs in over 10% of the cases. Wara et al. (141) and Sheline (125) have reported on their experience at the University of California. The majority of meningiomas occur in the fifth or sixth decade. No recurrences have been observed among a group of 84 patients with complete tumor removal, followed for periods of 20 years and beyond. Without irradiation following subtotal excision, only 12 of 58 patients remained alive and well, with 43 of 58 manifesting recurrence. In contrast, postoperative radiotherapy resulted in only 10 recurrences among a similar group of 34 subtotally resected cases, while 22 of the 34 remain alive and well for long periods (10 of the 22 beyond 10 years).

Doses of 5000-5500 rads/5-6 weeks to the area at risk are recommended. Treatment portal and techniques can confine the radiation within the area of demonstrable tumor including modest margins. Spread beyond the radiographic margins (usually very vascular and well defined on isotopic or CT scans) and seeding of the CSF are not considerations with this tumor type. If adequate postoperative irradiation is given (5000 rads or greater), the recurrence is only 22% as compared to 74% when radiotherapy is not administered. Occasionally, meningiomas are highly vascular and located in close proximity to the carotid artery, making even subtotal resection impossible. The role of definitive irradiation is not well defined but prolongation of the disease-free survival may be expected. Recurrences may become manifest after long intervals, even 10-20 years after initial therapy.

Pineal Region Tumors: Suprasellar Germinomas

Compared to the other tumor types discussed in this section, primary tumors in this region (pineal body and/or third ventricle) are rare, representing about 1.0% of all intracranial lesions. Irradiation is frequently administered without a biopsy, since attempts at surgical resection traditionally carry a high operative motality of 30-50% (7). More recent accounts in the neurosurgical literature report a considerably lower mortality rate of 5% (51). In any case, irradiation based on clinical parameters, CT findings, and neurological exam, without biopsy, seems justified. Only 2 of 52 (5%) of the cases reported by Derek et al. (29) were subsequently proven misdiagnosed.

Seeding, or direct extention of tumor within the ventricular system, is frequent enough to warrant whole-brain irradiation as an integral part of the radiotherapy plan. Salazar et al. (116) reviewed 9 published series and added their own 25 cases, examining routes of spread and causes of failure. They reported a one-third failure within the cranium compared to a modest 7% rate of spinal cord metastasis. Their diagrams document the fact that spinal seeding alone was never the sole cause of failure. The authors emphasize that 50% 10-year (NED) survival is not the best which can be achieved. Therapy to larger brain fields, including the posterior fossa where over 90% of all failures occur, should improve results, as should the routine administration of adequate doses (4500 rads/5-6 weeks + 1000 rads boost in adults). Irradiation to the entire spinal axis is not recommended routinely but should be considered when a malignant cytology is obtained from a millipore examination of the CSF. The reader is referred to the reports of Rubin and Kramer (108) and Maier and DeJong (75), for background and the more recent publications by Wara et al. (143), Mincer et al. (84), and Salazar et al. (116) for a more recent summary of radiotherapy results.

Oligodendrogliomas

These uncommon benign tumors are slow growing, frequently accompanied with a 10-year or greater history of symptoms. Five-year survivals with surgical removal and postoperative radiotherapy ranges from 53-85% (102, 121). Survival without postoperative radiotherapy is considerably lower in the range of 23-37% at 5 years. Although these series, summarized by Sheline (123), are not part of a controlled study, advanced, larger, or incomplete excised primaries tend to be referred for radiotherapy. Thus, the improvement in survival seen when irradiation is added to the surgical regimen cannot be disputed.

The doses required for control of the tumor and the optimal techniques to be applied are not established with certainty. Small-field techniques, to include a margin around gross tumor or "surgical bed," seem most justified without the need for whole-brain irradiation. Doses of 5000-5500 rads are probably required for control, however, precise time-dose response parameters have not been established within any degree of confidence.

Glioblastoma Multiforme

This term has been used to describe high grade (III-IV) malignant gliomas, although the prognosis for grade III tumors is considerably better than that experienced in grade IV (30% 5-year survival and 5% at 3 years, respectively) (113). The more malignant type (grade IV) is most common in the sixth and seventh decades and occurs almost twice as frequently in males. The value of specific radiation techniques and therapy of parameters has recently been analyzed by Salazar et al. (114). Traditional results attained by radiotherapy are summarized in Table 1. Unfortunately, the specific impact of such parameters as field size, tumor dosage, and grade (III vs. IV) are typically ignored in the published series. Concannon et al. (24) and Kramer (60) have shown conclusively that tumor extensions are frequently far distant from the apparent primary site, yet some radiotherapists continue to treat only partial brain fields.

The only prospective randomized trial comparing surgery alone and surgery plus postoperative radiotherapy utilized doses of only 4500 rads/4.5-5 weeks (4). Salazar (113) proved unequivocally that higher doses double median time to symptomatic relapse in grade IV astrocytomas, from 26-50 weeks as dosage increased from 5000-6000 rads to the 6000-8000 range.

Analysis of survival by field size and dosage shows only 1 survivor among 47 patients irradiated to either small fields (less than 200 cm^2) or low doses (less than 5000 rads). An improved survival was also reported by Marsa et al. (77) with whole-brain x-ray therapy compared to local irradiation in both grade III and grade IV tumors. The improvement in 2-year survival utilizing the whole-brain approach was 35% (15-50%) in grade III and 10% (5-15%) in the grade IV histological type.

Whether doses beyond 7000 rads (6000 rads whole brain + 1000 rads boost) adds to survival remains uncertain especially when considering the potential of late radiation necrosis upon normal brain.

The RTOG study # 74-01 of malignant gliomas has demonstrated no statistically valid survival benefit among patients receiving 6000 rads whole brain/6-7 weeks or an identical 6000 rads with a 1000 rad boost (98).

Neutrons have been utilized in an attempt to overcome the effects of tumor hypoxia and its associated radiation resistance; however, the early reports by Parker et al. (91) are far from encouraging. Perhaps pi-mesons and further neutron trials will prove more successful.

Urtasun and colleagues (139) reported a 4.5 month delay in relapse when the sensitizer agent metronidazole was added to modest doses of radiation (3000 rads, three fractions/week/18 days) under controlled conditions. Preliminary results from the RTOG pilot study using the more potent analog, misonidazole, appear mildly encouraging; however, the randomized study has not yet accumulated sufficient data to allow even a preliminary analysis of results.

The distinction between malignant glioma (grade III astrocytoma) and glioblastoma multiforme (grade IV astrocytoma) is frequently not considered important by neurosurgeons and pathologists. Stage and Stein (129), Kramer (64), Salazar et al. (113), and Sheline (124) have shown unequivocally the better survival among grade III tumors when separated from the broad glioblastoma category. Table 2 contrasts these grade III survival results with those reported in Table 1.

Whether total dosage and radiotherapy techniques for malignant gliomas (grade III) should mimic or vary from the glioblastoma (grade IV) histopathological type is unproven. The recommended dose for grade III tumors is that 6000 rads be given to the entire brain and that a local boost of 500-1000 rads be considered. Since the prospects for survival at 5 years are substantial, late radiation-induced changes (necrosis) should be avoided, but not at the expense of inadequate radiation doses. For additional information on tumor cell biology and kinetics the reader is referred to the reviews by Hoshino (47) and Jellinger (52).

CHEMOTHERAPY OF BRAIN TUMORS

Although a number of chemotherapeutic agents have demonstrated antitumor effect against malignant gliomas, only the most promising few will be mentioned. For additional detail, refer to summaries by Levin and Wilson (68), Wilson (147), and Lieberman and Ransohoff (71). The nitrosoureas (BCNU, CCNU) continue under intensive investigation by the Brain Tumor Study Group (BTSG). An early study (# 69-01) compared BCNU alone, radiotherapy alone, or the two in combination. Median survival was identical (35 weeks) among those receiving irradiation with or without the drug; however, BCNU alone was of no value (median survival 19 weeks). A later BTSG study (# 72-01) demonstrated a statistically significant survival benefit using the same drug (BCNU) in a more aggressive dosage regimen compared to the early study (median survivals of 52 weeks and 35 weeks, respectively). The BTSG has now embarked upon further investigation of a water-soluble nitrosourea (chlorozotocin), a methotrexate-like agent (trizinate), cis-platinum, and a combination of BCNU and 5-fluorouracil. Concurrently, another water-soluble nitrosourea, streptozotocin, is being investigated with these three additional regimen agents: hydroxyurea, epipodophylotoxin, and methyl-CCNU-procarbazine in combination.

BCNU and hydroxyurea have also been compared to BCNU alone (all patients also receiving radiation therapy) in a phase III trial reported by Levin et al. (68). Time to tumor progression and not survival, was the end point reported. A 4-month statistically valid increase in this end point was found by adding hydroxyurea to the glioblastoma multiforme treatment regimen. No further benefit was found among the nonglioblastoma cases when hydroxyurea was added to the BCNU-radiotherapy regimen.

The benefits attained from the chemotherapeutic agents currently available consist of an additional few weeks of survival and perhaps an improvement in the quality of that longevity. At worst, chemotherapeutic agents may increase patient costs and produce significant and occasional life-threatening side effects, on the bone marrow and GI systems, to worsen an already debilitated state. Each patient and family should discuss these goals with the oncology team, before embarking upon chemotherapy, to decide if the potential benefits counterbalance known liabilities. Of course, radiation therapy must be approached with exactly the same benefit-risk assessment.

FOLLOW-UP

The patient and family will equate completion of radiotherapy with end result. While serial CT exams are helpful in predicting clinical outcome, criteria for tumor control or progression are best determined by a combination of clinical parameters such as the neurological examination, the need for steroids, the functional status, and radiographic studies. Hoffman et al. (44) reported a relative lack of correlation between these parameters and actual tumor progression in the first 18 weeks following radiotherapy. One-third of the 25 patients with malignant gliomas judged worse at 18 weeks, actually improved their functional status in subsequent follow-up visits. These authors postulated that postirradiation deterioration may be related to transient radiation-produced demyelination.

If recurrence is suspected (low-grade astrocytomas, meningiomas, and oligodendrogliomas may recur even after 5 years), an assessment of retreatment possibilities must be made. Reirradiation to modest doses (3000-5000 rads) may produce temporary improvement, but its usage is far from routine and should be undertaken only if radiation necrosis is accepted as a likely sequelae after 12-18 months. Chemotherapy may improve the quality of life but significant prolongation of survival cannot generally be anticipated. Steroids, in doses of 16-32 mg dexamethasone/day will reduce brain edema sufficiently to allow improvement of neurological deficits and induce a general sense of well-being. Afra et al. (1) have reported upon 14 reoperations among 121 cases of supratentorial astrocytomas (initially low grade) and oligodendrogliomas. Those patients who were reoperated within relatively short periods experienced better results than did those following longer intervals, in spite of the frequent malignant transformation to glioblastoma. Whether reoperation is of similar value among failures of malignant gliomas is unknown, although surgery may be appropriate in highly selective cases with recurrence in noncritical areas.

CONCLUSIONS

The reader is reminded that new chemical agents (chemotherapy and radiation sensitizers) and experimental radiation beams (neutrons, mesons, protons) are under active investigation. The optimal treatment may ultimately include a combination of several modalities and adjuvants, with concomitant or sequential usage of each agent. Even hyperthermia, attempted by Sutton (132) with some reported success, may increase the survival results attained in the malignant gliomas.

REFERENCES

1. Afra, D., Muller, W., Benoist, Gy., Schroder, R.: Supratentorial recurrences of gliomas. Results of reoperations on astrocytomas and oligodendrogliomas. Acta Neurochirurgica 43:217-227, 1978.

2. Ambrose, J., Gooding, M.R., and Richardson, A.E.: An assessment of the accuracy of computerized transverse axial scanning (EMI Scanning) in the diagnosis of intracranial tumor: A review of 366 patients. Brain 98:569-582, 1975.

3. Cancer Facts and Figures, New York, American Cancer Society, 1978.

4. Anderson, A.P.: Postoperative irradiation of glioblastomas. Results in a randomized series. Acta Radiologica Oncology 17:475-484, 1978.

5. Andrew, D.S., Kerr, J.F.: Carcinoma of thyroid following irradiation for medulloblastoma. Clin. Radiol. 16:282-283, 1965.

6. Arnold, A., Baile, P., Harvey, R.A.: Intolerance of the primate brainstem and hypothalamus to conventional and high energy radiations. Neurology 4:575-585, 1954.

7. Aron, B.S.: Twenty years' experience with radiation therapy of medulloblastoma. Am. J. Roentgenol. 105:37-42, 1969.

8. Bailey, P. and Cushing, H.: Medulloblastoma cerebelli, common type of mid-cerebellar glioma of childhood. Arch. Neurol. Psychiat. 14:192-224, 1925.

9. Bamford, F.N., Morris-Jones, P., Pearson, D., Ribeiro, G.G., Shalet, S.M., and Beardwell, C.G.: Residual disabilities in children treated for intracranial space-occupying lesions. Cancer 37:1149-1151, 1976.

10. Barone, B.M. and Elvidge, A.R.: Ependymomas - A clinical survey. J. Neurosurg. 33:428-438, 1970.

11. Bloom, H.J.G.: Combined modality therapy for intracranial tumors. Cancer 35:111-120, 1975.

12. Bloom, H.J.G.: Recent results and research concerning the treatment of intracranial tumors. The Fifth Maurice Lenz Memorial Lecture. Presented at the Symposium on Tumors of the Brain and Eye - Modern Radiotherapy In Multidisciplinary Management. Columbia University, New York, May 24, 1979.

13. Bloom, H.J.G.: Medulloblastoma: Prognosis and prospects. Int. J. Radiat. Oncol. Biol. Phys. 2:1031-1033, 1977.

14. Bloom, H.J.G., Wallace, E.N.K., and Henk, J.M.: The treatment and prognosis of medulloblastoma in children - a study of 82 verified cases. Am. J. Roentgenol. 105:43-62, 1969.

15. Bloom, H.J.G. and Walsh, L.S.: Tumors of the central nervous system. In Cancer in Children - Clinical Management, edited by H.J.G. Bloom, New York, Springer-Verlag, 1975, pp. 93-119.

16. Bouchard, J.: Central nervous system. In Textbook of Radiotherapy, edited by G.H. Fletcher, Philadelphia, Lea and Febiger, 1973, pp. 366-418.

17. Bouchard, J. and Pierce, C.B.: Radiation therapy in the management of neoplasms of the central nervous system, with a special note in regard to children: Twenty years' experience, 1939-1958. Am. J. Roentgenol. 84:610-628, 1960.

18. Bradfield, J.S. and Perez, C.A.: Pineal tumors and ectopic pinealomas. Analysis of treatment and failures. Radiology 103:399-406, 1972.

19. Bray, P.F., Carter, S., and Taveras, J.M.: Brainstem tumors in children. Neurology 8:1-7, 1958.

20. Caveness, W.F.: Pathology of radiation damage to the normal brain of the monkey. Natl. Cancer Inst. Monogr. 64:57-76, 1977.

21. Chang, C.H., Housepian, E.M., and Herbert, C., Jr.: An operative staging system and a megavoltage radiotherapeutic technique for cerebellar medulloblastomas. Radiology 93:1351-1359, 1969.

22. Chang, C.H. and Wood, E.H.: The value of radiation therapy for gliomas of the anterior visual pathway. In Controversy in Ophthalmology, edited by R.J. Brockhurst, S.A Boruchoff, B.T. Hutchinson, and S. Lessell, Philadelphia, Saunders, 1977, pp. 878-886.

23. Chatty, E.M. and Earle, K.M.: Medulloblastomas. A report of 201 cases with emphasis on the relationship of histologic variants to survival. Cancer 28:977-983, 1971.

24. Concannon, P.J., Kramer, S., and Berry, R.: Extent of intracranial gliomata at autopsy and its relationship to techniques used in radiation therapy of brain tumors. Am. J. Roentgenol., Radium Ther. Nucl. Med. 84:99-107, 1960.

25. Cumberlin, R.L., Luk, K.H., Wara, W.M., Sheline, G.E., and Wilson, C.B.: Medulloblastoma - Treatment results and effect on normal tissues. Cancer 43:1014-1020, 1979.

26. Cummins, F.M., Taveras, J.M., and Schlesinger, E.B.: Treatment of gliomas of the third ventricle and pinealomas; with special reference to the value of radiotherapy. Neurology (Minneap.) 10:1031-1036, 1960.

27. Cushing, H.: Intracranial Tumors - Notes upon a Series of 2000 Verified Cases with Surgical Mortality, Percentages Pertaining Thereto, published by Charles C. Thomas, Springfield, Ill., 1932, p. 56.

28. Dayan, A.D., Marshall, A.H.E., Miller, A.A., Pick, F.J., and Rankin, N.E.: Atypical teratomas of the pineal and hypothalamus. J. Pathol. Bacteriol. 92:1-28, 1966.

29. Derek, R., Jenkin, T., Simpson, W.J., and Keen, C.W.: Pineal and suprasellar germinomas. Results of radiation treatment. J. Neurosurg. 48:99-107, 1978.

30. Deutsch, M., Scotti, L., Hardman, D.R., Reigel, D.H., and Scarff, T.B.: Myelography in patients with medulloblastoma. Radiology 117:467-468, 1975.

31. Dohrmann, G.J., Farwell, J.R., and Flannery, J.T.: Ependymomas and ependymoblastomas in children. J. Neurosurg. 45:273-283, 1976.

32. Evans, A.: Multimodal Therapy of Brain Tumor in Children. Presented at the Symposium on Tumors of the Brain and Eye - Modern Radiotherapy in Multidisciplinary Management. Columbia University, New York, May 23, 1979.

33. Fazekas, J.T.: Treatment of grades I and II brain astrocytomas. The role of radiotherapy. Int. J. Radiat. Oncol. Biol. Phys. 2:661-666, 1977.

34. Fienman, N.L. and Yakovac, W.: Neurofibromatosis in childhood. J. Pediatr. 76:339-346, 1970.

35. Fokes, E.C. and Earle, K.M.: Ependymomas: Clinical and pathological aspect. J. Neurosurg. 30:585-594, 1969.

36. Fragoyannis, S. and Yalcin, S.: Ependymomas with distant metastases - Report of 2 cases and review of the literature. Cancer 19:246-256, 1966.

37. Glaser, J.S., Hoyt, W.F., and Corbett, J.: Visual morbidity with chiasmal glioma. Arch. Ophthalmol. 85:3-12, 1971.

38. Greenberger, J.S., Cassady, J.R., and Levene, M.B.: Radiation therapy of thalmic, midbrain and brain stem gliomas. Radiology 122:463-468, 1977.

39. Greitz, T.: Computer tomography for diagnosis of intracranial tumors compared with other neuroradiologic procedures. In Computer Tomography of Brain Lesions, edited by T. Lindgren, Acta Radiol (Suppl. 346):14-20, 1975.

40. Gutin, P.: Corticosteroid therapy in patients with brain tumors. Natl. Cancer Inst. Mono. 46:151-156, 1977.

41. Harisiadis, L. and Chang, C.H.: Medulloblastoma in children: A correlation between staging and results of treatment. Int. J. Radiat. Oncol. Biol. Phys. 2:833-841, 1977.

42. Harter, D.J., Caderao, J.B., Leavens, M.E., and Young, S.E.: Radiotherapy in the management of primary gliomas involving the intracranial optic nerves and chiasm. Int. J. Radiat. Oncol. Biol. Phys. 4:681-686, 1978.

43. Hoff, J.T. and Ray, B.S.: Cerebral hemangioblastoma occurring in a patient with von Hippel-Lindau disease, case report. J. Neurosurg. 28:365-368, 1968.

44. Hoffman, W.F., Levin, V.A., and Wilson, C.B.: Evaluation of malignant gliomas patients during the post-irradiation period. J. Neurosurg. 50:624-628, 1979.

45. Hooper, R.: Intracranial tumors in childhood. Med. J. Aust. 1:624-627, 1976.

46. Hope-Stone, H.F.: Results of treatment of medulloblastoma. J. Neurosurg. 32:83-88, 1970.

47. Hoshino, T.: Therapeutic implications of brain tumor cell kinetics. Natl. Cancer Inst. Mono. 46:29-35, 1977.

48. Housepian, E.M.: Surgical treatment of unilateral optic nerve gliomas. J. Neurosurg. 31:604-607, 1969.

49. Hoyt, W.F. and Baghdassarian, S.A.: Optic glioma of childhood: Natural history and rationale for conservative management. Br. J. Ophthalmol. 53: 793-798, 1969.

50. Hudson, A.C.: Primary tumors of the optic nerve. R. Ophthalmol. Hosp. Rep. 18:317-439, 1912.

51. Jamieson, K.G.: Excision of pineal tumors. J. Neurosurg. 35:550-553, 1971.

52. Jellinger, K.: Glioblastoma multiforme: Morphology and biology. Acta Neurochirurgica 42:5-32, 1978.

53. Jenkin, R.D.T.: Radiotherapy of Astrocytoma and Ependymoma in Children. Presented at the Symposium on Tumors of the Brain and Eye - Modern Radiotherapy in Multidisciplinary Management. Columbia University, New York, May 23, 1979.

54. Jenkin, R.D.T.: Medulloblastoma in childhood: Radiation therapy. Can. Med. Assoc. J. 100:51-53, 1969.

55. Kapp, J.P., Paulson, G.W., and Odom, G.L.: Brain tumors with tuberous sclerosis. J. Neurosurg. 26:191-204, 1967.

56. Kessler, L.A., Dugan, P,, and Concannon, J.P.: Systemic metastases of medulloblastoma promoted by shunting. Surg. Neurol. 3:147-152, 1975.

57. Kim, Y.H. and Fayos, J.V.: Intracranial ependymomas. Radiology 124:805-808, 1977.

58. King, G.A. and Sagerman, R.H.: Late recurrence in medulloblastoma. Am. J. Roentgenol. Radium Ther. Nucl. Med. 123:7-12, 1975.

59. Koos, W.T. and Miller, M.H.: Intracranial Tumors of Infants and Children. St. Louis, C.V. Mosby Company, 1971, pp. 9-27.

60. Kramer, S.: Tumor extent as determining factor in radiotherapy of glioblastomas. Acta Radiol. 8:111-117, 1959.

61. Kramer, S.: The hazards of therapeutic irradiation of the central nervous system. Clin. Neurosurg. 15:301-318, 1968.

62. Kramer, S.: Radiation therapy in the management of brain tumors in children. Ann. NY Acad. Sci. 159:571-584, 1969.

63. Kramer, S. and Lee, K.F.: Complications of radiation therapy: The central nervous system. Semin. Roentgenol. 9:75-83, 1974.

64. Kramer, S.: Radiation therapy in the management of malignant gliomas. In Seventh National Cancer Conference Proceedings, Philadelphia, Lippincott, 1973, pp. 823-826.

65. Kretzscghmar, K., Aulich, A., Schindler, E., Lange, S., Grumme, T., and Meese, W.: The diagnostic value of CT for radiotherapy of cerebral tumors. Neuroradiology 14:245-250, 1978.

66. Kricheff, I.I., Becker, M., Schneck, S.A., and Taveras, J.A.: Intracranial ependymomas: Factors influencing prognosis. J. Neurosurg. 21:7-14, 1964.

67. Lampert, P.W. and Davis, R.L.: Delayed effect of radiation on the human central nervous system. Neurology 14:912-917, 1964.

68. Levin, V.A., Wilson, C.B., Davis, R., Wara, W.M., Pischer, T.L., and Irwin, L.: A phase III comparison of BCNU, hydroxyurea and radiation therapy to BCNU and radiation therapy for treatment of primary malignant gliomas. J. Neurosurg. 51:526-532, 1979.

69. Lee, F.: Radiation of infratentorial and supratentorial brain stem tumors. J. Neurosurg. 43:65-68, 1975.

70. Leibel, S.A., Sheline, G.E., Wara, W.M., Boldrey, E.B., Nielsen, S.L.: Role of radiation therapy in the treatment of astrocytomas. Cancer 35:1551-1557, 1975.

71. Lieberman, A. and Ransohoff, J.: Treatment of primary brain tumors. Med. Clin. N. Am. 63:835-848, 1979.

72. Lindgren, M.: Tolerance of brain tissue to roentgen irradiation. Acta Radiology (Suppl.) 17:46-70, 1958.

73. Lloyd, L.A.: Gliomas of the optic nerve and chiasm in childhood. Trans. Am. Ophthalmol. Soc. 71:488-535, 1973.

74. MacCarty, C.S., Boyd, A.S., and Childs, D.S.: Tumors of the optic nerve and optic chiasm. J. Neurosurg. 33:439-444, 1970.

75. Maier, J.G. and DeJong, D.: Pineal body tumors. Am. J. Roentgenol. Radium Ther. Nucl. Med. 99:826-832, 1967.

76. Marsa, G.W., Probert, J.C., Rubenstein, L.J., and Bagshaw, M.A.: Radiation therapy in the treatment of childhood astrocytic gliomas. Cancer 32: 646-655, 1973.

77. Marsa, G.W., Goffinet, D.R., Rubinstein, L.J., and Bagshaw, M.A.: Megavoltage irradiation in the treatment of gliomas of the brain and spinal cord. Cancer 36:1681-1689, 1975.

78. Marshall, L.F. and Langfitt, T.W.: Needle biopsy, high-dose corticosteroids, and radiotherapy in the treatment of malignant glial tumors. Natl. Cancer Inst. Mono. 46:157-160, 1977.

79. Martins, A.N., Severance, R.E., Henry, J.M., and Doyle, T.F.: Experimental delayed radiation necrosis of the brain. Part 1: Effect of early dexamethason treatment. J. Neurosurg. 51:587-596, 1979.

80. Matson, D.D.: Neurosurgery of Infancy and Childhood, 2nd ed., Springfield, Ill., Charles C. Thomas, 1969, pp. 403-643.

81. Mealey, J., Jr. and Hall, P.V.: Medulloblastoma in children - survival and treatment. J. Neurosurg. 46:56-64, 1977.

82. McCullough, D.C., Huang, H.K., DeMichelle, D., Manz, H.J., and Sinks, L.F.: Correlation between volumeric CT imaging and autopsy measurements of glioblastoma size. Computerized Tomography 3:133-141, 1979.

83. McFarland, D.R., Horwitz, H., Saenger, E.L., and Bahr, G.K.: Medulloblastoma - A review of prognosis and survival. Br. J. Radiol. 42:198-214, 1969.

84. Mincer, F., Meltzer, J., and Boststein, C.: Pinealoma. A report of twelve irradiated cases. Cancer 37:2713-2718, 1976.

85. Montgomery, A.B., Griffin, T., Parker, R.G., and Gerdes, A.J.: Optic nerve glioma: The role of radiation therapy. Cancer 40:2079-2080, 1977.

86. Nakagaki, H., Brynhart, G., Kemper, T.L., and Caveness, W.F.: Monkey brain damage from radiation in the therapeutic range. J. Neurosurg. 44:3-11, 1976.

87. Norman, D., Enzman, D.R., Levin, V.A., Wilson, C.B., and Newton, T.H.: Computed tomography in the evaluation of malignant gliomas before and after therapy. Radiology 121:85-88, 1976.

88. Onoyama, Y., Abe, M., Takahaski, M., Yabumoto, E., and Sakamoto, T.: Radiation therapy of brain tumors in children. Radiology 115:687-693, 1975.

89. Onoyama, Y., Ono, K., Nakajima, T., Hiraoka, M., and Abe, M.: Radiation therapy of pineal tumors. Radiology 130:757-760, 1979.

90. Panitch, H.S. and Berg, B.O.: Brain stem tumors of childhood and adolescence. Am. J. Dis. Child. 119:465-472, 1970.

91. Parker, R.G., Berry, H.C., Gerdes, A.J., Soronen, M.D., and Shaw,

C.M.: Fast neutron beam radiotherapy of glioblastoma multiforme. Am. J. Roentgenol. 127:331-335, 1976.

92. Patterson, E. and Farr, R.F.: Cerebellar medulloblastoma: Treatment of irradiation of whole central nervous system. Acta Radiol. (Ther.) 39:323-336, 1961.

93. Pay, N.T., Carella, R.J., Lin, J.P., and Kricheff, J.J.: The usefulness of computed tomography during and after radiation therapy in patients with brain tumors. Radiology 121:79-83, 1976.

94. Phillips, T.L., Sheline, G.E., and Boldrey, E.: Therapeutic considerations in tumors affecting the central nervous system: Ependymomas. Radiology 83:98-105, 1964.

95. Posner, M. and Horrax, G.: Tumors of the optic nerve. Long survival in three cases of intracranial tumor. Arch. Ophthalmol. 40:56-76, 1948.

96. Probert, J.C., Lederman, M., and Bagshaw, M.A.: Medulloblastoma - Treatment and prognosis. A study of seventeen cases in ten years. Calif. Med. 118:14-17, 1973.

97. Probert, J.C. and Parker, B.R.: Effects of radiation in bone growth. Radiology 144:155-162, 1975.

98. Progress report Malignant Gliomas, RTOG Protocol 74-01, presented at semi-annual RTOG meeting, June 21-23, 1978, Philadelphia, published by American College of Radiology, Philadelphia, 1978.

99. Phase III Study of Medulloblastoma. Radiation Therapy Oncology Group and Children's Cancer Study Group. February 1975.

100. Raventos, A. and Duszynski, D.O.: Thyroid cancer following irradiation for medulloblastoma. Am. J. Roentgenol. 89:175-183, 1963.

101. Redmond, J.S.: The roentgen therapy of pontine gliomas. Am. J. Roentgenol. 86:644-648, 1961.

102. Richmond, J.J.: Malignant tumors of the central nervous system. In Cancer, Vol. 5, edited by R. Raven, London, Butterworth, 1959, pp. 375-389.

103. Rider, W.D.: Radiation damage to the brain - A new syndrome. J. Can. Assoc. Radiol. 14:67-69, 1963.

104. Ringertz, N. and Redmond, A.: Ependymomas and choroid plexus papillomas. J. Neuropathol. Exp. Neurol. 8:355-380, 1949.

105. Rogli, V.L., Estrada, R., and Fechner, R.E.: Thyroid neoplasia following irradiation for medulloblastoma. Cancer 43:2232-2238, 1979.

106. Rubenstein, L.J.: Tumors of the central nervous system. In Atlas of Tumor Pathology, Washington, D.C., Armed Forces Institute of Pathology, 1972; pp. 130-253, medulloblastoma; pp. 104-126, ependymoma; pp. 269-284, pinealoma.

107. Rubin, P., Duthie, R.B., and Young, L.W.: Significance of scoliosis in postirradiated Wilms' tumor and neuroblastoma. Radiology 79:539-559, 1962.

108. Rubin, P. and Kramer, S.: Ectopic pinealoma: A radiocurable neuroendocrinologic entity. Radiology 85:512-523, 1965.

109. Rubin, P.: Extradural spinal cord compression by tumor. Part I: Experimental production and treatment trials. Radiology 93:1243-1248, 1969.

110. Rubin, P., Landman, S., Mayer, S., Keller, B., and Ciccio, S.: Bone marrow regeneration and extension after extended field irradiation in Hodgkin's disease. Cancer 32:699-711, 1973.

111. Ryoo, M.C., King, G.A., Chung, C.T., Yu, W.S., and Sagerman, R.H.: Irradiation of primary brain-stem tumors. Radiology 131:503-507, 1979.

112. Salazar, O.M., Rubin, P., Bassano, D., and Marcial, V.A.: Improved survival of patients with intracranial ependymomas by irradiation: Dose selection and field extension. Cancer 35:1563-1573, 1975.

113. Salazar, O.M., Rubin, P., McDonald, J.V., and Feldstein, M.L.: High dose radiation therapy in the treatment of glioblastoma multiforme: a preliminary report. Int. J. Radiation Oncology Biol. Phys. 1:717-727, 1976.

114. Salazar, O.M., Rubin, P., McDonald, J.V., and Feldstein, M.L.: Patterns of failure in intracranial astrocytomas after irradiation: analysis of dose and field factors. Am. J. Roentgenol. Radium Ther. Nucl. Med. 126:279-291, 1976.

115. Salazar, O.M.: Primary brain tumors of the posterior fossa. In Modern Radiation Oncology - Classic Literature and Current Management, edited by H.A. Gilbert and A.R. Kagan, New York, Harper & Row, 1978, pp. 125-143.

116. Salazar, O.M., Castro-Vita, H., Bakos, R.S., Feldstein, M.L., Keller, B., and Rubin, P.: Radiation therapy for tumors of the pineal region. Int. J. Radiat. Oncol. Biol. Phys. 5:491-499, 1979.

117. Schiefer, W., Hasenbein, B., and Schmidt, H.: Multicentric glioblastomas. Methods of diagnosis and treatment. Acta Neurochirurgica 42:89-95, 1978.

118. Schut, L. and Rosenstock, J.G.: Treatment of intracranial neoplasms in children. Semin. Oncol. 1:9-15, 1974.

119. Shalet, S.M., Beardwell, C.G., Morris-Jones, P., Bamford, F.N., Ribeiro, G.G., and Pearson, D.: Growth hormone deficiency in children with brain tumors. Cancer 37:1144-1148, 1976.

120. Shapiro, W.R.: Chemotherapy of primary malignant brain tumors in children. Cancer 35:965-972, 1975.

121. Sheline, G.E., Boldrey, E., Karlsberg, P., and Phillips, T.L.: Therapeutic considerations in tumors affecting the central nervous system: Oligodendrogliomas. Radiology 82:84-89, 1964.

122. Sheline, G.E.: Radiation therapy of tumors of the central nervous system in childhood. Cancer 35:957-964, 1975.

123. Sheline, G.E.: Radiation therapy of primary tumors. Semin. Oncol. 2:29-42, 1975.

124. Sheline, G.E.: Conventional radiation therapy of gliomas. In Recent Result in Cancer Research, Vol. 51, edited by J. Hekmatpanah, New York, Springer-Verlag, 1975, pp. 125-134.

125. Sheline, G.E.: Radiation therapy of brain tumors. Cancer 39:873-881, 1977.

126. Shuman, R.M., Alvord, E.C., and Leech, R.W.: The biology of childhood ependymomas. Arch. Neurol. 32:731-739, 1975.

127. Smith, C.E., Long, D.M., Jones, T.K., and Levitt, S.H.: Experiences in treating medulloblastomas at the University of Minnesota Hospitals. Radiology 109:179-182, 1973.

128. Smith, N.J., El-Mahdi, A.M., and Constable, W.C.: Results of irradiation of tumors in the region of the pineal body. Acta Radiol. (Ther.) 15:17-22, 1976.

129. Stage, W.S. and Stein, J.J.: Treatment of malignant astrocytomas. Am. J. Roentgenol. Radium Ther. Nucl. Med. 120:7-18, 1974.

130. Steinhoff, H., Grumme, T.H., Kazner, E., Lange, S., Lanksch, W., Meese, W., and Wullenweber, R.: Axial transverse computerized tomography in 73 glioblastomas. Acta Neurochirurgica 42:45-56, 1978.

131. Sung, D., Harisiadis, L., and Chang, C.: Midline pineal tumors and suprasellar germinomas: Highly curable by irradiation. Radiology 128:745-751, 1978.

132. Sutton, C.H.: Use of local hyperthermia in brain tumor therapy. Presented at the 68th annual meeting of the American Association of Cancer Research, 1977.

133. Svien, H.J., Mabon, R.F., Kernohan, J.W., and Craig, W.M.: Ependymoma of the brain: Pathologic aspects. Neurology 3:1-15, 1953.

134. Tarlov, I.M. and Davidoff, L.M.: Subarachnoid and ventricular implants in ependymal and other gliomas. J. Neuropathol. Exp. Neurol. 5:213-224, 1946.

135. Taveras, J.M., Mount, L.A., and Wood, E.H.: The value of radiation therapy in the management of glioma of the optic nerve and chiasm. Radiology 66:518-528, 1956.

136. Throuvalas, N., Bataini, P., and Ennuyer, A.: Les gliomes du chiasma et du nerf optique. L'apport de la radiotherapie transcutanee dans leur traitement. Bull. Cancer (Paris) 56:231-264, 1969.

137. Tym, R.: Piloid gliomas of the anterior optic pathways. Br. J. Surg. 49: 322-331, 1961.

138. Urtasun, R.C.: 60-Co radiation treatment of pontine gliomas. Radiology 104:385-387, 1972.

139. Urtasun, R., Band, P., Chapman, J.D., Feldstein, M.L., Mielke, B., and Fryer, C.: N. Engl. J. Med. 294:1364-1367, 1976.

140. Van Dyk, J., Jenkin, R.D.T., Leung, P.M.K., and Cunningham, J.R.: Medulloblastoma: Treatment technique and radiation dosimetry. Int. J. Radiat. Oncol. Biol. Phys. 2:993-1005, 1977.

141. Wara, W.M., Sheline, G.E., Newman, H., Townsend, J.J., and Boldrey, E.B.: Radiation therapy of meningiomas. Am. J. Roentgenol. Radium Ther. Nucl. Med. 123:453-457, 1975.

142. Wara, W.M., Richards, G.E., Grumbach, M.M., Kaplan, S.L., Sheline, G.E., and Conte, F.A.: Hypopituitarism after irradiation in children. Int. J. Radiat. Oncol. Biol. Phys. 2:549-552, 1977.

143. Wara, W.M., Fellows C.F., Sheline, G.E., Wilson, C.B., Townsen, J.J.: Radiation therapy for pineal tumors and suprasellar germinomas. Radiology 124:221-223, 1977.

144. Whyte, T.R., Colby, M.Y., and Layton, D.D.: Radiation therapy of brain-stem tumors. Radiology 93:413-416, 1969.

145. Wilson, C.B.: Medulloblastoma: Current views regarding the tumor and its treatment. Oncology 24:273-290, 1970.

146. Wilson, C.B.: Diagnosis and surgical treatment of childhood brain tumors. Cancer 35:950-956, 1975.

147. Wilson, C.B.: Current concepts in cancer. Brain tumors. N. Engl. J. Med. 300:1469-1471, 1979.

148. Wong, I.G. and Lubow, M.: Management of optic glioma of childhood - A review of 42 cases. In Neuro-ophthalmology, Symposium of University of Miami and Bascom Palmer Eye Institute, Vol. VI, St. Louis, C.V. Mosby, 1972, pp. 51-60.

149. Yamada, K., Bremer, A.M., and West, C.R.: Effects of dexamethasone on tumor induced brain edema and is distribution in the brain of monkeys. J. Neurosurg. 50:361-367, 1979.

chapter 4

HEAD AND NECK NEOPLASMS

C.C. Wang, M.D.

The head and neck area is considered to be one of the most productive fields of cancer management in terms of cure rates. Many of these cancers can be readily seen, palpated, evaluated, and biopsied with a relatively simple procedure. Because there is seldom a second chance to effect a cure, the choice of initial treatment must be the correct one made after careful consideration of all the clinical features in each individual patient. This clearly requires that surgeons and radiation therapists know the strengths and weaknesses of their disciplines and be thoroughly informed of the limitations of their specialty. It is the complimentary and cooperative efforts of this team wherein lies the welfare of patients with malignant disease.

Most of the malignant tumors originating in the mucous membranes of the aerodigestive tract are squamous cell carcinomas of varying malignant potential, ranging from in situ to poorly differentiated carcinomas. These are the diseases of middle and old age, occurring especially in patients having longstanding habits of cigarette smoking, alcoholism, and poor oral hygiene. Males are more often involved, although the incidence of female patients is rapidly increasing due to change in the life style of American women. Tumors of the salivary gland, lymph nodes, bone, and soft tissue also occur in the head and neck regions. These tumors are less common although they are by no means less important in the practice of modern oncology.

Cancers arising from the head and neck region are described and discussed under their anatomical groupings and cell types. These will be tumors in the oral cavity, oropharynx, hypopharynx, larynx, nasopharynx, paranasal sinuses, and salivary glands among others. In each of these anatomic sites, which are often subdivided into smaller areas, the tumor characteristics may be quite different. Each has its own natural history, different biological behavior, and separate mode of tumor growth and spread. The therapeutic management and results may differ greatly depending upon these factors.

For head and neck tumors, the American Joint Committee (AJC) for Cancer Staging and End Results Reporting developed and published a TNM staging system in 1977 (2). For tumors of the oral cavity and oropharynx, the T stage is determined primarily by the size of the lesion. For tumors of the nasopharynx, hypopharynx, and larynx, the T stage is determined by the involvement of anatomic sites and depth of invasion. Therefore, the stage is reflected in the mobility of the involved structures in laryngeal and hypopharyngeal cancers or invasion of bones or nerves in nasopharyngeal cancer. For cervical node disease, the N stage is uniform throughout in that the size, number, and bilaterality of nodes are the determinant factors. Fixation of an involved node, however, is not taken into consideration. M stage is determined by clinical and radiographic findings. The AJC N and M staging is as follows:

N0: no clinically positive node

N1: single clinically positive homolateral node less than 3 cm in diameter

N2a: single clinically positive homolateral node 3-6 cm in diameter

N2b: multiple clinically positive homolateral nodes; none over 6 cm in diameter

N3a: clinically positive homolateral node(s) one over 6 cm in diameter

N3b: bilateral clinically positive nodes

N3c: contralateral clinically positive node(s) only

M0: no distant metastasis

M1: distant metastasis

A variety of therapeutic measures are available for the management of cancers of the head and neck. These include surgical excision, radiation therapy, cryotherapy, laser excision, chemotherapy, immunotherapy, and others. The choice of treatment modalities is influenced by the cell type and degree of differentiation, site and extent of the primary lesion, metastatic nodal disease, gross characteristics of the tumor, i.e., exophytic, superficial vs. endophytic, invasive, presence of bone and muscle involvement, the likelihood of complete surgical resection, the possibility of preservation of speech and/or swallowing mechanisms, the physical condition, social status and occupation of the patient, and the experience and skill of both the surgeon and radiation therapist.

At the present time, cryotherapy and laser excision are used in experienced hands primarily for superficial, accessible tumors with limited success. Both chemotherapy and immunotherapy are used as an adjuvant procedure and have not found their place in the primary curative management of cancers of the head and neck.

Surgery and radiotherapy are equally effective in eradicating limited cancers in the head and neck region. Each of these modalities has its own merits, indications, and limitations. Radiation therapy has the advantage of being able to control the disease at the site thus avoiding removal of a useful and necessary part as well as preserving speech and/or swallowing functions. Therefore, it must be considered as the best tissue and organ sparing procedure presently available. On the other hand, for certain early lesions situated in less critical locations, surgery can be carried out expediently and effectively without significant functional and cosmetic mutilation and is, therefore, preferred.

In the management of advanced carcinomas, surgical failures are often due to inability to remove microscopic tumor extension at the periphery thus resulting in marginal recurrence. Tumor seeding in the wound and metastases via lymphatic or hematogenous routes are additional means to account for therapeutic failures after surgery. A tumor core greater than 150-180 μg often contains hypoxic cells which are insensitive to radiation therapy. In contrast, tumor cells at the periphery of the tumor mass are well oxygenated and well nourished and therefore are radioresponsive and controllable by radiation. Local failure from radiation therapy therefore is central rather than peripheral. Distant metastases through the lymphatic and hematogenous routes also constitute failures of local irradiation.

Radiobiologically, it is known that an approximately exponential relationship exists between the dose of ionizing radiation administered to a cell population and the surviving fraction of these cells. Experimental studies have demonstrated that relatively low doses will inactivate a vast number of cells in a tumor. This is in keeping with the clinical observation that small microscopic aggregates of tumor cells, which cannot be palpated on physical examination and yet by previous experience are histopathologically detectable, can be controlled with a dose of 4500-5000 rad/5 weeks in better than 90% of cases (17). However, for a larger tumor, higher doses such as 6000-7000 rads/7 weeks are required for inactivation or eradication of the entire cell population to increase the possibility of lasting cure. For such advanced stage tumors, radiation therapy is not only handicapped by excessive tumor cell population but also by the presence of a large number of radioresistant hypoxic cells. In such situations, the radiation dose level must be markedly increased, and sometimes beyond the limits of tolerance of the normal vasculoconnective tissues, thus resulting in radiation necrosis and making a lasting cure of such an advanced tumor highly improbable by radiation therapy.

Based on the presently available radiobiological knowledge and the mechanisms of treatment failures, the major strength of radiation therapy is therefore to eradicate the radiosensitive, actively growing, well-oxygenated, nourished cells in the periphery of the tumor or the subclinical disease implanted in the wound or in the lymph nodes. The strength of surgery on the other hand is to remove the centrally situated, radioresistant hypoxic tumor cells. For extensive tumors, which are rarely curable by either method alone, the logical approach at the present time is the combination of radiation therapy and surgery.

Attention must be paid to many important technical factors in the combined approach. The first of these is the dose and technique of administration of radiation therapy. In expert hands radiation therapy in moderate doses of 4000-5000 rads delivered over a period of 4-5 weeks can be delivered to an organ site without significantly increasing postoperative complications. Thus, the magnitude of the surgery can be based on the original extent of the tumor. In higher radiation dosages, i.e., 6000-6500 rads/7 weeks, which are considered cancerocidal in most epithelial cancers of the head and neck, the magnitude of surgery must be decreased in that only residual disease should be removed, i.e., nidusectomy.

Combined high-dose radical radiation therapy and radical surgical resection invariably invites excessive and at times unacceptable postoperative morbidity and mortality. Timing of the operation is also most important. Our clinical experience indicates that a dose of 4000-4500 rads/4-5 weeks should be followed by an interval of about a month prior to surgery. If an operation is undertaken earlier, it may be made technically more difficult because of edema and friability of tissues and excessive oozing of blood in the operative field. On the other hand, a delay beyond 8-10 weeks after radiation therapy may be accompanied by increasing fibrosis, making the operative procedure technically difficult and increasing postoperative complications. Two conceptual approaches to combined radiation therapy and surgery have emerged, i.e., pre- and postoperative radiation.

The aims of preoperative radiotherapy are to prevent marginal recurrences, to control subclinical disease in the primary site or in the lymph nodes, or to convert technically inoperable tumors into operable ones. This form of combined approach has been found to decrease iatrogenic scar implant, local recurrence, and the incidence of distant metastases.

The disadvantages of preoperative radiation therapy are (1) exact tumor extent is obscured due to shrinkage of the lesion prior to surgery; (2) delaying of surgery thus creating a great deal of anxiety on the part of some surgeons and patients; and (3) increase in postoperative complications. The dosage employed in this form of conventional preoperative radiotherapy program is subcancerocidal consisting of 4500 rads/1 month. This is followed in 1 month by radical surgery according to the original extent of the disease as though radiation therapy had not been given. The program is applicable to medium sized or advanced tumors of the oral cavity, such as oral tongue, floor of mouth, gum, hypopharynx, and larynx and is not associated with significant postoperative morbidity and mortality.

Low-dose, short-course preoperative radiation therapy, i.e., 1000 rads divided into four or five daily fractions followed immediately by radical surgery, has been used in other tumor sites such as bladder and colorectum and found effective in preventing scar implant and has shown decrease in distant metastases. This approach, however, has not been extensively employed in the management of head and neck tumors, but may be considered in certain selected patients.

In the so-called sequential postradiation resection, the dosage is cancerocidal, i.e., 6000-6500 rads/7 weeks delivered homogeneously to the primary site as well as the first-echelon lymph nodes. The treatment portal must be progressively reduced after 5000 rads/5 weeks. Contrary to a conventional subcancerocidal dose program, radiation therapy is followed by limited surgical resection and only the residual nidus of radioresistant hypoxic core of the primary lesion, mostly in the muscles or bone, is excised on the assumption that the radiosensitive peripheral, superficial disease has been controlled by high-dose radiation therapy. This approach is intended to avoid excessive functional and cosmetic mutilation following radical surgery and has been found useful in advanced lesions arising from the tonsillar region with involvement of the adjacent soft palate and base of tongue or gum. In expert hands the results thus far are quite satisfactory with minimally postoperative complications.

The aims of postoperative irradiation are to eradicate residual disease transected at the tumor margins and to control subclinical disease implanted in the wound or in regional lymph nodes. The procedure is usually carried out approximately 3-4 weeks after surgery when the wound is healed. Generally, a dose of 5500 rads/6 weeks is planned if the surgery is radical in extent. On the other hand, if the surgery is primarily a debulking procedure with gross residual disease remaining, high-dose radiotherapy must be given, i.e., 6500 rads/7 weeks through a shrinking field technique to the area of known disease.

The decision for preoperative vs. postoperative radiation therapy should be made on individual basis, personal preference, and experience. Theoretically, preoperative therapy performed with the cancer cells in their maximum stage of oxygenation possesses a possible advantage over irradiation in the postoperative hypoxic condition (30). Therefore, preoperative irradiation is often preferred. There are, however, times when postoperative treatment is definitely advised. These include patients with extensive tumors of the larynx and hypopharynx in whom emergency tracheostomy is required. In such circumstances, the infected larynx and tumor would be better removed first so that radiation therapy can be expediently carried out without the complications of pain, aspiration, and pulmonary infection which are often present when laryngectomy is not done primarily. Patients with extensive disease requiring laryngo-pharyngo-esophagectomy and extensive, complicated reconstruction would be better treated by postoperative radiation therapy in the belief that preoperative therapy would add further difficulties to the already increased operative complications after such extensive surgery. In addition, all patients with advanced T2, T3, and T4 lesions who were treated by primary excision and found at histiological examination to have tumor extension to the resection margins or outside the capsule of the lymph node would benefit from postoperative radiation therapy.

The management of metastatic nodes in the neck from a primary arising in the head and neck region depends upon the size, number of nodes, and the cell type and location of the primary lesion. Radiotherapy is highly curative for small, metastatic nodes with primary tumors arising from Waldeyer's ring, i.e., nasopharynx, faucial tonsil, and base of tongue. Therefore, for such N1 and early N2 lesions, radiation should be given for cure and surgery is reserved for salvage. For metastatic nodes with primaries arising from the oral cavity and larynx in advanced stage, a combination of radiation therapy and surgery is the treatment choice. i.e., radical neck dissection either preceded by or followed with radiation therapy (21). A dose of 4500 rads/4 weeks as a preoperative procedure and 5500 rads/5.5 weeks as a postoperative procedure would be planned. For inoperable metastatic nodes in the neck, high-dose radiotherapy is necessary for local control. A dose of 7500-8000 rads often is needed for N3 disease. This treatment program may result in painful fibrosis of the neck.

MODALITIES OF RADIATION THERAPY

Undue emphasis is often placed on the equipment of radiation therapy, but as in all medicine, the knowledge and skill of the radiation therapist are the determinants of success of a given treatment rather than the hardware. Nevertheless, the armamentarium of modern radiation therapy does make possible techniques previously unavailable. This may result in improvement in cure rates and reduction of undesirable complications and local side effects.

The tools of radiation therapy used in the management of cancers of the head and neck primarily are megavoltage radiations with energies of several million volts and radioactive isotopes. These megavoltage radiation energies possess certain inherent physical advantages such as skin and bone sparing, sharply defined beam, and increased depth dose. Skin sparing is reflected in the fact that often a full course of curative radiation therapy can be given without causing significant radiation dermatitis. Sharp beam and increase in depth dose make it possible to deliver maximal amount of homogeneous radiations to accurately encompass the individual lesions, thus minimizing unnecessary damage to adjacent normal tissue. The bone sparing effect is due to lesser differential absorption between soft tissue and bone, thus resulting in a lesser incidence of osteoradionecrosis as compared to kilovoltage radiations.

The present-day means of generating x- or gamma radiations or photons in the megavoltage range for the treatment of head and neck tumors are the telecobalt and x-ray machines and isotopes. The telecobalt "bomb," though technically not an x-ray machine, is used in the same manner and for all practical purposes is a megavoltage x-ray machine. The source of ionizing rays, in this case gamma rays, is several thousand curies of radioactive ^{60}Co and is housed in a shielded container, with collimating devices and electrical circuits. It is a common and practical machine for treatment of head and neck tumors. The most commonly used x-ray machines are linear accelerators. These accelerators, commonly known as linacs or clinacs, provide a reliable source of ionizing radiations. Either x-rays or electrons of energies in the range of 4-40 million electron volts can be produced. Linear accelerators have the advantage of high output and compactness and have been very popular in the major cancer centers. Kilovoltage radiations, as generated by the 100-250 x-ray machines may be used for treatment of carcinoma of the skin and lip, otherwise, they have no place in the primary management of carcinoma of the head and neck. Most lesions suitably treated by kilovoltage machines can now be satisfactorily managed by electron beam therapy.

Energetic electrons can be generated by a linear accelerator or a betatron. According to the depth of the lesions, varying energies ranging from 6-18 MeV or above, can be selected for optimum irradiation of the head and neck tumors. The characteristic of an electron beam is sharp dose fall off beyond the 50-80% isodose for the specified energy applied, thus structures immediately beyond the treatment target receive a relatively low dose. The principal areas of application suitable for electron beam therapy include lesions of the skin, lip, primary lesions situated at 2-5 cm depth, parotid tumors, metastatic cervical nodes, and anteriorly situated oral lesions treated by transoral cone, and others. Frequently, electron beam therapy is given in conjunction with photon irradiation.

Radioactive isotopes are important sources to provide gamma rays for the management of cancer of the head and neck, and are primarily used interstitially either as a temporary or permanent implant. In the past, ^{226}Ra was a time-honored isotope, and was used in the form of needles. Because of its inherent hazards of radiation exposure to the staff, afterloading devices using angiocath and ^{192}Ir have been developed and extensively used in lieu of radium needles (45). The implants are removed after delivering a prescribed dose to the tumor, frequently in 2-3 days. Radon, a gaseous decay product of radium contained in a seed capsule, was used extensively in the past as a permanent interstitial implant, but has been largely replaced by ^{198}Au or ^{125}I grains.

The modern practice of radiation therapy for head and neck tumors demands extreme technical sophistication. By using various treatment modalities and techniques such as wedge filters or rotation or combination of photons and electrons, most of the irreparable radiation injuries of the bone and soft tissues, which were commonly seen in the past kilovoltage era, are greatly reduced. Radical surgery often can be performed subsequently without significant postoperative complications.

TREATMENT PLANNING

After radiation therapy is elected, treatment should be carefully planned and executed. In the modern practice of radiation therapy, treatment planning is based on the nature, size, and location of the tumor, the volume of tissue to be encompassed, the normal structures to be spared, and intent of treatment, whether curative or palliative. It is carried out with the aid of a simulator and dedicated computer prior to actual treatment. This procedural preparation for radiotherapy must be as thorough as the preparation of a patient who is to undergo surgery. All workups should be complete, including evaluation of the extent of the primary lesion by inspection, palpation, and various diagnostic means such as radiographs, polytomes, xerograms, contrast studies, and, when indicated, ultrasonic and CT scans. This is mandatory in order to determine the exact tumor volume for optimum direction of the treatment beams. Since most of the lesions of the head and neck region are accessible for biopsy, a histological confirmation of malignancy must be obtained prior to radiation therapy. Needless to say, a complete physical examination, including blood and urine studies and liver profile for appraisal of patient's physical status, is highly desirable. Anemia, weight loss, poor dental hygiene, or electrolyte imbalance should be corrected.

THE INTENT OF RADIATION THERAPY

The intent of radiation therapy can be divided into curative, palliative, or as adjunctive to combined modality treatment.

Radical radiation therapy with intent to cure is not without morbidity and should be performed with both care and justification. In curative therapy, the treatment course is usually prolonged and physically taxing. Painful radiation reactions in the oropharyngeal mucosa may be quite severe resulting in dysphagia and impairment of nutrition. As a matter of fact, the discomfort suffered by the patient from curative therapy is no less and is sometimes more than that of radical surgery. It is generally observed that old patients or alcoholics tolerate radical surgery procedures, i.e., partial glossectomy or total laryngectomy for advanced disease, far better than they tolerate a radical course of radiation therapy extending for 6-7 weeks or with interstitial implant.

With massive primary tumor or cervical nodal metastases, the condition is rarely curable and palliative radiotherapy for symptomatic relief would be the aim. Pain, bleeding, ulceration, and oropharyngeal obstruction may be alleviated by radiation therapy but unfortunately, for effective palliation for most of the carcinomas of the head and neck, the dose of radiation is generally high, approaching 5000 rads or more in 6 weeks, if lasting effects are to be obtained. This palliative radiation dose may produce symptomatic reactions if one is not careful. Therefore, for patients with far advanced but relatively asymptomatic lesions in a terminal stage, the best treatment may be human kindness, morphine, and good nursing care.

In radiation therapy as in surgery, the first choice of treatment must be the correct one. If the lesion recurs after therapy, it may have acquired resistance to further irradiation because of impairment of local blood supply and formation of more radioresistant hypoxic cells due to changes in cellular component. Consequently, in most instances when a full course of radiation has been given, reirradiation with intent to cure generally is of little value and is less likely to be successful. Such recurrences should be treated by surgery if there is still a chance of cure. The exceptions to this rule, however, are nasopharyngeal cancer (48) and glottic cancer (35) where reirradiation has salvaged a few otherwise inoperable and incurable patients.

Radiation therapy is frequently used as an adjuvant procedure given either before or after surgery for advanced cancer of the head and neck. The rationale, aims, and treatment concepts have been previously discussed.

GENERAL GUIDELINES OF MANAGEMENT OF HEAD AND NECK CANCERS

Oral Cancer

Oral cancer is a relatively common malignancy of the head and neck (40). The TNM staging system for oral cancer as recommended by the American Joint Committee in 1977 is as follows:

T1: tumor 2 cm or less in greatest diameter

T2: tumor greater than 2 cm but not greater than 4 cm in greatest diameter

T3: tumor greater than 4 cm in greatest diameter

T4: massive tumor greater than 4 cm in diameter with invasion of adjacent structures such as bone, soft tissue, etc.

The majority of cancers of the oral cavity are squamous cell carcinomas. As a general rule, when the location of the lesions is further away from the lips toward the oropharynx, the tumors tend to be less differentiated. Since squamous cell carcinomas represent dysplastic mucosal membrane, there is almost always some degree of mucosal changes associated with the tumor. The lesions show some bleeding, especially after detailed examination and scraping with tongue depressors. Early mucosal lesions may appear as only superficial granularity or an indurated nodule or as a shallow ulceration which may have minimal subjective symptoms. Advanced tumors often extend deeply into the underlying muscles or bone causing fixation of the organ and resulting in difficulty in speech and deglutition. Metastases commonly occur to the ipsilateral subdigastric, upper and mid jugular nodes, although cross-metastases to the opposite neck may also occur with lesions across the midline of the oral cavity or lesions arising from the tip of the tongue and floor of mouth. The incidence of cervical lymph node metastasis for early lesions, T1, ranges from 10-20%; for the intermediate lesions, T2, 25-30%; and advanced lesions, T3 and T4, 50-70%. Distant metastases below the clavicle are uncommon and occur late in the course of the disease.

The use of radiation therapy in the management of squamous cell carcinoma of the oral cavity, as is true for most squamous cell carcinoma of the head and neck, is based on the following principles:

1. Carcinomas of the head and neck are radioresponsive, and in early stages highly radiocurable.

2. The more differentiated the tumors, the less the radiation response. Thus, verrucous carcinoma and in situ carcinoma require very high dose of radiation for their permanent control.

3. Exophytic and well-oxygenated tumors are more radioresponsive than ulcerative, deeply infiltrative, and hypoxic ones.

4. Squamous cell carcinomas, when limited to the mucosa, are highly radiocurable. Bone or muscle involvement adversely alters the radioresponsiveness of carcinomas, and subsequently decreases the radiocurability.

5. Early advanced cervical metastatic nodes are treatable by irradiation only and advanced metastatic nodes are, when possible, treated by combined surgery and radiotherapy.

The treatment of carcinoma of the oral cavity is mostly by low megavoltage or ^{60}Co radiations with interplay of interstitial isotope implants. In general, external beam therapy is suitable for most lesions and in many instances is the procedure of choice. The radiotherapy treatment program should include the primary and regional nodes, especially in patients with lesions associated with propensity to nodal metastases. The irradiated volume is therefore large and often associated with some radiation sequelae.

Interstitial isotope implant is only suitable for lesions situated in the anterior portion of the oral cavity such as lip, buccal mucosa, floor of mouth, and oral tongue. The irradiated volume of the implant is generally small but the radiation dosage is intense. The implant procedure requires skill, experience, and good judgment on the part of the radiation therapist, and is often used as a boost to the primary lesion. There are, however, inherent dosimetric difficulties in implants in that inhomogeneity of dose distribution is invariably present, and results in "hot" and "cold" spots. Interstitial implants are not suitable for lesions invading or adjacent to the mandible due to the high risk of osteoradionecrosis or for lesions involving the tonsillar region or base of tongue.

Results of radiation therapy for carcinoma of the oral cavity are related to the size of the primary lesion and the presence or absence of metastatic nodes (3, 4, 16). In early lesions (T1), the 3 year NED (no evidence of disease) rates should approach 75-80% and for the intermediate lesions, T2, 50-60%. The radiotherapeutic results of advanced carcinomas, T3 and T4, generally approximate 10-20%. For the lesions without nodes, the 3 year NED rates range between 50-70%, while the presence of nodes reduces the cure rates from one-half to one-third.

From the standpoint of anatomic origin, cancer of the oral cavity can be further subdivided as follows: lip, oral tongue, floor of mouth, retromolar trigone and anterior tonsillar pillar, buccal mucosa, alveolar ridge, and palate. A brief discussion of each of these lesions is presented below:

Lip

The AJC staging for lip carcinoma is as follows:

T1: tumor less than 1 cm in size
T2: tumor 1-3 cm in size
T3: tumor greater than 3 cm in size
T4: massive tumor with or without bone and muscle involvement

Most of the carcinomas of the lip are well-differentiated squamous cell carcinomas and are less than 1 cm in size. Basal cell carcinoma does not occur in the lip per se but may originate in the skin with secondary involvement of the lip. Squamous cell carcinoma of the lip occurs mostly after the fifth decade of life and predominantly in a males (90%). The tumor is more commonly seen in patients with outdoor occupations, having heavy exposure to sunshine. Pipe smokers have a high predilection for lip cancer. Most lesions originate in the lower lip midway between the midline and commissure. Less than 15% of the lesions occur in the upper lip. For the carcinomas located in the lateral third of the lip or commissure, metastases occur primarily to the submental and prevascular submandibular nodes, rarely across the midline and usually late in the stage of the disease. For the upper lip lesions, metastases may occur in the preauricular and upper cervical as well as in the submandibular nodes. It is rare for the metastases to skip these nodal groups and go to the inferior jugular nodes. Distant metastases are extremely rare. The lesser differentiated lesions tend to metastasize more frequently than the well-differentiated lesions, i.e., for grade I lesions the incidence of metastases is 7%; grade II, 22%; and grade III, 35%. Likewise, the incidence of metastases increases with increase of the primary stage and in recurrent lesions after repeated surgical procedure.

As a rule, therapy is directed to the primary lesion if there are no palpable nodes. A small carcinoma of the lip can be dealt with expediently and successfully by "V" excision and the procedure will not result in cosmetic or functional deformity. Radiation therapy can produce excellent cure rates and cosmesis for superficial cancers involving half of or the entire lip and for tumors involving the lip commissure. Recurrent tumors after prior excision or patients who refuse surgery should have the benefit of curative radiation. Surgical excision is mandatory for radiation failures, for extensive cancers which involve the mandible, or cancer associated with significant soft tissue destruction that will require major reconstruction after the lesion is controlled by radiation therapy. Since radiation therapy or surgery has yielded extremely high cure rates for the small, limited cancers, i.e., 3-year NED rate of 90%, selection of treatment modality must depend upon the cosmetic result which follows the treatment procedure. Radiation therapy for the superficial small tumor (T1) consists of low-energy x-rays, such as 250 kV or low-megavoltage electrons. For the extensive tumors (T2, T3) combined external beam therapy of x-rays or electrons and interstitial isotope implant yields excellent cure rates and cosmetic results. For far advanced tumor, x-rays with energy of a few million volts or ^{60}Co radiations are used to include the primary and the metastatic nodes. When metastatic nodes are present in the neck, N2b disease, adjuvant preoperative or postoperative radiotherapy to the whole neck should be given with a dose of 5000 rads/5 weeks.

Oral Tongue

Squamous cell carcinoma of the oral tongue (anterior two-thirds of the tongue) is a common type of oral cancer and includes the lesions arising from the mobile portion of the tongue in front of the circumvallate papillae. It frequently invades the underlying muscle early, and tends to spread along the muscle plane with poorly defined margins, causing fixation of the organ. Palpation helps in assessing the degree of submucosal extension. It is attended by a high incidence of cervical lymph node metastases. Because of the rich supply of lymphatics, approximately 50% of the entire group, 20-30% of T1 and T2 lesions and 70-80% of T3 and T4 lesions, when diagnosed have clinical lymph node metastases to ipsilateral cervical nodes. Approximately 10-15% of these patients have bilateral nodal involvement. This tumor is difficult to manage by either radiation therapy or surgery due to the high incidence of local recurrence and propensity to nodal involvement. Surgical resection is indicated for extremely small cancers, T1, which can be expediently excised without resulting deformity or tumor involving the tip of the tongue. Surgery alone can sometimes be used for large infiltrative lesions, T3 and T4, which are associated with a great deal of muscle involvement. Surgery is often used as a salvage procedure for residual or recurrent disease following failure of radical radiation therapy.

The superficial exophytic T1 and T2 lesions without a great deal of muscle involvement are amenable to radiation therapy with high local control and excellent cosmetic results. In certain moderately infiltrative lesions, less than 2 cm muscular invasion, a course of radiotherapy of 4500 rads/4.5 weeks can be given, followed by interstitial implant or coned-down external beam therapy to 6500-7000 rads. Surgery can be used if salvage is necessary. For large, advanced, infiltrative T2, T3, and T4 lesions, a planned course of combined irradiation and surgery is the treatment of choice.

Floor of the Mouth

Carcinoma of the floor of the mouth is commonly located in the anterior portion of the floor adjacent to Wharton's duct orifice. It may extend to the adjacent tongue and gum and later invade the mandible (9). In extensive lesions, the tumor may present as a continuous mass from the floor of the mouth onto the submandibular triangle. When the tumor is limited to the mucosa, it is highly curable by radiation therapy alone. Although bone involvement compromises treatment results, radiation therapy for such lesions is possible when bone is eroded but not infiltrated by tumor. It is therefore necessary to obtain good radiographs of the mandible if the lesion is found to be adherent to the gum. In general, small lesions of the floor of the mouth are treated by external beam therapy first followed by either electron beam boost through an intraoral cone or by interstitial implant. In extensive lesions with involvement of the adjacent tongue and mandible preoperative radiotherapy of 4500 rads/4.5 weeks can be given prior to planned surgery. When this is done, the margins of the tumor are tattooed prior to radiation therapy in order to define the extent of the surgery later required. Although nodal metastases are quite low in T1 lesions, i.e., less than 10%, extensive tumors such as T2 and T3 are associated with high incidence of lymph node metastases ranging from 50-75%, respectively. Of these, 20% are bilateral. The commonly involved nodes are submandibular and subdigastric groups. Submental nodes are rarely involved. The treatment of extensive nodal disease can be by combined radiation therapy and neck dissection.

Retromolar Trigone and Anterior Faucial Pillar

Squamous cell carcinomas arising from the retromolar trigone and anterior faucial pillar are generally under one heading for discussion and should not be confused with carcinoma of the tonsil. These lesions may spread to adjacent soft and hard palate, gingiva, or adjacent buccal mucosa, as well as to the tonsillar fossa, and inferiorly to the base of the tongue and floor of the mouth. Advanced lesions may extend to the pterygoid fossa resulting in trismus. Most of these tumors are well differentiated and the superficial lesions can be successfully treated with external beam therapy. Primary radical surgery generally is attended by marked facial deformity and impairment of swallowing mechanism and often results in a high incidence of marginal recurrence. Since these lesions tend to remain localized, salvage surgery is frequently able to affect a lasting cure at the cost of cosmetic and functional mutilation if radiation therapy fails to eradicate the entire lesion. Most common sites of failure after radiation therapy are the base of the tongue and adjacent mandible infiltrated by tumor. Residual disease after high-dose radiotherapy is best managed by limited resection, i.e., nidusectomy. Large, infiltrative lesions (T3 and T4), with or without pterygoid invasion, are best treated by combination of high-dose, limited-field radiation therapy and composite resection.

Buccal Mucosa

Carcinoma of the buccal mucosa is usually well-differentiated squamous cell carcinoma, frequently associated with areas of leukoplakia. Because the mucous membrane adheres closely to the muscle of the cheek, early invasion of the masseter muscle can occur and produce trismus. Once the deeper muscles are involved, there is an increased likelihood of cervical lymph node metastases. Primary surgical removal of the small, superficial lesions is preferred. For the intermediate lesions (T2), radiotherapy may result in a high cure rate with good functional and cosmetic results. If the buccogingival sulcus is not involved by tumor, the best results of therapy have been achieved by combined external photon, electron beam therapy and interstitial implant. The cure rates for extensive T3 and T4 lesions with deep muscular invasion by radiation therapy alone are extremely poor. In most instances, en bloc excision of such lesions and neck dissection with adjuvant radiotherapy is preferred.

Gingival Ridge

Carcinoma of the gingival ridge usually arises in the posterior portion of the lower dental arch and is associated with leukoplakic changes. Since the mucous membrane adheres to the periosteum of the mandible, tumor arising from the gingival ridge is likely to invade underlying bone in its early stage of development. Most of these tumors are well-differentiated squamous cell carcinoma. Carcinoma of the upper gingiva is an uncommon disease but should not be confused with tumors which originate from the maxillary sinus, secondarily extending to the gingiva. Radiograph of the paranasal sinuses is helpful in differential diagnosis, and also allows careful evaluation of the extent of the bony involvement. Treatment of the gingival ridge depends upon the extent of the lesion, degree of bony involvement, and the status of the cervical lymph nodes. Special note should be made between smooth, erosive pressure defect which results from a slowly expanding tumor and the moth-eaten type of bone destruction which is caused by tumor infiltration. The latter lesion cannot be successfully treated by radiation therapy, whereas the former can. The small, T1, exophytic cancer without bone involvement can be successfully managed by external beam therapy alone (24). For advanced lesions associated with destruction of the mandible with or without metastases, radical surgery is preferred since partial mandibulectomy with radical neck dissection provides good survival rates (8). Since local spread of the disease along the subperiosteal lymphatics may occur, radiation therapy is often given prior to or following resection of the advanced tumors in order to reduce local recurrence.

Because of the eccentric location of both the primary lesion and its regional nodes, radiation therapy is delivered either by photons with lateral wedge, or electron beam technique. Radium mould was once used but has been entirely replaced by modern megavoltage irradiation. Due to the proximity of bone to the tumors, interstitial implant for this disease often results in osteoradionecrosis and is not advised.

Palate

The palate is divided into the hard and soft palate. The hard palate is the most common site for occurrence of minor salivary gland tumors in the oral cavity. Squamous cell carcinomas arising from this site are quite rare and are usually ulcerative and generally invade the underlying bone. Early lesions without bone involvement can be treated satisfactorily by radiation therapy alone with surgery reserved for radiation salvage. The advanced, deeply infiltrative lesions with bone destruction are rarely curable by radiation therapy and are better treated by combined therapy; the resulting defect can be corrected by a prosthesis. Malignant salivary gland tumors are traditionally treated by surgery and have been recently treated with increasing frequency by combination of surgery and postoperative radiation therapy. Some inoperable malignancies of the minor salivary glands in the oropharynx have been successfully controlled by high-dose radiotherapy.

Most malignant tumors of the soft palate and uvula are well-differentiated squamous cell carcinomas and are included with the oropharyngeal cancer in the American Joint Committee staging publication. They are invariably ulcerated lesions with poorly defined borders and biologically and radiotherapeutically behave like carcinomas of the oral cavity and therefore are discussed herein. Surgical resection of such lesions is unsatisfactory and often results in marginal recurrences. Even when surgery is successful, impaired swallowing and speech mechanism often ensues unless prosthetic support is available. Because of the relatively superficial nature of most T1 and T2 lesions, good local control has been achieved by megavoltage radiation therapy (18). For T3 and T4 lesions, often associated with cervical nodal metastases, the results of radiotherapy are generally poor and such lesions, at the present time, are being considered inoperable and are treated by palliative radiotherapy, chemotherapy, or cryotherapy. If the lesions are borderline operable, after high-dose therapy, surgery should be carried out in hopes of improving the cure rate.

Oropharynx

The oropharyngeal lesions, according to the American Joint Committee staging, include tumors arising from the faucial tonsil, base of the tongue, pharyngeal wall, and faucial arch. The term faucial arch tumors refers collectively to lesions arising from various anatomic structures with different biological behavior, including soft palate and anterior and posterior pillars. Except for the latter, these tumors would best be included under the discussion of oral cavity lesions because of their similarity to oral cancers in terms of tumor growth, spread, and prognosis. In contrast to carcinoma of the oral cavity, oropharyngeal carcinomas are generally poorly differentiated, including a special variant, so-called lymphoepithelioma. The staging for oropharyngeal carcinomas is the same as staging of oral cancer. These lesions are characterized by a high incidence of cervical lymph node metastases, irrespective of the stage of the primary lesion, ranging between 50-75% at the time the diagnosis is made. Over half of the lesions with cervical node metastases from the base of the tongue present with bilateral involvement (28).

Radiation therapy for this disease is primarily external beam therapy. Technically, it is extremely difficult to obtain a satisfactory interstitial implant in lesions situated in the base of the tongue or tonsillar fossa. Owing to the unusually high incidence of nodal metastases, radiation therapy must include the primary tumor as well as the first-echelon lymphatic areas in a common portal even in patients with clinically N0 necks. Radiotherapeutic results for carcinoma of the oropharynx were considered to be notoriously unfavorable. Studies at the Massachusetts General Hospital and the Massachusetts Eye and Ear Infirmary indicate that in tumors of comparable stages the cure rates for oropharyngeal cancer are comparable to those for carcinomas of the oral cavity. With early lesions, T1, the 3-year NED rate ranges from 75-85% and intermediate lesions, T2, 50-60%. For extensive lesions, T3 and T4, the cure rate by radiotherapy is approximately 10-20%. Contrary to squamous cell carcinoma of the oral cavity, the presence of N1 nodal metastasis does not appear to effect the prognosis significantly, and many lesions with such early metastatic disease can be controlled by radiotherapy alone.

Tonsil

Squamous cell carcinoma of the faucial tonsil, as previously noted, is different from that which originates from the retromolar trigone and anterior tonsillar pillar. These lesions are prone to spread posteriorly to the lateral pharyngeal wall and base of tongue and superiorly to the soft palate (31). Most of the carcinomas of the tonsil are radiosensitive and in early stages, highly curable. For such early lesions, radiotherapy is the treatment of choice (15,18). Advanced tumors of the tonsil with invasion of the base of the tongue are best treated by combined therapies (29). This includes high-dose external beam therapy through shrinking field technique to a total dose of approximately 6000 rads to be followed by limited surgery with removal of the residual disease commonly present in the base of the tongue or adjacent mandible (39). Any residual disease in the neck following high-dose radiotherapy is dealt with by neck dissection.

Base of Tongue

This is the fixed portion or posterior third of the tongue starting anatomically from the circumvallate papillae posteriorly toward the epiglotticopharyngeal folds. In order to evaluate the extent of this disease, in addition to indirect laryngoscopy, digital palpation of the base of the tongue is required as a routine procedure. Treatment of this disease is primarily by external beam therapy with limited surgery being reserved for residual disease. Unfortunately, most of the cancers of the base of the tongue are so situated that appropriate surgery will have to include excision of the entire tongue and laryngectomy. Such aggressive surgical procedure with resultant mutilation often is unrewarding because of the dismal cure rates and makes a bad situation worse. For small, T1 and T2 lesions, the 3-year NED rates are as high as 80 and 60%, respectively, by radiation therapy alone. The T3 and T4 lesions currently are considered inoperable and incurable and palliation is all that can be hoped for.

Pharyngeal Wall

The pharyngeal wall includes the lateral and posterior walls and posterior tonsillar pillar. Primary lesions arising from the posterior tonsillar pillar alone are extremely rare. Squamous cell carcinomas arising from these sites tend to be ulcerative and their exact extensions upward or downward are difficult to determine. Therefore, lateral soft tissue xerograms are essential to detect the extent of the tumor. Because of the strategic location, surgery is unlikely to be successful due to high frequency of local recurrences. These tumors are better treated by external beam therapy which must include the entire pharynx from the nasopharyngeal vault down to the pyriform sinus (37). Because of the proximity of the tumor to the spinal cord, care must be exercised to avoid excessive irradiation of the cord. Owing to the high sensitivity of the mucosa of the posterior pharyngeal wall, patients generally experience rather severe painful radiation reaction with dysphagia and odynophagia, with consequent impairment of nutritional status, and therefore radiation therapy must be carried out with great caution. Any residual disease limited to the lateral pharyngeal wall after a course of radiotherapy occasionally may be dealt with by laryngopharyngectomy although cure rates generally are poor (14).

Hypopharynx

Hypopharyngeal tumors include lesions arising from the pyriform sinus, posterior pharyngeal wall, and postcricoid area. The T staging system is defined by tumor extension to the adjacent sites and status of the mobility of the larynx, if involved, and is as follows:

- T1: tumor confined to the site of origin
- T2: extension of tumor to adjacent region or site without fixation of the hemilarynx

T3: extension of tumor to adjacent region or site with fixation of hemilarynx
T4: massive tumor invading bone or soft tissues of neck

Owing to the lack of severe symptoms, carcinoma arising from these sites tends to be extensive, frequently with extensive cervical lymph node metastases, often bilateral. These tumors are moderately undifferentiated, with poorly defined borders, and tend to infiltrate to the adjacent structures and involve the underlying cartilage and musculature. Treatment either by surgery or radiotherapy is unsatisfactory due to difficulty in controlling disease at the primary site and in cervical lymph nodes. Recently, except in carcinoma of the posterior pharyngeal wall, combination radiation therapy and surgery are carried out for these tumors with improved results.

Pyriform Sinus

Carcinoma of the pyriform sinus is characterized by an extensive primary lesion and frequently cervical nodal metastases. More than half of the patients when first seen present with T3 and T4 disease and two out of three patients present with cervical metastases. Distinction must be made between the lesions arising in the medial and lateral walls of the pyriform sinus from the apical portion of the pyriform sinus. The tumor arising from the upper walls of the mouth of the pyriform sinus tends to be exophytic and is curable by radiation therapy. The tumor arising from the apical portion of the pyriform sinus is often infiltrative with extensive involvement of adjacent cartilage, larynx, and upper trachea and is not likely to be radiocurable. Such a lesion would best be dealt with by a combination of irradiation and surgery. The overall 3-year NED rate for carcinoma of the hypopharynx treated by radiotherapy is approximately 20%. The cure rates have doubled by combined treatment with radiotherapy and surgery (49). The majority of therapeutic failures are due to uncontrolled nodal disease in the neck, cervical esophagus, or base of the skull, and recurrence in the base of the tongue or tracheal stoma. A small number of patients die with distant metastases.

Posterior Pharyngeal Wall

Carcinoma of the posterior pharyngeal wall is an infrequent tumor. The most common symptoms are dysphagia and sore throat with foreign body sensation. Most of the lesions are flat but exophytic and often quite large and may extend laterally to involve the lateral pharyngeal wall inferiorly to the cervical esophagus. Therefore, a xerogram of the lateral pharynx and a barium swallow are minimal investigative procedures. Approximately one-half of the patients, when first seen, have cervical lymph node metastasis.

Like carcinoma of the nasopharynx, posterior pharyngeal wall cancer is considered totally inoperable and would best be treated by radiation therapy. Neck dissection is used if there are residual nodes postirradiation. For the early T1 and T2 lesions, the radiotherapeutic results are approximately 50%. Advanced tumors carry an approximately 10% cure rate after radiation therapy (37).

Larynx

Anatomically and therapeutically, the larynx can be divided into three separate portions: supraglottic, glottic, and subglottic. The supraglottic tumors include the lesions arising from the laryngeal surface and rim of the epiglottis, aryepiglottic fold, arytenoid, false cord, and laryngeal ventricle. The glottic tumors originate from the vocal cord and anterior and posterior commissures. The subglottic lesions arise from the area approximately 1 cm inferior to the true cord down to the lower margin of the cricoid cartilage. The most common cancer of the larynx is squamous cell carcinoma of varying degrees of malignant potential. This cancer is predominantly a disease of the male in the fifth, sixth, and seventh decades of life. The T staging system for laryngeal cancer is as follows:

Supraglottis:

T1: tumor confined to region of origin with normal mobility
T2: tumor involving adjacent supraglottic site(s) or glottis without fixation
T3: tumor limited to larynx with fixation and/or extension to involve postcricoid area, medial wall of the pyriform sinus, or preepiglottic space
T4: massive tumor extending beyond the larynx to involve the oropharynx soft tissues of neck or destruction of cricoid cartilage

Glottis:

T1: tumor confined to vocal cord(s) with normal mobility (including involvement of anterior or posterior commissures)
T2: supraglottic and/or subglottic extension of tumor with normal or impaired cord mobility
T3: tumor confined to larynx with cord fixation
T4: massive tumor with thyroid cartilage destruction and/or extension beyond the confines of the larynx, or both

Subglottis:

T1: tumor confined to the subglottic region
T2: tumor extension to vocal cords with normal or impaired cord mobility
T3: tumor confined to larynx with cord fixation
T4: massive tumor with cartilage destruction or extension beyond the confines of the larynx, or both

Supraglottis

This ranks second to glottic carcinoma in incidence and generally is associated with a poorer prognosis. Usually, the tumor is poorly differentiated squamous cell carcinoma. Owing to the abundant supply of lymphatics in this anatomic site, supraglottic carcinoma is characterized by a high incidence of lymph node metastases, reportedly as high as 50%. Because of frequent extension across the midline, bilateral cervical lymph node metastases are common and occur in 20-50% of patients. The incidence in some series has been reported as high as 90% for tumors arising from the base of the epiglottis, false cord, and ventricle. Treatment of this disease must therefore include management of the primary lesion as well as lymph node metastases in the neck. The results of radiotherapy for supraglottic carcinoma are less satisfactory than for glottis tumors (5,19). The 5-year NED rates following radiation therapy vary depending upon the extent of the primary tumor and the status of the cervical nodes (41). For a superficial, exophytic, early lesion, T1 or T2 with normal mobility of the laryngeal structures, cure rate by radiotherapy alone is quite high, ranging from 70-90%. For such lesions irradiation should be considered as the initial method of treatment. This is particularly true for the exophytic tumors arising from the tip of the epiglottis and free margins of the aryepiglottic fold. If the primary lesion is extensive and deeply ulcerative with fixation of the laryngeal structures and/or with cervical lymph node metastases, i.e., T3 or T4, N1 or N2, the 5-year NED rates following radiotherapy are approximately 20-25%. These advanced lesions are presently managed by planned combined approach (32), i.e., 4500 rads/5 weeks followed by total laryngectomy and concomitant neck dissection with improved results (49). Should the patient experience laryngeal stridor requiring emergency tracheostomy, it is recommended that the patient have laryngectomy first, followed by postoperative radiotherapy. This should include the entire neck, tracheal stoma, and upper mediastinum to a dose of approximately 5500 rads/6 weeks and should be carried out approximately 3-4 weeks after surgery.

Glottis

The most common form of laryngeal cancer is well-differentiated squamous cell carcinoma of the vocal cord. Owing to its manifestations of disease by hoarseness of voice, glottic carcinoma is often discovered early and is readily curable either by radiation therapy or surgery. With tumor confined to the cord with normal mobility, the incidence of nodal metastases is extremely low, ranging from 0-2%. Therefore, the treatment of early glottic carcinoma does not include treatment of cervical nodes.

Radiation therapy is considered to be the treatment of choice for the T1 and T2 tumors with normal cord mobility (20,25). It not only provides excellent control of disease, being in the neighborhood of approximately 90% (42) 5-year NED, but also preserves a good, useful voice in approximately 95% of patients. There is no doubt that a significant number of patients with laryngeal cancer in the early stage can be cured by primary surgery alone (27); but total laryngectomy for early cancer with mobile cord should be condemned. Conservation surgery, such as laryngofissure and cordectomy or partial laryngectomy, in experienced hands can control early glottis lesions in highly selected patients, but the functional results are inferior to those of radiation therapy because of the residual permanent hoarseness of voice following surgery. For T2 lesions with impaired cord mobility, a trial course of radiotherapy is initially given. If the tumor shows good regression and/or return of normal cord mobility after a dose of 4500 rads/4.5-5 weeks, radiation therapy may be continued to a curative dose level of about 6500 rads/6.5-7 weeks. Salvage surgery is then reserved for failure. The extensive T3 and T4 lesions with completely fixed cord are rarely curable by radiation therapy alone and are currently treated by planned combination of radiotherapy and surgery. Lymph node metastases from laryngeal cancer indicate advanced disease and are managed by neck dissection and or radiation therapy.

Subglottis

This tumor is less than 1% of all laryngeal cancers. Early tumors can be successfully dealt with by radiation therapy. Unfortunately, most lesions are silent and extensive and are often heralded with laryngeal stridor requiring tracheostomy. Therefore, they would best be dealt with by laryngectomy first, followed by postoperative radiotherapy.

Nasopharynx

Anatomically, the nasopharynx is considered to be a blind spot for routine clinical examination. Many metastatic carcinomas found in the neck without a primary are from occult primary lesions arising in this area. Most of the carcinomas of the nasopharynx are undifferentiated carcinomas including subtypes of lymphoepithelioma and transitional cell carcinoma. Asymptomatic mass in the neck, unilateral impairment of hearing and otitis media, nasal obstruction, epistaxis and diplopia due to cranial nerve involvement are the common manifestations of this disease and should arouse the suspicion of nasopharyngeal carcinoma. Evaluation of the extent of the lesion should include inspection and palpation of the lesion by direct or indirect nasopharyngoscopy and digital examination. X-ray examinations include soft tissue films and polytomes of the nasopharynx and base of the skull in various projections for evaluation of the tumor and evidence of bone destruction. CT scans are extremely useful to detect the presence or absence of intracranial extension of the lesion.

The T staging of carcinoma of the nasopharynx is as follows:

T1: tumor one site or positive biopsy
T2: tumor involving two sites
T3: tumor extending to nasal cavity or oropharynx
T4: massive tumor invading bone, cranial nerve, or soft tissues of neck

Owing to the rich lymphatic supply and undifferentiated nature of the tumor, carcinoma of the nasopharynx is known to have a high incidence of cervical lymph node metastases, ranging from 60-80% irrespective of T stage. Therefore, in the management of carcinoma of the nasopharynx, similar to carcinoma of the oropharynx and supraglottis, treatment must be directed to both the primary site and neck, even in the N0 neck. Owing to its inaccessible location, primary surgery has no place in the curative management of this disease (26). Because the nasopharynx is surrounded by many vital structures and organs, treatment of this disease by radiotherapy calls for careful techniques. High-dose radiation is required for control of the primary. For small, T1 and T2 lesions without nodes, the radiotherapeutic results are 50% NED at 5 years (11,44). Even among patients with advanced disease with cranial nerve involvement, about one-quarter may survive for 5 or more years although some will have residual disease (47). Since these lesions tend to recur locally after external therapy, routine supplementary therapy with intracavitary cesium implant as part of the overall treatment program for T1 and T2 lesions has been found to reduce the incidence of local recurrence from 30% to less than 10% (47). Persistent nodal disease in the neck following radiotherapy is dealt with by neck dissection although the majority of the metastatic nodes can be controlled by irradiation alone.

Paranasal Sinus

Squamous cell carcinoma arising from the paranasal sinuses generally is a silent tumor and early diagnosis can rarely be made. Most lesions, when first diagnosed, already present evidence of bone destruction. The maxillary and ethmoid sinuses are commonly involved. Tumors arising from the sphenoid or frontal sinuses alone are rare. Detailed evaluation of this disease requires careful radiographic examination including polytomes and CT scans of the paranasal sinuses in AP and lateral projections (7).

The T staging system for tumor of the maxillary antrum is as follows:

T1: tumor confined to the antral mucosa of the infrastructure with no bone erosion or destruction

T2: tumor confined to the suprastructure mucosa without bone destruction or to infrastructure with destruction of medial or inferior bony walls only

T3: more extensive tumor invading skin of cheek, orbit, antrum, ethmoid sinuses, pterygoid muscle

T4: massive tumor with invasion of cribriform plate, posterior ethmoids, spenonasopharynx, pterygoid plates or base of skull.

Treatment of this group of lesions, except for early mucosal carcinomas, is a combination of radiation therapy and surgery. Although most tumors are advanced lesions, the incidence of lymph node metastases is approximately 20% of all cases. Routine radical neck dissection or elective neck irradiation is not recommended in patients without nodes. For most operable cases, radical surgery is performed first to remove the bulk of the tumor and to establish drainage of the infected sinuses and followed by postoperative radiotherapy of 5500-6000 rads/6 weeks. For some extensive, inoperable lesions, radiation therapy with a dose of 5000 rads/5 weeks is generally given first to be followed by maxillectomy and ethmoidectomy in approximately 1 month. Further radiation may be given postoperatively to any area of residual disease with boost technique.

In spite of advanced stages of carcinoma of the paranasal sinuses, the therapeutic results following combined radiotherapy and surgery are still reasonably good (12). Approximately one-third of the patients of the entire group can be cured. For the early lesions, better than one out of two patients enjoy freedom from recurrence for 5 or more years. Radical neck dissection is indicated only when the metastatic nodes in the neck become apparent.

Salivary Glands

Malignant tumors of the salivary glands are comprised of mucoepidermoid carcinoma, squamous cell carcinoma, acinic cell carcinoma, adenocystic carcinoma, adenocarcinomas, and others (22). The majority of the tumors occur in the parotid gland and a few in the oral cavity and oropharynx. The growth usually manifests as a painless swelling. The first therapeutic approach is surgical removal. Radiotherapy is indicated only in inoperable lesions, incomplete surgical removal with known residual disease and/or difficulty with clearance of the resection margin, tumor extension beyond the capsule found during histological examination, extensive perineural involvement, high-grade malignant tumors, tumors with one or more local recurrences after previous surgery, or patients refusing surgery. Generally a dose of 6500 rads/6.5 weeks is given for inoperable lesions or those with known residual disease. Localized microscopic disease requires a dose of 5500 rads/5.5 weeks. In parotid tumors, treatment can be carried out by a combination of external photon therapy and wedge technique for about 4500 rads/4.5 weeks to be followed by electron beam boost or interstitial implant for 2000 rads if accessible. When there are gross residual lesions in the oral cavity and oropharynx, external photon therapy is employed with a dose of 6500-7000/6.5-7.5 weeks. Experience has shown that following irradiation of this magnitude, the local recurrence rate is less than 10%.

Miscellaneous Tumors

Malignant lymphoma, other than Hodgkin disease, may arise from the oral cavity (38), Waldeyer's ring (36), and the paranasal sinuses (38). These tumors, so-called extranodal malignant lymphomas, tend to involve multiple adjacent sites. If localized, they may be highly curable by radiation therapy. Such extranodal lymphomas must be appropriately evaluated from the standpoint of systemic disease by bipedal lymphograms, abdominal CT, blood, liver profile, bone marrow biopsy, etc. If the disease is localized (stage I and stage II), radical irradiation is the treatment of choice. On the other hand, if the lesion is found to be generalized in nature, chemotherapy will have to be the treatment of choice and radiation therapy is reserved for localized systemic relief.

The classification of head and neck lymphoma is the same as for lymphoma in general, and is briefly as follows:

Stage I: limited to primary site

Stage II: lesion limited to the primary site with involvement of adjacent lymph nodes, limited above the diaphragm

Stage III: presence of generalized involvement with disease above and below the diaphragm.

Radiotherapy of stage I and stage II lymphomas of Waldeyer's ring, i.e., faucial, lingual, and nasopharyngeal tonsils, consists of 4500-5000 rads/4.5-5.5 weeks to the entire Waldeyer's ring and upper cervical nodes. Elective radiation to the lower neck and supraclavicular area is also given with 4500 rads/1 month. For lymphomas arising from the oral cavity, localized irradiation with generous margins is necessary. Similarly, lymphoma involving the paranasal sinuses requires large-field irradiation covering the entire hemiparanasal sinuses with a total tumor dose of 5000 rads/5 weeks. For lesions arising in the oral cavity, paranasal sinuses, the incidence of regional lymph node metastases is low and therefore elective neck irradiation does not appear to be indicated. The results of treatment of extranodal lymphoma of the head and neck, stage I and stage II, shows three of four and one of two patients being cured following radical radiotherapy. For lesions arising from the oral cavity and paranasal sinuses, the 5-year survival rate is equally satisfactory with 65% for stage I and 33% for stage II lesions. No 5-year survivors with lesions spreading below the clavicle are recorded.

Solitary plasmacytoma of the upper air and food passages is a rare tumor. It is generally not a manifestation or herald of multiple myeloma. If systemic disease does develop in a patient with soft tissue plasmacytoma, it may occur years later and run a prolonged course. This is in contrast to the course of this disease in patients who develop multiple myeloma de novo and usually are dead within 2-3 years.

These tumors may recur as late as 10 years after treatment and are compatible with long survival. Treatment of this disease is by radiation therapy. Primary radical surgery is not justified in the light of the radioresponsiveness and radiocurability of this tumor. Surgery may be used in the management of recurrences after irradiation. For localized solitary tumor, a dose of 5000 rads/5 weeks is adequate. No elective neck irradiation is advised. The radiotherapeutic results indicate that approximately one out of two patients is free of disease for 5 or more years after adequate irradiation (23).

Glomus tumor or chemodectoma occurs in the temporal bone. Most of the lesions are treated by temporal bone resection followed by postoperative radiotherapy. Although some clinicians feel that radiation therapy has not been demonstrated to be a curative procedure, patients with this disease may survive free for many years after a course of radiation therapy. A dose of 5000-5500 rads/5-6 weeks is adequate and should not be exceeded if temporal bone necrosis is to be avoided (46).

Squamous cell carcinoma arising from the nasal vestibule is relatively rare. There is no official staging system for this lesion. For the purpose of classification, the following stages have been proposed:

T1: lesion is limited to the nasal vestibule, relatively superficial, involving one or more sites within

T2: lesion has extended from the nasal vestibule to its adjacent structures, such as the upper nasal septum, upper lip, philtrum, skin of the nose and/or nasolabial fold, but not fixed to the underlying bone

T3: lesion has become massive with extension to the hard palate, buccogingival sulcus, large portion of the upper lip, upper nasal septum, turbinate and/or adjacent paranasal sinuses, fixed with deep muscle and bone involvement

These tumors behave quite differently from squamous cell carcinoma of the skin and present problems in therapeutic management both to the surgeons and to the radiation therapists. The small, T1 lesions can be treated either by surgery or by radiation therapy alone with a satisfactory cure rate (43). The choice of treatment modality depends upon the cosmetic result following the procedure. If significant deformity or mutilation will result following surgery, radiation therapy should be the treatment of choice.

Radiation therapy for these lesions calls for a high dose to a small volume of tissue. For the T1 and early T2 lesions, radiation therapy can be delivered by a combination of external beam orthovoltage therapy, or electron beam therapy, and interstitial implant without significant radiation complications. For the extensive T3 lesions, radical surgery with or without preoperative radiation therapy employing megavoltage technique is preferred.

Nodal metastases are treated by preoperative radiation therapy and radical neck dissection. Because of the relatively low incidence of nodal metastases for the small, limited lesions (approximately 10%), elective neck irradiation or dissection is not warranted.

The radiotherapeutic results show that for T1, T2, and T3 lesions the 3-year NED rates were 83, 71, and 50% respectively.

Squamous cell carcinoma of the skin of the face and of the nose and eyelids may metastasize to the preauricular lymph nodes. Surgical treatment of these metastatic nodes generally is unsatisfactory often resulting in marked mutilation with failure to control the disease locally. Treatment of preauricular lymph node metastasis by radiation therapy can be rewarding. In general, if the node is solitary, it should be treated by excisional biopsy followed by external photon therapy of approximately 4000 rads/4 weeks followed by additional 3000 rads/3 weeks either by electron beam or interstitial implant. Because preauricular lymph node metastasis generally indicates the aggressive nature of the primary lesion, elective cervical irradiation is in order, 5000 rads/5 weeks. No meaningful statistics are available as to the results of treatment due to the small number of cases treated. Local control in our experience has been accomplished in two out of three patients so treated.

COMPLICATIONS OF RADIATION THERAPY

Since radiations affect both normal and abnormal biological tissues, certain effects of therapy are expected, such as abnormal facial growth in children and epilation of the irradiated part. Long-term effects of radiation-induced malignancy, particularly in childhood, have been observed, but the incidence of such malignant transformation is extremely low and should not be seriously taken into consideration in the selection of radiation therapy for life-threatening malignant tumors.

Minor side effects such as xerostomia, loss of taste, and dental caries are relatively common following radiation therapy to the oropharynx and salivary glands and can usually be managed by supportive measures in addition to careful oral and dental hygiene. Most of the unpleasant side effects relative to taste and dry mouth are temporary, though in some instances the effects may be long lasting. Carious teeth should be extracted prior to radiation in order to minimize later infection of the mandible. Most sound teeth can survive radiation therapy and need not be extracted if the dosages are kept within the limits of tolerance of the mandible. A meticulous dental hygiene program, such as frequent fluoridation of teeth, should be maintained after irradiation.

Major complications include soft tissue ulceration, orocutaneous fistulas, and osteoradionecrosis of the mandible and hard palate (6,13,46). These may be related to curative radiations but may be coincidental to unusually aggressive therapy or faulty treatment technique. Important factors in the occurrence of complications include treatment modalities employed, the time-dose-fraction program, the size of the irradiated portals, the magnitude of radiation dosages, the extent of the disease and its location, as well as the patient's age and nutritional status. The incidence is further exaggerated following combined radiation therapy and surgery due to an excessive impairment of local blood supply and secondary infection. This is particularly true when curative doses of radiation are given first to tumors followed by radical surgical procedure. In such an environment, the postoperative morbidity and mortality could be exceptionally high and at times, unacceptable in modern practice of oncology. Other uncommon radiotherapeutic complications are radiation-induced hypopituitarism, hypothyroidism, and cataract formation. However, these complications and unpleasant sequelae of treatment should be accepted as a risk in the management of extensive tumors but may be minimized by observing careful radiotherapeutic and surgical techniques and principles. Radiation-induced transverse myelitis fortunately is extremely rare and should be avoided at all costs.

SUMMARY

Squamous cell carcinomas of the head and neck are potentially curable cancers. When the tumor is diagnosed and treated in its early stages (T1), the cure rate achieved either by radiation therapy or surgery is high. The choice of treatment modality is extremely complex and demands full knowledge of the biology of the tumors, advantages and disadvantages of various disciplines, expectant therapeutic and cosmetic results, and sympathetic understanding on the part of the physician and the patient. The T2 tumors may be better treated by radiation therapy first since satisfactory control of the disease can be achieved with preservation of normal function and anatomic part. Surgery can then be reserved for radiation failures as a salvage procedure. The extensive lesions, T3 and T4, often associated with bone and/or muscle involvement and cervical lymph node metastases, are treated by combined radiation therapy and surgery, if the lesion is surgically resectable. If the lesions are obviously incurable by any means, palliative radiation therapy may offer some symptomatic relief. The management of cervical metastatic nodes depends upon the primary site, the size and number of nodes. The limited metastatic nodal disease (N1 and N2) from primaries arising from Waldeyer's ring can be satisfactorily controlled by radiation therapy alone in a high percentage of cases, and any residual in the neck nodes is dealt with by salvage surgery. The large metastatic nodes (N2b, N3a) from oral cavity, hypopharynx, and larynx are better treated by radical neck dissection with adjuvant radiation therapy. At the present time, chemotherapy is used as an adjuvant procedure, or for palliation in patients with incurable cancers, including nonepithelial malignancies.

Although malignant tumors of the head and neck are considered to be among the most curable neoplasms, the therapeutic results for advanced tumors are still far from ideal. The need for early diagnosis and treatment cannot be too strongly emphasized. It is hoped that the newer treatment modalities such as heavy charged particulate (33) and high LET neutron radiations (10), radiation potentiators and sensitizers (1), or hyperthermia with radiation therapy (34) will one day come to fruition with further improvement in cure rates. Indeed, it is the full cooperation and efforts between surgeon and radiation therapist, as among all clinicians and researchers, which ultimately benefits the patients afflicted with malignant disease.

REFERENCES

1. Adams, G.E.: Chemical radiosensitization of hypoxic cells. Br. Med. Bull. 29:48-53, 1973.

2. Manual for Staging of Cancer, 1977, American Joint Committee for Cancer Staging and End Results Reporting, Chicago, American Joint Committee, 1977.

3. Ash, Clifford L.: Oral cancer: A twenty-five year study, Janeway lecture, 1961. Am. J. Roentgenol. 87:417-430, 1962.

4. Ballantyne, A. J. and Fletcher, G. H.: Management of residual or recurrent cancer following radiation therapy for squamous cell carcinoma of the oropharynx. Am. J. Roentgenol. 93(1):29-35, 1965.

5. Bataini, J.P., Ennuyer, A., Poncet, P., and Ghossein, N.A.: Treatment of supraglottic cancer by radical high dose radiotherapy. Cancer 33:1253-1262, 1974.

6. Bedwinik, J.M., Shukovsky, L.J., Fletcher, G.H., and Daley, T.E.: Osteonecrosis in patients treated with definitive radiotherapy for squamous cell carcinoma of the oral cavity and naso- and oropharynx. Radiology 119(3):665-667, 1976.

7. Boone, M.L., Harle, T.S., Higholt, H.W., and Fletcher, G.H.: Malignant disease of the paranasal sinuses and nasal cavity: Importance of precise localization of extent of disease. Am. J. Roentgenol. 102:627-636, 1968.

8. Cady, B. and Catlin, D.: Epidermoid carcinoma of the gum: A 20-year survey. Cancer 23:551-569, 1969.

9. Campos, J.L., Lampe, I., and Fayos, J.V.: Radiotherapy of carcinoma of the floor of mouth. Radiology 99:677-682, 1971.

10. Catterall, M. and Vanberg, D.D.: Treatment of advance tumors of head and neck with fast neutrons. Br. Med. J. 3:137-143, 1974.

11. Chen, K.Y. and Fletcher, G.H.: Malignant tumors of the nasopharynx. Radiology 99:165-171, 1971.

12. Cheng, V.S.T. and Wang, C.C.: Carcinomas of the paranasal sinuses: a study of sixty-six cases. Cancer 40(6):3038-3041, 1977.

13. Cheng, V.S.T. and Wang, C.C.: Osteoradionecrosis of the mandible resulting from external megavoltage radiation therapy. Radiology 112:685-689, 1974.

14. Cunningham, M.P. and Catlin, D.: Cancer of the pharyngeal wall. Cancer 20:1859-1866, 1967.

15. Fayos, J.V. and Lampe, I.: Radiation therapy of cancer of the tonsillar region. Am. J. Roentgenol. 111:85-94, 1971.

16. Fayos, J.V. and Lampe, I.: Treatment of squamous cell carcinoma of the oral cavity. Am. J. Surg. 124:493-500, 1972.

17. Fletcher, G.H.: Elective irradiation of subclinical disease in cancers of the head and neck. Cancer 29:1450-1454, 1972.

18. Fletcher, G.H. and Lindberg, R.D.: Squamous cell carcinomas of the tonsillar area and palatine arch. Am. J. Roentgenol. 96(3):574-587, 1966.

19. Flynn, M.B., Jesse, R.H., and Lindberg, R.D.: Surgery and irradiation in the treatment of squamous cell cancer of the supraglottic larynx. Am. J. Surg. 124:477, 481, 1972.

20. Horiot, J.C., Fletcher, G.H., Ballantyne, A.J., and Lindberg, R.D.: Analysis of failures of early vocal cord cancer. Radiology 103:663-665, 1972.

21. Jesse, R.H. and Fletcher, G.H.: Treatment of the neck in patients with squamous cell carcinoma of the head and neck. Cancer 39 (2 suppl):868-872, 1977.

22. Kadish, S., Goodman, M., and Wang, C.C.: Treatment of minor salivary gland malignancies of upper food and air passage epithelium. Cancer 20:1021-1026, 1972.

23. Kotner, L. and Wang, C.C.: Plasmacytoma of the upper air and food passages. Cancer 30:414-418, 1972.

24. Lampe, I.: Radiation therapy of cancer of the buccal mucosa and lower gingiva. Am. J. Roentgenol. 73:628-638, 1955.

25. Lederman, M.: Cancer of the larynx. I. Natural history in relation to treatment. Br. J. Radiol. 44:569-731, 1971.

26. Lederman, M. and Mould, R.F.: Radiation treatment of cancer of the pharynx: With special reference to telecobalt therapy. Brit. J. Radiol. 41:251-274, 1968.

27. Leroux-Robert, J.: Indications for radical surgery, partial surgery, radiotherapy and combined surgery and radiotherapy for cancer of the larynx and hypopharynx. Ann. Otol. 65(1):137-153, 1956.

28. Lindberg, R.: Distribution of cervical lymph node metastases from squamous cell carcinoma of the upper respiratory and digestive tracts. Cancer 29:1446-1449, 1972.

29. Perez, C.A., Lee, F.A., Ackerman, L.V., Ogura, J.H., and Powers, W.E.: Non-randomized comparison of preoperative irradiation and surgery vs. irradiation alone in the management of carcinoma of the tonsil. Am. J. Roentgenol. 126(2):248-260, 1976.

30. Powers, W.E. and Palmer, L.A.: Biological basis of preoperative radiation treatment. Am. J. Roentgenol. 102:176, 1968.

31. Rider, W.D.: Epithelial cancer of the tonsillar area. Radiology 78:760-765, 1962.

32. Silverstone, S.M., Goldman, J.L., and Ryand, J.R.: Combined high dose radiation therapy and surgery of advanced cancer of the laryngopharynx. Frontiers Radiat. Ther. Oncol. 5:106-122, 1970.

33. Suit, H.D., Goitein, M., Tepper, J.E., Verhey, L., Koehler, A.M., Schneider, R., and Gragoudas, E.: Clinical experience and expectation with protons and heavy ions. Int. J. Radiat. Oncol. Biol. Phys. 3:115-125, 1977.

34. Suit, H.D. and Shwayder, M.: Hyperthermia: Potential as an anti-tumor agent. Cancer 34:122-129, 1974.

35. Wang, C.C.: Radical re-irradiation for carcinoma arising from the previously irradiated larynx. Laryngoscope 77:2189-2195, 1967.

36. Wang, C.C.: Malignant lymphoma of Waldeyer's ring. Radiology 92:1335-1339, 1969.

37. Wang, C.C.: Radiotherapeutic management of carcinoma of the posterior pharyngeal wall. Cancer 27:894-896, 1971.

38. Wang, C.C.: Primary malignant lymphoma of the oral cavity and paranasal sinuses. Radiology 100:151-154, 1971.

39. Wang, C.C.: Management and prognosis of squamous cell carcinoma of the tonsillar region. Radiology 104:667-671, 1972.

40. Wang, C.C.: Role of radiation therapy in the management of carcinoma of the oral cavity. Otolaryng. Cl. of No. Am. 5:357-363, 1972.

41. Wang, C.C.: Megavoltage radiation therapy for supraglottic carcinoma. Radiology 109:183-186, 1973.

42. Wang, C.C.: Treatment of glottic carcinoma by megavoltage radiation therapy and results. Am. J. Roentgenol. 120:157-163, 1974.

43. Wang, C.C.: Treatment of carcinoma of the nasal vestibule by irradiation. Cancer 38:100-106, 1976.

44. Wang, C.C.: Treatment of carcinoma of the nasopharynx by irradiation. Ear Nose Throat J. 56(3):97-101, 1977.

45. Wang, C.C., Boyer, A.L., and Mendiondo, O.: Afterloading interstitial radiation therapy. Int. J. Radiat. Oncol. Biol. Phys. 1:365-368, 1976.

46. Wang, C.C. and Doppke, K.: Osteoradionecrosis of temporal bone - Consideration of Nominal Standard Dose. Int. J. Radiat. Oncol. Biol. Phys. 1:(9-10):881-883, 1976.

47. Wang, C.C., Little, J.B., and Schulz, M.D.: Cancer of the nasopharynx: Its clinical and radiotherapeutic considerations. Cancer 15:921-926, 1962.

48. Wang, C.C. and Schulz, M.D.: Management of locally recurrent carcinoma of the nasopharynx. Radiology 86:900-903, 1966.

49. Wang, C.C., Schulz, M.D., and Miller, D.: Combined radiation therapy and surgery for carcinoma of the supraglottis and pyriform sinus. Laryngoscope 82:1883-1890, 1972.

RECOMMENDED READINGS

1. Ackerman, L. and del Regato, J.: Cancer: Diagnosis, Treatment and Prognosis, 5th edition, St. Louis, C.V. Mosby, 1977.

2. Buschke, F. and Parker, R.G.: Radiation Therapy in Cancer Management, New York, Grune and Stratton, 1972.

3. Cararett, A.P.: Radiation Biology, Englewood Cliffs, N.J., Prentice-Hall, 1968.

4. Textbook of Radiotherapy, 2nd edition, edited by Fletcher, Gilbert, Mungerford, Philadelphia, Lea & Febiger, 1973.

5. Hall, E.J.: Radiobiology for the Radiologist, 2nd edition, Hagerstown, Md., Harper & Row, 1978.

6. MacComb, W.S. and Fletcher, G.H.: Cancer of the Head and Neck, Baltimore, Williams & Wilkins, 1967.

7. Moss, W.T., Brand, W.N. and Battifore, H.: Radiation Oncology, 5th edition, St. Louis, Mosby, 1979.

8. Rubin, P. and Casarett, G.: Clinical Radiation Pathology, 2 vols., Philadelphia, Saunders, 1968.

chapter 5

LUNG CANCER

Frederick W. George III, M.D.

Since first identified in 1812, lung cancer or bronchopulmonary carcinoma (BPC) has truly become "Captain of the Men of Death," with an annual mortality far greater than any other neoplasm. Efforts to stem this lethal tide have been marked by consistent and almost paradoxical failures. BPC is a largely preventable cancer, yet its incidence is skyrocketing at a steeper and steeper rate. It has also failed totally to yield to screening measures so that we must rely on management approaches to improve its prognosis today and in the foreseeable future. Unfortunately, treatment as generally administered has also yielded discouraging results. From the time of diagnosis, the average overall survival is 6-9 months with only 20% of patients living over 1 year. With the annual death toll now exceeding 100,000 per year, the disease has taken on the dimension of a national calamity.

Radiotherapy has become the mainstay and most used form of treatment because so many patients (80%) are not surgical candidates when first seen. While this approach is rational, it is uncommon for either radiotherapy or surgery to save the patient with lung cancer.

For example, even in the well-designed Veterans Administration Lung Cancer Group (VALG) studies, 95% of the patients have died by the end of the second year. These and similar figures give rise to the popular belief that lung cancer once diagnosed will invariably be fatal. However, much carefully recorded data, from experience with a great volume of lung cancer patients, provides us with explanations for the dismal results with these past methods and points the way to successful approaches for the future.

Too often, influenced by systemic symptoms even with limited thoracic disease, the radiotherapist may be intimidated by the grim prognosis so that he treats a patient with doses that are far too low and portals that are far too small to achieve more than limited palliation. The data now available suggest that as many as 75% of the patients with squamous cell carcinoma and 50% of large cell and adenocarcinoma die of intrathoracic tumor without systemic involvement. This sharply contradicts the widely held impression of early systemic dissemination in this disease. Such data suggest that the majority of patients could be salvaged with effective cancericidal locoregional therapy, and that most current regimens are not effective in achieving local control.

For management with curative intent, in addition to local control, it has long been advocated by some workers that adequate radiotherapy portals include nodal draining areas. Therefore, the mediastinosupraclavicular areas have often been included. However, in the past, evaluation and treatment of the upper abdomen have almost invariably been omitted. Observations, both at surgery and at postmortem examinations, show a high percentage of involvement of the brain and upper abdomen. Elective brain irradiation has been adovated for treatment of brain metastases. Today such treatment may be facilitated and targeted by CT and scans, lymphograms, interventional angiography with biopsy, scintigrams with gallium and other radionuclides.

These and similar sensitive and specific techniques are identifying an increasing percentage of newly diagnosed BPC patients as ineligible for definitive resection. This increases the burden of responsibility for the radiotherapist to demonstrate efficacious treatment in a larger percentage of the total number of patients.

Fortunately, many new modalities and techniques are now available to enhance the planning and delivery of treatment. Some of these will be discussed in the pages that follow, but a few more words about the current status of lung cancer are submitted to put the increasingly important role of radiation management in the appropriate context. The central role which the radiotherapist must now assume in this disease makes a broad view and comprehensive approach essential to him at this time.

INCIDENCE AND MORTALITY

Carcinoma of the lung is more common in those exposed to fibrogenic pulmonary insults (e.g., coal miners). The average age at onset is approximately 60 years, the peak incidence is from 50-60 years. Although recent statistics include much younger men, less than 1% of cases occur under the age of 30, 10% of the cases occur over the age of 70.

The incidence of lung cancer has shown a very dramatic and rapid rise in the past several years. For example, in 1976, there were an estimated 93,000 new cases diagnosed, 73,000 males and 20,000 females. Only 4 years later, in 1980, there were 117,000 new cases of lung cancer. Its incidence, for the first time, has exceeded colorectal cancer. Thus, lung cancer is now the most common deep cancer, exceeded only by that of skin cancer. To make matters worse, the overall 5-year survival rate has remained unchanged since its diagnosis was first accurately recorded in 1913.

This lethality is grimly testified to by the 101,300 deaths in 1980. The death rate in men has risen steeply since 1945, from 14 per 100,000 to 76 per 100,000, and is doubling every 10 years. In women, the rate began to rise steeply in 1965 and is now about where it was for men in 1950, foreboding ill for the future unless dramatic advances are made.

ETIOLOGY AND PREVENTION

The risk of epidermoid, large or small cell bronchopulmonary carcinoma in male smokers exceeds the risk in nonsmokers by a factor of 20. Adenocarcinoma was, at one time, not thought to be related to smoking. However, male smokers have been found to have increased risk.

Thus, tobacco is causally associated with most forms of lung cancer. More specifically, cigarettes are reputed to be responsible for 95% of squamous cell and 90% of oat cell carcinomas. Squamous cell carcinoma is rarely encountered in nonsmokers. Though cigarette smoke is itself a carcinogen, other etiological factors (e.g., asbestos) can interact with it to produce additive and synergistic effects.

Other carcinogens include arsenic, chromates, radon (and other radioactive materials), coke gas, nickel, iron ore, bis-chloromethyl ether, isopropyl oil, petroleum mists, and mustard gas. Atmospheric pollution has also been implicated in view of the higher incidence of lung cancer in urban areas.

The intercalation of two or more factors may produce a risk much greater than the sum of the individual risks combined. For example, among asbestos workers, one death out of five is due to lung cancer. The risk to these workers is 6-19 times greater than in the general population and increases to 92 times greater for heavy smokers as compared to nonsmokers not exposed to asbestos.

The incidence of smoking by teenage girls is a grave concern today. According to a 1979 survey, nearly 13% of teenage girls between the ages of 12 and 18 are smokers, a rate 2% higher than that for teenage boys. This represents a marked change from the 1950s-mid-1970s when girls were less likely to start smoking than boys, and those who did, started at a later age. More than half of the girls in the 1979 study reported smoking before the age of 13. The cancer risk is higher and the onset earlier for those who start smoking at an early age.

DETECTION AND SCREENING

Many lung cancer screening studies have been conducted here and abroad. Sputum cytologies have also been used to screen for occult lesions. If cytology is positive and radiographs negative, these patients have received bronchial wash-out studies for localization. Such studies in high-risk groups have been shown to detect occult, presumably curable cancers. However, none of these studies, here or abroad, have demonstrated an improvement in survival over screened as opposed to control patients. In fact, there is concern and some data which indicate that there may be an increased morbidity and mortality associated with the diagnostic interventions in false positive patients.

Many biological markers (e. g., immunoactive ACTH) have been identified which correlate well with BPC, also offering promising new tools for screening as well as posttreatment monitoring. These and similar techniques have important long-range potential but offer no immediate solutions for today's lung cancer patients. It may well be that the seeming ineffectiveness of screening studies to improve survival may be more an indictment of the therapy subsequently administered than the efficacy of the screening. The American Cancer Society currently recommends against screening approaches, even in high-risk populations. Instead, it stresses the use of preventive measures such as the use of low-tar cigarettes. Ironically, recent reports of an adverse health potential of flavor enhancing additives in such cigarettes may result in repudiation of this approach as well.

The setbacks in prevention and screening programs underscore the importance of optimizing patient management to reduce the mortality in the patient population encountered today and in the immediate future. In point of fact, there is evidence that if every smoker gave up cigarettes tomorrow the lag time in the appearance of undetected lesions already in an irreversible stage would provide vast numbers of victims requiring definitive treatment for years to come.

HISTOPATHOLOGY

Most clinical management decisions in the past have only required differentiation between small cell and nonsmall cell BPC. The terminology of the World Health Organization (WHO) has been widely utilized for record purposes and consequently, has demonstrated significant differences in clinical behavior and natural history based on histological characteristics.

The major WHO categories may be briefly summarized as follows:

1. Squamous cell carcinoma: well differentiated to poorly differentiated

2. Adenocarcinoma (includes bronchioalveolar cell carcinoma): well differentiated to poorly differentiated

3. Large cell anaplastic carcinoma

4. Small cell anaplastic carcinoma: includes oat cell

5. Other rarer types include: mesothelioma, sarcoma, melanoma, and other but not thymoma or lymphoma

The histopathological criteria for these categories have been established by WHO. However, there is considerable interobserver disagreement in the more anaplastic group (80%) and between repeat observations by single observers. These inconsistencies in the correlation of the WHO have been recorded by many workers. Therefore, they have recommended the use of the Working Party for Lung Cancer Therapy (WP-L) classification. Portions of both are compared in Table 1.

Because of these disagreements and controversies a group is now considering a number of major changes in the WHO classification. Modification of the radiotherapeutic approach based on sophisticated histopathological classification is a potentially important new direction, since data has accumulated which indicates patterns of spread are significantly different for different histologies. For example, solitary cranial metastases are found in large cell BPC in a much higher percentage than other histologies (possible justification for elective cranial radiotherapy in large cell carcinoma). Therefore, refinement in histopathology between simple small cell and nonsmall cell histologies will become increasingly meaningful in the near future.

For purposes of completeness the remainder of the WHO classification is presented below:

V. Combined epidermoid and adenocarcinomas

VI. Carcinoid tumors

VII. Bronchial gland tumors
   1. Cylindromas
   2. Mucoepidermoid tumors
   3. Others

Table 1. Comparison of the Histopathological Classifications Established by the World Health Organization and the Working Party for Lung Cancer Therapy

WHO Classification	WP-L Classification
I. Epidermoid carcinoma	10. Epidermoid carcinoma
	11. Well differentiated
	12. Moderately differentiated
	13. Poorly differentiated
II. Small cell anaplastic carcinoma	20. Small cell anaplastic carcinoma
1. Fusiform	21. Lymphocyte-like (oat cell)
2. Polygonal	22. Intermediate cell (fusiform, polygonal, others)
3. Lymphocyte-like (oat cell)	
4. Others	
III. Adenocarcinoma	30. Adenocarcinoma
1. Bronchogenic	31. Well differentiated
a. Acinar	32. Moderately differentiated
b. Papillary	33. Poorly differentiated
2. Bronchioalveolar	34. Bronchioalveolar/papillary
IV. Large cell carcinoma	40. Large cell carcinoma
1. Solid tumors with mucin	(40/30) with much protection
2. Solid tumors without mucin	(40/10) with stratification
3. Giant cell	41. Giant cell
4. Clear cell	42. Clear cell

VIII. Papillary tumors of the surface epithelium
1. Epidermoid
2. Epidermoid with goblet cells
3. Others

IX. "Mixed" tumors and carcinomas
1. "Mixed" tumors
2. Carcinosarcomas of the embryonal type
3. Other carcinosarcomas

X. Sarcomas

XI. Unclassified

XII. Mesotheliomas
1. Localized
2. Diffuse

XIII. Melanomas; benign lesions of the lung mimicking malignant tumors
1. Sclerosing hemangiomas
2. Plasma cell granulomas
3. Pseudolymphomas

ANATOMY AND ROUTES OF SPREAD

Primary Site

The mucosa of the bronchus is the usual site of origin of cancer of the lung. The right and left main bronchus divide into lobar bronchi for the upper, middle, and lower lobes on the right, and the upper and lower lobes on the left. Fifty percent of lung cancers occur in the upper lobes, 20% in the lower lobes, 5% in the right middle lobe, and 25% are hilar or involve two lobes. Peripheral nodules tend to be adenocarcinomous, while squamous and small cell cancer tend to cause central masses. Squamous cancer can undergo central cavitation. Adenocarcinomas may more likely arise at the site of old scars. Calcification may occur in both benign and malignant lesions.

Nodal Stations and Lymphogenous Spread

The principal pathways in the dissemination of lung cancer in the order of frequency are the lymph drainage system, the blood vascular system, and direct tumor invasion. By far the most common spread is through the lymphatic vessels to the regional lymph nodes. The first-station lymph nodes are intrapulmonary, peribronchial, and hilar. Second-station lymph nodes are those in the mediastinum. Scalene and more distant nodes are considered distant metastases.

The pulmonary lymph capillaries drain into the hilar nodes, to the mediastinal nodes, and to the supraclavicular and jugular nodes. The right-sided lymph nodes drain the left lower lobe (LLL) as well as the entire right lung. Therefore, care must be taken to include the right supraclavicular area in radiotherapy for LLL lesions. The left-sided lymph nodes drain the left upper lung and the lingula. The lymphatics from the lower lobes course through the substance of the upper lobes. Hilar node metastases occurs in about 60% of right upper lobe (RUL) and right middle lobe (RML) lesions, and in approximately 75% of tumors arising in the remainder of the lung. Mediastinal adenopathy is found in 40-50% of operative specimens, except with RML lesions, where it is less common. Supraclavicular node metastasis predominates on the ipsilateral side with an incidence of up to 30% in RUL, RML, and left upper lobe (LUL) tumors.

Influence of Histology on Patterns of Spread

1. Squamous cell carcinoma: These lesions tend to remain localized to the thorax, but may metastasize to bone, liver, kidney, adrenals, and brain. Involvement of hilar and mediastinal lymph nodes is common, as well as spread to the pleura, the diaphragm, the opposite lung and cardiovascular system. Forty-six percent of patients have no spread outside of the thorax at autopsy.

2. Adenocarcinomas: As compared to epidermoid, these lesions tend to metastasize more widely to the regional nodes, adrenals, liver, bone, kidney, and central nervous system. However, these lesions may also remain intrathoracic, particularly bronchioalveolar histologies.

3. Small cell anaplastic carcinomas: A very high percentage of these lesions tend to be disseminated at the time of diagnosis. Bone marrow is involved in the majority of cases. Metastases will be found in regional nodes, abdominal nodes, opposite lung, pancreas, liver, adrenals, bone, central nervous system, and endocrine organs. The longest survivors in the NCI registry, however, are early-stage patients treated surgically in this entity, usually not considered appropriate for surgical management.

4. Large cell anaplastic carcinomas: These lesions tend to metastasize in patterns similar to those of adenocarcinomas with a predilection for mediastinal nodes, pleura, liver, adrenals, cardiacs, bone, and central nervous system. There is an unusual tendency to metastasize in the mucosa and submucosa of the gastrointestinal tract. Solitary metastasis to the brain is most common in this group.

Metastases by Way of the Blood Vascular System

The most recent frequent site of blood-borne metastasis may be the adrenal gland. In a necropsy study of 676 patients, 296 (43.8%) had metastases to the adrenal glands. The next most frequent site was the liver (289 cases or 42.7%). Anaplastic or oat cell cancers metastasized to the liver in over half the cases, adenocarcinomas (42%) and squamous cell. The incidence of adrenal and liver metastases underscores the need for careful assessment of patients for surgical resection or radiation therapy.

Patterns of Spread in Irradiated Patients

In 48 autopsied cases of irradiated, apparently localized lung cancer, metastasis was found in the liver in 35%, the bones in 33.3%, the adrenals in 28%, the kidneys in 18.7%, and the brain in 8.7% (Table 2).

The peripancreatic nodes and the nearby paraaortic nodes were a particularly notable area of involvement. The upper abdomen between the thoracic cavity and the pelvic brim (diaphragm included) was the seat of malignant disease in 25 patients (52%). In 14 of these, the tumor cells were confined to the thorax and the upper abdomen, while in 10 cases they were associated with bone metastases, and in 1 spread to the brain. A similar pattern of metastatic spread has been reported in other series.

Table 2. Comparison of the Mode of Metastasis in Different Series

	Abadir (%) (2)	Galluzzi (%) (81)	Ochsner (%) (125)
Liver	35.5	39.3	33.3
Adrenal	20.8	33.5	20.3
Kidney	18.7	15.4	17.5
Brain	8.7	25.7	16.5
Bones	33.3	14.6	21.3

CLINICAL SIGNS AND SYMPTOMS

A change in pulmonary habit is the most significant harbinger of lung cancer. It is hardly necessary to review the presenting symptoms of BPC since the frequency of this disease constantly reinforces them in the mind of the radiation oncologist. Although squamous and large cell cancers usually present with symptoms due to intrathoracic spread, there is a persistent tendency to assume that occult spread has already occurred. This is in large part due to systemic toxicity and paraneoplastic syndromes so often associated with the disease. These, taken together with its grim prognosis, may persuade the radiotherapist to withhold comprehensive evaluation and aggressive radiation in order to spare the patient morbidity and the next of kin financial burden. It is unlikely that the present mortality rate will improve if this philosophy continues. As mentioned in some series, up to 75% of squamous cell BPC patients are found to have disease limited to the thorax on biopsy. Small cell and adenocarcinoma more often present well-defined symptoms of distant metastases, but here again, clinical manifestations are varied and mimic other pulmonary (and nonpulmonary) conditions.

Local disease and intrathoracic extension may commonly be associated with cough, hemoptysis, and excessive pinkish sputum, while hoaraseness results from recurrent nerve palsy. Pain in the lateral chest may be due to pleural nerve or rib involvement, while with the upper chest lesions neuritic radiation to the homolateral upper extremity may occur. Horner syndrome (ptosis, miosis, and anhydrosis) is classically associated with superior sulcus tumor. Obstruction with superior vena caval symptoms or phrenic nerve palsy with elevated diaphragm may occur with disease limited to the thorax. Symptoms ordinarily attributed to extrathoracic disease, such as weight loss, fatigue, dyspnea, convulsions, headache, nausea, personality changes, and even pathological fractures may all occur with intrathoracic lesions due to toxicity or paraneoplastic syndromes.

It is well documented that these manifestations in lung cancer may reflect the high percentage of patients with paraneoplastic syndromes in great variety. These syndromes are due to the systemic effects often associated with localized tumors rather than to systemic metastases. Therefore, patients who present with systemic symptoms must not be assumed to be incurable patients with disseminated cancer. Often radiation treatment of the primary tumor will lead to reversal of these syndromes. Some of the more common paraneoplastic syndromes include:

1. Hypercalcemia associated with parathormone or prostaglandin production is a life-threatening condition which is all too often seen in untreated squamous cell BPC and may be refractory to systemic measures. When it occurs, fatal outcome is not uncommon.

2. Hypercorticism due to ACTH production (Cushing syndrome, pigmentation, obesity, osteoporosis, hypokalemia, impaired glucose tolerance, hypertension, with increased urinary excretion of 17-hydroxy corticoids and 17-ketosteroids, suppressed by corticosteroids) is most common in small cell BPC.

3. Gynecomastia associated with HCG production is more frequent in large cell BPC.

4. Migratory thrombophlebitis, nonbacterial endocarditis and disseminated intravascular coagulation (DIC) are examples of grave cardiovascular manifestations.

5. Dermatomyositis and acenthosis negricans are examples of dermatological syndromes.

6. Encephalopathy and peripheral neuropathy are potentially reversible neurological syndromes.

7. Inappropriate antidiuretic hormone syndrome is not uncommon in small cell BPC.

8. Myasthenic (Eaton-Lambert) syndromes are not as well known as some of the foregoing, and may be more subtle in onset, particularly in a patient with prior symptoms of systemic toxicity.

9. Hypertrophic pulmonary osteoarthropathy because of its dramatic radiological bony changes and physical findings is the best known syndrome.

It is important to differentiate between these syndromes and cerebral metastases, common enough that a chest film is mandatory to rule out BPC.

Immunological depression is also very common with even localized disease and is more impaired in this cancer than others. This depression is reflected in skin tests to recall antigens (PPD, mumps, varidase, candida, PHA blastogenesis in vitro, sensitization to DNCB) and in absolute lymphocyte count. Immunoreactive ACTH levels may be depressed. Because most prospective and retrospective studies show a strong correlation between patient survival and the initial performance status (IPS) of the patient (or host) several systems have been used to record the patient's activity and symptoms. The most common are summarized in Table 3.

STAGING CLASSIFICATIONS

The classification and staging system currently advocated for use in the United States is that promulgated by the American Joint Committee (AJC) (1978) (13). This differs in some respects from the system formerly recommended which was devised by the International Union Against Cancer (UICC). It should be noted particularly that there is no T4 category in the AJC system, nor is there an N3 or N4 category. The former T4 category as been absorbed by the present T3, and metasis to the supraclavicular nodes is now considered to be metastatic (M) rather

Table 3. Initial Performance Status

AJCC	ECOG/Zubrod Scale (161)	Karnofsky Scale (%) (108)
H0: Normal activity	0	90-100
H1: Symptomatic but ambulatory, cares for self	1	70-80
H2: Ambulatory more than 50% of the time, occasionally needs assistance	2	50-60
H3: Ambulatory less than 50% of the time, needs nursing care	3	30-40
H4: Bedridden, may need hospitalization	4	10-20

than nodal (N) disease. The American Joint Committee for Cancer Staging (AJCCS) includes a surgical and pathologic staging system as well. The clinical staging system is summarized below, the detailed system is available in the American Joint Committee for Cancer Staging (1978) manual (13).

Abbreviated definitions of T (tumor), N (node), and M (metastases) categories for carcinoma of the lung and the associated stage grouping according to the AJCCS (139) are summarized below (Tables 4-6), with the RTOG modifications (98) (Table 7) in use for the advanced stages, on the pages that follow, since the majority of radiotherapy patients are advanced categories for which the AJCCS is not adequate.

Table 4. Classification and Staging of Primary Tumors (T)

	T1	T2	T3
Size	< 3 cm	< 3 cm	Any
Location	Lobar bronchus or beyond	Lobar bronchus or more than 2 cm from carina	May be less than 2 cm from carina
Atelectasis/ pneumonitis	None	Less than entire lung	May be entire lung
Pleural involvement	None	Visceral pleura no effusion	Pleural effusion
Extrapulmonary extension	None	None	Any

Table 5. Classification and Staging of Regional Nodes (N)

	N0	N1	N2
Peribronchial and hilar nodes	-	+	-
Mediastinal nodes	-	-	+

Table 6. Stage Grouping

Stage 1
T1N0M0
T2N0M0
T1N1M0

Stage 2
T2N1M0

Stage 3
T3 any N or M
N2 any T or M
M1 any T or N

Simplified Staging for Small Cell Bronchopulmonary Carcinoma

Stage A, localized: solitary nodule or regional; resectable. Stage B, limited disease (LD): unresectable but limited to one hemithorax (may involve scalene nodes). Stage C, extensive disease (ED): extrathoracic spread. Recent recommendations advocate a shift to the AJCC or its RTOG modification for better classification of small cell BPC. For example, Shields et al. (149) indicate that "The American Joint Committee has suggested that patients with undifferentiated small cell tumors should not be classified by this schema, since all such patients have a poor prognosis regardless of the extent of the disease." However, recent data reported by Higgins (97) and Stott (154) suggest that patients with peripheral small cell tumor classified as T1N0M0 may achieve satisfactory long-term survival after resection. Further, the data from the various chemotherapy studies reviewed by Bunn and his colleagues (33,34,35) show that patients with undifferentiated small cell carcinoma and limited disease (stages I, II, and limited Stage II disease) have a higher incidence of complete response than those with extensive (disseminated) stage II disease. Therefore, it is appropriate to tentatively classify even the patients with undifferentiated small cell carcinoma by this schema.

Table 7. RTOG Stage Grouping of Carcinoma of the Lung

Stage 0:	T-X, N-0, M-0	An occult carcinoma based upon positive cytology.
Stage I:	T-1, N-0, M-0	A tumor that can be classified T-1 without any spread to nodes or distant metastases.
Stage II:	T-2, N-1, M-0 T-2, N-0, M-0 T-2, N-1, M-0	A T-2 pulmonary intrathoracic tumor or spread to the ipsilateral hilar nodes only (N-1) or both T-2 and N-1.
Stage III:	T-3, N-0, N-1 N-2, with T-1 T-2, T-3, M-0	Any extrapulmonary extrathoracic tumor spread to the lymph nodes in the mediastinum.
Stage IV:	T-4* with any N, N-3** with any T M*** of any category	Extensive extrapulmonary invasion into the viscera and bone with extrathoracic but no regional spread, metastases may also be present.
* T-4	Extrapulmonary, intrathoracic extensive: a very extensive lesion, into the chest wall, viscera, and/or deep mediastinal structures. This does not include extrathoracic visceral metastasis.	
** N-3	Supraclavicular or biopsied scalene nodes.	
*** M-1	Solitary, isolated metastasis confined to one organ or anatomic site. This also applies to cervical, axillary, or abdominal celiac nodes.	
M-2	Multiple sites in one organ	
M-3	Multiple organ sites	

Source: Modified from Ref. 11.

STAGING WORKUP AND TREATMENT PLANNING

The refinement of diagnostic procedures and the advent of new technology has revolutionized our approaches to patient evaluation. These are probably the most significant new directions in the radiation management of BPC. Failures to adequately define the extent and location of the tumor and the physical status of the patient are almost inevitably associated with therapeutic failure. Staging workup has been arbitrarily divided into three phases, which ordinarily should occur in sequence (and for which the AJCC has developed appropriate protocols) as follows:

Clinical-diagnostic staging: This should be based on the anatomic extent of the disease that can be detected by examination before thoracotomy or the implementation of any treatment. Such an examination may include a medical history, physical examination, routine and special roentgenograms, endoscopic examinations including bronchoscopy, esophagoscopy, mediastinoscopy, mediastinotomy, thoracentesis, or thoracoscopy and any other examinations, including those used to demonstrate the presence of extrathoracic metastasis.

Surgical evaluative staging: This should be based on all of the data obtained for the clinical diagnostic classification and on information obtained at the time of exploratory thoracotomy, including biopsy but not including that information obtained by complete examination of a therapeutically resected specimen.

Postsurgical treatment-pathologic staging: The surgical pathology report, and all other available data, should be used to assign a postsurgical treatment classification to those patients who have a resection.

Retreatment staging: In the course of follow-up examinations, a patient may manifest evidence of progressive disease indicating treatment failure. Before initiating further treatment, the extent of tumor should be carefully reassessed, using all available information, and the patient should again be staged under the retreatment classification.

Autopsy staging: In case of death of a lung cancer patient, the extent of the cancer, if any found at autopsy, may be recorded by the TNM system and an autopsy stage may be reported.

Clinical-Diagnostic Staging and Evaluation

The procedures recommended for clinical evaluation subsequent to targeted history taking and physical examination with specific attention to the unique features of this disease are as follow.

Conventional Radiographic Procedures

PA and lateral chest films with selective skeletal studies as indicated.

Special Radiologic Procedures

Fluoroscopy, conventional tomography, bronchography, and angiography may be used to further define the nature and extent of involvement demonstrated by conventional radiography. Tomograms (55 degree oblique views of the hilum) are valuable for determining the extent of the primary tumor, particularly valuable in radiation treatment planning. But it is in the area of interventional radiologic procedures in the form of either percutaneous angiographic or transcutaneous approaches directly to the area of interest (e.g., a peripheral nodule) that some of the most significant advances are occurring. Percutaneous angiographic techniques can demonstrate the site, location, and extent of tumors, the degree of tumor vascularity, and the possibilities for hyperthermia in hypervascular tumors. Selective transarterial occlusion with hyperthermia, selective beta radiation membrane sensitizing, and chemotherapeutic agents are therapeutic modifications of this technique.

Sputum Cytology

Lung cancers detected when occult (chest x-ray negative, sputum cytology positive) have the highest cure rates. Early diagnosis of lung cancer rests on accurate sputum cytology by the Papanicolaou technique. Adequate methods of induced sputum collection, the blending and centrifugation of sputum, and the making of smears is essential to diagnose lung cancer early in high-risk individuals. A clearly positive cytology is probably 95% accurate. A negative one cannot be relied upon, but when optimal procedures are followed, it may be positive and as high as 85% accurate with bronchopulmonary carcinoma when early morning deep expectoration is used. Routine bronchial washings at the time of bronchoscopy do not yield as good results as the sputum examinations performed after bronchoscopy.

Bronchoscopy or Rigid Bronchoscopy

1. Conventional fiberoptic or rigid bronchoscopy: Selective bronchiolar washout techniques with fiberoptic scopes can identify even occult lesions. Bronchoscopy is done in most cases unless the lesion is peripheral, in which case percutaneous needle biopsy is preferable. An accessible metastatic lesion may be biopsied for diagnosis as well as staging. For bronchial brush biopsies a controllable brush and a new controllable guide have been developed. Selective bronchial catheterization, done like arterial catheterization, has returned a positive tissue diagnosis in 81% (35 of 41) of suspected cases. This procedure is applicable to small and peripheral nodules.

2. Serial bronchoscopy: Serial bronchoscopy evaluation during the course of radiotherapy is advocated for assessing the response of small cell BPC, since local failures have been reported with the time-dose regimens employed in several series. It has also been advocated by some workers in nonsmall cell BPC to evaluate response to conventional regimens, particularly with bronchostenosing lesion associated with atelectasis in which reversal of atelectasis is sought.

3. Fluorescence fiberoptic bronchoscopy: Diagnosing occult lung cancers by fiberoptic bronchoscopy has been difficult, necessitating differentially brushing the many lobar bronchi. Twenty-five to fifty percent of occult cancers will not be visualized by routine fiberoptic bronchoscopy. Bronchoscopic examination with extensive selective brushings of numerous segments and lobes may have to be repeated, even up to four or five times. This problem in localization has led to the development of fluorescence bronchoscopy. Fluorescence bronchoscopy offers distinct advantages, and is sensitive and accurate in (1) the diagnosis of lung cancer early and (2) determining the extent of the carcinoma, and thus, allowing the oncologist to make better decisions regarding therapy. In this technique hematoporphyrin derivative is injected intravenously (2 mg/kg). The patient is bronchoscoped at 72 hr, by means of a two-channel bronchoscope. One channel contains a quartz fiber capable of conducting violet light (400 mm). Small bronchial cancers fluoresce, emitting red light, and are observed through an image intensifier attached to the eyepiece of the bronchoscope. This is due to the fact that hematoporphyrin is retained in the cancer cells at a greater concentration and for a longer period of time than normal cells. There is a contrast background upon exposure to violet light. Fluorescence bronchoscopy has the potential to localize a small cancer plaque 1-1.5 mm in diameter and 100 μm thick, similar to the size of a small area of carcinoma in situ.

With the advent of fiberoptic and fluorescent bronchoscopy, better localization and visualization of the endobronchial involvement is now possible and a schematic notation of the findings should be recorded using the AJCCS mapping nomenclature of the bronchopulmonary segment to delineate the extent of pulmonary involvement.

Scalene Biopsy

This should be done if a node is palpable, and, if positive, is classified as M1 (AJCC-N3 RTOG) and generally considered to show unresectability unless adjuvant radiation is planned. It yields positive findings of metastases in 20-30% of the cases. As mentioned above, the right scalene fat pad drains the right lung and left lower lobe. The left scalene fat pad drains the lingula and upper left lobe. If the scalene fat pad biopsy contains metastatic cells, thoracotomy without radiation treatment is contraindicated. If nothing is palpable in the supraclavicular area, a positive rate of 10% makes biopsy unrewarding.

Mediastinoscopy or Mediastinotomy

Mediastinoscopy affords a method of obtaining intrathoracic tissue for microscopic study without thoracotomy. Mediastinal lymph node involvement, which might be detected by mediastinoscopy, is present in 75% of the patients.

Ordinarily, indications for surgical mediastinal involvement either by cervical mediastinoscopy or mediastinotomy include the presence of a large undifferentiated peripheral tumor, an abnormal hilar or mediastinal shadow, a hilar or mediastinal shadow obscured by the tumor or associated with parenchymal changes, and positive mediastinal gallium scan.

Mediastinoscopy should be done before a thoracotomy, unless other signs of unresectability are present. Involvement of interlobar nodes does not markedly affect prognosis, but mediastinal involvement does. The 5-year survival is almost 40% if the mediastinum is free of tumor but less than 10% when it is involved (unless postresection irradiation is used). In addition, contralateral involvement is common, especially with cancer of the left lung and with poorly differentiated cancers. If a tumor is found in the contralateral nodes, thoracotomy is contraindicated. The procedure can cause bleeding, pneumothorax, and mediastinal emphysema, but mortality is rare.

Percutaneous Needle Biopsy

This technique is particularly valuable for peripheral nodules. The risks of seeding needle tract and pneumothorax, and of hemorrhage are low in the hands of an experienced surgeon or radiologist. Histological confirmation of diagnosis may be forthcoming only after exploration and direct biopsy of the tumor or of its metastases. A preoperative microscopic diagnosis is made in approximately 50% of cases. The percutaneous technique is also being used for intralesional BCG injection.

Radionuclide Scintigraphy

Some workers (58), feel that radionuclide studies such as ^{67}Ga scans of the thorax and mediastinum are routinely indicated. In the absence of clinical findings their clinical use to discover occult metastases is not considered to be indicated by others. We feel these studies are essential to determine the status of the lung, mediastinum, brain, liver, adrenal, and skeleton. If the skeletal scan is positive, then a search for specific targeted lesions can be made by specific site by detailed radiography, rather than doing skeletal surveys by conventional radiographs.

Evaluation of Hematological, Electrolyte, Nutritional, and Immunological Statuses

Hematological, electrolyte, nutritional and immunological statuses have been shown to be important independent prognostic factors in many lung cancer studies. Their evaluation is important in that they define specific management problems, many of them life threatening, and furnish guidance for nutritional medical support.

Hematological studies ordinarily consist of RBC, WBC, hematocrit, differential, and platelets. Total blood lymphocyte counts also yield information in regard to immunological status. Hemoglobin below 10 and hematocrit below 30 are usually managed by transfusion.

The nutritional status of the muscle compartment can be assessed by the 24-hr urine creatinine and the nutritional status of the visceral compartment by the serum albumins and iron-binding protein levels.

Nutritional evaluation should also include documentation of weight and history of weight loss (more than 10 lb is an adverse prognostic sign) and performance status (less than 60 is also an adverse sign).

Immunological testing may include recall skin tests, immunoglobulin quantification by immunodiffusion (IgG, IgA, IgM), B cell quantitation (sIg and EAC), T cell quantitation (E rosettes), and mitogen-induced lymphocyte transformation (PHA, ConA, PWM). These and total lymphocyte counts may be an important means of demonstrating immunosuppression which is prevalent.

It is likely that the prognostic effect of weight loss is mediated via effects on body protein nutritive status. Nutritional support with or without anabolic agents may reverse negative nitrogen balance and immunological parameters. Dietary supplements, enteric and parenteric hyperalimentation (peripheral and central), and other approaches to patient support including psychosocial measures may be employed.

However, in studies where nutritional repletion with intravenous hyperalimentation (IVH) was undertaken, those patients with initial cell-mediated immunoincompetent responses had greater body weight loss, lower serum albumin concentration and total lymphocyte count, and had a decreased response to treatment or an increase in treatment morbidity and mortality when compared with patients who initially had cell-mediated immunocompetent responses.

Bioassays and Tumor Markers

A number of circulating substances (some of them hormonal) may be found in lung cancer. They may aid in detecting recurrence and in following the response of the disease to therapy. CEA is currently regarded as the most important. It is elevated in about half of the patients with advanced lung cancer, its level correlates with the stage of the disease, and it can be elevated in all histological types (but infrequently in large cell).

Placental alkaline phosphatase may be present. Hormones including HCG and HPL (more common in large cell cancer) may be associated with gynecomastia. Parathormone and prostaglandin (more common is squamous cell cancer) may be associated with hypercalcemia.

A variety of products have been reported in small cell cancer. These include normal and "big" ACTH (may cause Cushing syndrome), ADH, renin (may cause hypokalemia), serotonin, and related compounds. Histaminase, erythropoiesis suppressor (causing pure red carcinoid syndrome), l-dopa-decarboxylase, and others. These small cell markers may vary between lesions and patients, thus limiting their usefulness at present.

Bone Marrow Biopsy

Bone marrow biopsies produce a 50% positive result in oat cell cancers at diagnosis in contrast to 20% for other types. This is a mandatory procedure for patients with small cell carcinoma before treatment planning is begun.

Pulmonary Function and
Radionuclide Imaging Studies

With increasing use of upper hemibody irradiation, levamisole, misonidazole, and polyagent chemotherapy, pulmonary function and toxicity have become the dose-limiting factor in many radiotherapy regimens. Fatal pulmonary toxicity has been reported at dose levels now in use. Pulmonary reactions are the most common reason for terminating levamisole treatment. A long list of other pulmonary toxic agents are regularly employed in management. Tailoring of portals and techniques to spare functional rather than nonfunctional pulmonary tissue cannot be accomplished with conventional chest x-rays, since carcinoma of the bronchus may alter both ventilation and perfusions. These tumors derive their blood supply from the bronchial arteries, so that they appear as defects on perfusion scans. Small tumors (less than 2 or 3 cm in diameter) are not usually detected, unless they involve vessels at the hilum. Larger tumors produce perfusion defects that correspond to the size of the tumor, or the involved segment or lobe or even the entire lung. The larger the perfusion defect in relation to the size of the tumor, the greater the involvement of the hilar vessels by the tumor. Such involvement may be due to metastatic spread to the lymph nodes, direct invasion of the mediastinum, or, less commonly, invasion and thrombosis of the pulmonary veins, or still more rarely of the pulmonary arteries.

Pulmonary function studies are an essential part of a patient's evaluation prior to surgical evaluation by thoracotomy. The maximum voluntary ventilation (MVV) with a forced expiratory volume in 1 sec ($FEV/_1$) is the more useful predictor of ability to undergo surgery. Abnormalities for carbon dioxide are more important than for oxygen. Pulmonary resection is usually possible if the FEV_1 is greater than 50% of the total forced capacity, or greater than 2 L if the MVV is greater than 50% of the predicted and if the partial pressure of carbon dioxide is normal.

In patients who have borderline pulmonary status, further studies could include split pulmonary function testing by bronchial spirometry, radioactive xenon, radiospirometry, or xenon scanning, together with right heart catheterization with temporary unilateral pulmonary arterial occlusion. The criteria of operability in these individuals would be a mean pulmonary artery pressure after occlusion and exercise of less than 35 mm Hg and a predicted postpneumonectomy FEV_1 of greater than 8/20L.

Following radiation treatment for cancer of the bronchus some return of perfusion may be seen in about 40% of patients. The remainder show either no change or progressive reduction in perfusion. Ventilation tends to return earlier and more frequently. The restoration of blood flow is of no prognostic significance. Perfusion also decreases in radiation pneumonitis, which may result in severe damage to the pulmonary vasculature.

Computed Axial Tomography in
Clinical Evaluation and Follow-Up

Computed tomography has found wide acceptance in the evaluation of lung cancer patients. Such scans may help determine resectability, particularly in looking for enlarged hilar or mediastinal nodes. CT scan data leads to a change in the radiation portal in a high percentage of patients. In addition, CT scans of the upper abdomen can spare some patients a thoracotomy. This is because the incidence of metastasis in the upper abdomen is particularly high in lung cancer patients.

Surgical and Pathological Evaluation

Thoracotomy remains an important component of evaluation and staging in bronchopulmonary carcinoma, as well as the first step in definitive surgical treatment for the limited number of patients who are eligible for operation (15-20%); and thereafter, depending on thoracotomy findings, the even smaller number who may proceed to complete or partial resection.

In the past, thoracotomy, in the patients clinically staged as apparently localized or regionally extended disease, was thought to be contraindicated under the following circumstances: (1) when the lesion is within 2 cm of the carina; (2) nonresectable pulmonary metastases; (3) when the physiological or actual age is more than 70 years for pneumonectomy and 75 years for lobectomy; (4) when the pulmonary reserve is insufficient for the patient to tolerate loss of lung tissue required for curative resection; (5) when the anesthetic risk is great for other reasons, such as myocardial infarction or uncontrolled heart failure; (6) paralysis of the recurrent or phrenic nerves; and (7) cerebral, hepatic, or renal insufficiency. However, with today's new surgical techniques, radiation techniques, and combinations, thoracotomy may be carried out even when a number of those circumstances exist.

For example, one may now carry out thoracotomy (with preoperative radiation) in certain stage III patients including those with superior sulcus tumors, peripheral lesions with chest wall involvement, tracheocarinal lesions in which tracheobronchial reconstruction is planned, and patients with limited pulmonary function where sleeve lobectomy or intraoperative interstitial implantation, without definite resection, is envisioned for patients with inadequate pulmonary function.

About half of the patients present with tumors judged clinically to originate in the hilar region. Twelve percent are in the main bronchus, 34% are peripheral, and 7% apical tumors. The most favorable prognosis overall is seen for patients with tumors originating in a peripheral location. Squamous cell carcinoma originating in the main bronchus has a less favorable outcome than tumors in other locations. Unfortunately, over two-thirds of patients with squamous cell carcinoma presented with tumors on the hilus or main bronchus. Adenocarcinoma also has a bad prognosis in a central location; in this lesion 43% present as peripheral lesions and about 40% as hilar tumors.

Progressive erosion of survival expectations is evident as the disease extends to involve the first- and second-stage lymph nodes. Forty-eight percent of patients with no lymph node involvement survived 5 years. When the disease extends or metastasizes to involve lymph nodes within the lung, the survival dropped to 35%.

Further spread to the mediastinal lymph nodes is indicative of poor prognosis. Long-term survival is achieved by less than 10% of these patients even though all known disease has been resected, unless postresection radiation is employed.

Of patients with squamous cell carcinoma with hilar lymph node involvement, 40% survived. For patients with adenocarcinoma, the proportion that survived dropped to 24% and a similar observation was made in large cell carcinoma. The adverse effect of mediastinal lymph node involvement is evident in all cell types. However, the survival achieved for patients with squamous cell carcinoma and large cell carcinoma following definitive resection clearly exceeds the average surgical mortality. Thirteen percent of the patients with squamous cell carcinoma and 11% of those with large cell carcinoma survived 5 years. By contrast, only 2% of the patients with adenocarcinoma with this level of disease had long-term survival. For this reason, unless adjunctive treatment is planned, these patients with adenocarcinoma are not considered candidates for definitive resection.

About 12% of patients present with pleural effusion, which indicates a very poor prognosis, more so if the malignant cells are identified. For this reason, surgery is not considered a valid option in these T3 cases. Unresectable patients who may be eligible for intraoperative interstitial implantation are those with findings at thoracotomy of involvement of the great vessels, trachea, esophagus, limited chest wall, pleura, and pericardium.

All clinical stage I and II patients, who are physiologically able, are candidates for definitive resection. Those patients with regional extension of disease included in these categories have a disease classification of T1N1, or T2N1. The survivals for these groups following apparent complete resection are 52 and 31%, respectively. In many cases, however, attempted resections do not demonstrate lung cancer or are not carried to completion. Minet (121) in Liege analyzed 845 patients who were subjected to thoracotomy and found only 704 (83%) were histologically confirmed. Sixty-seven percent had a diagnosis of squamous cell carcinoma, 10% of adenocarcinoma, and 22% of small cell carcinoma. Of 472 squamous cell carcinomas resected, he found only one-third had complete resection while two-thirds had incomplete resections. For fully resected patients, the median survival was 17 months, while for unresected patients the medial survival was 8 months. All patients with incomplete resections were irradiated. Fifty percent of the complete resections were irradiated as borderline resectable patients (the decisions were made by the surgeon). The survivals are presented in Tables 8 and 9.

Taken in the context of the experience of Minet in which even "complete resections" showed residual disease 1 month or less after autopsy, a compelling need for effective postoperative radiation is demonstrated. Of the N1 and N2 patients, 25% were resected of which 75% of the partially resected patients were irradiated (again, those who, in the opinion of the surgeon were poor-risk patients).

Selected patients with certain stage III lesions are also considered candidates for definitive resection as mentioned above. Surgical therapy is considered a valid option in these patients where complete resection of all known tumor is anticipated, and in which there are biologically favorable signs. The survival overall is 16% at 5 years for these groups of patients if the surgery is combined with preoperative and/or postoperative radiation therapy. Also in this category are included the resected patients demonstrated to have positive lymph nodes.

Table 8. Median Survivals in Patients with Complete and Incomplete Resections

Procedure	Median Survival (Mo)
Complete resection	28
Complete resection plus no RT	26
Incomplete resection	17
Incomplete resection plus RT	48

Table 9. Median Survivals in Patients with Incomplete Resections and Inoperative Patients

Procedure	Median Survival (Mo)
Resected	30
Inoperative	6
Incomplete resection plus RT	14
Incomplete resection plus no RT	4

With unresectable lesions, interstitial implantation therapy may be done at thoracotomy and may be a more effective method than thoracotomy alone, particularly if followed by postoperative external irradiation to treat locoregional extension of disease.

An attractive feature of the intraoperative implantation process is that it converts a diagnostic or staging procedure for exploratory thoracotomy into a therapeutic one. Some of the advantages cited for intraoperative implantation are:

1. The radiation dose can be precisely localized.

2. Higher doses can be delivered to the tumor by the implant.

3. The dose is adaptable to the tumor shape and falls off rapidly outside the implanted volume, thus reducing damage to normal tissue.

4. The treatment time is much shorter; a permanent implant requires only a single procedure, whereas a complete course of radiation therapy requires 5-6 weeks. If preoperative or postoperative radiation therapy is used, the total number of treatments is lessened.

When interstitial implantation is carried out during the thoracotomy, if total resection has been performed, the entire tumor bed is implanted. If only partial resection or no resection is done, the entire tumor volume, including any positive lymph nodes, is implanted. Source used are ^{125}I seeds, in most cases, generally employing the Mick implantation gun. The minimum dose to the entire tumor volume is 12,000-16,000 rads over 1 year; the maximum dose is 18,000-20,000 rads over 1 year.

PREOPERATIVE IRRADIATION

Bloedorn et al. (23) reported no recognizable tumor cells at the primary site in 54% of a group of 26 patients treated with 6000 rads in 6 weeks preoperatively. The mediastinal nodes failed to show any cancer in 92% of the cases. Rubin (141) showed improved 1-year survival in patients with more than 5000 rads compared with patients treated with lower doses; on the other hand, Roswit (138,139) reported no difference in the survival rates of patients receiving doses of 5000-6000 rads in comparison with others treated with lower doses.

This group includes patients with a primary tumor classification of T3 and whose tumors are amenable to surgical treatment such as (1) those with peripheral tumors having direct extension into the parietal pleura and invasion of the intercostal muscle or ribs; (2) superior sulcus tumors with painful apical syndrome; (3) patients with small tumors located less than 2 cm from the carina, with no metastasis, that are amenable to tracheal-bronchial resection and reconstruction; (4) patients with peripheral lesions with direct invasion of the chest wall; and (5) technically resectable T3 lesions and N2 lesions where the extent of lymph node involvement is limited to the ipsilateral tracheobronchial area and/or subcarinal space.

The report of Paulson (127,128) on an extensive experience with surgical treatment of superior sulcus tumors illustrates that a combined treatment plan of preoperative irradiation and extended en bloc resection can provide meaningful long-term survival for patients with these T3 lesions. The overall survival on 100 patients was 33%. None of the patients with nodal involvement survived much more than 1 year, whereas nearly 50% of those whose disease was classified as N0 survived over 3 years.

The effectiveness of sleeve resection procedures for tumors in either stem bronchus or in the lower trachea has been reported. Survival for 85 patients who underwent sleeve lobectomy was 36% at 5 years in Jensik's series (106).

Patients who are candidates for tracheal sleeve pneumonectomy are those with centrally lying tumor obliterating the tracheobronchial angle or tumor extending to the carina or upward along the lateral wall of the trachea.

There is a high incidence of local persistence as well as dissemination and incisional recurrence in patients with peripheral lesions which invade the chest wall when not treated with adjunctive irradiation. This high incidence precludes addressing such lesions without preoperative and postoperative radiotherapy.

As shown earlier, stage II patients with N2 disease who have epidermoid (squamous cell) or large cell carcinoma and intranodal mediastinal involvement that is limited to the nodes of the tracheobronchial angle and/or subcarinal space have a more favorable prognosis following definitive resection. However, adjuvant therapy should be a part of the treatment plan either preoperative, postoperative, or pre- and post- (sandwich) radiation therapy.

Patients who are operable but technically unresectable and in whom intraoperative radiotherapy is under serious consideration have been discussed in the section on thoracotomy and will be further addressed in the section on Intraoperative Radiotherapy.

INTRAOPERATIVE RADIOTHERAPY OF BRONCHOPULMONARY CARCINOMA

Hilaris and Martini (94) report that interstitial implantation was first used in conjunction with a pneumonectomy in 1933 by Graham and Singer. At about the same time, Ormerod, from England, treated unresectable lung tumor by radon seeds introduced into the tumor by bronchoscope.

Although the results of interstitial implantation at thoracotomy have been encouraging, this form of treatment was limited to a few institutions for two reasons: (1) the technique of interstitial implantation required that the radiotherapist develop surgical experience in addition to the knowledge of radiotherapy, and (2) radiation exposure from high-energy radionuclides, such as ^{222}Rn, ^{198}Au, and ^{192}Ir was high and discouraged many radiotherapists. The introduction of low-energy ^{125}I sources in 1976 at Memorial Hospital removed some of these obstacles to interstitial implantation.

Clinical Considerations

The patient should tolerate anesthesia and thoracotomy with little or no risk. Preoperative assessment of the cardiac status and pulmonary reserve is essential. Age, in and of itself, is not a contraindication.

Nonsmall cell BPC, squamous cell, and adenocarcinoma are the main histological variants of lung cancer suitable for intraoperative radiation management.

The best results with interstitial radiation are achieved in small- to medium-sized tumors, not exceeding 6-7 cm in average dimension. Larger tumors involving more than one lobe or extending into the chest wall or mediastinum can also be implanted, provided partial or total resection is also done (7 cm without debulking). Patients with pleural effusion are generally not good candidates.

Methods of Implantation

The methods available today are either for permanent or temporary implantation at bronchoscopy. Temporary implants with ^{192}Ir were explored at Memorial Hospital for a short period from 1960-1961. The usefulness of this method is being reevaluated and since early 1977 has been used by us in nearly 50 patients. Endobronchial implants have been used for tracheal involvement as well as for recurrent tumor in major bronchi after resection and external radiotherapy and these results have been reported.

The permanent afterloading technique developed by Henschke (96) has been used at thoracotomy to treat unresectable lung cancer in all patients:

1. Permanent ^{125}I (thoracotomy, endobronchial)
2. Afterloading (1960-1961, 1977-1980 greater than 50 cases).

Tumors are exposed through a posterolateral thoracotomy. The total activity to be implanted is based on multiplying the average dimension in centimeters by a constant, which is 5.0 for ^{124}I. More recently, the activity has been read from a nomogram for which larger volumes results in activities larger than five times the average dimension. A spacing nomogram is also available which specifies the appropriate interval between uniformly spaced seeds.

From 1956-1973, 375 patients had unresectable lung cancer at the time of thoracotomy; 340 had no evidence of metastases outside of the chest at the time of treatment; and 35 patients had no metastases to cervical nodes prior to the planned thoracotomy. Some patients were treated with implantation only for cervical lymph nodes, or for other distant sites through bronchoscopy, or through an intact chest wall under radiographic guidance.

Results

External beam irradiation to the mediastinum and to the primary site was added only if: (1) all gross tumor could be implanted, (2) there were positive mediastinal lymph nodes, and (3) the implant dose distribution was deemed unsatisfactory.

Of 340 patients 17 died within 30 days of treatment, a postoperative mortality of 5%. Of the remaining 323 patients, 141 (41%) were alive at 1 year and 57 (17%) at 2 years from treatment; 24 patients (7%) lived 5 years or more. Of 13 patients, 6 (40%) with stage I unresectable carcinoma lived 5 years or more; there were no 5-year survivors in patients with stage II disease. Of 322 patients with stage III disease 18 (6%) were alive at 5 years.

Thirty-five patients were explored for palliative treatment with implantation although they had known metastases in supraclavicular nodes prior to thoracotomy. Of 35 patients 14 (40%) were alive 1 year after treatment, 5 (14%) at 2 years, and 2 (6%) at the end of 3 years.

The overall 20-day mortality was 5% (17 of 375). This compares well with the mortality rate of thoracotomy without implantation. Forty-three percent of 13 patients with stage I unresectable lung cancer survived 5 years or more. Although the number of patients is small, the results suggest that interstitial implantation is a successful alternative to surgery for patients with small lesions and negative nodes and who cannot tolerate resection. The observed locoregional failures (3 of 13) are due mainly to inadequate implantation and can be reduced by refinements in interstitial techniques as have taken place in recent years.

Locoregional control was achieved in nearly 70% of the treated patients with minimal impairment in the lung functions by radiation fibrosis. The poorest results were observed in patients who also had regional lymph node metastases. Both local recurrence and distant metastases were frequent in this group of patients. In an attempt to improve the outcome of these patients, we have recently combined partial resection with or without node dissection with permanent interstitial implantation of the residual primary tumor and temporary iridium implantation of the ipsilateral mediastinum. Postoperatively, these patients receive routine external beam radiation to the regional nodes and are given chemotherapy. It is too early to draw conclusions from this approach. Preliminary results suggest prolongation (Tables 10-14) of the median survival time but follow-up periods are still short.

DEFINITIVE IRRADIATION

The role of radiation therapy in the palliative treatment of lung cancer is unquestionable; its role in the definitive treatment of the disease remains controversial.

Table 10. Determinate Survival According to Histopathologic Findings Following Regional Node Dissection

Histological Findings	Patients at Risk	Determinate Survival (Year)				
		1	2	3	4	5
N0	182	88	41	28	22	19 (10%)
N1	10	5	3	2	0	0
N2	148	48	13	6	5	5 (3%)

Table 11. Distribution of Patients with Unresectable Lung Cancer Treated by Interstitial Radiation (1956-1973)

Surgical Stage	Surgical TNM	Number of Patients	%
I	T1N0M0	2	
	T2N0M0	10	3.5
	T1N1M0	1	
II	T2N1M0	5	1.3
III	T3N0M0	170	
	T3N1M0	4	
	T1N2M0	3	85.9
	T2N2M0	22	
	T3N2M0	123	
	Any T, N, M1	35	9.3

Total number of patients 375

Table 12. Determinant Survival According to Stage

Surgical Stage	Patients at Risk	Determinate Survival (Years)				
		1	2	3	4	5
I	13	10	8	6	6	6 (46%)
II	5	2	2	2	0	0
III	322	129	47	28	21	18 (6%)
I-III	340	141 (41%)	57 (17%)	36 (11%)	27 (8%)	24 (7%)

Table 13. Determinate Survival According to Histologic Type

Histologic Type	Patients at Risk	Determinate Survival (Years) 1	2	3	4	5
Epidermoid CA	270	111	43	27	21	18 (7%)
Adenocarcinoma	63	26	11	7	5	5 (8%)
Spindle and giant cell CA	7	4	3	2	1	1 (14%)

Table 14. Treatment Failures According to Stage

Surgical Stage	Patients at Risk	Locoregional Recurrences	Distant Metastases	Locoregional and Distant Failures
I	13	3	3	0
II	5	1	4	0
III				
(N0)	170	34	47	16
(N1)	4	1	3	0
(N2)	148	30	53	25
Total	340	69	110	41
		(20%)	(32%)	(12%)

Rationale

There has long been evidence that radiation therapy is potentially curative in patients with bronchopulmonary carcinoma (BPC) limited to the thorax and adjacent lymph node stations. Smart in 1956 reported a 23% 5-year survival after treatment with 4000-5000 rads (151). Guttman (89) during this same period reported a 57% 1-year survival and 17% 3-year survival with 5000 rads, although the figures at 4 years and 5 years fall off to 10 and 8% probably representing uncontrolled disease in the chest. The median survival was lengthened in treated patients to 27 months, compared to 6 months in untreated patients. The success of these series is related in large part to adequate radiation dose levels and careful patient evaluation. Since that time, many new modalities have been developed and applied in small cell bronchogenic carcinoma (SCBC), but actual treatment has changed little for the patients with squamous cell carcinoma, large cell carcinoma, and adenocarcinomas that account for 80% of all cancer of the lung. Only a small proportion of these patients (15-20%) are eligible for operative intervention for purpose of resection. This proportion has become smaller as preoperative diagnostic methods, such as computerized tomography (CT), become more sophisticated. As a result, approximately 25,000 patients each year are demonstrated to have localized but unresectable nonsmall cell cancer.

Until recently, early distant metastases were almost invariably held to be the major cause of poor survival in lung cancer, and this misconception is still present. Several recent reports, however, indicate that the major cause of failure in this disease is the inability to control the primary intrathoracic tumor in spite of aggressive radiation therapy. RTOG studies indicate that while 60% of patients treated with over 5000 rads fail with cancer, over one-half of these failures result from locoregional recurrence. Cox et al. (50) report that up to 75% of squamous cell patients die with disease limited to the thorax. Clearly, a need and opportunity exists to improve survival through improvements in radiation treatment.

Unfortunately, many tumors in the lung are large and doses may be needed in the range of 6000-7000 rads in 6-7 weeks, ordinarily above the tolerance of the dose-limiting structures. Therefore, it is not surprising that most dose schedules have utilized suboptimal tumor doses to avoid prohibitive normal tissue damage.

The upper dose that can be given is limited by the need to protect sensitive transit tissues and by the development of symptomatic esophagitis. The optimal dose of radiation necessary to sterilize squamous cell carcinoma with conventional fractionation is thought to be in the range of 5000-6500 rads or more for tumors larger than 3 cm although Bromley and Szur (27) noted in 1955 that localized cancer could be eradicated in about 40% of the cases with doses of 4700 rads.

RADIATION TREATMENT APPROACHES FOR IMPROVED LOCAL CONTROL AND NORMAL TISSUE SPARING

Split-Course Radiation

Split-course radiation has been claimed to give better local control of disease, and some unconventional fractionations have been reported to be more effective than conventional five times a week fractionation; but, no significant improvement in long-term survival has been demonstrated yet.

Lee (117) reported on a randomized trial of 188 cases of unresectable but potentially curable bronchogenic carcinoma treated with either a split or continuous course of 4500-5000 rads. The survival rates were similar.

Holsti's prospective study of 5500 rads split-course treatment compared with 5000 rads continuous daily fractionated treatment demonstrated no difference in survival or disease-free survival between the groups or the histological subgroups (squamous carcinoma, small cell carcinoma, or anaplastic carcinoma). The continuously treated responders did slightly better than the split-course treated responders (99,100).

These studies are in agreement with the reports of Levitt (118), Hazra (93), and others. On the other hand, a clear increase in survival was reported by Salazar with a moderately intensive split-course method (142). In a selected squamous cell carcinoma group, Aristizabal and Caldwell reported an excellent 16% 5-year survival with split-course therapy (16).

Also, Abramson and Cavanaugh compared patients given 6000 rads/6 weeks with those given a split course of 2000 rads/1 week, 3 weeks' rest, 2000 rads/1 week. The 1-year survival was better in the split course (43%) as compared to the continuous course (14%), although the 2-year survival was only 30% and the 3-year survival fell to 7%. Seventy-five percent of each group received relief of symptoms, but the split-course patients got relief sooner. The split course was better tolerated, and the complications were equal. Local control was achieved in 60% of the split-course patients (3,4).

For further evaluation, several RTOG lung studies have employed one or more split-course arms. In those analyzed to date, the continuous arms are equal or superior to the split course in response rate, local control, survival, and toxicity. The best fractionation schedules for irradiation in nonsmall cell lung cancer have not been established. For example, a randomized RTOG study number 75-01 comparing 4000 rad split course with 4000, 5000, and 6000 rads continous course was closed in August 1978 (140). The survival rates for the continuous regimens (45% 1-year survival and 25% 2-year survival) are superior in the split dose, the incidences of intrathoracic failure are: thirty-three percent of patients receiving 6000 rads failed in the chest, compared with 30% receiving 5000 rads, 49% receiving 4000 rads continuous course, and 44% receiving 4000 rads split course.

Multiple Daily Fractions (MDF)

Twice daily radiation treatment sessions of 120 rads each, at least 3 hr but no more than 6 hr apart have been studied in squamous cell upper respiratory lesions and in the thorax (esophagus) in RTOG study protocols. Experimental evidence and preliminary clinical experience indicates hyperfractionation can give better normal tissue tolerance and improve the therapeutic ratio. Specific application to NSCBC is in planning by Petrovich and others and holds promise for enhancing tolerance in extended fields to include upper abdominal disease extensions.

Extended Fractionation with High-Dose Increments

Mohiuddin et al. (122) tried an extended fractionation protocol in 30 patients, giving 6600 rads/10 weeks to see if a different approach, using more extended fractionation, would allow delivering the high doses necessary to obtain more consistent control of these large tumors, while at the same time keeping the normal tissue damage to the lungs within tolerance levels. In 90% of the patients there was more than 50% tumor size regression on chest x-ray. Complications were acceptable.

Extended fractionation was planned so that the large initial priming doses of irradiation would result in accelerated initial regressions and subsequent three times a week fractionation would allow a greater degree of reoxygenation of the tumor between fractions, thereby making the treatment more effective. It was felt that because of the long cell cycle time of these tumor cells (72 hr), repopulation of the tumor between 48 hr fractions would not be a significantly negative factor.

Preliminary results indicated that the extended fractionation schedule allowed delivery of high doses to lung tumors with an improvement in local response of these tumors. The treatment was tolerated well and had no side effects or complications. The normal tissue reactions were within tolerance levels of the lung parenchyma.

The local response rate is shown in Table 15 and compared with the results from the best arm (continuous dose 1000 rads/week) of the recent RTOG 73-01 study. In 27 of 30 (90%) of patients, greater than 50% regression of tumor occurred. In the majority of these patients (46 of 60 or 76%) regression was greater than 75% of the tumor; 7 of 30 (23%) of patients had a complete response.

Table 15. Local Response

	Present Series		Best Arm of RTOG 73-01 Study	
	No.	%	No.	%
Complete regression	7	23	12	24
>75% response	16	53		
50-75% response	4	14	19	39
<50% response or no change	3	10	14	29
Progression	0	0	2	4
Unknown	0	0	2	4
Local tumor (complete + partial) regression response rate	27/30	90	31/49	63

Table 16. Relief of Symptoms

	No.	%
Cough	22/78	79
Hemoptysis	9/9	100
Dyspnea	19/26	73
Pain	7/7	100
Superior vena caval obstruction	2/3	66

Table 16 lists the degree of relief from symptoms. Subjective response to treatment was as good as with any conventional approach to fractionation and treatment.

Survival of patients who had localized intrathoracic disease appears in Table 17 and compares favorably with other published results. A median survival of 44 weeks was obtained in the 18 patients with stage III disease.

Extended Fractionation With Low Daily Increments

Our experience with 219 postresection patients of whom 94 were observed and 125 received fractionation irradiation with low daily increments also confirmed the efficacy of this approach for enhanced local control and tissue sparing. Patients received 160 rads/day, 5 days/week for a total dose projected at 6000 rads. Telecobalt radiation at 100 cm was directed in all cases to a field including the hilar, mediastinal, and supraclavicular regions. No effort was made to block the cord or use crossfired portals, and only one field (anterior or posterior) was treated each

Table 17. Survival in Localized Intrathoracic Disease

Series	> 6 mo (%)	⩾ 12 mo (%)	Medial Survival (wk)
Jefferson (122)	94	44	44
Roswit et al. (138)	44	22	28
Radiation (302 pts)			
Roswit et al. (139)	37	16	26
Control (240 pts.)			
Salazar et al. (142)	88	44	49
(approx. 75 pts.)			
RTOG # 73-01 (140)	78	40	44

day. Portals were reduced as dose levels were achieved at off-axis sites. With tumor extension to the visceral pleura the region of the primary was included in the field.

No severe complications involving the heart, spinal cord, esophagus, or other sites were encountered. Pneumonitis and pulmonary fibrosis was restricted to the boundaries of the treatment portal.

Of the 219 patients 78 had positive intrapulmonary, hilar, or mediastinal nodes. Positive-node patients receiving no irradiation had a 5-year survival of 3%, while of those irradiated 35% survived 5 years. In view of the mixture of histologies (squamous cell carcinoma, adenocarcinoma, and anaplastic carcinoma) this 35% would seem to closely approximate the number of patients in whom disease limited to the irradiated areas might be expected. Radiation at other sites (e.g., whole brain) may be necessary to enhance survivals above this level in node-positive patients. The extended length of the treatment regimen (7-8 weeks) was well accepted by the patients and offered an opportunity to monitor patients and supervise nutritional, psychosocial, and general medical support.

Few studies of extended fractionation exist in the literature but many radiation oncologists use similar fractionation and report excellent patient tolerance; however, pending their results, these extended techniques may be desirable in clinics whose complex techniques may be unfeasible to implement. Further clinical trials of extended fractionation should be planned.

Electron Beam Therapy

Anterior electron beam portals may be used to reduce spinal cord dose. Schumacher attempted to improve local control and survival in bronchogenic carcinoma using high-dose-per-fraction radiotherapy with electron beams from a high-energy Betatron. He found that single, large fractions in the range of 500-800 rads delivered weekly over a prolonged time period appear to improve survival (145). This experience was the basis of a protocol performed by the Lung Working Party that was never completed because of the inactivation of that group. Their experience indicated that the regimen was acceptable from the radiation toxicity standpoint and that response was apparently at least as good as with conventional fractionation.

Radiosensitizers and High Linear Energy Transfer Particles

Both physical (hyperthermia) and chemical radiosensitization is being extensively employed in lung cancer to enhance the response of larger, more radioresistant tumors. Hypoxic cells are known to be present in solid tumors in man and animals, and are known to be more resistant to the ionizing effects of radiation than aerated cells. Whether or not the radioresistance of such tumors is a limiting factor in the local control of solid tumors treated with radiotherapy is the subject of much investigation. Attempts to improve the killing of such hypoxic cells have involved the use of hyperbaric oxygen, hyperthermia, high linear energy transfer particulate irradiation, and hypoxic cell sensitizers. Of the compounds tested to date as hypoxic cells sensitizers, the nitroimidazoles appear to have the greatest potential. Among these, metronidazole (Flagyl) and misonidazole (Ro-07-0582), and desmethylmisonidazole, a newer analogue, are in clinical evaluation in a broad series of RTOG protocols. Neurotoxicity is the most serious side effect of misonidazole, but this is expected to lessen with desmethylmisonidazole. In any case, early results are most promising with this new modality.

Hyperthermia

A striking synergism between radiation therapy and hyperthermia has been observed. Hyperthermia is a potent modifier of the response of tumors to radiation and can be tumoricidal. Further, the effects appear potentiated via a low pH. Heat appears to damage the vasculature of tumors but not of normal tissue. Heat appears to inhibit the radiation-induced DNA injury. Hyperthermia enhances the killing of tumor cells by selected chemotherapeutic agents.

Methods of heating tumors have generally applied energy from outside (immersion, ultrasound, RF, and microwave modalities) or have been surgical procedures (perfusion). All these methods have one or more of the following deficiencies: long induction times (up to 3 hr), maximum temperature of only 42°C, long treatment times, necessity of using anesthesia, inability to penetrate deeply, reflection of energy, preferential energy absorption in inappropriate tissue (fat, bone, etc.), inability to heat adequate volumes, and so forth. The hyperthermia research currently being done for lung cancer focuses primarily on regional hyperthermia.

Ultrasound techniques are not appropriate for intrathoracic lesions because they cannot be used near large bones or in the areas of large air space, because the sound waves are reflected by bone and travel relatively inefficiently through air. There are, however, several modalities being used for heating chest lesions, including microwaves, radiofrequency waves, and local radiofrequency and local radiofrequency currents. There are advantages and disadvantages to each of these modalities and areas where the application of one has advantages over that of a competing modality.

Commercially available devices for deep heating include the Tronado unit, Clinitherm, the BSD system with annular phased array, and the Henry Electronics Magnetrode, while devices such as the USC Localized Current Frequency System (LCF) are developed internally at the institution in which used. Few details are available on most commercial systems except the BSD Annular Phased Array which is said to utilize the principle of phase reinforcement to produce an electrical field within the body that heats from the inside out. Sixteen radiating elements surround the patient and radiate RF energy through him. In this regard, it resembles the Tronado. Reinforcement occurs because all elements are driven simultaneously and with identical phase and polarization at a frequency such that the body diameter approximates one-half wavelength (60 MHz). The resultant energy deposition pattern favors the center of the body up to diameters of at least 33 cm. Hyperthermia above 42°C may be expected with short induction times of 15 min or less. Monitoring of tumor and adjacent normal tissues is critically important. Nonperturbing probes have been designed for use on microwave fields which do not perturb, nor are they perturbed by the field, thus providing accurate temperature information throughout the treatment if positioned correctly within the body.

They are flexible and slender (1.1 cm) enough to be inserted into tissues with an angiocatheter at various tissue depths and surface positions. These temperature probes are part of the automatic closed-loop system which regulates the power entering the subject and this controls normal tissue temperature. Typically, tumor temperatures may be expected to selectively and automatically rise to temperatures 1 or more degrees higher than adjacent normal tissues presumably because of the poor blood flow. LaVeen, using localized radiofrequency current, Holt, using the Tronado, and Storm, using the Magnetrode have reported tumor response in intrathoracic lesions (116,101,153).

The RTOG and North American Hyperthermia Group have several ongoing protocol studies which address questions regarding the efficacy of hyperthermia in primary and metastatic lung cancer with and without radiation. Interested radiation oncologists may participate by affiliation with RTOG radiation oncology centers.

High LET Particle Radiation

These radiation modalities (neutrons, pi-mesons, and heavy ions), which present another alternative for large anoxic tumors, are available to radiation oncologists and their patients throughout the United States with travel support and funds frequently provided.

1. Neutrons: Several centers (University of Washington, MDAH, Fermilab) are comparing (RTOG 79-07) neutrons, x-rays, and "mixed beam" (neutrons and photons in nonsmall cell bronchopulmonary carcinoma. These studies have yielded most encouraging early results and hold great promise in the view of the study chairman (Griffin). New cyclotron facilities are being built at the MDAH, University of Washington, UCLA, and the University of Pennsylvania (DT generator).

2. Helium heavy ions: The Northern California Oncology Groups (NCOG) and the Bay Area Heavy Ion Association (Bahia) are assessing heavy ions (argon, neon, etc.) in large radioresistant lesions. The NCOG has pioneered an important new direction in cancer management: the development of regional networks in association with advanced major modality (heavy ion) radiation facilities.

3. Pi-mesons: Complete responses and extended survivals with locally advanced lesions have been reported in lung cancer. The development of the PIGMI (Pion Irradiation Generator for Medical Installations) device at the Los Alamos Scientific Laboratories (LASL) holds promise of the availability of these particles in large metropolitan areas.

TECHNICAL CONSIDERATIONS IN DEFINITE IRRADIATION

Treatment Portals and Volume For Curative Radiation Therapy

Radiation fields for the primary lesion include a margin of at least 2 cm of normal-appearing tissue, and to the mediastinum to 5-6 cm below the carina for upper and middle lobe lesions or the diaphragm for lower lobe lesions. The mediastinal field should be 8 cm wide or wide enough to cover the hilar shadows with a small margin.

The supraclavicular areas are treated

1. when they are clinically involved,
2. when the tumor is apical, or
3. when there is an unfavorable site or histology.

To prevent subsequent supraclavicular adenopathy 4500 to 5000 rads is sufficient. Emami et al. (68) treated the supraclavicular area electively in 79 patients, only 1 of whom subsequently developed adenopathy. Of 153 patients who did not receive supraclavicular field (SCF) irradiation, 14% developed evident metastatic involvement there. When supraclavicular nodes were clinically involved on presentation, a dose of 5000 rads, uncorrected for source to skin distance (SSD), was effective in controlling the SCF disease in 96% of 27 patients.

Spinal Cord Shields

Spinal cord tolerance has tended to be the dose-limiting factor in many regimens although dose levels achieved in the pericardium and esophagus figure prominently in treatment planning. The most obvious approach to this problem is the use of spinal cord shields.

Anterior Loading, Oblique or Lateral Crossfired Portals

Alternatives to spinal cord shields are the use of 3:2 anterior loading or oblique/lateral crossfired portals to achieve boost dose levels above acceptable doses for critical sensitive structures (spinal cord, 4500 rads; heart, 4000 rads; esophagus, 5000 rads). Anterior loading does not spare anterior structures so that in most RTOG studies posterior oblique portals with 30-45 degree wedges are advocated. Multilevel CT computer treatment planning in conjunction with the use of such oblique portals underscores serious problems with incorporating the primary and high-risk nodal areas in oblique portals without crossfiring sensitive structures at some level above or below the central ray. Since Lambert and others have indicated that radiation myelopathy is often associated with the interdigitation of multiple portals, great care must be used in the planning and implementation of this technique.

Compensating Absorbers

With the use of radiosensitizers and high total and split-course fractionation, the need for precision compensating absorbers becomes critical to obtain a uniform dose at depth with external beam radiation treatment. This is particularly important with coplanar opposing fields, to make allowances for the surface tomography of the patient and to compensate for "missing tissue." Different institutions at different times use various materials such as aluminum blocks, styrofoam filled with wax and lead sheets.

Recently, replacement of aluminum block compensators by lead sheet compensators and the introduction of automatic computation into certain aspects of the design has been accomplished. This change should lead to equivalent or better compensating. There will be easier checking for accuracy available at various stages of the design and construction, and improved documentation for patient record purposes.

Direct measurements are taken at a rectangular matrix of points of the depth of the patient's surface which is perpendicular to the central ray. These measurements together with relevant patient data and structural data are fed into a computer program which produces full-scale drawings of the shapes of the lead sheets from which the compensator is to be constructed, together with indicators of how the sheets should be placed (position and orientation) with respect to the central ray of the treatment machine.

POSTRESECTION IRRADIATION

Today a still unresolved controversy exists in the minds of many physicians and the public as to the desirability of postresection irradiation and the timing of its initiation. It is important to summarize at the outset some of the overwhelming evidence in support of its timely initiation and aggressive administration in the immediate postoperative period.

Only a small fraction of the lung cancer patients who are surgical candidates (15-20%) can be cured by surgery. Mountain reports 37% of curatively resected patients survive 5 years with squamous cell lesions and even a smaller number (27%) of large cell and adenocarcinoma patients. When mediastinal nodes are involved, this 5-year survival figure drops to 8%, then to less than 2% for such patients with adenocarcinoma (123).

Therefore, surgery can no longer be considered the mainstay in definitive treatment. Conventional wisdom has dictated that surgical failures occur from occult distant metastasis present at diagnosis and therefore the major therapeutic enhancement should be accomplished with adjunct chemotherapy and immunotherapy. Regrettably, controlled studies have failed to show improved survival with these techniques. Current justification for the use of postresection radiation therapy stems from these failures and new data, such as the autopsy experience which suggests that many patients have an orderly progression of disease from local to regional to distant spread, and that local failure, not distant spread, is the principal cause of failure in many squamous cell cancer patients.

M.J. Matthews reviewed the autopsy experience of 202 patients who died within a 30-day period after curative resection (120). One-third with epidermoid carcinoma had locally persistent disease (Table 18). Of these, 60% had tumors limited to bronchial stump and/or regional lymph nodes. It is of particular significance that the surgical impression of these patients was that they had left no residual disease. The pattern of failure for adenocarcinoma was predominantly distant metastasis. Spjut and Mateo's (102) autopsy study showed one-third of the patients who died within 1 month of surgery had mediastinal lymph node involvement. The incidence of recurrent disease in the hemithorax remained uniformly high with a peak of 60% in patients surviving 6 months (152). P.S. Rasmussen's autopsy study of patients dying 2 months or longer after pulmonary resection showed 20 of

Table 18. Distribution of Lung Cancer as Found at Autopsy in Patients Dying Within 1 Month of Lung Resection Presumed to be Curative

Histology	No. Pts.	No. Persistent Disease	No. Distant Metastases	Site of Distant Metastasis
Squamous cell	131	44 (33%)	22 (17%)	Distant nodes, 6; adrenals, 5; liver, 5; other, 3
Small cell	19	13 (70%)	12 (62%)	Liver, 7; nodes, 6; brain and kidney, 2; adrenals, 3
Adenocarcinoma	30	13 (43%)	12 (40%)	Adrenals, 7; brain, 5; lymph nodes, 4; vertebrae, 3
Large cell	22	3 (17%)	3 (14%)	Kidney, 3; adrenals, liver, and other, 3
Total	202	73 (35%)	49 (24%)	Adrenals, 18, liver, 16; lymph nodes, 17, kidney and others, 6

64 with local recurrence alone, 34 of 64 with local recurrence and distant metastasis, and 10 of 64 with distant metastasis alone (134). T. W. Shields et al. (149) reported a very disappointing 17% 5-year survival for patients with hilar lymph node metastasis and 9% for those with mediastinal lymph node metastasis in patients who did not receive postresection irradiation. N. P. Bergh and Scherten (19) stressed the importance of perinodal tumor growth: 9 of 15 patients with intranodal metastasis survived 5 years, whereas only 2 of 84 with perinodal spread survived 5 years. The implications of these surgical experiences are that patients with resected regional disease may often have persistent regional disease and do not invariably have occult distant metastases. The studies of Eisert et al. (66), Perez et al. (131, 132), and others also emphasize that these patients fail regionally and come to autopsy in more than 50% of the cases with disease limited to the thorax.

Still not fully answered is the quest on of whether postresection irradiation to the hemithorax, hilum, and mediastino upraclavicular area will salvage more patients. Patterson and Russell (129) re ported randomized studies and concluded there was no benefit. However, Patte son treated only the hilum and adjacent mediastinum. Bangma (17) employed a wide variety of radiotherapy techniques. Neither analyzed their results according to the presence or absence of lymph node metastasis. Recently Kirsch et al. (111) reported a nonrandomized experience of patients who underwent mediastinal lymph node dissection and received postoperative irradiation. Five-year survival was 34% for squamous cell carcinoma and 11.8% adenocarcinoma.

Kirsch noted in an unrandomized series that patients with histologically proven, confirmed squamous cell carcinoma and mediastinal metastases following resection and postoperative radiation therapy of 5000-5500 rads, there was a 5-year survival of 19.4% while there were no survivors reported among the patients treated with surgery only (110). Pavlov et al. (130) reported on 16 patients with a 24% 5-year survival for surgery only and 38% for surgery and postoperative radiation therapy (4000-5000 rads). Israel et al. (104) reported on randomized studies in which 50 patients with lymph node metastasis from epidermoid carcinoma for the lung had local failure in 44% after treatment by surgery only and 26% of 38 patients treated by postoperative radiation therapy. On the other hand, Shields et al. (149) advocated resection of the primary tumor and metastatic nodes when possible, but did not advocate postresection irradiation, the 5-year survival rate of patients with nodal metastases in his series was 11%. Green's et al. (87) experience revealed a 5-year survival, postresection with positive hilar or mediastinal nodes of 35% if extended field, high-dose postoperative radiation therapy was given (Table 18).

Of 287 patients who underwent thoracotomy, 219 had resectable tumors confined to the lung; 142 underwent lobectomy, 77 had pneumonectomy. One hundred twenty-four patients had squamous cell carcinoma, 46 had adenocarcinoma, and 49 anaplastic carcinoma. Eighteen patients had interlobar node metastases, 46 had hilar node metastases, and 32 patients had metastases in mediastinal lymph nodes. One hundred twenty-five patients received postresection irradiation. In all cases the treatment fields included the hilar, mediastinal, and supraclavicular regions. In patients with tumor extension to the visceral pleura, the region of the primary tumor was included in the treatment field. A tumor dose of 5000-6000 rads was planned at a rate of 800 rads/week, 200 rads/treatment (some patients received a lower tumor dose because of declining health).

Comparison of the patients treated by surgery alone and by surgery with postoperative irradiation showed important differences in survival according to the absence or presence of nodal metastases. In patients without node metastases, 22% (14 of 64) of the patients treated by surgery alone and 27% (16 of 59) of the patients treated by surgery plus irradiation survived 5 years. In contrast, in patients with node metastases, 3% (1 of 30) of the patients treated by surgery alone and 35% (23 of 66) of the patients treated by surgery plus irradiation survived. The improvement in survival with postoperative irradiation was significant ($p = 0.01$) (Table 19).

RADIOCHEMOTHERAPY AND NEW MODALITIES IN NONSMALL CELL BRONCHOPULMONARY CARCINOMA (NSC BPC)

The remarkable accomplishments with the integration of chemotherapy and radiation in small cell bronchopulmonary carcinoma (SCBPC) have not been duplicated in nonsmall cell BPC. The failure rate after curative treatment including surgery and/or radiotherapy is about 80%. Since a large portion of lung tumors are inoperable at the time of diagnosis, effective chemotherapy could be an important palliative treatment. Single-drug chemotherapy is largely ineffective, and combination chemotherapy has a failure rate of 50% or more in adenocarcinoma and large cell anaplastic carcinoma. Results generally obtained with squamous cell carcinoma are disappointing. In squamous cell and large cell carcinoma the response is lower with the combined modalities than with radiotherapy alone (Sealey) (147). There is a statistically significant difference in median survival in patients

Table 19. Comparison of 5-Year Survival Rates for Carcinoma of the Lung With and Without Postoperative Irradiation

Histology	Treatment	
	Surgery Alone	Surgery Plus Irradiation
Patients without node metastasis		
Squamous cell carcinoma	10/37 (27%)	12/43 (28%)
Adenocarcinoma	3/16 (19%)	2/8 (25%)
Anaplastic carcinoma	1/11 (9%)	2/8 (25%)
Total	14/64 (22%)	16/59 (27%)
Patients with node metastasis		
Squamous cell carcinoma	1/16 (6%)	6/28 (21%)
Adenocarcinoma	0/6 (0%)	10/16 (62%)
Anaplastic carcinoma	0/8 (0%)	7/22 (27%)
Total	1/30 (3%)	23/66 (35%)
Final total	15/94 (16%)	39/125 (31%)

Table 20. Agents with Proven Activity in Primary Lung Cancer

Mechlorethamine (HN2)
Cyclophosphamide (CPA)
(Other alkylators)
Mitomycin C (MMC)
CCNU 1-2 (Chloroethyl)-3-cyclohexyl-1-nitrousurea
Procarbazine (PCZ)
Hexmethylmelamine (HMM)
Cis-platinum (DDP)
Etoposide (VP-16)
Vincristine (VCR)
Vindesine (DVA)
Methorexate (MTX)
Bleomycin
Adriamycin (ADM)

with squamous cell carcinoma in favor of radiotherapy alone (Table 22). The problem in assessing combined modalities is further compounded by doubts regarding the favorable effects of chemotherapy alone (Table 23).

Table 20 lists agents with some proven activity in primary lung cancer. It is probable that nitrogen mustard and cyclophosphamide as well as other alkylating agents have a similar degree of activity. There are at least 13 active agents that are pharmacologically distinct. Unfortunately, none of these agents gives a response rate above 20%.

Table 21. WP-L 73.31 Study: Treatment-Related Complications

Treatment	Degree of Toxicity (No. of Pts.)			
	Mild	Moderate	Pronounced	Life Threatening
Radiotherapy	19	11	5	1
Radiotherapy and chemotherapy	3	21	24	6

Table 22. Radiotherapy vs. Supportive Therapy in Inoperable Carcinoma of the Lung*

Investigator	Medial Survival (days)	
	RT	Control
Durant (61)	249	252
Green (87)	180	150
Roswit (139)		
Squamous cell carcinoma	180	135
Adenocarcinoma	225	180
Scheer (144)	120	120
Wolf (159)	165	150

* Agents used included ACD = actinomycin D, CTX = cyclophosphamide, FU = fluorouracil, HN2 = nitrogen mustard, HYD = hydroxurea, MTX = methotrexate, PCZ = procarbazine, VLB = vinblastine.

Table 23. Chemotherapy vs. Supportive Therapy in Nonsmall Cell Carcinoma of the Lung*

Investigator	Chemotherapy	Median Survival	
		Chemotherapy	Control
Green (88)	HN2	210	120
Laing (113)	PCZ	190	220
	HN2, VLB, PCZ and Prednisone	75	
Scheer (144)	HYD	115	120
Durrant (61)	HN2	261	252

* Agents used included ACD = actinomycin D, CTX = cyclophosphamide, FU = fluorouracil, HN2 = nitrogen mustard, HYD = hydroxyurea, MTX = methotrexate, PCZ = procarbazine, VLB = vinblastine.

Cyclophosphamide is the best single agent. Procarbazine (Matulane) has produced objective remission of 20-25%. Methotrexate leads the list for epidermoid cancers with a 25% response rate. Adriamycin (Doxouricin), CCNU, and vinblastine have occasional good responses and are utilized in combination with the aforementioned agents because of a lack of cross-resistance. Bleomycin, because of a lack of hematologic toxicity, has been utilized with a response rate of 13%.

Alexander found a shortening in survival with a chemotherapy regimen combining the use of actinomycin D and methotrexate. Results of Sealey's ST 53 study mirror this experience and these deleterious effects point to the importance of defining (1) appropriate chemotherapy and (2) radiation dose levels.

Dose levels above 4000 rads have been most commonly used (Table 25) with chemoradiotherapy. With these high-dose regimens, the average median survival following radiation therapy was 218 days, which, compared to the low-dose average of 169 (Table 24), supports the use of higher doses.

However, with higher doses, substantially greater toxicity is seen in the combined modality patients as compared to radiation alone in the WPL 73.31 study (Table 21) comparing 5000 rads alone with 5000 rads and polyagent chemotherapy. Median survival, on the other hand, was the same. An RTOG study (73-02) to evaluate the effect of cytoxan after palliative radiation in inoperable SCBPC suspended randomization to cytoxan because of toxicity.

More recently, 78 patients with inoperable lung cancer of various histological types were treated by Schulz with split-course 6 MeV x-ray therapy to the primary and mediastinal and supraclavicular nodal areas and combination chemotherapy with CCNU, adriamycin, and vinblastine (146).

Table 24. Radiotherapy and Chemotherapy vs. Low-Dose Radiotherapy in Inoperable Small Cell Bronchopulmonary Carcinoma*

Investigator	Treatment		Median Survival	
	Radiotherapy	Chemotherapy	RT	RT + CT
Alexander (11)	3000	HN2	150	120
	3000	MTX + ACD		60
Cohen (42-45)	2000	FU	206	186
	4000		175	
Fingerhut (74)	3000	FU	105	
Gollin (83)	4000		150	
	3400	FU		294
Hendry (95)	1600	CTX	162	128
Langdon (115)	3500	FU	186	186
Tucker (155)	3000	MTX	240	270
Velasco (156)	1800	AB 132		110
	4000		110	

* Agents used included ACD = actinomycin D, CTX = cyclophosphamide, FU = fluorouracil, HN2 = nitrogen mustard, HYD = hydroxyrea, MTX = methotrexate, PCZ = procarbazine, VLB = vinblastine.

Table 25. Radiotherapy and Chemotherapy vs. Large Dose of Radiotherapy in Inoperable Small Cell Carcinoma of the Lung*

Investigator	Treatment		Median Survival	
	Radiotherapy	Chemotherapy	RT	RT + CT
Benninghoff (18)	4000	FU	270	270
Bergsagel (20)	4500	CTX	223	327
Coy (48)	4000	VLB	195	195
Durrant (61)	4000	HN2	255	264
Hill (90)	5000	FU	136	133
		ACD		150
Holsti (99,100)	6400	FU	405	402
Horowitz (102)	5000	Chlorambucil	147	228
Host (103)	5000	CTX	300	300
Krant (112)	4000	HN2	105	105
Kuang (109)	5000	CTX	154	147
Landgren (114)	5000	PCZ	330	180
Sandison (143)	5000	FU	210	291
		PCZ	330	180
		Chromycin		150
Scheer (144)	5000	HYD	120	150

* Agents used included ACD - actinomycin D, CTX = cyclophosphamide, FU = fluorouracil, HN2 = nitrogen mustard, HYD = hydroxyrea, MTX = methotrexate, PCZ = procarbazine, VLB = vinblastine.

Radiotherapy Technique

A split-course approach was the standard procedure (2 x 2000 rads/11 fractions, 5 fractions/week with a 2-week split). Reduction of field sizes during the second course of radiation was always attempted and was usually possible.

About 50-60% of long-term survivors developed a slight paramediastinal fibrosis which was asymptomatic. Four patients developed a transient pneumonitis requiring steroids.

Chemotherapy tolerance was good, and much of the chemotherapy was given on an outpatient basis. The combined radiotherapy and chemotherapy was well tolerated.

Seventy-four percent of nonsmall cell patients responded to therapy. The median survival time was 11 months; 21% of patients survived more than 2 years mostly free of disease.

No broad and unequivocal evidence exists to support the hypothesis that combination of radiotherapy and chemotherapy is beneficial in the treatment of regional nonsmall cell lung cancer. At the present it appears that other modalities under study, including radiosensitizers such as misonidazole and hyperthermia, offer a potentially more effective means for enhancing local control.

Operable but unresectable patients may respond to preoperative and intraoperative radiation with and without surgical debulking which offers great promise as do high LET particles.

Extrathoracic extensions may respond to extended radiation fields or upper hemibody radiation with boost doses to specific sites (e.g., liver, bone, and brain). Disseminated disease may respond to radiolabeled tumor-specific antibodies and immunostimulators (e.g., levamisole). Table 26 is a tabular listing of the several RTOG studies using the new modalities in a matrix according to the relevant RTOG stage grouping. Notwithstanding, the foregoing efficacious chemotherapeutic agents would clearly be of value in patients with systemic disease. More comprehensive patient support programs, such as those being studied with intensive combination therapy in SCBPC, should be employed in nonsmall cell radiochemotherapy (RCT) to improve responses and reduce toxicity. Altered time-dose regimens, including protraction and multiple daily fractions (MDF), may also be utilized to enhance systemic and local tolerance.

Table 26. Radiation Therapy Oncology Group Summary of Lung Protocol Eligibility

	N0	N1 (Hilar nodes)	N2 (Mediastinal nodes)	N# (Supraclavicular nodes)
Tx	RTOG 78-11**			
T1	RTOG 78-11** RTOG 81-03**	RTOG 78-11** RTOG 79-27* RTOG 81-03**	RTOG 79-17** RTOG 79-27** RTOG 81-03**	RTOG 79-25**
T2	RTOG 78-11** RTOG 81-03**	RTOG 78-11** RTOG 79-27* RTOG 81-01**	RTOG 79-17** RTOG 79-27* RTOG 81-03**	RTOG 79-25**
T3	RTOG 78-11** RTOG 81-03**	RTOG 78-11** RTOG 79-27* RTOG 81-03**	RTOG 79-17** RTOG 79-27* RTOG 81-03**	RTOG 79-25**
T4	RTOG 79-25** RTOG 81-03**	RTOG 79-25** RTOG 81-03**	RTOG 79-25** RTOG 81-03**	RTOG 79-25**

List of Protocols (140)

RTOG 78-11
Phase III levamisole
(inoperable patients)

RTOG 79-17
Phase III Misonidazole
(inoperable patients)

RTOG 79-25
Phase III Misonidazole
(inoperable patients)

RTOG 79-27
Phase III Postoperative
± Levamisole

RTOG 81-03
Phase I Antiferritin
(inoperable patients)

* Postoperative patients
** Inoperable patients

RADIOIMMUNOTHERAPY

Unfortunately, many BPC patients succumb to metastatic disease sometimes unassociated with local control. The need to eradicate occult metastases in association with additional regional therapy would be desirable. An approach to treating microscopic disseminated disease as well as the primary site of the tumor has been to stimulate the immune system. Manipulation of the patient's immune status may prevent recurrence of tumor and prolong survival. A living vaccine, the Calmette-Guerin bacillus (BCG) strain of microbacterium tuberculosis bovis or its methanol-extracted residue (MER) has been administered in a single postoperative intrapleural dose as a pulmonary resection for lung cancer (119). This form of regional immunotherapy is reasonably well tolerated if the vaccine is given in a limited dose and if a follow-up course of isoniazid (INH) is administered. The preliminary findings in a small randomized prospective clinical trial indicate that patients with stage I lung cancer are significantly improved by the treatment, but patients with more advanced disease do not benefit.

Levamisole is also in use for a number of studies for immunostimulation; although toxicity is not severe, patients do not object to flulike syndromes which are common with this modality. It has been used extensively as an antihelminthic; Renoux et al. (135) demonstrated in 1972 that it possessed immunotropic properties. Levamizole appears to restore inefficient or impaired host defense mechanisms. It has been shown to induce an immunostimulatory response and enhance the effect of antitumor drugs resulting in greater survival. The greatest prolongation of life span by levamisole has been seen when tumor reduction is maximal.

A double-blind, placebo-controlled trial of levamisole in resectable BPC by Amery (15) indicates that recurrences in the levamisole-treated group are about half as frequent (10 of 51) as in the patients receiving placebo after resection (20 of 60). The greatest benefit of levamisole was seen in patients with larger tumors. Recurrence in distant sites (bone, brain, and liver) were less frequent in the levamisole-treated group than with the placebo ($p + 0.06$). The Southwestern Oncology Group is comparing radiotherapy, chemotherapy, and levamisole; the British Medical Research Council is comparing the effects of levamisole pre- and postoperatively.

Dellon et al. (57) have shown decreased T-cell peripheral blood levels in patients irradiated for bronchogenic carcinoma. Those on whom some recovery for the T cells was noted had a better prognosis than the patients without recovery. Based on the foregoing experience, an evaluation of the immunostimulatory effect of levamisole in nonoat cell BPC is being undertaken by the Radiation Therapy Oncology Group, in two studies, one for resectable (79-11) and one for nonresectable (79-17), nonsmall cell BPC. The objective is to test whether nonspecific levamisole immunostimulation delays or reduces the appearance of local recurrence or distant metastases following postsection radiotherapy for SCBPC. Patients receive 5000 rads/5 weeks plus a 1000 rad boost to the primary and placebo or levamisole 2.5 mg/kg p.o. on day 1 and 2 for a weekly dose of 5 mg/kg. No significant differences in median survival have been demonstrated but a surprisingly high number of patients object to the flulike symptoms associated with the levamisole. Tumor-specific radioimmunotherapy for nonresectable squamous cell and large cell BPC is the subject of a phase I study (RTOG 81-03) comparing ^{131}I isotopically labeled antiferritin immunoglobulin with the ^{125}I-labeled antibody 3 weeks after 5100 rads (300 rads x 10 in 2 weeks, two weeks rest then 300 rads x 7).

The localization in tumors or radioimmunoglobulin directed against tumor-associated antigens has been established in several clinical facilities using anti-ferritin antibody. Proteins associated with metabolism involved in the proliferation of malignant tissue may also be targeted by antibody. A particularly prominent example is ferritin, a tumor-associated antigen in nonoat cell lung cancer. Ferritin has been described as a major antigen in nonsmall cell cancer of the lung.

The use of antibody of known tumor-associated specificity radiolabeled with ^{131}I is within the conventional experience in radiation therapy in that isotopic therapy was administered in thyroid cancer where doses of 100-200 mc of ^{131}I were common. The relationship of the effective half-life in the tumor (7.5-7.8 days) and the physical half-life of ^{131}I (8 days) suggests that ^{131}I is a useful agent.

The shorter range of ^{125}I and the reduction in both total body dose and scheduling requirements as well as the potentially tumoricidal effectiveness without the need for prolonged hospitalization makes ^{125}I-labeled antiferritin antibody attractive. If used as an adjuvant in lung cancer to deal with disseminated disease, it would require mainly outpatient commitment rather than extensive hospitalization. If for any reason the unexpected half-life is associated with unexpected toxicity, this ^{125}I arm will be dropped and the study will continue with ^{131}I antiferritin only.

SMALL CELL BRONCHOPULMONARY CARCINOMA

Small cell bronchopulmonary carcinoma (SCBPC) accounts for 15-20% of all bronchogenic cancers. Less than a decade ago, it was just one of several diseases that comprised "lung cancer." The median survival for untreated patients was very poor: 5 weeks for those with extensive disease and 12 weeks for those with limited disease. Attempts to perform curative resection in a few individuals with resectable disease did not alter the gloomy picture, although median survival figures approached 6 months. However, in contrast to the other forms of BPC, the decade of the 1970s has seen much progress in the delineation of the actual history of SCBPC as well as in treatment. Whereas during the 1960s SCBPC was almost invariably fatal (1), there are now certain groups of patients who have long survival free of disease (2), and the overall median survival has increased from about 2 months to greater than a year (3). Long-term survivors (greater than 2.5 years) now have become frequent enough that a case study registry for such patients has been established, and greater than 106 documented cases have been entered to date (4).

These results are attributed mainly to the incorporation of effective combination chemotherapy regimens in treatment programs with or without other modalities. During the last few years, the main therapeutic approach for patients with SCBPC has shifted from RT to systemic CT. Several important reasons led to this change in therapeutic strategy: (1) SCBPC is usually disseminated from its early stages and is regarded as a systemic disease from diagnosis; (2) the local effectiveness of thoracic irradiation does not influence the metastatic component and, therefore, does not improve survival; (3) effective combination chemotherapy became available which yielded responses in metastatic as well as local disease. These programs have become increasingly aggressive and have applied effective oncologic principles such as systemic staging and thorough searches for occult metastases, intensive induction therapy, noncross-resistant drug combinations, and radiation of the primary tumor and of "sanctuary" tumor sites such as the brain. A maximal effort has been made to increase complete remission (CR) rates and to prolong survival in an analogous fashion to what has been accomplished in the treatment of leukemia and lymphoma.

The staging procedures used in most reported series include physical examination, chest roentgenogram, bone marrow examination, and radionuclide liver and brain scans, radionuclide bone scans and bone radiographs (36,37). Liver biopsy (either percutaneously or by peritoneoscopy) is also employed. Limited disease is found in approximately 30% of patients. Liver and bone are the most common sites of metastatic disease detected by staging evaluation. Tumor dissemination to bone marrow, central nervous system, and soft tissue is also frequent.

Simplified Staging for SCBPC

In the recent past, most patients have been staged using the following simple system:

1. Stage A: Solitary nodule or regional (resectable)
2. Stage B: Limited (unresectable), one hemithorax (may involve scalene nodes)
3. Stage C: Extensive extrathoracic spread

In patients with limited disease, supraclavicular node involvement has been described as a poor prognostic sign. This possibility could require revision of the present staging system in order to improve its clinical utility, perhaps by incorporating the number of sites of metastases or some other measure of overall tumor burden. Recent recommendations advocate a shift to the AJCCS or its RTOG modification for better classification of SCBPC, since more precise correlations with initial extent of disease were needed.

Whether irradiation of the local chest tumor improves survival in SCBPC is presently uncertain, but review of the sites of intrathoracic failure in irradiated patients may prove useful for identifying means by which the delivery of radiotherapy could be made more effective. Sequential chest roentgenograms and mediastinoscopy were also employed for restaging. Fifteen of 21 patients found to be pathologically free of disease after this restaging process are alive without evidence of tumor 6 to 25+ months after discontinuation of chemotherapy. Such aggressive restaging procedures could prove useful in deciding whether to terminate therapy in an individual patient.

Chemotherapy

The effectiveness of thoracic irradiation depends upon the time-dose-volume factors employed. When these are curtailed, such as when portals do not encompass an adequate margin surrounding the primary disease and the entire mediastinum, or when the total dose delivered is decreased to 1400 rets (4000-5000 rads of conventional fractional RT), the only hope of achieving total control of the primary depends on the supplementary antitumor effect of the cytotoxic agents.

Ajaikumar and Barkley studied 163 bronchogenic patients with small cell undifferentiated carcinoma treated over two periods of time (7). Earlier patients received radiation alone or radiation plus single-agent chemotherapy, while the later patients were treated with multiagent chemotherapy plus radiation therapy. The latter group of patients had median time of survival extended about 4 weeks at the cost of much morbidity and occasional mortality. At autopsy, however, only 5 out of 30 were free of disease in the treatment portals, and all of these had received more than 4000 rads tumor dose independent of adjuvant therapy.

On the other hand, improved local control was reported by Rissanen, using doses of 4800-6250 rads (136). Of 7 radiation patients, 6 showed no intrathoracic tumor at autopsy. While in 14 consecutive autopsies of patients who had received only multiagent chemotherapy without radiation, visible tumor was present in the primary and regional lymphatics in all 14 patients. Holoye and Samuels report only 1 of 16 patients with limited disease, who received 4500-6000 rads on a split course with chemotherapy, had a relapse in the thorax (98).

Local Radiation Therapy for Stage B Limited Disease (LD)

Five groups have reported on RT and RT + CT. In all series, total tumor doses of 4500-5000 rads were delivered in 4-8.5 weeks. Three of the five groups have claimed a significant increase in median duration of response and mean survival time (MST) for those patients that were treated with combined modality therapy. One series that randomized patients to RT or CT reported an overall increase in response in MST for RT-treated patients. Another series that randomized between surgery and RT reported that RT yielded better MST and overall survival.

Toxicity has been minimal with local radiation alone for limited SCBPC: no treatment-related fatalities have been reported; life-threatening complications have been less than 3%; severe complications have been less than 5%, and these usually were transitory.

Combined RT and CT in Stage B Limited Disease SCBPC

Twenty-five groups of investigators have reported their results on combined modality therapy (CT and RT) for patients with SCBPC limited to the thorax. Most series are not comparable for many reasons, e.g., the inclusion or exclusion of supraclavicular nodal metastases in the limited disease category and variations in the number and doses of drugs employed.

The average patient was treated with an induction CT regimen consisting of three drugs: cyclophosphamide (CTX) in combination with either adriamycin (ADR) or oncovin (VCR) or lomustine (CCNU) and methotrexate (MTX). The average patient was treated with local RT 5.5 weeks after the initiation of CT. A total dose of 4005 rads was delivered with 15 fractions/5 weeks. In 14 of these 25 groups, a split-course radiation therapy regimen was used with rest periods of 2-7 weeks.

In eight groups, radiation therapy was delivered concomitantly with CT. In the remaining 17 groups RT followed induction CT.

Combined RT and CT in Stage C Extensive Disease SCBPC

Although the major emphasis in treating patients with extensive SCNPC has been with chemotherapy, there is an increasing use of localized or extended-field radiation therapy. The average patient is treated with an induction CT consisting of more than three drugs and receives regional RT 6 weeks after the induction of CT. A total dose of 3300 rads is delivered with 12 fractions in 3.1 weeks. A split-course radiation therapy regimen may be used with rest periods which range from 2-4 weeks. The average treatment consisted of 2750 rads/2 weeks, a rest period of 1 week, and the 550 rads/2 days. The time-dose relationships yield NSD dose of 1280 ret. A total of 9 weeks elapses from the initiation of CT to the completion of RT. RT is delivered either concomitantly with CT or following induction CT.

The best results in the treatment of extensive SCBPC patients utilized combined modality RT plus CT approaches. The induction CT regimen used was cyclophosphamide, adriamycin, vincristine (CAV).

Discussion

There is an appreciable increase in responses and median survival time when more intensive CT is given. However, very few patients with extensive SCBPC survive beyond 2 years. Consolidation with radiation therapy of previously involved tumor areas which have responded completely to induction therapy seems a logical approach.

The use of very intensive CT results in severe, even life-threatening and fatal toxicity. The intensification of RT doses, especially when combined with multidrug CT (particularly with adriamycin) also may result in severe permanent complications.

Radiation Therapy Toxicity

The recall phenomenon occurs when adriamycin is used after radiation, and results in frequent recurrent esophagitis. Interaction between bleomycin and radiation occurs in the lung where 5-13 patients in one study developed severe pulmonary fibrosis and 3 died. A RTOG study reports three cases of life-threatening pneumonitis, apparently due to adriamycin or adriamycin combinations after failure of initial therapy from a combination of chemotherapy and radiation. It is important to decide whether to accept an increase in fatal and life-threatening toxicity if more patients are not being cured.

Elective Brain Irradiation (EBI) in SCBPC

Two to ten percent of patients with SCBPC present with brain metastases at diagnosis, and an additional 20-30% will develop this complication during the course of the disease; at autospy, the incidence of brain involvement is as high as 28-55%.

Most studies have used 3000 rads/2 weeks, but Cox reports successful prophylactic brain irradiation using only 2000 rads/2 weeks (49). If patients are treated therapeutically (i.e., after the brain metastasis occurs), rather than prophylactically, the treatment is not nearly so successful: one-half of these patients will die of brain metastases. There is no survival difference between patients treated therapeutically and patients treated prophylactically to the whole brain.

If EBI significantly reduces the incidence of brain metastases, but does not yield improvements in median survival, it implies that patients are dying of disease elsewhere.

Upper Hemibody Irradiation (UHBI)

Preliminary studies show that a single dose of 600-800 rads of upper hemibody irradiation has achieved approximately a 16% CR and 75% PR for a total response rate that exceeds 90%.

HBI is a systemic form of radiation which can supplement cytotoxic agents for the control of distant metastases. It is also a local treatment which can be supplemented with local chest irradiation for the control of the primary disease and draining nodes. The major limitations of HBI are the determination of its safest and most effective dose and its pulmonary toxicity.

It has been effectively used in metastatic patients who failed with conventional therapies. Half-body irradiation has achieved good objective tumor responses (14% CR and 71% PR) in advanced SCBPC patients. In addition to reducing the size of massive tumor growths, HBI alleviates cancer-related pain. This treatment modality can be used as a systemic consolidation technique in patients with extensive SCBPC, which is a radiosensitive tumor. Patients consolidated with radiation therapy receive chemotherapy between the sixth and eleventh week. After consolidation with radiation therapy, maintenance chemotherapy is started on the twelfth week.

Patients consolidated with radiation therapy receive chemotherapy between the sixth and eleventh week. After consolidation with radiation therapy, maintenance chemotherapy is started on the twelfth week.

Upper Hemibody Irradiation and Localized Chest Irradiation (LCI)

All consolidation radiotherapy is done between the sixth and eleventh week. The program consists of delivering UHBI with parallel opposed field arrangement which delivers a single midplane dose of 600 rads at a rate of 30-40 rads/min. No corrections are made for increased dose absorption in the lungs. One week later LCI begins with anterior and posterior fields that encompass the primary tumor (with a margin >2 cm), the entire mediastinum, and both supraclavicular areas. A total local dose of 2000 rads is delivered with five fractions of 400 rads each week. Radiation is given with megavoltage photon equipment; patients are treated at a source-axis-distance (SAD) of 100 cm for LCI and over 200 cm for UHBI.

Symptomatic radiation therapy may be added: superior vena caval obstruction (2000 rads/1 week with local portals); palliation of extremely symptomatic liver metastases (1500 rads/1 week); or palliation of painful brain and bone metastases (3000 rads/2 weeks). Supplementary radiation is given with five fractions/week. No patients progressed or developed new metastatic areas during the 6-week interval of radiation therapy during which chemotherapy was interrupted.

Toxicity

There was no fatal or life-threatening hematologic toxicity in the nine consolidated patients during the 4-5 weeks after UHBI. Only one patient exhibited severe toxicity (WBC of 1000-2000) 2 weeks after UHBI. None of the patients developed radiation pneumonitis, severe fibrosis, esophageal strictures or fistulae, severe esophagitis, or mucositis.

A total combined-therapy approach would have implied delivering lower HBI, however, an additional 5-6 weeks of rest would have been required for bone marrow recovery. At the present time, two other groups are testing HBI coupled with LCI as a primary or adjuvant therapy for both limited and extensive SCBPC.

Discussion

The primary therapeutic approach for patients with SCBPC is currently systemic chemotherapy. The major contribution of thoracic RT to the management of SCBPC has been and is local tumor control. Radiation therapy has been proven effective in decreasing the incidence of brain metastases when used prophylactically. Other forms of RT such as hemibody irradiation coupled with thoracic irradiation are beginning to emerge as helpful and hopeful consolidation approaches after systemic chemotherapy induction. It is important to reemphasize that the morbidity of the therapeutic approaches and the compromise of the patients' quality of life cannot and should not outweigh the therapeutic benefits for this or any other disease in oncology. However, the importance of local control and its influence on survival is emphasized by a retrospective analysis of patients treated with local field irradiation plus chemotherapy. Patients whose tumors were controlled locally had improved median survival compared to those whose tumors were not controlled.

Since at the present time the vast majority of patients with SCBPC die from this disease, it is quite possible that median survival figures may not change dramatically, although significant gains may be achieved in the plateau phase (the "tail" on the survival curve). Those series using radiotherapy have the best complete response rates and the majority of 2 year relapse-free survivals (Table 27). Radiotherapy should not be withheld in this entity, since it contributes to palliation, local control, and survival.

CONCLUSIONS

We have reviewed the current status of lung cancer in the United States with an emphasis on divining new directions in radiation management.

It is clear that in spite of explosive growth of biomedical technology, no progress has been made in the last decade in reducing the incidence or mortality of lung cancer or increasing the number of patients eligible for curative surgery.

In fact with the rapid advances in the sensitivity, and precision of newer diagnostic and evaluative techniques, increasing numbers of patients are identified as too extensive for curative surgical resection.

Even those few who are eligible for resection with curative intent in most cases cannot be cured by surgical means. Fortunately, postresection irradiation has been clearly demonstrated to substantially enhance survival. Also clearly demonstrated are consistently poor results with polyagent chemotherapy as a surgical or radiation adjuvant in inoperable nonsmall cell carcinoma as well as in the local control of small cell carcinoma in spite of dramatic improvements in median survival of small cell patients.

These development place the primary burden on the radiotherapist in the great majority of these patients. The enormity of this responsibility may be underscored most succinctly by pointing out that in 1980 nonsmall cell cancer was the first most common cause of death from cancer in the United States. Fortunately many new developments in prevention, screening, and radiation management have passed from the biomedical research laboratories to clinical trials and application. Tragically for the many thousands of lung cancer victims, most patients go to their graves with no opportunity to benefit from these advances.

These circumstances cry out for the assumption of broad responsibilities by the radiotherapist in coordination of the lung cancer management effort from detection, prevention, delineation of the extent of disease, as well as for timely therapeutic interventions. The unique patient population of the radiotherapist includes a large number of lung and head and neck cancer patients, all of whom are at risk

Table 27. Actual Relapse-Free Survival of 2 Year or Longer in Stage A Limited SCBPC

Investigator	Therapy*	No. of Patients	Complete Response (%)	Number Relapse-Free 2 Years or Longer
Holoye-M.D. Anderson Hospital (98)	CTX, VCR, RT	16	50	3
Einhorn-Indiana University (65)	CTX, ADR, VCR, RT, CCNU, MTX, BCG	19	89	5
Israel-Centre Hospitalier (104)	CTX, ADR, CCNU, MTX, VCR, BLEOMYCIN, 20 Emetine, C parvum	20	70	4
Jackson-Bowman Gray (105)	CTX, ADR, VCR, CCNU, MTX, RT	12	-	2
Hansen-Copenhagen (91)	CTX, CCNU, MTX, VCR, RT	110	-	12
Brereton-National Cancer Institute (28)	CTX, ADR, VCR, RT	10	100	4
Eagan-Mayo Clinic (62-63)	CTX, VP-16, RT ADR, VP-16, RT	12 9	40 33	4 1
Cohen NCI-VA+ (42-45)	CTX, MTX, CCNU, ADR, VCR, PROCAR	19	74	3
Bitran-University of Chicago (21)	CTX, ADR, VCR, MTX, RT	12	100	2
Greco-Vanderbilt University (86)	CTX, ADR, VCR, RT, HEXA, VP-16, MTX	16	94	2
Total		255	72	42

* Agents used included ACD = actinomycin D, CTX = cyclophosphamide, FU = fluorouracil, HN2 = nitrogen mustard, HYD = hydroxyurea, MTX = methotrexate, PCZ = procarbazine, VLB = vinblastine.

for second tumors at nonirradiated sites. Regular monitoring of these patients may detect and eliminate early lesions, using new fiberoptic laser endoscopic techniques, or provide opportunity to prevent them through nutritional and psychosocial support. In the past, preoccupation with cost containment and attempts to minimize morbidity by withholding diagnostic and therapeutic procedures has handicapped the radiation oncologist and has certainly not proved successful in terms of controlling lung cancer mortality. Our priority today need no longer be to save costs but to save lives.

Fortunately a broad range of diagnostic and therapeutic modalities are now available to every radiation oncologist either directly or through affiliation with nearby major radiation oncology centers. The timely implementation of state of the art radiation management in this disease should see immediate enhancement in local control, survival, and palliation.

An important task exists for each radiation oncologist and the radiotherapy community as a whole to transmit this message to the referring clinicians and the public so we may realize the successes now possible in the radiation management of lung cancer.

Taken together with careful record keeping and pooling of data, the rapid accumulation of further information will permit the radiation oncologist to move forward effectively in evolving a broad range of radiation regimens increasingly effective in every stage and histological entity. Since most patients are treated in the community hospital setting, it is the community radiation oncologist who will implement such a program and it is the current high caliber of community radiation oncology that makes this in every way possible.

REFERENCES

1. A Collective Study: Preoperative irradiation of lung cancer: Final Report of a therapeutic trial. Cancer 36:914-925, 1975.

2. Abadir, N. and Muggia, F.M.: Irradiated lung cancer. Radiology 114:427-430, 1975.

3. Abramson, N. and Cavanaugh, P.J.: Short-course radiation therapy in carcinoma of the lung. Radiology 96:627-630, 1970.

4. Abramson, N. and Cavanaugh, P.J.: Short-course radiation therapy in carcinoma of the lung: A second look. Radiology 108:686-687, 1973.

5. Abelof, M.D., Ettinger, D.S., and Khouri, N.: Intensive induction therapy for small cell carcinoma of the lung (SCC). Proc. Am. Soc. Clin. Oncol. 20 (Abstract C-144):366, 1979.

6. Ackerman, L.V. and del Regato, J.A.: Cancer: Diagnosis, Treatment and Prognosis. 4th Edition, St. Louis, Mosby, 1970.

7. Ajaikumar, B. S. and Barkley, H. T.: The role of radiation therapy in the treatment of small cell undifferentiated bronchogenic cancer. Int. J. Radiat. Oncol. Biol. Phys. 5:977-981, 1979.

8. Alberto, P.: Remission rates, survival, and prognostic factors in combination chemotherapy for bronchogenic carcinoma. Cancer Chemo. Rep. 4:199-206, 1973.

9. Alberto, P., Berchtold, W., Sonntag, R.W., Barrelet, L., Jungi, F., Martz, G., and Obrecht, P.: Sequential versus simultaneous use of cell cycle specific and cycle non-specific chemotherapeutic agents in the treatment of anaplastic small cell lung carcinoma. Submitted to Cancer Chemother. Pharmacol.

10. Alberto, P., Brunner, K.W., Martz, G., Obrecht, J.P., and Sonntag, R. W.: Treatment of bronchogenic carcinoma with simultaneous or sequential combination chemotherapy, including methotrexate, cyclophosphamide, procarbazine and vincristine. Cancer 38:2208-2216, 1976.

11. Alexander, M., Glatstein, E.J., Gordon, D.S., and Daniels, J.R.: Combined modality treatment for oat cell carcinoma of the lung: A randomized trial. Cancer Treat. Rep. 61:1-6, 1977.

12. American Joint Committee for Cancer Staging and End Result Reporting (AJCCS), Task 2 Force on the Lung: Manual Classification of Cancer by Site, Chicago. AJCCS, 1977, pp. 56-67.

13. American Joint Committee for Cancer Staging and End Results Reporting (AJCCS), Task Force on the Lung, C. F. Mountain, Chairman: Cancer of the lung. Manual for Staging of Cancer, Chicago, AJCCS, 1978, pp. 59-65.

14. American Joint Committee for Cancer Staging and End Results Reporting D.T. Carr, Chairman: Fascicle for Staging of Lung Cancer, Chicago, AJCCS, 1979.

15. Amery, W.K.: Immunopotentiation with levamisole in respectable bronchogenic carcinoma: Double-blind controlled trial. Br. Med. J. 3:461-463, 1975.

16. Aristizabal, S.A. and Caldwell, W.L.: Radical irradiation with split-course technique in carcinoma of the lung. Cancer 37:2630-2635, 1976.

17. Bangma, P.J.: II Postoperative radiotherapy. In Modern Radiotherapy Carcinoma of the Bronchus, edited by T. Deeley, London, New York, Appleton, 1971, 163-170.

18. Benninghoff, D. L. and Alexander, L. L.: Treatment of lung carcinoma. Radiation versus radiation combined with 5-fluorouracil. N.Y. State J. of Med. (Part 1) 68:532-534, 1967.

19. Bergh, N.P. and Scherten, T.: Bronchogenic carcinoma. A follow-up study of a surgically treated series with special reference to the prognostic significance of lymph node metastases. Acta Chir. Scand.(Supp. 347):1-42, 1965.

20. Bergsagal, D.E., Jenkin, R.D.T., Pringle, J.F., White, D.M., Fetterly, J.C.M., Klaasen, D.J., and McDermot, R.S.R.: Lung Cancer: Clinical trial of radiotherapy alone vs. radiotherapy plus cyclophosphamide. Cancer 30:621-627, 1972.

21. Bitran, J.D., Desser, R.K., DeMeester, T.R., Colman, M., Evans, R., Griem, M., Rubenstein, L., Shapiro, C., and Golomb, H.M.: Cyclophosphamide, adriamycin, methotrexate and procarbazine (CAMP)-Effective four-drug combination chemotherapy for metastatic non-oat cell bronchogenic carcinoma. Cancer Treat. Rep. 60:1226-1230, 1976.

22. Bleehan, N.M.: Role of radiation therapy and other modalities in the treatment of small cell carcinoma of the lung. In Lung Cancer: Progress in Therapeutic Research, Vol. 2, edited by F.N. Muggia and M. Rozencweig, New York, Raven Press, 1979, pp. 567-574.

23. Bloedorn, F.G., Cowley, R.A., Cuccia, C.A., Mercado, R., Wizenberg, M.J., and Linberg, E.J.: Preoperative irradiation in bronchogenic carcinoma. Am. J. Roentgenol. 92:77-87, 1964.

24. Bloedorn, F.G.: Rationale and benefit of preoperative irradiation in lung cancer. JAMA 196:340-341, 1966.

25. Bloomer, W.D. and Hellman, S.: Normal tissue responses to radiation therapy. N. Engl. J. Med. 293:8-83, 1975.

26. Bodey, P., Lagakos, S.W., Guiterrez, A.C., Wilson, H.E., and Salawry, O.S.: Therapy of advanced squamous carcinoma of the lung. Cyclophosphamide versus "COMB." Cancer 39:1026-1031, 1977.

27. Bromley, L.L. and Szur, L.: Combined radiotherapy and resection for carcinoma of the bronchus: Experiences with 66 patients. Lancet 2:937-941, 1955.

28. Brereton, H.D., Kent, C.H., and Johnson, R.E.: Chemotherapy and radiation therapy for small cell carcinoma of the lung: A remedy for past therapeutic failure. In Lung Cancer: Progress in Therapeutic Research, Vol. 11, edited by F.M. Muggia and M. Rozencweig, New York, Raven Press, 1979, pp. 575-586.

29. Broder, L.E., Cohen, M.H., and Selawry, O.S.: Treatment of bronchogenic carcinoma II - small cell. Cancer Treat. Rev. 4:219-260, 1977.

30. Broder, L.E. Selawry, O.S., Bagwell, S.P., Silverman, M.A., and Charyulu, K.N.: A controlled testing two non-cross resistant chemotherapy regimens in small cell carcinoma (SCC) of the lung. Proc. Am. Assoc. Cancer Res. 19:71, 1978.

31. Broder, L.E., Selawry, O.S., and Johnson, M.K.: Treatment of small cell carcinoma (SCC) of the lung utilizing mutually non-cross resistant chemotherapy regimens. Proc. Am. Assoc. Cancer Res. 20 (Abstract 1126), 278, 1979.

32. Brunner, K.W., Veraguth, P., Obrecth, P., Hunig, R., Martz, G., and Horst, W.: Radio or chemotherapy or combined treatment in inoperable locoregional lung cancer. Proc. Am. Soc. Clin. Oncol. 19 (Abstract C-436):415, 1978.

33. Bunn, P.A., Cohen, M.H., Ihde, D.C., Fossieck, B.E., Matthews, M.J., and Minna, J.D.: Advances in small cell bronchogenic carcinoma. Cancer Treat. Rep. 61:333-342, 1977.

34. Bunn, P.A., Nugent, J.L., and Matthews, M.J.: Central nervous system metastases in small cell bronchogenic carcinoma. Sem. Oncol. 5:314-322, 1978.

35. Bunn, P.A., Cohen, M.H., Ihde, D.C., Shackney, S.E., Matthews, M.J., Fossieck, B.E., and Minna, J.D.: Review of therapeutic trials in small cell bronchogenic carcinoma of the lung. In Lung Cancer: Progress in Therapeutic Research, edited by F.M. Muggia and M. Rozencweig, New York, Raven Press, 1979, pp. 549-558.

36. Cahan, W.G. and Beattier, E.S.: Lymph node dissections in lung cancer. Clin. Bull. Memorial Sloan-Kettering Cancer Center 1:123, 1972.

37. Carr, D.T., Childs, D.S., and Lee, R.E.: Radiotherapy plus 5-FU compared to radiotherapy alone for inoperable and unresectable bronchogenic carcinoma. Cancer 29:375-380, 1972.

38. Casper, E.S., Grall, R.J., and Colbey, R.B.: Vindesine (DVA) and cis-dichloradiammineplatinum II (DDP) combination chemotherapy in nonsmall cell lung cancer (NSCLC). Proc. Am. Soc. Clin. Oncol. 20:337, 1979.

39. Chernak, E.S., Rodriquez-Antunez, A., Jelden, L., Dhallival, R.S., and Lavik, P.S.: The use of computed tomography for radiation therapy treatment planning. Radiology 117:613-614, 1975.

40. Choi, D.H. and Carey, R.W.: Small cell anaplastic carcinoma of lung - reappraisal of current management. Cancer 29:375-380, 1972.

41. Choi, C.H., Gardiello, M. and Grillo, H.: Postoperative or preoperative radiotherapy in the management of bronchogenic carcinoma. Int. J. Radiat. Oncol. Biol. Phys. (Supp. 2) 4:73, 1978.

42. Cohen, M.H.: Lung Cancer: A status report. J. Natl. Cancer Inst. 55:505-511, 1975.

43. Cohen, M.H., Creaven, P.J., Fossieck, B.E., Broder, L.E., Selawry, O.S., Johnston, A.V., Williams, C.L., and Minna, J.D.: Intensive chemotherapy of small cell bronchogenic carcinoma. Cancer Treat. Rep. 61:349-354, 1977.

44. Cohen, M.H., Ihde, D.C., Fossieck, B.E., Bunn, P.A., Matthews, M.J., Shackney, S.E., Johnston, A.V., and Minna, J.D.: Cyclic alternating combination chemotherapy of small cell bronchogenic carcinoma (SCBC). Proc. Am. Soc. Clin. Oncol. 19:359, 1978.

45. Cohen, M.H., Ihde, D.C., Bunn, P.A., Fossieck, B.E., Matthews, M.J., Shackney, S.E., Johnston-Early, A., Mukuick, R., and Minna, J.D.: Cyclic alternating combination chemotherapy for small cell bronchogenic carcinoma. Cancer Treat. Rep. 63:163-170, 1979.

46. Cook, J.E., West, H.J., Kraft, J.W.: The treatment of lung cancer by split-dose irradiation. Am. J. Roentgenol. 103:772-777, 1968.

47. Concannon, J.P., Dalbow, M.H., Davis, W., Hodgson, S.E., Mitchell, J., and Markopoulos, E.: Immunoprofile studies for patients with bronchogenic carcinoma-III. Multivariate analysis of immune tests in correlation with survival. Int. J. Radiat. Oncol. Biol. Phys. 4:225-261, 1978.

48. Coy, P.: A randomized study of irradiation and vinblastine in lung cancer. Cancer 26:803-807, 1970.

49. Cox, J.D., Byhardt, R.W., Wilson, J.F., Komaki, P., Eisert, D.R., and Greenburg, M.: Dose-time relationship and the local control of small cell carcinoma of the lung. Radiology 128:205-207, 1978.

50. Cox, J.D., Eisert, D.R., Komaki, R., Mietlowski, W., and Petrovich, Z.: Patterns of failure following treatment of apparently localized carcinoma of the lung. In Lung Cancer: Progress in Therapeutic Research, Vol. 11, edited by Muggia, F.M. and M. Rozencweig, New York, Raven Press, 1979, pp. 279-288.

51. Creech, R.H., Seydel, H., Mietlowski, W., Salazar, and Perez, C.A.: Radiation therapy and chemotherapy of localized small cell carcinoma of the lung. Proc. Am. Soc. Clin. Oncol. 20 (Abstract C-94):313, 1979.

52. Cutler, S.J. and Ederer, F.: Maximum utilization of the life table method in analyzing survival. J. Chron. Dis. 8:699-713, 1958.

53. Dawson, J.M., Hall, T.C., Schneiderman, M.A., Schnider, B.I., Ownes, A.H., Andrews, J.R., Baxer, D.H., Brenner, S., Hunter, C., Levene, M.B., Sheehan, R., and White, G.: Objective evaluation of change in tumor size in lung cancer patient with non-measurable disease. Cancer 19:415-420, 1966.

54. Deeley, T.J.: A clinical trial to compare two different tumor dose levels in the treatment of advanced carcinoma of the bronchus. Clin. Radiol. 17:299-301, 1966.

55. Deeley, T.J. and Singh, S.P.: Treatment of inoperable carcinoma of the bronchus by megavoltage x-rays. Thorax 22:562-566, 1967.

56. Deeley, T.J.: Modern Radiotherapy - Carcinoma of the Bronchus, New York, Appleton-Century-Crofts, 1971, pp. 206-207.

57. Dellon, A.L., Provin, C., and Chretien, R.B.: Thymus-dependent lymphocyte levels during radiation therapy for bronchogenic and esophageal carcinoma: Correlations with clinical course in responders and nonresponders. Am. J. Roentgenol. 123:500-511, 1975.

58. DeMeester, T.R., Bekerman, G., Joseph, J.G., Toscano, M.S., Golomb, H., Bitran, J., Gross, N.J., and Skinner, D.B.: Gallium-67 scanning for carcinoma of the lung. J. Thorac. Cardiovasc. Surg. 72:699-708, 1976.

59. Dinse, G.E. and Lagakos, S.W.: The analysis of partially-censored data from a first-order semi-Markov model. J. Stat. Com. Sim. (accepted for publication).

60. Dombernowsky, P., Hansen, H.H., Sorenson, S., and Osterlind, K.: Sequential versus non-sequential combination chemotherapy using 6 drugs in advanced small cell carcinoma. A comparative trial including 146 patients. Proc. Am. Assoc. Cancer Res. 20 (Abstract 1123):277, 1979.

61. Durrant, K.R., Berry, R.J., Ellis, S., Ridehalgh, F.R., Black, J.M. and Hamilton, W.S.: Comparison of treatment policies in inoperable bronchial carcinoma. Lancet 2:715-719, 1971.

62. Eagen, R.T., Maurer, L.H., Forcier, R.J., and Tulloh, M.: Combination chemotherapy and radiation therapy in small cell carcinoma of the lung. Cancer 32:379, 1973.

63. Eagen, R.T., Ingle, J.N., Frytak, S., Rubin, J., Dvols, L.K., Carr, D.T., Coles, D.T., and O'Fallon, J.R.: Platinum-based polychemotherapy versus dianhydrogalacitol in advanced non-small cell lung cancer. Cancer Treat. Rep. 61:1339-1345, 1977.

64. Edmondson, J.H., Lagakos, S.W., Selawry, O.S., Perlia, C.P., Bennett, J.M., Muggia, F.M., Wampler, G., Brodovsky, H.S., Horton, J., Colsky, J., Mansour, E.G., Creech, R., Stolbach, L., Greenspan, E.M., Levitt, M., Israel, L., Ezdinli, E.Z., and Carbone, P.P.: Cyclophosphamide and CCNU in the treatment of inoperable carcinoma and adenocarcinoma of the lung. Cancer Treat. Rep. 60:925-932, 1976.

65. Einhorn, L.H., Bond, W.H., Hornback, N., and Joe, B.T.: Long-term results in combined modality treatment of small cell carcinoma of the lung. Sem. Oncol. 5:309-313, 1978.

66. Eisert, D.R., Cox, J.D., and Komaki, R.: Irradiation for bronchial carcinoma: Reasons for failure. Cancer 37:2665-2670, 1976.

67. Ellis, F.: Dose, time and fractionation: A clinical hypothesis. Clin. Radiol. 20:1-7, 1967.

68. Emami, B., Lee, D.J., and Munzenreder, J.E.: The value of supraclavicular area treatment in radiotherapeutic management of lung cancer. Cancer 41: 1240-1297, 1978.

69. Engelman, R. and McNamara, W.: Bronchogenic carcinoma: Statistical review of 234 autopsies. J. Rhor. Surg. 27:227-237, 1954.

70. Ennuyer, A.: L'irradiation du medistin apres pnemectomie pour cancer ronchique. Poumon et Coeur 19:1093-1098, 1963.

71. Epp, E.R., Boyer, A.L., and Doppke, K.P.: Underdosing of lesions due to lack of electronic equilibrium in upper respiratory air cavities irradiated by 10 MVX-rays. Int. J. Radiat. Oncol. Biol. Phys. 2:613-620, 1977.

72. Ettinger, D.S., Abeloff, M.D., Karp, J.E., Burke, P.J., and Braine, H.C.L.: Intensive chemotherapy for small cell carcinoma of the lung. Proc. Second Natl. Cancer Inst. Conference on Lung Cancer Treatment, Abstract 16, 1977, p. 14.

73. Feld, R., Pringle, J., Evans, W.K., Kean, C.W., Quirt, I.C., Curtis, J.E., Baker, M.A., Yeah, L., and Deboer, G.: Combined modality treatment of small cell carcinoma of the lung (SCCL). Proc. Am. Soc. Clin. Oncol. 20 (Abstract C-88):312, 1979.

74. Fingerhut, A.G. and Barnett, M.B.: X-ray therapy and combined therapy (x-ray and 5-fluorouracil) in the treatment of cancer of the lung. Dis. Chest. 49: 393-395, 1966.

75. Fisher, R.A.: The logic of inductive inference. J.R. Stat. Soc. 98:39-54, 1935.

76. Fitzpatrick, P.J. and Rider, W.D.: Half-body radiotherapy. Int. J. Radiat. Oncol. Biol. Phys. 1:197-207, 1976.

77. Fletcher, G.H.: Textbook of Radiotherapy, 3rd edition, Philadelphia, Lea and Febiger, 1980.

78. Fryer, D.J.H., Fitzpatrick, P.J., Rider, W.D., and Poon, P.: Radiation pneumonitis: Experience following a large single dose of radiation. Int. J. Radiat. Oncol. Biol. Phys. 4:931-936, 1978.

79. Fox, W. and Scadding, J.G.: Medical research council comparative trial of surgery and radiotherapy for primary treatment of small celled or oat celled carcinoma of bronchus. Lancet 2:63-65, 1973.

80. Fullerton, G., Sewchand, W., Payne, J., and Levitt, S.: CT determination of parameters of inhomogeneity. Corrections in radiation therapy of the esophagus. Radiology 126:167-171, 1978.

81. Galluzzi, S. and Payne, P.M.: Bronchogenic carcinoma: A statistical study of 741 necropsies with special reference to distribution of blood borne metastases. Br. J. Cancer 9:511-521, 1955.

82. Ghossein, N.A., Ager, P.J., Ragins, H., Turner, S.S., De Luca, F., Alpert, S. and Lowy, S.J.: The treatment of locally advanced carcinoma of the colon and rectum by a surgical procedure and radiotherapy postoperatively. Surg. Gynecol. Obstet. 148:916, 1979.

83. Gollin, F.F., Ansfield, F.J. and Vermund, H.: Clinical studies of combined chemotherapy and irradiation in inoperable bronchogenic carcinoma. Am. J. Roentgenol. Rad. Ther. Nucl. Med. 92:88-95, 1964.

84. Golomb, H.M. and DeMeester, T.R.: Lung Cancer, CA 29:258-275, 1979.

85. Gordon, D.S.: Studies on the in vivo and in vitro effects of levamisole in a murine chemo-immunotherapy model. Second conference on "Modulation of Host Resistance in the Prevention and Treatment of Induced Neoplasia" (in press).

86. Greco, F.A., Brereton, H.D., Kent, H., Zimbler, H., Merrill, J. and Johnson, R.E.: Adriamycin and enhanced radiation reaction in normal esophagus and skin. Ann. Int. Med. 85:294-296, 1976.

87. Green, N., Kurohara, S.S., George, F.W., and Crews, Q.E.: Postresection irradiation for primary lung cancer. Radiology 116:405-407,

88. Green, R.A., Humphrey, F., Close, H. and Patro, M.E.: Alkylating agents in bronchogenic carcinoma. Am. J. Med. 46:516-525, 1969.

89. Guttmann, R.J.: Results of radiation therapy in patients with inoperable carcinoma of the lung whose status was established at exploratory thoracotomy. Am. J. Roentgenol. 93:99-103, 1965.

90. Hall, T.C., Derrick, M.M., Chalmers, T.C., Krant, M.J., Shnider, B.I., Lynch, J.J., Holland, J.F., Ross, C., Koons, R., Owens, A.H., Frie, E., Brindley, C., Miller, S.P., Brenner, S., Hosley, H.F. and Olson, K.B.: A clinical pharmacologic study of chemotherapy and x-ray therapy in lung cancer. Am. J. Med. 43:186-193, 1967.

91. Hansen, H.H., Selawry, O.S., Simon, R., Carr, D.T., van Wyk, C.E., Tucker, R.D. and Sealy, R.: Combination chemotherapy of advanced lung cancer. A randomized trial. Cancer 38:2201-2207, 1976.

92. Hayes, T.P., Danis, L.W., and Raventos, A.: Brain and liver scans in the evaluation of lung cancer patients. Cancer 27:362-363, 1971.

93. Hazra, T.A., Chandrasekaran, M.S., Colman, M., Prempree, T. and Inalsingh, A.: Survival in carcinoma of the lung after a split-course of radiotherapy. Br. J. Radiol. 47:464-466,

94. Hilaris, B.S. and Martini, N.: Interstitial brachytherapy in cancer of the lung. Int. J. Radiat. Oncol. Biol. Phys. 5:1951-1956, 1979.

95. Hendry, G.A.: M.D. Thesis, University of Aberdeen. Quoted by W.M. Ross in: Modern Radiotherapy: Carcinoma of the Bronchus, edited by T.J. Delley, pp. 201-221, Butterworths, London, 1970.

96. Henschke, U.K., Hilaris, B.S. and Mahan, G.D.: Afterloading in interstitial and intracavitary radiation therapy. Am. J. Roentgenol. Rad. Ther. Nucl. Med. 90:386-389, 1963.

97. Higgins, G.A. and Beebe, G.W.: Bronchogenic carcinoma: Factors in survival. Arch. Surg. 94:539-549, 1967.

98. Holoye, P.Y. and Samuels, M.L.: Cyclophosphamide, vincristine and sequential split course radiotherapy in the treatment of small cell lung cancer. Chest 67:675, 1975.

99. Holsti, L.R. and Vourinen, P.: Radiation reaction in the lung after continuous and split course megavoltage radiotherapy of bronchial carcinoma. Br. J. Radiol. 42:280-284, 1967.

100. Holsti, L.R.: Alternative approaches to radiotherapy alone and radiotherapy as part of a combined therapeutic approach for lung cancer. Cancer Chemother. Rep. (Part 3) 4:165-169, 1973.

101. Holt, J.G. and Laughlin, J.S.: A practical method of obtaining density distribution within patients. Radiology 93:161-166, 1969.

102. Horowitz, H., Wright, T.L., Perry, H. and Barrett, C.M.: "Suppressive" chemotherapy in bronchogenic carcinoma. Am. J. Roentgenol. Rad. Ther. Nuc. Med. 93:615-638, 1965.

103. Host, H.: Cyclophosphamide (NSC-26271) as adjuvant to radiotherapy in the treatment of unresectable bronchogenic carcinoma. Cancer Chemother. Rep. (Part 3) 4:161-164, 1973.

104. Israel, L., Bonadonna, B., Sylvester, R., and members of the EORTC Lung Cancer Group: Controlled study with adjuvant radiotherapy, chemotherapy, immunotherapy and chemo-immunotherapy in operable squamous carcinoma of the lung. Progress in Cancer Research and Therapy, Vol. 11, edited by M. Rozencweig and F.M. Muggia, New York, Raven Press, 1979.

105. Jackson, D.V., Cooper, M.R., Richard, F., Ferree, C., Muss, H.B., White, D.R. and Spurr, C.L.: The value of prophylactic cranial irradiation in small cell carcinoma of the lung. A randomized study. Proc. Am. Soc. Clin. Oncol. 18:319, 1977.

106. Jensik, R.J., Penfield, F.L., Milloy, F.J. and Amato, J.J.: Sleeve lobectomy for carcinoma. J. Thorac. Cardiovasc. Surg. 64:400-412, 1972.

107. Jones, J.D., Kern, W.H., Chapman, N.D., et al.: Long-term survival after surgical resection for bronchogenic carcinoma. J. Thorac. Cardiovasc. Surg. 54:383-391, 1967.

108. Karnofsky, O.: Evaluation of chemotherapeutic agents. In: Clinical Evaluation of Chemotherapeutic Agents in Cancer, p. 191, Columbia Univ. Press, N.Y., 1949.

109. Kaung, D.T., Wolf, J., Hyde, L. and Zelen, M.: Preliminary report on the treatment of nonresectable cancer of the lung. Cancer Chemother. Rep. 58:359-364, 1974.

110. Kirsh, M.M., Kohn, D.R., Gago, O., Lampe, I., Fayas, J.V., Prior, M., Moores, W.Y., Haight, C., and Sloan, H.: Treatment of bronchogenic carcinoma with mediastinal metastases. Ann. Thorac. Surg. 12:11, 1971.

111. Kirsh, M.M., Prior, M., Gago, O., Moores, W.Y., Kahn, D.R., Pellegrini, R.V., and Sloan, H.: The effect of histologic cell type on the prognosis of patients with bronchogenic carcinoma. Ann. Thorac. Surg. 13:310, 1972.

112. Krant, M.J., Chambers, T.C., Dederick, M.M., Hall, T.C., Levene, M.B., Muench, H., Shnider, B.I., Gold, G.L., Hunter, C., Bersack, S.R., Owens, A.H., deLeon, N., Dickson, Brindley, R.J., Brace, K.C., Frei, E., Gehan, E. and Salvin, L.: Comparative trial of chemotherapy and

and radiotherapy in patients with nonresectable cancer of the lung. Am. J. Med. 35:363-373, 1963.

113. Laing, A.H. and Berry, R.J.: Treatment of inoperable carcinoma of the bronchus, Lancet 2:1161-1164, 1975.

114. Landgren, R.C., Hussey, D.H., Samuels, M.L. and Leary, W.V.: A randomized study comparing irradiation alone to irradiation plus procarbazine in inoperable bronchogenic carcinoma. Radiology 108:403-406, 1973.

115. Langdon, E.A., Ottoman, R.E., Rochlin, D.B. and Smart, C.R.: Early results of combined radiation and chemotherapy in the treatment of malignant tumors. Radiology 81:1008-1013, 1963.

116. La Veen, H.: Tumor irradiation by radiofrequency therapy. JAMA 235: 2198-2200, 1976.

117. Lee, R.E.: Radiotherapy of bronchogenic carcinomas. Semin. Oncol. 1: 245-252, 1974.

118. Levitt, S.H., Bogardus, C.R., Jr., and Ladd, G.: Split-dose intensive radiation therapy in the treatment of advanced lung cancer: A randomized study. Radiology 88:1159-1161, 1967.

119. McNeally, M.F., Maller, C.M., Alley, R.D., Kansel, H.W., Older, T.M., Foster, E.D., and Lininger, L.: Regional immunotherapy of lung cancer using intrapleural BCG-Summary of a four-year randomized study. In Progress in Cancer Research and Therapy, Vol. 11, edited by M. Rozencweig and F.M. Muggia, New York, Raven Press, 1979.

120. Matthews, M., Kanhouwa, S., Pickrer, J. and Robinette, D.: Frequency of residual and metastatic tumor in patients undergoing curative surgical resection for lung cancer. Cancer Chemo. Rep. 4:63, 1973.

121. Minet, P.: Que peut attendre le medecin practicien du traitment d'un patient cancereux au Service du Radiotherapie de l'Universite de Liege? Rev. Med. Liege 34:776-784, 1979.

122. Mohiuddin, M., Rouby, E. and Kramer, S.: Results of a pilot study with extended fractionation in treatment of lung cancer. Int. J. Radiat. Oncol. Biol. Phys. 5:2039, 1979.

123. Mountain, C.F., and Hermes, K.E.: Management implications of surgical staging studies. In Progress in cancer research and therapy. Vol. 11, edited by F. M. Muggia and M. Rozencweig, Raven Press, N.Y., 1979.

124. Nealon, T.F.: Choice of operation and technique for carcinoma of the lung. In Proceedings of the Sixth National Cancer Conference, Philadelphia, Lippincott, 1970.

125. Ochsner, A. and DeBakey, M.: Symposium on cancer. Primary pulmonary malignancy. Surgery Gynec. Obstet. 68:435-451, 1939.

126. Overholt, R.H., Oliynk, P.N., and Cady, B.: The current status of primary carcinoma of the lung. Prog. Clin. Cancer 4:211, 1970.

127. Paulson, D.L., Shaw, R.R., Kee, J.T., Mallams, J.T., and Colmer, R.E.: Combined preoperative irradiation and resection for bronchogenic carcinoma. J. Thorac. Surg. 44:281-294, 1962.

128. Paulson, D.L., Urschel, H.C., McNamara, J.J., and Shaw, R.R.: Bronchoplastic procedures for bronchogenic carcinoma. J. Thorac. Cardiovasc. Surg. 12:11, 1971.

129. Patterson, R. and Russel, M.H.: Clinical trials in malignant disease. Part IV - Lung Cancer. Value of postoperative radiotherapy. Clin. Radiol. 13: 141-144, 1962.

130. Pavlov, A., Pirogov, A., Trechtenberg, A., Volkova, M., Maximov, T., and Matveeva, T.: Results of combination treatment of lung cancer patients: Surgery plus radiotherapy and surgery plus chemotherapy. Cancer Chemo. Rep. 4:133, 1973.

131. Perez, C.A., et al.: A prospective randomized study of various irradiation doses and fractionation schedules in the treatment of inoperable non-oat cell carcinoma of the lung. Cancer 45:2744-2753, 1980.

132. Perez, C.A.: Radiation therapy in the management of carcinoma of the lung. Cancer 39:901-916, 1977.

133. Pouillart, P., Palangie, T.H., Hugvenin, P., Morin, P., Gautier, H., Lededonte, A., Baron, A., and Matho, G.: Adjuvant nonintrapleural BCG. Progress in cancer research and therapy, Vol. 11, edited by M. Rozencweig and F.M. Muggia, New York, Raven Press, 1979.

134. Rasmussen, P.S.: Metastases in lung cancer. A study based on a series of pulmonary resections. Dan. Med. Bl. 11:60, 1964.

135. Renoux, G. and Renoux, M.: Antigenic competition and nonspecific immunity after rickettsial infection in mice: Restoration of antibacterial immunity by hyl-imidothiazole treatment. J. Immunol. 109:761, 1972.

136. Rissanen, P.M., Tikka, U. and Holsti, L.R.: Autopsy findings in lung cancer treated with megavoltage radiotherapy. Acta Radiol. (Ther.) 7:433-442, 1968.

137. Rosenow, E.C. and Carr, D.T.: Bronchogenic carcinoma. CA 29(4):233-245, 1979.

138. Roswit, B., Patno, M.E., Rapp, R., Veinberg, A., Feder, B., Stuhlbarg, J. and Reid, C.B.: The survival of patients with inoperable lung cancer. Radiology 90:688-697, 1968.

139. Roswit, B., Higgins, G.A., Shields, W. and Keehn, R.J.: Preoperative radiation therapy for carcinoma of the lung: Report of a national VA controlled study. In Frontiers of Radiation Therapy and Oncology, Vol. 5, edited by J.M. Vaeth, pp. 163-176, University Park Press, Baltimore, 1970.

140. RTOG Protocol Abstracts, American College of Radiology, Philadelphia, September, 1980.

141. Rubin, P.: Panel report: Radiotherapy for lung cancer. Cancer Chemother. Rep. 4:311-315, 1973.

142. Salazar, O.M., Rubin, P., Brown, J.E., Feldstein, M.L. and Keller, B.E.: The assessment of tumor response to irradiation of lung cancer: Continuous versus split-course regimens. Int. J. Radiat. Oncol. Biol. Phys. 1:1107-1118, 1976.

143. Sandison, A.G., Falkson, G., Fichardt, T. and Savange, D.J.: A statistical evaluation of the treatment of 215 patients with advanced bronchial cancer managed by telecobalt therapy alone and in combination with various cancer chemotherapeutic agents. S. Afr. J. Radiol. 5:21-27, 1967.

144. Scheer, A.C., Wilson, R.F. and Kalisher, L.: Combined radiotherapy and hydroxyuria in the management of lung cancer. Clin. Radiol. 25:415-418, 1974.

145. Schumacher, W.: The use of high-energy electrons in the treatment of inoperable lung and bronchogenic carcinoma. In High-Energy Photons and Electrons: Clinical Applications in Cancer Management, edited by S. Kramer, N. Suntharalingam and G.F. Zinninger. John Wiley & Sons, New York, 1976.

146. Schulz, M.D.: Results of radiotherapy in cancer of the lung. Radiology 69: 494-498, 1957.

147. Sealy, R.: Some aspects of combined radiotherapy and chemotherapy in non-oat cell bronchogenic carcinoma. Abstract. Proceedings of Second National Cancer Institute Conference on Lung Cancer Treatment, Arlie House, Virginia, 1977.

148. Seydel, H.G., Chait, A., and Gmelich, J.T.: Cancer of the Lung. John Wiley & Sons, Inc., New York, 1975.

149. Shields, T.W.: General Thoracic Surgery, p. 808, Lea & Febiger, Philadelphia, 1971.

150. Slawson, R.G. and Scott, R.M.: Radiation therapy in bronchogenic carcinoma. Radiology 132:175-176, 1979.

151. Smart, J.: Can lung cancer be caused by radiation alone? JAMA 195:1034, 1966.

152. Spjut, H.J. and Mateo, L.E.: Recurrent and metastatic carcinoma in surgically treated carcinoma of the lung. An autopsy survey. Cancer 18:1462-1466, 1965.

153. Storm, E. and Israel, H.I.: Photon cross sections from 1 kev to 100 MeV for elements Z-1 to Z-100. In Los Alamos Sci Laboratory, Nuclear Data Tables, Vol. 7, No. 6, Academic Press, New York, 1970.

154. Stott, H., Steven, R.J., Fox, W. and Roy, D.C.: 5-year follow-up of cytotoxic chemotherapy as an adjuvant to surgery in carcinoma of the bronchus. Br. J. Cancer 34:167-173, 1976.

155. Tucker, R.D., Sealy, R., Van Wyk, C., Soskoline, C.L. and LeRoux, P.L.M.: A clinical trial of methotrexate (NSC-740) and radiation therapy for squamous cell carcinoma of the lung. Cancer Chemother. Rep. (Part 3) 4:157-158, 1973.

156. Velasco, H.A., Ross, C.A., Webster, J.H., Sokal, J.E., Stutzman, L. and Ambrus, J.L.: Combined use of AB-132 (Meturedepa, Turloc) and x-irradiation in the management of advanced bronchogenic carcinoma. Cancer 17:841-849, 1964.

157. Warram, J.: Preoperative irradiation of cancer of the lung: Final report of a therapeutic trial. A collaborative study. Cancer 36:914, 1975.

158. Watson, W.L.: Ten-year survival in lung cancer. A study of 56 cases. Cancer 18:133-134, 1965

159. Wolf, J., Patno, M.E., Roswit, B. and D'Esopo, N.: Controlled study of survival of patients with clinically inoperable lung cancer treated with radiation therapy. Am. J. Med. 40:360-367, 1966.

160. Yamamura, Y.: Immunotherapy of lung cancer with BCG cell-wall-skeleton and related compounds. In Progress in Cancer Research and Therapy, Vol. 11, edited by M. Rozencweig and F.M. Muggia, New York, Raven Press, 1979.

161. Zubrod, C.G., Schneiderman, M., Frei, E., Brindley, C., Gold, G.L., Shnider, B., Oneido, R., Gorman, J., Jones, R., Jonsson, U., Colsky, J., Chalmer, T., Ferguson, B., Dederick, M., Holland, J., Selawry, O., Regelson, W., Lasagna, L. and Owens, A.H.: Appraisal of methods for the study of chemotherapy of cancer in man. J. Chronic Dis. 11:7-33, 1960.

chapter 6

MALIGNANT LYMPHOMAS

A.M. Jelliffe, M.D., B.S.

The malignant lymphomas have been divided into two major groups, Hodgkin disease and the non-Hodgkin lymphomas. This division is fully justifiable in that there are major differences between the two groups in their histological recognition, clinical manifestations, patterns of spread, most relevant investigations, and in their possibilities of cure. This classification will be followed here.

HODGKIN DISEASE

Hodgkin disease is, in general, a radiosensitive condition which has always been potentially curable by irradiation. This fact was clearly recognized by Gilbert (29) whose pioneer work was studiously ignored by the medical profession in general. Kaplan (47) refers to the arguments which were constantly used to denigrate reports favoring any attempt at radical treatment by irradiation. These arguments were as follows: (1) Relapse of the disease within radiotherapeutically treated regions was the rule rather than the exception. (2) The spread of Hodgkin disease was unpredictable. (3) The disease was systemically distributed at its inception. (4) Instances of apparent cure may be discounted as diagnostic mistakes. (5) Since some patients with known active Hodgkin disease may survive for many years, so called cures in this condition may be regarded as a selection of relatively benign cases in which recurrence of the disease may be expected eventually, providing the patient does not die of some other cause before this can happen. The obvious outcome of a consultation between a pessimistic patient and pessimistic doctor is referred to by Easson (25). However, this negative attitude by the medical profession persisted until the late 1960s in spite of reports by Peters (64), Nice and Stenstrom (61), Jelliffe and Thomson (39), Peters and Middlemiss (65), Kaplan (46), Easson and Russell (24), Craven (19), Jelliffe (40), and others, all of which indicated that up to about 40% of patients with localized Hodgkin disease might be cured by radiotherapy. With the present day acceptance that some patients may be curable has come a greater interest in this uncommon disease, and this new optimistic approach has coincided with a better understanding of the histological interpretation of lymphomas, greatly improved investigative procedures, and the availability of more effective radiotherapy and chemotherapy, all of which have contributed to a higher cure rate of Hodgkin disease. The general acceptance of the Lukes and Butler (55) classification has proved extremely helpful in the management of Hodgkin disease and in particular, permits comparison of results between centers. This is one of the many differences between Hodgkin disease and the non-Hodgkin lymphomas.

However, certain points which may be of importance in the management of Hodgkin disease are beginning to emerge. The recognition of the nodular sclerotic type of Hodgkin disease has been of the greatest value, but the situation has been confused by the inclusion in this category of a presclerotic type of Hodgkin disease which is characterized by the lacunae cells typically found in the fully established nodular sclerotic form, but without established fibrotic bands. Whether the presclerotic type carries the good prognosis of the fully established nodular sclerotic picture is as yet unproven. The lymphocytic predominant group includes cases showing a background cell pattern which is predominantly histiocytic rather than lymphocytic. Some of these patients may not carry the good prognosis recognized as typical of true lymphocytic predominant disease. The inclusion of both these variants in these two main groups may be diluting their good prognosis.

For many years a few biochemical investigations such as liver function studies have been carried out routinely in the assessment of patients with Hodgkin disease. It is probable that investigations of this type are of little use. The first real breakthrough in the investigation of Hodgkin disease came with the introduction of the lymphogram (12,38). This remains an effective and relatively safe method of demonstrating intraabdominal spread which can also be useful in treatment planning and for follow-up as long as lipiodol persists in the nodes.

Historically, the next group of investigations to provide reliable information in the study of Hodgkin disease were various methods of radioactive isotope organ scanning. In 1969 the introductions of diagnostic laparotomy (30) as a method of determining the extent of Hodgkin disease revolutionized its management. It also allowed a more critical evaluation of procedures such as lymphography and isotope scanning of the spleen and liver. In the early days of diagnostic laparotomy, many patients whose livers demonstrated unexpected microscopic changes were incorrectly diagnosed as having stage IV disease. As is always the case, the true value of a new investigative procedure requires time for its full evaluation.

Over the last few years, the wide acceptance of ultrasound and the more recent introduction of computerized tomographic (CT) scanning have increased the range of investigative procedures even further. Simultaneously, there has been a great improvement in techniques of isotope scanning. Although the value of these newer methods may at times appear obvious, their full evaluation requires more time and at present many authorities cannot yet see any way of completely abandoning diagnostic laparotomy especially in apparently early cases. Splenic involvement is particularly difficult to detect without this procedure.

Radiotherapy

Assuming that the cure of Hodgkin disease by irradiation depends upon its direct effects on the lymphomas, the initial problems to be solved were the tumoricidal dose level and the volume requiring irradiation.

Early publications (39,40) suggested that although lower doses could lead to local control of the disease, the best chance of local cure was provided by a dose of between 3500-4000 rads/3.5-4 weeks. This was confirmed by Kaplan (47) whose review of his own cases and of the literature showed that the probability of local cure could be related closely to the local dose, reaching a 95% cure rate with 4000 rads.

The volume requiring irradiation remains a subject of discussion. The work of Gilbert (29), of Peters (64), and of Kaplan (46) suggested the prophylactic wide-field irradiation was necessary to cure Hodgkin disease, but all this work was carried out before the introduction of diagnostic laparotomy, which has made such a difference in our understanding of the distribution and accurate localization of disease. With accurate staging it is likely that more localized radiotherapy can be as curative as widefield irradiation. The work of the British National Lymphoma Investigation (BNLI) (9) has shown that patients with PS I, IIA (upper half) Hodgkin disease in whom the extent of the disease has been confirmed by a diagnostic laparotomy can be cured by relatively localized irradiation and there is no need to contemplate total nodal irradiation (TNI) with its greater morbidity (Fig. 1). Without a diagnostic laparotomy, subdiaphragmatic relapse occurs with distressing frequency, particularly in the male, and relapse of this type carries a high risk of dying from Hodgkin disease. Patients investigated without a diagnostic laparotomy require more energetic treatment either by widefield irradiation or with additional chemotherapy (42).

When lymph nodes are involved in both halves of the body, widefield irradiation is necessary. The use of supervoltage irradiation has obviously simplified the radiotherapists' task and reduced the patients' burden. Indeed it is unlikely that many patients would be treatable in this fashion without the technological advances that have become generally available over the last decade.

Cytotoxic Drugs

Although this article is concerned primarily with the treatment of lymphomas by radiotherapy, it is impossible to avoid referring to the highly effective cytotoxic drugs which may be used either in preference to, or as alternatives to, irradiation or in combination with radiotherapy.

The first effective chemotherapeutic agent to be introduced into clinical practice was nitrogen mustard (33). Over the following 20 years new agents were introduced in increasing numbers with some improvement in the percentage of patients achieving complete remission (CR). Just over 10 years ago, pulsed combination chemotherapy was introduced in the management of Hodgkin disease (50) and reached a peak of efficacy with the introduction of nitrogen mustard, vincristine sulphate (Orcorin), procarbazine hydrochloride, prednisone (MOPP) (22). The results reported by DeVita and his colleagues 10 years ago have never been surpassed despite the trials of many other combinations of effective drugs. It is obviously impossible to consider radiotherapy as a method of treatment for Hodgkin disease in isolation and in the subsequent sections both methods of treatment will be compared when necessary. It is worth considering briefly certain general aspects of each method of treatment when comparing their usefulness in the different stages of Hodgkin disease. The ultimate objective of treatment is cure of the greatest number of patients with the least possible interference with their normal lives and the avoidance of complications either immediate or late. If cure is impossible, the next best alternative is the maximum prolongation of life without distressing symptoms. Both methods of treatment are potentially harmful and capable of producing severe side effects. Radiotherapy is effective in localized disease. Complications are in general also localized and their avoidance provides the main limiting factor to this treatment modality. When large volumes have to be irradiated then systemic side effects become increasingly severe and debilitating. Cytotoxic drug therapy benefits widespread disease and may be extremely effective with either macroscopic or microscopic deposits. Obviously the side effects which it may produce are generalized. Bone marrow depression, severe vomiting induced at regular intervals with production of a Pavlovian response with severe psychological complications, and alopecia are some of the more common distressing possible side effects. More recently, less obvious and dramatic but potentially serious are the effects on gonadal functions (17) and the production of second primaries.

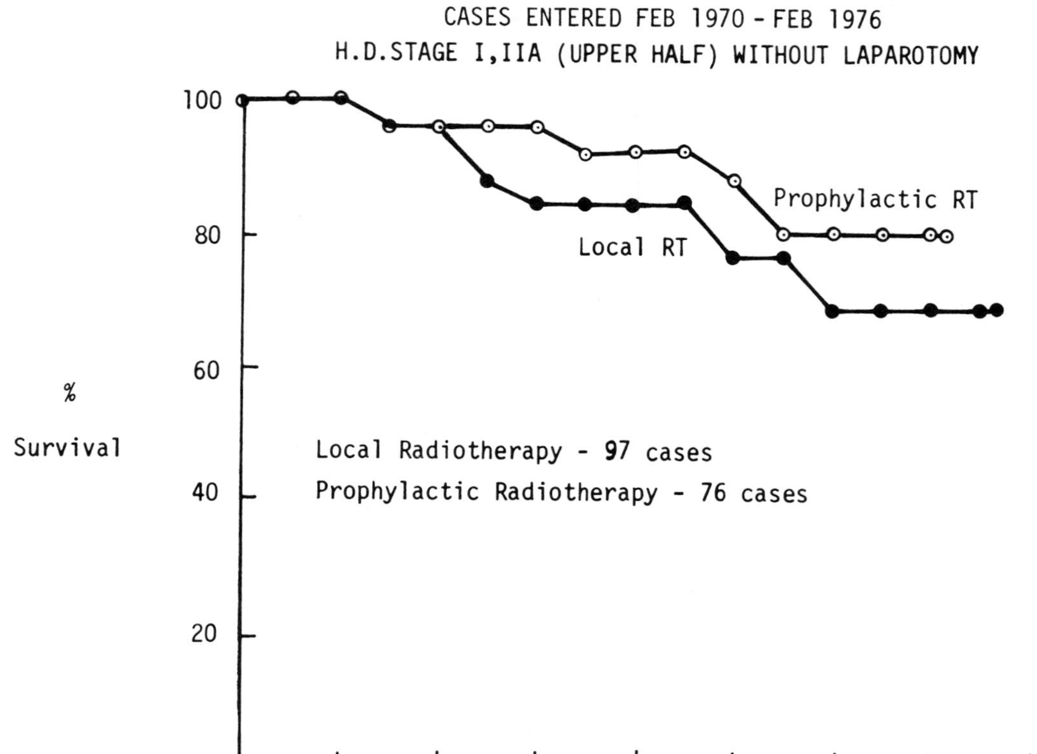

Figure 1. Hodgkin disease, stage I, IIA (upper half of body). Cases entered in the BNLI between February 1970 and February 1976, investigated with or without a diagnostic laparotomy: Analysis performed in 1978. Treatment consisted of either local radiotherapy or irradiation of the full mantle type (prophylactic). There is no obvious difference in survival between the two groups of patients. However, there is an obvious difference between those staged without laparotomy (A) and those staged with laparotomy (B). It is not possible to compare these groups directly as obviously the laparotomy has removed from the second group a number of patients with more advanced disease. These "removed" patients have been analyzed. It is interesting to see the excellent results of treating early advanced disease (C). If the second and third groups are added together, it is possible to compare them with the first group of nonlaparotomized patients in order to see the effect of diagnostic laparotomy on the survival rate (D). There is as yet no statistically significant difference between these survival rates. (Reported with acknowledgements to colleagues in the British National Lymphoma Investigation).

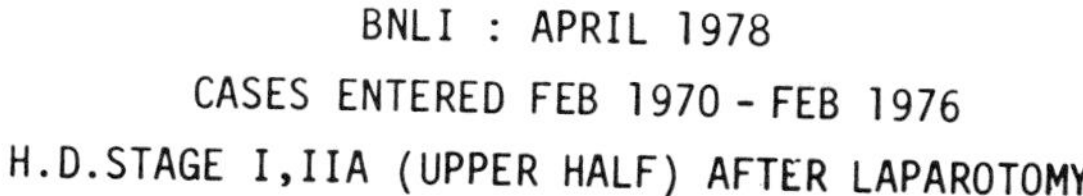

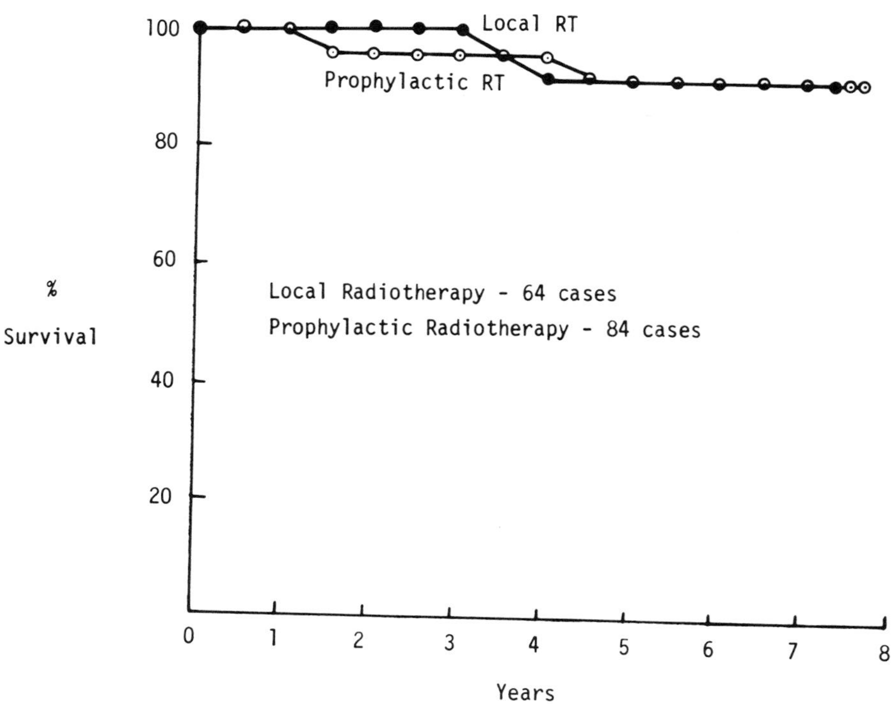

Figure 1.B.

INVESTIGATION OF PATIENTS WITH HODGKIN DISEASE AND OTHER LYMPHOMAS

As indicated already, the logical management of a patient with Hodgkin disease is totally dependent upon correct investigation. It is sensible to investigate all patients with a suspected lymphoma in a sequential fashion, starting with the simplest, cheapest, and least invasive procedures and progressing logically through the list down to the most potentially unpleasant and expensive investigations which include a diagnostic laparotomy. This sequential approach which was originally recommended for the investigation of patients with non-Hodgkin lymphomas (45) has obvious advantages in the management of all lymphomas where such an approach is ethically permissible because the patient is not acutely ill. A suggested sequential investigation ladder is shown in Table 1.

Complete examination of the patient must include all clinically demonstrable lymph node regions with particular emphasis on Waldeyer's ring. This is rarely involved in Hodgkin disease but frequently affected in non-Hodgkin lymphoma. The presence of B symptoms (14) may indicate the need for a totally different therapeutic approach. It is important to question the patient carefully to ensure that B symptoms are indeed true B symptoms. In particular, night sweats may be difficult to evaluate accurately. It is suggested that a true night sweat should be one that wakes the patient during the night, leaving the night clothes soaked. Night

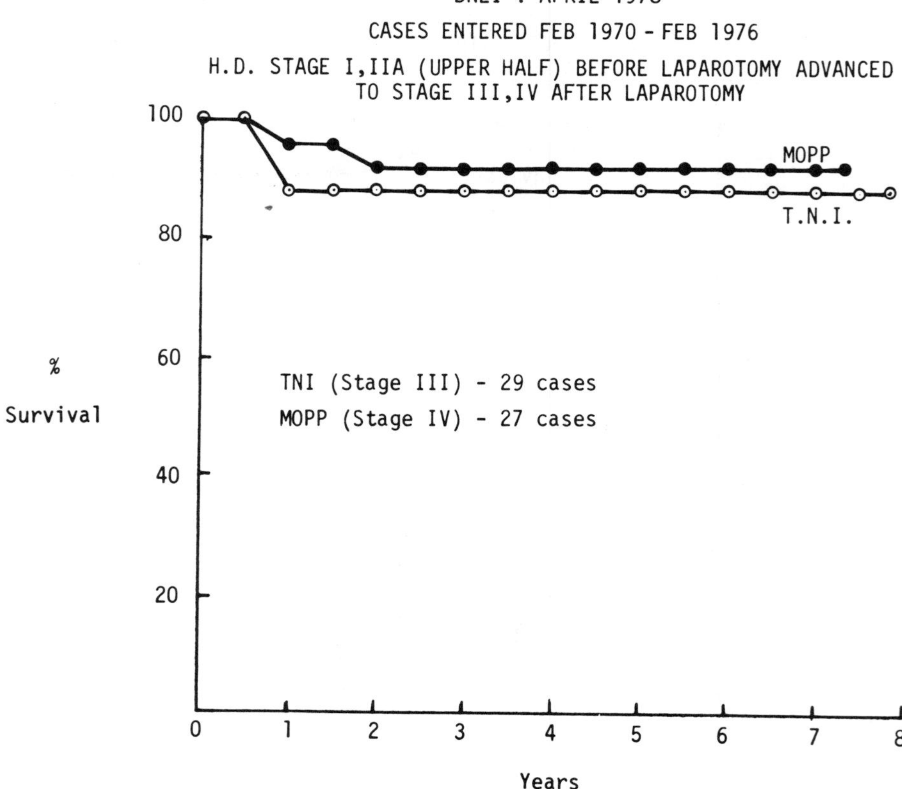

Figure 1.C.

sweats in sensitive individuals who are aware of the details of their illness may be simulated by such simple procedures as the purchase of warmer pajamas. It is, of course, very difficult to evaluate B symptoms developing for the first time after the patient has started investigations, some of which are quite capable of producing side effects indistinguishable from true B symptoms.

Lymphomas are often difficult to recognize and classify even by experts and the pathologist's task must not be made more difficult by the presentation of an inadequate specimen. Preferably a whole lymph node should be removed. If this is not possible, a large segment of a node which is likely to represent the pattern of the whole gland provides an acceptable alternative. Inadequate biopsies from extranodal lymphomas are particularly common. Little fragments snipped from the surface of an enlarged tonsil will not necessarily be representative of the whole mass.

Poor fixation of a biopsy specimen is a common failing. This often follows the removal of a large piece of tumor, which is placed in fixing fluid without incisions being made into it to allow adequate permeation. Such a specimen left overnight before reaching the pathologist will often provide sections which cannot be diagnosed accurately.

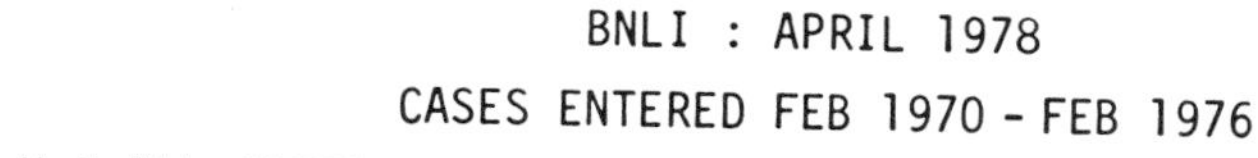

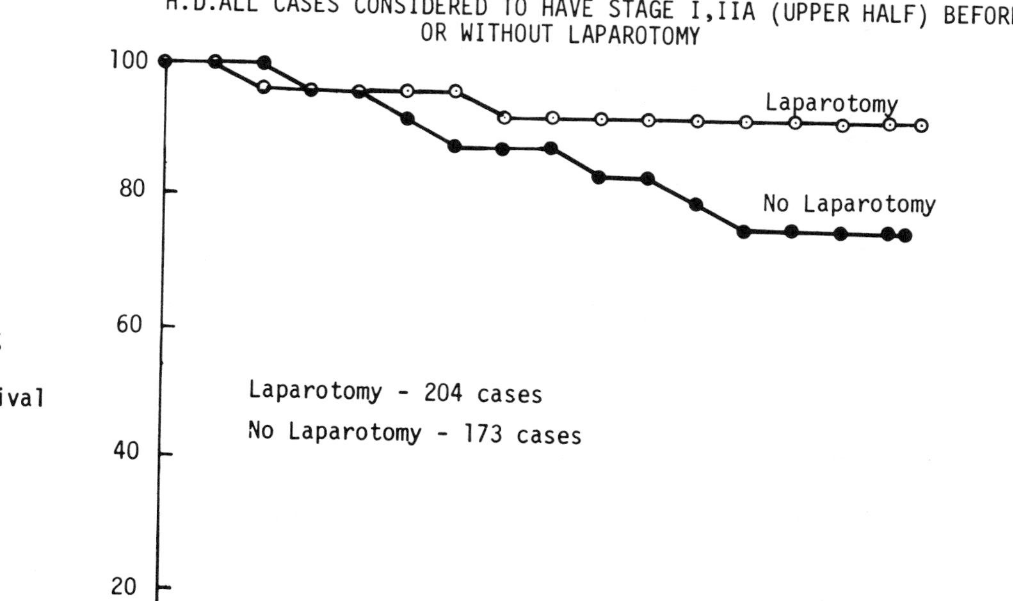

Figure 1.D.

A routine complete blood count is obviously important as it may offer an early indication of possible generalization of the disease, or a failing marrow, or hemolytic anemia which may affect treatment. The erythrocyte sedimentation rate (ESR) remains an extremely useful and inexpensive indication of disease activity, especially in Hodgkin disease. It is, of course, entirely nonspecific, but a persistently raised ESR in a patient with apparently controlled disease is not uncommonly the first sign of a relapse which may not become obvious for many months or even years.

Liver and kidney function tests are of value partly as indications of possible diseased sites but even more so in the general management of a patient who may be retreated with cytotoxic drugs which are eliminated from the body by either organ. The uric acid is frequently raised with lymphomas with a high rate of cell production and hypercalcemia is occasionally found, particularly in Hodgkin disease. Both findings may affect treatment. Plasma protein abnormalities occasionally may affect the diagnosis and, when present, they may provide markers which can be followed as the patient is treated. Bone marrow aspirate and trephine biopsy, preferably using the Jamshidi needle, are mandatory in the investigation of non-Hodgkin

Table 1. Lymphomas: Routine Sequential Investigation (BNLI)*

Biopsy(ies)
History, clinical examination
Waldeyer's ring
Full blood count, ESR
Blood biochemical survey
Immunoglobulins
Bone marrow
Abdominal lymphogram
Intravenous pyelogram
Ultrasound scans
Isotope scans
CT scans
Closed liver biopsy
Laparoscopy
Diagnostic laparotomy
Further special tests

* A suggested routine sequential approach to the investigation of patients with suspected lymphoma. The investigations become progressively more invasive or more expensive, and at the same time, less often necessary when earlier tests reveal abnormalities. For example, the discovery of a positive bone marrow will establish the diagnosis of stage IV disease, making further investigation of academic interest only. Organ imaging using isotope, ultrasound, and computerized tomography is increasingly valuable, but the final place of each technique remains to be seen. Further special tests include examination of the gastrointestinal tract and cerebrospinal fluid in patients with non-Hodgkin lymphomas, as well as projects or investigational methods which may be used at a specific center.

lymphoma. The lower rate of involvement in Hodgkin disease makes examination of the bone marrow less profitable; nevertheless, it is strongly recommended because the presence of normal bone marrow may be important in treatment.

The value of lymphangiography is now well established. The initial fear that the presence of lipiodol would prevent the correct histological interpretation of lymph nodes removed subsequently during a diagnostic laparotomy has been disproven with increased experience. The finding of grossly abnormal lymph nodes in the presence of a confirmed lymphoma elsewhere may be taken as a definite indication of intraabdominal spread, but of course abnormal intraabdominal glands alone may be due to many causes. With abnormal glands lipiodol may persist for many months providing an easily measurable marker of the response to treatment. There are rarely any serious complications provided that there is no known pulmonary impairment: special care is necessary if prior irradiation has been given to the lungs. Sensitivity reactions to lipiodol, or more commonly to patent blue, are potentially dangerous but fortunately rare. Lymphography seems likely to remain as a routine investigation for many patients with Hodgkin disease. It is less likely to remain a routine procedure in the non-Hodgkin lymphomas where intra-abdominal nodal involvement is more likely to involve nodes other than those in the retroperitoneal regions. CT, isotope, and ultrasound scanning may prove to be of greater value in this group of patients.

Visualization of the renal tract has advantages. Renal infiltration, obstruction to the renal outflow, and pressure on the bladder are not uncommon in the lymphomas and will obviously effect treatment policies. In addition, if abdominal irradiation is contemplated, the position of the kidneys must be determined precisely. For repeated studies of renal function a renogram (11) provides an inexpensive and less unpleasant investigation. An intravenous pyelogram should be carried out normally after an abdominal lymphogram, as the investigations may be complimentary when performed in this order.

Isotope scans of established value are those of the skeleton and liver. It is now generally accepted that bone scanning will often demonstrate tumor involvement before this can be seen on routine radiographs, and an isotope scan of the whole skeleton is less expensive than a radiographic skeletal survey. In the lymphomas in general, a positive bone scan is less common than a positive bone marrow. But, when it is found to be positive in patients with otherwise localized disease, the management becomes different immediately.

Because liver involvement is often diffuse, liver scans are again not commonly found to provide definite evidence of invasion in apparently early disease and all too often the report is equivocal. However, occasionally gross filling defects may be demonstrated with, again, obvious effects on treatment policy.

Lymph node isotope scanning is not yet a uniformly reliable procedure, and splenic scanning, except in extreme cases, is frequently totally misleading and therefore, valueless. However, the introduction of emission scanning and other recent developments may completely alter this state of affairs and may greatly increase the scope of isotope organ imaging.

Constant improvements in ultrasound organ imaging have lead to the development of an apparatus which is capable of producing remarkably accurate definition of disease processes in many parts of the body. For example, pericardial involvement with or without an effusion can be demonstrated with a high degree of reliability, which cannot be matched by other scanning methods, and many workers believe that ultrasonography provides the most reliable method of demonstrating early liver involvement with malignant disease. One obvious and important advantage of ultrasonography is that the apparatus required is inexpensive when compared with that required for isotope or CT scanning. Its disadvantage is that the most reliable results are obtained when the scan is carried out by a highly experienced operator who is fully aware of the patient's medical condition and the aims of the investigation, and highly trained operators who are fully oriented medically are not yet widely available. In expert hands, enlarged nodes and other involved organs may be clearly demonstrated, but without considerable expertise, misinterpretation is all too easy.

The importance of CT scanning is widely recognized and need not be emphasized here. Certain features are worth mentioning when comparing this investigational modality with other scanning methods. First, the equipment is very expensive and its maintenance costs and high staffing requirements place a heavy burden on the hospital service. Clearly if this expensive piece of equipment is to be used to its maximum advantage, the radiologist in charge must be largely or totally committed and prepared to do far more than just interpret scans which are presented to him by technicians, however expert they may be. Second, the CT scanner has the enormous advantage of presenting to the clinician the information that he requires in a form with which he is totally familiar which makes clinical decision making much less emotionally demanding. Third, in the management of tumors and in particular the lymphomas, facilities already exist for the transfer of CT scan results to automated treatment planning equipment which allows the organization of effective radiotherapy with a minimum waste of time. Finally, the progress of lymphomas under treatment can be visualized directly by the clinician in charge of the case.

Aspiration biopsy of the liver has been in use as a routine investigative procedure for many years. When performed with routine precautions by an expert it carries negligible risks but it is not of equal value in all types of lymphoma. In Hodgkin disease where hepatic infiltration is often patchy, a normal biopsy does not exclude involvement of this organ. In the non-Hodgkin lymphomas hepatic infiltration is more likely to be diffuse with a much greater chance that a blind liver biopsy will demonstrate involvement. Under these circumstances, a negative result is of greater significance.

In Great Britain laparoscopy has not become generally accepted as a routine method of investigation and staging of lymphomas, as opposed to the United States where it is frequently included in the assessment of patients, particularly with non-Hodgkin lymphomas. At laparoscopy it is possible to obtain needle biopsies of the liver under direct vision. The possible value of this procedure in staging is indicated by a series of patients described by Chabner et al. (16). Of 49 patients in whom a percutaneous liver biopsy had shown no liver involvement, 18% (9) were found to have infiltration of this organ at laparoscopy. Laparoscopy should certainly be considered in the older patient who is not thought to be suitable for a full staging laparotomy.

It is generally accepted that a full staging laparotomy must include a splenectomy, lymph node biopsies from all accessible regions, and at least two deep needle and two wedge biopsies of the liver. While the patient is anesthetized, it is reasonable to consider also the removal of any other enlarged superficial lymph nodes, and also an open bone marrow biopsy using a Stryker saw. In young women, it is customary to consider the possibility of moving the ovaries away from their normal position, to a site where they can be protected more easily during abdominal irradiation using the inverted Y technique (3). In many cases it is impossible to know definitely whether or not there is involvement with lymphoma before the specimens are examined histologically, and for this reason it may be preferable to move only one ovary, leaving the other in its normal position near the fallopian tube. In this way, fertility will not be greatly reduced if inverted Y irradiation proves to be unnecessary.

Since its introduction in 1969 by Glatstein and colleagues (30), staging laparotomy has become generally accepted in many centers as routine in the staging of patients with Hodgkin disease (9,28,41,48,51). It is less acceptable in the management of patients with non-Hodgkin lymphomas, partly because widespread disease is more often demonstrated by simpler procedures such as bone marrow examination, partly because the findings at laparotomy are less likely to influence the treatment policy, and partly because the patient is more commonly in an older age group. The place of laparotomy in non-Hodgkin lymphomas in their staging, and the value of the procedure when compared with laparoscopy and bone marrow examination have been examined in detail recently (7,72). Both these reports confirm the widespread extranodal involvement of most cases of non-Hodgkin lymphoma. The work of the Milan group (7) also emphasizes the frequency of gastrointestinal involvement.

Staging of Patients with Lymphomas

The internationally accepted Ann Arbor classification (Table 2) designed for the staging of Hodgkin disease has proved to be valuable.

Table 2. Ann Arbor Staging System*

I:	Involvement of a single lymph node region (I) or of a single extralymphatic organ or site (IE).
II:	Involvement of two or more lymph node regions on the same side of the diaphragm (II) which may be accompanied by localized involvement of an extralymphatic organ or site (IIE).
III:	Involvement of lymph node regions above and below the diaphragm (II) which may be accompanied by localized involvement of organ or site (IIIE).
IV:	Diffuse or disseminated involvement of extranodal organs, with or without lymph node involvement. (In this system, Waldeyer's ring and the spleen are regarded as lymph node sites and not as extranodal extensions.)
A:	The absence of weight loss of more than 10%
B:	The presence of (1) fever above 38°C, (2) night sweats

* The above symptoms must have no other discernible cause. The exact definition of a night sweat may be difficult. The BNLI define a night sweat as a phenomenon by which the patient is woken up in discomfort by the sweating which is so heavy that it is usually necessary to change the bed clothes.

Whether or not a diagnostic laparotomy has been performed is indicated by the prefixes CS (staging based on clinical investigations) or PS (staging based on pathological findings after diagnostic laparotomy).

Involvement of special organs may be indicated by various suffixes as follows: H, liver; S, spleen; L, lung; M, marrow; P, pleura; O, osseous; D, skin. If lymph node involvement is confirmed histologically at laparotomy, this may be indicated by the suffix N. Using this nomenclature the pre- and postlaparotomy staging findings may be summarized as shown in this example:

CS IIA, PS IV, N + S + H + M + D -

The same classification has been adopted for the staging of the non-Hodgkin lymphomas with more difficulty because of the frequency of extranodal involvement and the variation in organ involvement even with apparently localized disease. Bonadonna and colleagues (7) emphasized the need for very careful examination and often the blind biopsy of suspicious areas of Waldeyer's ring, gastrointestinal radiological examination, and gastroscopy, and lumbar puncture in children and young adults. It seems certain that it is necessary to separate nodal from extranodal non-Hodgkin lymphomas when comparing results.

Experience has shown that this staging may be too simple, particularly when comparing results of treatment of Hodgkin disease between centers. For example, survival after combination chemotherapy is much better with early stage IV Hodgkin disease demonstrated only at laparotomy than with clinically obvious stage IV disease. Evidence is accumulating that the prognosis may be related more precisely to the total tumor mass, as has been shown with myeloma (23). Certainly evidence is accumulating that in Hodgkin disease the extent of splenic involvement may be related to the outlook and therefore the need for more aggressive treatment.

Radiotherapy in Hodgkin Disease

Stage I, IIa, Upper Half of Body

The importance of a staging laparotomy in demonstrating microscopic disease below the diaphragm is widely accepted. When the abdomen is shown to be free after an adequate laparotomy, irradiation can be confined to the supradiaphragmatic regions with little fear of relapse below the diaphragm at a later date. Initial relapse below the diaphragm after diagnostic laparotomy was reported in only 4% of a total of 196 patients (42). Examination of the same series of patients studied in the British National Lymphoma Investigation showed no difference in survival between those treated with prophylactic (mantle-type) and local irradiation, provided a diagnostic laparotomy had been carried out (Fig. 1). However, 9% of patients receiving only local irradiation had initial relapses in an adjacent site which would have been irradiated if a full mantle technique had been used. All three relapses were subsequently controlled completely, usually by further irradiation, with no fatalities. At the present time, the choice between local and mantle-type irradiation is a matter of personal choice, but it may be that with the gradual accumulation of more patients into this study, indications for mantle-type irradiation may become apparent.

The evolution and the technique of mantle irradiation have been described by Kaplan (48) and by Smithers and Freeman (77). The technique consists basically of the irradiation in continuity of all the lymph node regions in the upper half of the body, usually with opposing fields. Shielding of the lungs may be accomplished by the use of various combinations of lead blocks of adequate thickness, but if a large number of patients are to be treated, time can be saved by the use of prepared templates shaped to the contours of the mediastinal and hilar lymphadenopathies. An elegant technique has been devised in which holes are cut to the desired shape in a thick polystyrene block with a hot wire and subsequently filled with lead shot (26,82) or cerobend.

Normally the upper border of the mantle field is a line between the top of the chin and the occipital protuberance (Fig. 2). In some centers it is considered essential to routinely irradiate Waldeyer's ring: this can be accomplished by adding two opposed lateral fields, the lower border of which must closely match the upper border of the mantle field to which they are, of course, at right angles. The rarity of Hodgkin disease originating in Waldeyer's ring makes this procedure of doubtful value as a routine, as it produces considerable morbidity, but it may be irradiated prophylactically if there is high-cervical or preauricular lymph node involvement.

The lower border of the mantle field varies according to different authorities. Kaplan (48) refers to "a level in the body, approximately the eleventh or twelfth dorsovertebral level at which there are relatively few lymph nodes." Others take the lower border down to the second lumbar vertebral (40). First, this is the point above which it is not possible to visualize lymph nodes by a lymphogram, and second, the spinal cord ends at this level. In some centers certain patients are treated

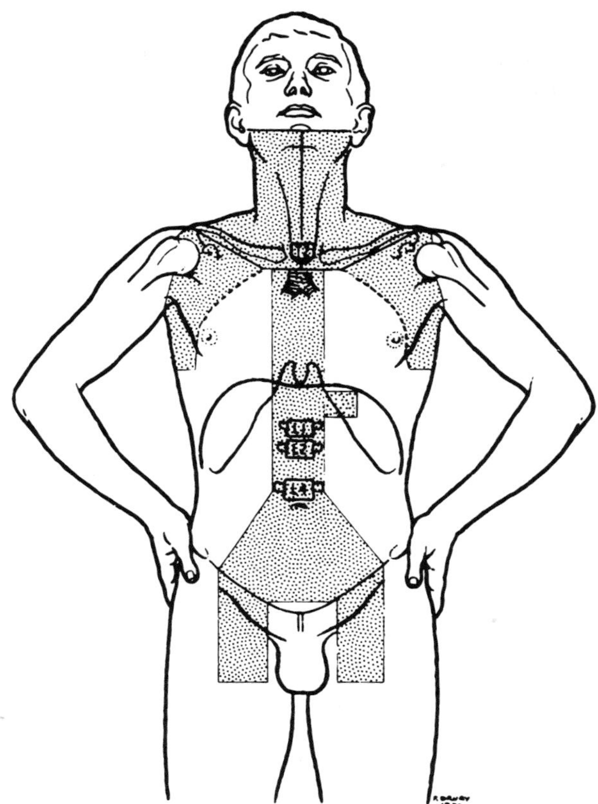

Figure 2. Diagrammatic representation of fields used in total node irradiation. TNI consists of mantle irradiation added to an inverted Y field. Some authorities include the liver if there is microscopical evidence of splenic involvement. The upper border of the mantle is normally a line drawn between the top of the mandible and the occipital protuberance. The upper border of the lung shielding blocks runs along the lower border of the fourth rib posteriorly. The minimal width of the mediastinal and paraaortic fields is 8 cm. A small field projects to the left below the diaphragm to cover the splenic pedicle. Wider fields will obviously be necessary in order to encompass any lymph node masses.

with an anchor field which covers the paraaortic nodes down to the level of the fifth lumbar vertebra (77). Whichever level is used, it is extremely important that it is permanently recorded on the patient's skin by tattooing so that any later treatment that might prove necessary can be carefully matched without risk of overlapping and overtreating normal tissues, especially the spinal cord.

A suggested technique for mantle irradiation is described in Fig. 2. As is so common in medicine, a compromise has to be reached between achieving a uniform dose of 4000 rads/4 weeks to the whole block of tissue included in the irradiation field and the overirradiation of sensitive normal tissues. With stage I, IIa (upper half) Hodgkin disease, one is treating a group of patients of whom it is hoped that well over 90% will be living normal lives 10 years later, and the very greatest care is necessary to avoid or reduce late postradiation sequelae.

Protection of the lung has been referred to already. With the advent of CT scanning it has become easier to detect minimal pulmonary infiltration and thus avoid overshielding of lungs which may, in fact, require treatment. Well aware of this risk, Kaplan (48) advocated the use of "thin lung blocks" which partially shield the whole lungs but allow the administration of 1500 rads to both lungs during routine mantle irradiation. The upper edge of lung blocks may be aligned along the lower border of the fourth rib posteriorly. The lymph nodes along the medial edge of the scapula are moved laterally into the irradiation fields either by placing the hands on the hips and rotating the elbows anteriorly, or by placing the hands behind the head, or simply elevating the hands above the head.

The spinal cord is the other structure in the upper half of the body which requires special protection. Protection of the spinal cord using a mantle field technique can be achieved only as a compromise. It is generally accepted that the absolute maximum radiation dose that can be tolerated safely by a long section of the spinal cord is 4000 rads spread over a period of 4 weeks (48) in daily dose of about 200 rads. Most authorities recommend a mantle technique using two opposing fields. With two opposing fields, a midline dose of 4000 rads will give a larger dose to the spinal cord which is normally between 5 and 7 cm deep to the skin of the back. Using two opposing fields it is necessary to shield the spinal cord when treating posteriorly, when cord tolerance has been reached. Shielding the cord in this way will reduce the dose to the center of the tumor mass.

Another treatment method which avoids this difficulty may be used, especially with the thinner patient. This technique is dependent upon the fact that in Hodgkin disease the main bulk of the tumor lies in the anterior mediastinum, and much less commonly extends into the posterior half of the thorax. Particularly with a linear accelerator, the depth dose is such that in very thin individuals treatment can be given entirely from an anterior field. Obviously one of the limiting factors, in this situation, would be the dose received by the pericardium and anterior heart muscle. Thus, it is advisable to add a posterior field to the thorax if it is necessary to give more than 5000 rads to the anterior pericardium.

The advent of megavoltage radiotherapy has changed radiotherapy completely but has introduced an additional source of error in the treatment of some tumors and none more so than in Hodgkin disease. The anterior mediastinal siting of this disease has been referred to already. Modern investigations, in particular the CT scanner, show that the tumor masses may not only lie immediately behind the anterior chest wall but there may also be actual invasion of the structures of the chest wall, including the sternum. Using a linear accelerator it is very easy to underirradiate the anterior chest wall as well as anteriorly situated cervical nodes, unless adequate buildup is provided.

Stage I, IIa, Lower Half of Body

The standard irradiation technique for treatment of lymph nodes in the lower half of the body is usually referred to as an inverted Y. Well described by Kaplan (48) and Smithers and Freeman (77) the technique needs no general description. If there is no gross lymph node enlargement, then a field 8 cm wide will encompass the central axis, paraaortic nodes, and at the same time avoid unnecessary irradiation to the kidneys. With younger women it is customary to move the ovaries out of the direct irradiation field (68). With young men, complete protection of both testicles is impossible. A reduced sperm count is common after treatment and it is common practice nowadays to recommend sperm storage for young males before either inverted Y irradiation or chemotherapy.

If the spleen has not been removed during the patient's investigations, it should be included in the treatment volume. One of the reasons originally put forward for diagnostic laparotomy and splenectomy was that this operation removed the need for splenic irradiation with the risk of irradiation of the left kidney. Le Bourgeois et al. (52) refer to 75 patients studied since 1972 following irradiation to the left kidney during irradiation to the spleen. The midline dose to the spleen was 4000 rads/4 weeks, and the amount of the left kidney included in the treatment volume varied between 30-80%. In spite of the finding of cortical atrophy of the upper pole of some kidneys, there was no evidence of biochemical or blood pressure changes, suggesting that perhaps earlier anxieties regarding renal complications may have been unduly alarmist.

Stage IIIA

Total nodal irradiation (TNI) is an established technique for the initial management of stage IIIa Hodgkin disease. Basically it consists of mantle irradiation, followed or preceded by inverted Y irradiation (Fig. 2). It is usual to irradiate first that half of the body which is productive of more symptoms or disease. Each half receives 4000 rads/4 weeks and a gap of about 4 weeks is allowed between the two halves to permit bone marrow recovery and to give the patient a short break in what is often a very taxing course of treatment. The technique and its problems have been well described (48, 77).

The main problem with this technique lies in the obvious danger of overlapping and overdosing the spinal cord. Great care must be taken to avoid this, particularly as 85% of stage IIIa patients may be expected to survive 5 years. One obvious way in which this possibility can be avoided is to match the upper and lower fields at the second lumbar vertebra below the spinal cord. Unfortunately this technique involves the patient in much greater strain during the mantle irradiation, and it is sometimes necessary to prolong the interval before proceeding to the inverted Y.

Another technique which has been introduced more recently makes a deliberate attempt to avoid this well-recognized complication. At the Memorial Hospital, Nisce and D'Angio (63) have developed what they describe as the "3 and 2" technique (Fig. 3). Using this technique, the whole of the main lymph node regions in the upper and lower half of the body are irradiated during the same course of treatment, dividing the volume first into 3 and then into 2. Moving the junctions in this way lessens the chance of overlap and serious overdosage. The usual dose delivered to the lymph nodes by this technique is 4000 rads in about 12 weeks.

As an alternative to TNI, initial treatment for stage IIIa Hodgkin disease, especially when the extent of the disease has not been confirmed by a diagnostic laparotomy, may be with combination chemotherapy. The most commonly used combination is that generally known as MOPP. Highly effective, it is a very reasonable alternative to TNI but its use is associated with more upsetting side effects than TNI, including gonadal effects which have been reported recently by Chapman et al. (17) and increased second primaries. A paper published in 1976 suggested that the likelihood of achieving CR initially was greater with TNI than with MOPP (10), but because of the excellent salvage treatment at present available, the long-term survival rates were identical with either method of treatment.

Adjuvant chemotherapy after TNI may be of value in the long-term control of stage IIIa Hodgkin disease, but obviously this combination of both treatment

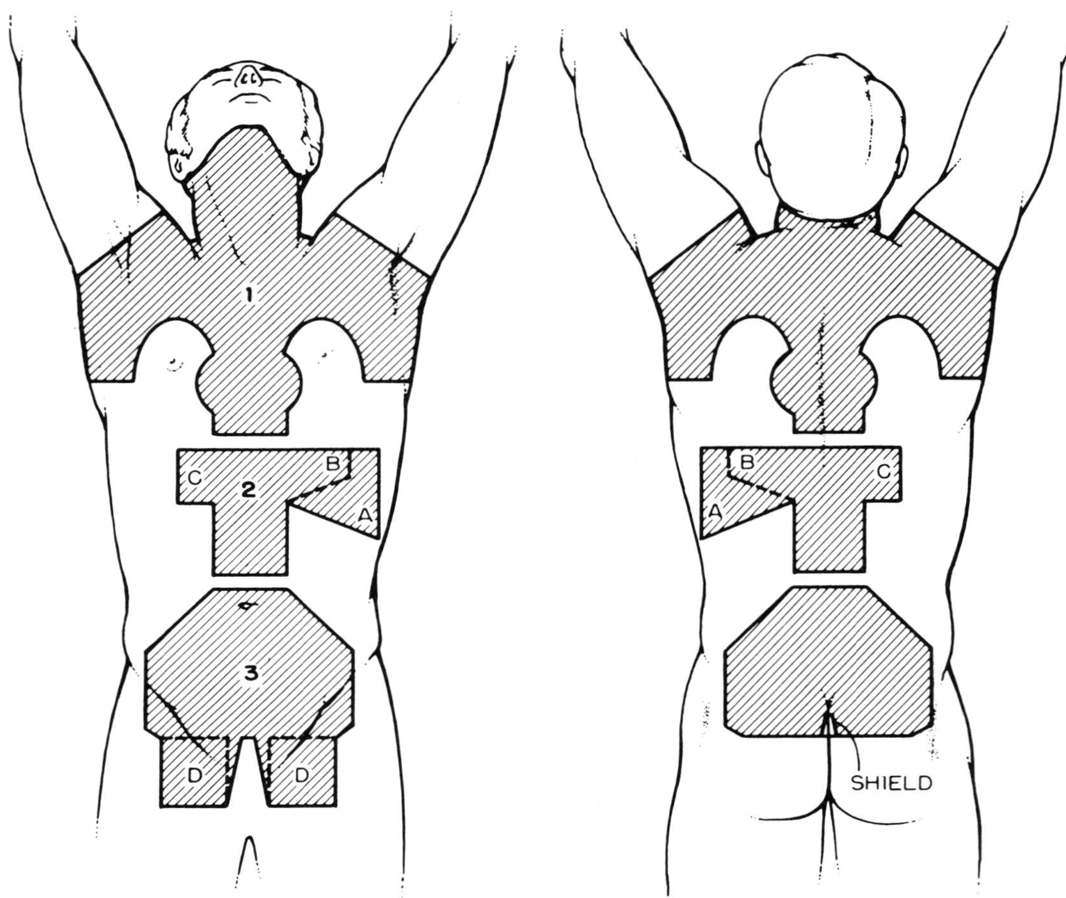

3-2 TECHNIQUE - FIRST PHASE

Figure 3. "3 and 2" technique as described by Nisce and D'Angio (63). The radiotherapy course takes place in two phases. In phase 1, the lymph node areas are divided into three groups (A). Each of the three groups is irradiated sequentially to 2000 rads in an overall period of 4. 5 weeks, with daily increments of 250 rads. There is no rest period between the segments. After a rest period of 3-4 weeks, phase 2 is commenced. Using two fields (B) 1800-2000 rads in 3. 5 weeks is given to each of the two fields. No rest period is given between fields. Patient tolerance is better than with conventional two-field TNI and the dosimetry is superior, avoiding hot and cold spots. (Nisce and D'Angio, 1976. Reproduced with acknowledgements to the authors and publishers.)

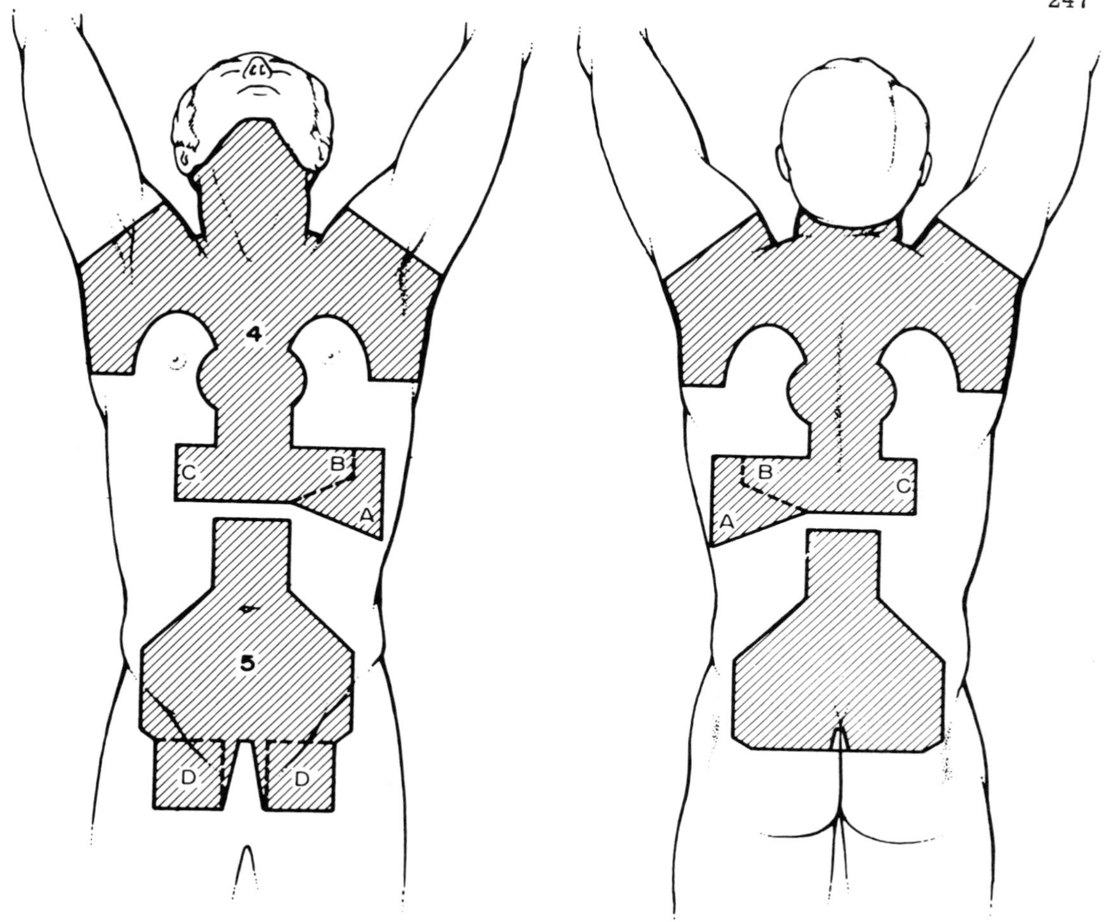

3-2 TECHNIQUE - SECOND PHASE
Figure 3.B.

methods, one after the other, will interfere with a patient's normal life for up to a year depending on bone marrow and psychological tolerance. The BNLI is at present comparing the treatment of patients with stage IIIa Hodgkin disease using TNI or TNI followed by six courses of chlorambucil, vincristine, procarbazine, and prednisone LOPP (10) (Table 3). This drug combination is almost identical with that reported by McElwain and colleagues (58) as being of equal efficacy as MOPP with far less side effects, due to the substitution of oral chlorambucil in place of intravenous nitrogen mustard. It is too early as yet to know if the addition of this drug combination improves the prognosis, but it is certainly well tolerated and to date there have been fewer relapses in those patients receiving adjuvant LOPP. In PS IIIa, Kaplan (49) advises additional hepatic irradiation when the spleen is shown to be involved microscopically and adjuvant chemotherapy when there is massive spleen or nodal involvement (Table 4). The current BNLI study will provide an opportunity to confirm the view that splenic involvement is an indication for additional treatment.

PS IB, IIB, IIIB

It has been recognized for many years that patients with systemic manifestations carry a worse prognosis than patients whose disease is of a similar extent,

Table 3. LOPP*

Chlorambucil	10 mg/m^2	p.o.	Days 1-10
Vincristine	1.4 mg/m^2 (maximum 2 mg)	i.v.	Days 1 + 8
Procarbazine	100 mg/m^2	p.o.	Days 1-10
Prednisone	25 mg/m^2 (maximum 60 mg)	p.o.	Days 1-14

* The usual interval between courses is 3 weeks from day 8, depending on the blood count. The platelet count should be 100,000 or above and the total white count should be 4000 or above.

but who are without B symptoms. TNI alone may be very effective, as is recommended by Kaplan (49), with lymphocytic predominance or nodular sclerotic pathology, when the disease is limited to stage I or II with or without localized extranodal spread. When the disease is more extensive and histological examination reveals either mixed cellularity or lymphocytic depletion, the same author recommends a combined approach, starting with TNI and continuing with combination chemotherapy or in alternating sequency, beginning with two courses of chemotherapy when the disease involves both halves of the body.

The early experience of the BNLI with radiotherapy as the initial treatment method in patients with B disease was disappointing, and current practice with this group of patients is to commence treatment with combination chemotherapy. One reason for adopting this approach is that it provides rapid relief for the patient from those B symptoms which are usually the most distressing part of the illness. After complete remission has been produced and consolidated with chemotherapy, irradiation to the original sites of bulk disease may help to prevent relapse.

In patients with stages I, II, and III disease where the extent has been carefully confirmed by a diagnostic laparotomy, bulk disease (before chemotherapy) has been clearly defined and there is little doubt as to the radiation fields required. The value of bulk irradiation of this type has not as yet been evaluated and the BNLI is carrying out a comparative prospective study with this in mind.

When the exact extent of the disease has not been confirmed by a diagnostic laparotomy, then bulk disease irradiation cannot be less than TNI which must of course include the spleen, and probably also the liver. Such treatment is obviously of much greater magnitude than simple bulk disease irradiation and may prove to be poorly tolerated by the patient. These patients may be better treated as stage IV disease.

Stage IVA, B

When Hodgkin disease is widespread and involves extranodal tissues, there is general agreement that initial treatment should be with combination chemotherapy. Some authors consider that irradiation to sites of bulk disease should be introduced early, to alternate with chemotherapy (49) or later, after complete remission has been obtained and consolidation chemotherapy has been given.

Table 4. Treatment Recommendations in Previously Untreated Patients

Stage	Histological Type	Description	Recommended Treatment
1. (a) PSIA	LP or NS	Limited to one upper cervical region; negative lymphangiogram and laparotomy	Local cervical supraclavicular (involved field) or minimantle and Waldeyer field radiotherapy only
(b) PSIA	MC or LD	Same as 1 (a)	Total lymphoid radiotherapy
2. CSIA	NS	Limited to mediastinal nodes; clinically negative cervical supraclavicular nodes, negative lymphangiogram	Mantle field radiotherapy only
3. (a) PSIA	LP or NS	Limited to one inguinal femoral region; negative lymphangiogram and laparotomy	Inverted Y (pelvis, paraaortic, and splenic pedicle) field radiotherapy only
(b) PSIA	MC or LD	Same as 3 (a)	Total lymphoid radiotherapy
4. (a) PSIA	LP or NS	Limited to one lower cervical supraclavicular region; negative lymphangiogram and laparotomy	Subtotal lymphoid radiotherapy only (mantle and spade fields; Waldeyer field also when upper cervical nodes involved)
(b) PSIIA	LP or NS	Involvement of two or more lymph node regions above the diaphragm; negative lymphangiogram and laparotomy	Same as 4 (a)
(c) PSIA	MC or LD	Same as 4 (a) or (b)	Total lymphoid radiotherapy
5. (a) PSIIA	LP	Involvement of two or more lymph node regions below the diaphragm; negative spleen, liver, and bone marrow	Subtotal lymphoid radiotherapy only (full inverted Y and minimantle fields)
(b) PSIIA	NS, MC or LD	Same as 5 (a)	Total lymphoid radiotherapy (including mediastinal and hilar nodes)

Table 4 (Cont'd)

Stage	Histological Type	Description	Recommended Treatment
6. PSIB	LP or NS	As in 1-5, but with constitutional symptoms	Total lymphoid radiotherapy (mantle and full inverted Y fields; Waldeyer field also when upper cervical nodes involved)
7. PSII$_e$A, B	LP or NS	As in 4, 5, or 6, but with one or two localized extralymphatic site(s) of involvement	Total lymphoid radiotherapy plus local irradiation of the extralymphatic lesion(s): if lymphadenopathy is massive, this may be followed (after a 6-8 week rest period) by six cycles of combination chemotherapy (omitting prednisone)
8. PSIB, IIB	MC or LD	As in 6 or 7	Combined modality therapy: total lymphoid radiotherapy (mantle and full inverted Y fields, Waldeyer field also when upper cervical nodes involved) and combination chemotherapy in an alternating sequence, starting with radiotherapy to the involved region
9. PSIIIA, III$_s$A, III$_e$A, III$_{es}$A	Any	Involvement of nodes above and below diaphragm, with or without spleen; no marrow or liver involvement; constitutional symptoms only	Total lymphoid radiotherapy (plus local irradiation of E lesion(s), if present); when spleen is involved, hepatic field irradiation in addition; with massive spleen or nodal involvement, adjuvant combination chemotherapy is indicated

10. PSIIIB, III_sB, III_eB, $III_{es}B$	Any	As in 9, but with constitutional symptoms	Combined modality therapy: total lymphoid radiotherapy (mantle, paraaortic/hepatic, and pelvic fields) and combination chemotherapy in a split course or alternating sequence, beginning with two cycles of chemotherapy
11. $PSIV_{h+}A$, $IV_{h+}B$	Any	Biopsy-proven liver involvement with spleen and node involvement	Alternating combined modality therapy: two to three cycles of combination chemotherapy, then paraaortic/hepatic field radiotherapy; two more cycles of chemotherapy (omitting prednisone) and ending with pelvic field radiotherapy
12. (a) CS or $PSIV_{Lp}$	Any	Multiple bilateral pulmonary lesions, or pulmonary and biopsy-proven pleural lesions	Combination chemotherapy (three to six cycles) followed by low to moderate dose (2000-3000 rads) radiotherapy to regions of initially bulky lymph node involvement, and three to six consolidation cycles of chemotherapy; no maintenance chemotherapy
(b) CS or $PSIV_o$	Any	Multiple disseminated lesions of bone	
(c) $PSIV_{m+}$	Any	Biopsy-proven bone marrow involvement	
(d) CS or PSIV	Any	Stage IV lesions other than the above	

Source: Ref. 48.

The need for additional irradiation is probably very real in certain cases but the problem is their definition. Since the introduction of MOPP, complete remission rates of between 60 and 80% have been reported with advanced Hodgkin disease and the original results reported by De Vita and colleagues (22) in 1970 have never been bettered, despite the introduction of many different combinations of active drugs. Of those patients achieving CR, about one-half relapse subsequently and most of these unfortunates die of their disease, in spite of repeated treatments which may often produce very satisfactory temporary remissions. If it is possible to predict those patients who are likely to relapse, then additional irradiation would be even more justifiable. When comparing the results reported by different centers, certain factors should be remembered. The first is the selection of cases which is included in the reported series. The effect of sex and age upon the prognosis in Hodgkin disease is generally recognized and has been accepted for at least 25 years. The complete remission rate for patients with advanced disease treated by combination chemotherapy is greater if patients are under 45. It is probable that bulk disease irradiation is more necessary in older men and less so in young women.

The exact method of definition of the extent of the disease is also important. For example, if a patient is defined as having stage IVB disease largely as a result of clinical examination following nonpathological investigations, the patient probably has very extensive, bulky disease. Bulk irradiation after successful chemotherapy is then likely to be especially helpful, but the exact extent of the sites requiring bulk irradiation may be difficult to define, in the absence of a previous laparotomy. Bulk irradiation in the absence of exact definition becomes a matter of probabilities and clinical judgment. In extreme cases it will approximate to total-body irradiation.

At the opposite end of the spectrum is stage IV disease which has been discovered accidentally, following a diagnostic laparotomy for clinical stage I, IIa (upper half) disease. In this situation the stage IV disease is microscopical, and a complete response is almost certain following adequate combination chemotherapy. The precise definition of the extent of disease provided by the operation certainly permits very accurate bulk irradiation, but additional treatment of this type is of doubtful value and, indeed, in view of the excellent results of treatment with chemotherapy alone, its value, if any, becomes impossible to assess.

Finally, the efficacy of combination chemotherapy is changing as new methods of assessment of progress of the disease are introduced. The usual approach with chemotherapy is to continue until complete remission has been achieved, following which a certain number of courses of consolidation treatment will be given. The amount of treatment given depends largely on the demonstration of complete remission. Modern investigative procedures including CT scanning have demonstrated that intraabdominal lymphoma may persist for longer than was appreciated previously. It is possible that some of the previous chemotherapy failures were due to premature treatment cessation, and it will be very difficult to compare the value of bulk irradiation in older and current series.

While combination chemotherapy is the cornerstone of treatment with stage IV Hodgkin disease, bulk irradiation with truly advanced stage IV disease is likely to improve the prognosis. However, it is becoming increasingly recognized that the risks of combination chemotherapy and widefield irradiation are additive, and there is real need to determine the exact place of irradiation in patients with advanced disease.

The Management of Relapse in Hodgkin Disease

Because Hodgkin disease is generally extremely responsive to both radiotherapy and chemotherapy, it is one of a very small group of tumors where retreatment after relapse is often followed by complete remission and, in some patients, by permanent cure. Obviously, the management of such a patient will be related closely to the treatment previously given. The following principles are suggested. A relapse should be treated as generalized if B symptoms are present.

Diagnosis of Relapse

With all lymphomas there is a real danger that almost any new development in the patient's life may be attributed to reactivity of the original disease. It is essential that a patient with a relapse must be investigated thoroughly and, whenever possible, histological confirmation of the relapse must be obtained. The risks of repeated treatment greatly exceed those of repeated biopsies. When relapse has been confirmed, the patient must be restaged as thoroughly as if the case was being studied initially, because the extent of the relapse will affect the treatment. The recommendations below assume that the patient has been completely restaged and the extent of the relapse has been carefully delineated.

Local Relapse in Previously Irradiated Lymph Nodes

Occasionally when the relapse is strictly limited in extent, reirradiation may be considered reasonable, and this may be followed by long-term control. Obviously this is reasonable only when normal local tissue tolerance can be exceeded without serious risk to the patient. Usually relapse in lymph nodes previously irradiated to a dose of about 4000 rads/4 weeks is best treated by combination chemotherapy. The most commonly used combination is MOPP.

Local Relapse in Nodes Adjacent To Those Previously Irradiated

Irradiation to a dose of 4000 rads/4 weeks may be curative. The importance of permanently marking the edge of irradiation fields is obvious if adjacent treatment is to be given safely. Another reasonable approach would be to consider irradiation to all the previously unirradiated node regions in the body.

Relapse in Previously Unirradiated Lymph Node Regions in the Opposite Half of the Body

Irradiation to a dose of 4000 rads/4 weeks is the method of choice. Usually this will involve treating the lower half of the body (inverted Y) in a patient who has previously received mantle irradiation. The importance of the junction line between the upper and lower fields is obvious, as this often overlies the spinal cord. If the lower edge of the upper field has not been recorded exactly, and there is a risk of overirradiating the cord, combination chemotherapy may be considered to be safer treatment.

Generalized Relapse After Previous Irradiation
To Lymph Nodes (e.g., Mantle, TNI)

Combination chemotherapy is the mainstay of treatment, most commonly with MOPP. Local bulk disease irradiation may be considered, especially for patients whose disease is not showing a marked response by the third course. Bulk disease irradiation may be taken to 4000 rads/4 weeks except when this is precluded by previous irradiation or by normal tissue tolerance. For example, the normal dose to the whole lungs should not exceed 1500-2000 rads/4 weeks.

Generalized Relapse After Previous Response
To Chemotherapy for Generalized Disease

These patients may be considered in several main groups: (1) Relapse after response to a single agent: This should never be seen nowadays, as treatment with a single agent can be regarded as totally inadequate. The complete remission rate with single agents is in the order of 30% and permanent cure after treatment of this type is almost unknown. Treatment of the relapse should be initially with a recognized combination of drugs, particularly nitrogen mustard, vincristine, procarbazine and prednisone (MOPP) or (MVPP). Unfortunately the response of this group is disappointing and only 35% of patients achieve complete remission as opposed to the usual 60-80% CR rate reported after initial treatment with an effective combination (62). (2) Relapse a long interval after response to an effective drug combination: The disease in these patients can be considered to have responded to the combination used, and it is reasonable to use it again, with or without bulk radiotherapy, as recommended by Kaplan (49). It is possible that treatment was not continued for long enough and that true CR was not recorded. Perhaps this will become less common with the introduction of modern, more efficient imaging techniques. (3) Relapse soon after response to an effective drug combination: Relapse may be seen within a few weeks or months after a well-recorded CR and adequate consolidation chemotherapy. Other cases may have shown an initial response and then relapse, while the same adequate treatment continues. This group is a very difficult one to treat: eventual success has been reported by some authors, switching over to alternative regimes, such as ABVD (adriamycin, bleomycin, vincristine, and dicarbazine), thought not to be cross-resistant. Santoro and Bonadonna (74) reported CR in 62% of patients resistant to MOPP. Unfortunately this successful outcome has not been obtained by others (79) and, in the experience of the author, these unfortunate patients are all destined to die of their disease. Successful response may be obtained by other combinations but, in general, they are never maintained and further relapse occurs. Bulk radiotherapy may be combined with chemotherapy combinations, or local radiotherapy used for effective local palliation, and sometimes single agents, such as vinblastine or cis-dichlorodiammineplatinum (18) may produce long remissions, but the eventual outcome is predictable. These patients require the greatest care if they are to be given the longest, most enjoyable life that is possible. Treatment with combination chemotherapy allows little time for the enjoyment of a normal existence and opportunist infections occur with particular frequency in these unfortunates.

NON-HODGKIN LYMPHOMA

Classification

Over the year, the heterogenous group of lymphomas now referred to as non-Hodgkin lymphomas have been classified morphologically in many different ways.

The system that was developed by Robb Smith over a period of 30 years (69) proved generally unacceptable to most pathologists and clinicians in Europe, who continued to refer to the simpler classification of four main groups of lymphomas: (giant) follicular lymphoma, (lymphocytic) lymphosarcoma, lymphoblastic lymphosarcoma, and reticulum cell sarcoma. This was not due to just complacency. To a clinician a disease classification is of value only if it helps in the management of his patients. Twenty years ago it was generally accepted that patients with lymphoreticular neoplasms were incurable, and it seemed pointless to use a much more complicated nomenclature which would not affect the issue. This simple European classification referred to above gave the clinician a reasonable idea as to the length of life left to the patient and was, therefore, adequate. The acceptance that Hodgkin disease could be cured renewed interest in the classification and treatment of non-Hodgkin lymphomas. It was assumed that a better understanding of this group of diseases would lead to their better management.

The first new classification was that of Rappaport (67) which became widely accepted and is the most widely used. Since then fundamental changes in our understanding of the behavior of the reticuloendothelial system have occurred. It is now accepted that there are at least two main groups of lymphocytes which differ morphologically and functionally. It is also accepted that many tumors, composed of so-called reticulum cells - originally classified by Rappaport as histiocytic - are in fact composed of transformed lymphocytes. Probably the most forward looking classification of the non-Hodgkin lymphomas is that advocated by Lukes and Collins (56,57) which divides lymphomas into B or T lymphocytic, U (uncommitted) lymphocytic, true histiocytic, or unclassifiable. Most non-Hodgkin lymphomas are of the B-cell type and usually of follicular origin. Tumors with a follicular pattern usually consist mainly of cleaved cells inside the follicles, which are difficult to recognize as such with normal histiological preparations. When tumor cells are found in the blood, the cleaved nature of the cells becomes more obvious. The presence of occasional blood-borne cells does not appear to affect the good prognosis of follicular tumors. When the majority of the follicular cells are large, the prognosis may be worse. When the follicular pattern is lost and when the tumor is composed largely of either large, cleaved or large, uncleaved cells, the tumors often behave in a highly malignant fashion. Some of these tumors exhibit marked immunological abnormalities or have occurred in patients with recognized immunological disorders such as rheumatoid arthritis. These are recognized by Lukes and Collins as immunoblastic sarcomas. This modern approach is supported by the work of the Lennert group (78), but there are difficulties associated with both these classifications, which are dependent on special immunological investigations.

Immunological investigations of this type are not always available and also their results are affected by a wide range of factors (80). Techniques such as these offer enormous possibilities for the future, but are not necessarily available as routine investigations. It is probable that morphological classifications will remain the most important method of routinely assessing the non-Hodgkin lymphomas. A useful morphological classification of this type should be easily understood by the clinicians and offer guidance as to the patient management, taking into account recent immunological concepts and utilizing recently acquired ultrastructural information so that on-going studies can be undertaken, which may allow improvements in management as material and knowledge accumulates. From the clinician's point of view it is preferable to avoid confusing and complicated neologisms. Such a morphological classification, which also utilizes modern concepts, was presented initially by Bennett and colleagues (5) at a workshop held at the University of Chicago in 1973. This classification has been used by the British National Lymphoma Investigation (BNLI) and has been published in detail (15,35). It can be used by the routine histopathologist using a light microscope (Table 5).

Table 5. British National Lymphoma Classification (Non-Hodgkin)*

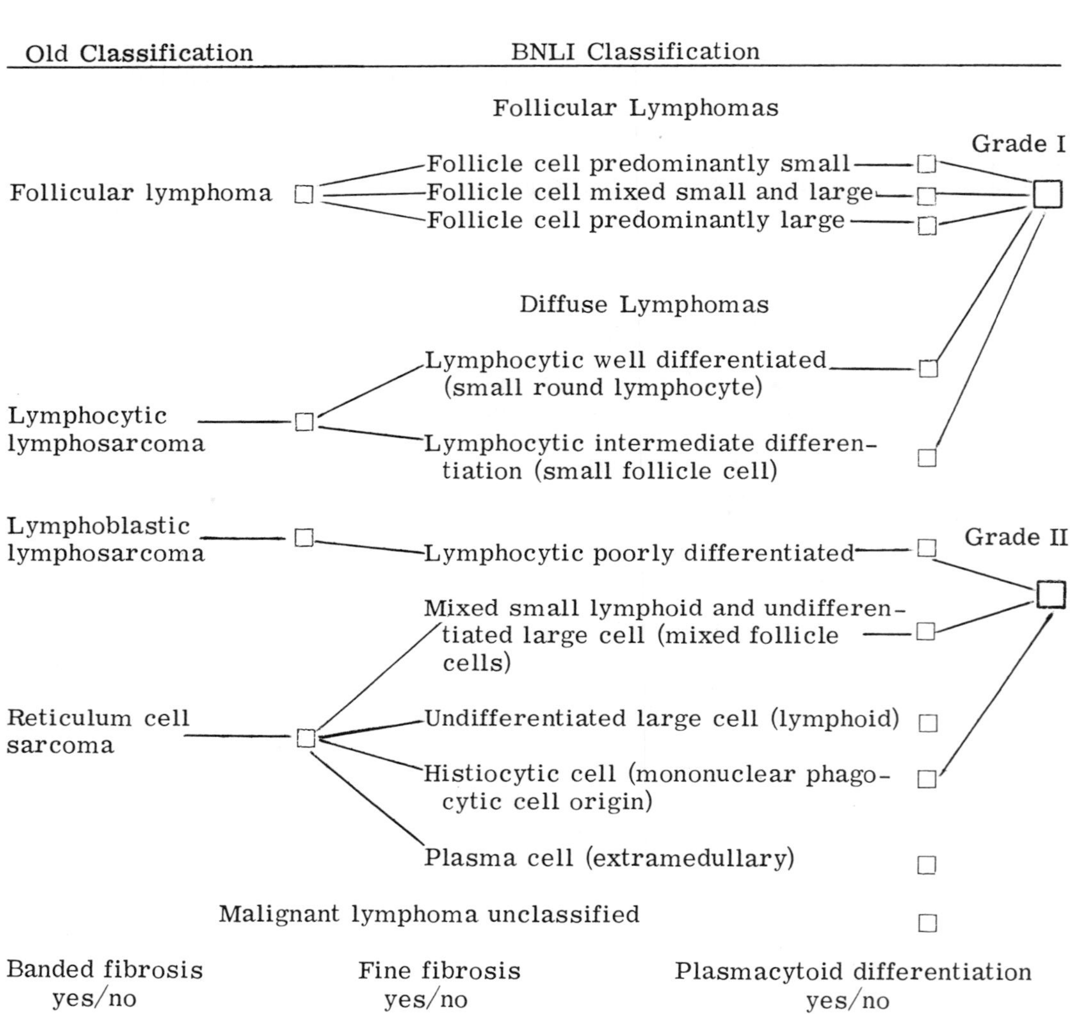

* This classification was presented at the Workshop on Classifications of Non-Hodgkin's Lymphomas (9) in Chicago in 1973 and has been used by the BNLI since its earliest studies on this group of diseases. Certain of its features should be noted. It is possible to relate the modern subdivisions to the old European classification. After subgrouping, patients can be placed in two main histological grades which can be closely related to the prognosis. In general, the terminology used is easy to understand and neologisms have been avoided. Fibrosis and plasmacytoid differentiation may occur in many of the subgroups and are therefore recorded in every case. Special subdivisions for these features would add unnecessary complications. The lymphocytic poorly differentiated group includes the anterior mediastinal convoluted lymphocyte ("chicken foot-print) of T-cell lymphoma of Lukes and Collins (55, 56) Burkitt lymphoma, and non-Burkitt lymphomas. The mixed cell tumor contains a mixture of true follicle cells. An admixture of reactive small lymphocytes can be seen with

Follicular Lymphoma

This group may be considered as a separate entity carrying a relatively good prognosis but may be divided into three types according to the proportion of small and large cells within the follicle. The prognosis appears to be marginally worse when these cells are predominantly large. Cleaving is rarely visible in normal tissue sections. Nodes with a minimal follicular pattern are still classifiable as follicular lymphomas because recent analysis has indicated that the presence of areas of diffuse replacement does not affect the prognosis (27).

Diffuse Lymphomas

The prognosis of this group varies enormously.

1. Diffuse lymphocytic well differentiated (DLWD) (small round cell): The normal lymph node structure is diffusely replaced with small round lymphocytes with minimal cytoplasm and darkly staining nuclei, identical with those in the blood in chronic lymphatic leukemia. Occasionally there is plasmacytoid differentiation and there may be a monoclonal gammopathy, which can be used as a tumor marker.

2. Diffuse lymphocytic intermediate differentiated (DLID) (small follicle cell): This is the diffuse counterpart of the predominantly small cell follicular lymphoma. The small lymphocytes have darkly staining, irregularly contoured nuclei and cleaving is very difficult to demonstrate. The use of the term differentiated, as opposed to undifferentiated, bears no relation to the functional development of the lymphocyte. The work of Lukes and Collins and others indicates that the large undifferentiated forms have been transformed from the smaller, less active forms. However, to the clinician the words "differentiated" and "undifferentiated" are related to the tempo of the disease and therefore the prognosis; they have been retained in this classification as it is considered that they would be helpful in the management of these tumors.

3. Diffuse lymphocytic poorly differentiated (DLPD): This is a composite group of tumors. Burkitt tumor contains sheets of large lymphocytes (lymphoblasts) with scattered, large macrophages producing the classical "starry sky" appearance. The non-Burkitt type typically does not demonstrate this starry sky appearance. A third subgroup consists mainly of poorly differentiated tumors presenting in the anterior mediastinum of children and young adults. The nucleus of the tumor cell is convoluted giving a pattern which has been described as having a "chicken's foot" appearance. This lymphoma is considered to be of T-cell origin. The association of this tumor with acute lymphocytic leukemia and meningeal infiltration is well recognized.

Table 5 (Cont'd)

many larger-celled lymphomas, and this finding must not be misinterpreted as a true mixed follicle cell lymphoma. The undifferentiated large-cell tumor may be composed of large, cleaved or noncleaved cells: the management and prognosis of either type of tumor is so similar that differentiation is unnecessary from the clinician's viewpoint. Since 1973, the BNLI has recognized true histiocytic and extramedullary plasma cell lymphomas, and these subgroups are becoming generally accepted.

4. Diffuse lymphocytic mixed (DLMX) (mixed follicle cells): A true tumor of this type is composed of both small and large follicle center cells and is the diffuse counterpart of the mixed-cell follicular lymphoma.

5. Diffuse undifferentiated large cell (DUL) (large lymphoid cell): The basic cell is the large lymphoid cell, with a smooth nuclear outline, and one or more prominent nucleoli. Sometimes there may be plasma-cytoid differentiation. These large cells are transformed lymphocytes or immunoblasts and use of the word "undifferentiated" is justified by the clinical behavior of these tumors rather than by their evolutionary stage. Sometimes these tumors contain atypical bizarre cells, including giant cells resembling Reed-Sternberg cells, and scattered macrophages may present a starry sky appearance. Not uncommonly eosinophils and many small lymphocytes are present. If there is also diffuse fibrosis (6), it is not surprising that these tumors are sometimes misdiagnosed as lymphocyte-depleted Hodgkin disease.

6. Histiocytic cell (mononuclear phagocytic cell): The original studies leading to the recognition of this group of tumors were made with the electron microscope, but they are not recognizable by routine morphological methods (36). Well-differentiated, true histiocytic tumor cells closely resemble normal histiocytes. Sometimes they may be composed of less well-differentiated large cells, with lumpy lobulated nuclei, often multinucleate, with foamy, granular, or eosinophilic cytoplasm. The cell margin is less well defined than is the margin of the diffuse undifferentiated large cell tumors. Fine sclerosis may be present and sometimes the cytoplasm is markedly pyrinophilic.

7. Plasma cell tumors: Extramedullar plasmacytomas involving lymphatic tissue, particularly in the neck, have been reported, but they were considered to be rare. It has become recognized recently that primary lymphomas of the gastrointestinal tract may include a high proportion of plasma cell tumors (36). Typical tumors of this type may be recognized by a perinuclear halo which can be enhanced by methyl green-pyronin. The chromatin arrangement typical of plasma cells is retained even when the tumor cells are less well differentiated.

8. Unclassified: Using the BNLI classification, this group is a small one.

Another feature of many of the varieties of the non-Hodgkin lymphomas is fibrosis. This phenomenon was first reported by Bennett and Millett (4) and later by Rosas-Uribe and Rappaport (71). The presence of fibrosis appears to improve the prognosis, whatever the basic tumor cell type and pattern (6). From the clinician's point of view the final division in the BNLI classification into two grades is of value because there is a difference between the prognosis and the management of grade I and grade II tumors.

Radiotherapy in Non-Hodgkin Lymphoma

Patients with non-Hodgkin lymphomas should be investigated as already described. They are usually staged according to the Ann Arbor classification. After full investigation certain obvious differences emerge when the results are compared with those in Hodgkin disease.

At least four out of every five patients with non-Hodgkin lymphoma depending upon the center concerned, can be shown to have widespread disease after full investigation. In the abdominal cavity mesenteric node involvement is common and throughout the whole body extranodal involvement of many sites rarely involved in

Hodgkin disease is frequent, including in particular Waldeyer's ring, the gastrointestinal tract, the liver, and bone marrow. This difference in distribution is an important factor in the treatment of non-Hodgkin lymphomas. The frequency of extranodal involvement is emphasized by many authors. Bonadonna and colleagues (7) refer to the need for blind biopsy of Waldeyer's ring, gastrointestinal radiological examination, gastroscopy, and lumbar puncture in children and young adults.

When considering the treatment of patients with non-Hodgkin lymphoma it is necessary to consider not only the stage and histological grade of the tumor but also, with localized extranodal disease, the exact primary site.

There is less information available as to the ideal dose of irradiation required to produce permanent local control of the non-Hodgkin lymphomas than there is for Hodgkin disease. This is partly because the non-Hodgkin lymphomas embrace a broader spectrum of disease and partly because only recently has it been appreciated that such a large proportion of patients with this group of lymphomas already have widely disseminated disease and failure of local control may in the past have been more commonly due to reseeding of the sterilized volume from as yet undetected foci elsewhere. It is generally accepted that a large number of patients with localized grade I non-Hodgkin lymphomas can be controlled with a dose of 3500-4000 rads/4 weeks, but some lymphomas of grade II histology are more radioresistant and complete disappearance of local disease may require a dose as high as 6000 rads/6 weeks.

Stage I, II, Grade I (Primary Nodal)

When, after full investigation, the patient with grade I non-Hodgkin lymphoma (NHL) is found to have localized disease, a case can be made for local irradiation to a maximum dose of 3500-4000 rads. Where there is evidence that Hodgkin disease often progresses systematically to involve, in turn, adjacent groups of lymph nodes, most authorities agree that in most patients with NHL, when the disease progresses it does so in an unpredictable fashion, often skipping adjacent lymph node regions. For this reason it seems illogical to consider prophylactic irradiation of the mantle type as is used with Hodgkin disease. Long-term survival after local irradiation for localized NHL has been reported by many investigators (35, 53, 66, 70, 81).

It is recommended that stage I, II, grade I NHL arising in the upper half of the body should be treated initially with wide local radiotherapy up to 4000 rads/4 weeks. The value of adjuvant chemotherapy with this type of patient is as yet unproven. Prospective comparative trials are at present being undertaken by the British National Lymphoma Investigation; to date, adjuvant chemotherapy offers no advantages.

With stage I, II, grade I NHL localized to the lower half of the body, the problem is more complicated. If no diagnostic laparotomy has been carried out, it is especially difficult to exclude involvement of mesenteric and other node regions which cannot be demonstrated by lymphography. Although modern investigational methods including CT and ultrasound scanning may solve this problem, at the present time it seems logical that local irradiation to localized disease in the lower half of the body should include irradiation of the whole abdomen and its contents. A very elegant and apparently safe and effective technique has been evolved at Stanford University (32). This method uses a four-field box arrangement which delivers 4400 rads to the whole abdomen, but protects the liver and kidneys from excessive irradiation by shrinking the irradiation ports when the tolerance dose to these organs has been achieved.

Stage I, II, Grade II (Primary Nodal)

Again, as with grade I tumors, a case can be made for local radiotherapy, but the therapist must be prepared to take the dose to a higher level as some of these lymphomas are relatively radioresistant. When local cure can be obtained, survival without relapse for about 5 years may be regarded as evidence of complete cure. In an earlier series (59) only eight patients were found to have localized grade II NHL and of these only three survived 5 years. However, all three patients then survived for 11-17 years and still remain disease free today, a further 10 years later, after radiotherapy alone.

Unfortunately modern investigations demonstrate widespread disease in more than 80% of patients, and there are very few cases where radiotherapy alone appears to provide reasonable treatment. However, the possibility that they have truly localized disease is greatly increased by these investigations. Adjuvant chemotherapy with this type of case is of unproven value as yet, but prospective comparative trials are being undertaken.

In this group of poor-histology tumors there is probably a much greater need for adjuvant chemotherapy, partly because control by chemotherapy is more difficult to achieve with macroscopic tumors of this grade and partly because the growth rate of many of these lymphomas is notoriously rapid. It may be that better control will be obtained if all patients are treated initially by combination chemotherapy followed by local radiotherapy to bulk disease.

Stage I, IIE (Primary Extranodal)

Local involvement of an extranodal structure is indicated by the letter "E." Non-Hodgkin lymphomas have been reported as arising from almost every part of the body. Some sites are commonly affected and some rarely so. From the practical point of view, they may be divided into extranodal lymphomas arising in the head and neck, extranodal lymphomas apparently originating in the intraabdominal gut, and those arising in other organs.

All patients should, of course, be completely investigated, as already indicated. There is no evidence that NHL originating in the tonsil, for example, is less likely to generalize than a tumor which is histologically identical but which originates in a cervical lymph node. When generalized disease is discovered, the patient is managed as any patient with stages III and IV disease.

Extranodal: Head and Neck

Although Waldeyer's ring is included as a primary lymphatic structure in the Ann Arbor classification, all NHL arising in the head and neck, excluding those involving only the lymph nodes, will be considered together under this heading. Lymphomas of the orbit itself and intracranial primary lymphomas are rare. Between one-quarter and one-third of all primary extranodal lymphomas arise in the head and neck region. The number of cases seen by the clinical oncologist will depend upon the closeness of links with ENT colleagues, who see most patients initially. Most commonly, NHL arise in Waldeyer's ring. Other primary sites include the parotid and submandibular salivary glands, the antrum and paranasal sinus, the palate and buccal surfaces, the lacrymal gland, and the thyroid gland. The histological picture is that of a grade II tumor in at least three out of four patients. Of the remainder most are grade I and a small number of plasmacystomas.

These tumors are most commonly managed by irradiation, treating the primary site with a field arrangement that varies according to the site. Usually, the patient is treated as if the primary tumor was a poorly differentiated carcinoma and the arrangement used is similar. In most centers the primary site and the lymph nodes in both sides of the neck, whether clinically involved or not, are treated to a dose of 3500-4000 rads/4 weeks, which is the tolerance limit for the spinal cord as well as the mucosa in the head and neck when the whole volume is irradiated. The treatment is then changed so that a further 2000-2500 rads is given to the primary site only, for example the nasopharynx or the tonsillar bed. This technique gives an excellent chance of destroying local disease. The poor results following radiotherapy of this type that have been published in the past are with patients who have been underinvestigated.

At present there is no factual evidence that adjuvant chemotherapy will improve the prognosis in those patients who have been fully investigated before receiving treatment as having localized disease. There may be a greater place for treatment of this type when the lymphoma is of grade II histology, and especially when the patient is young (see below).

Extranodal: Gastrointestinal

This group includes NHL arising in the gut below the diaphragm. The most common primary sites are the terminal part of the small bowel, the stomach, and the large bowel. The problem is totally different from that encountered in NHL arising in the head and neck. In an attempt to produce a better understanding of the management of these tumors, Crowther and Blackledge (20) have suggested a staging system which appears to be closely related to the prognosis (Table 6). When the lymphoma is limited to the bowel or has spread no further than immediately adjacent lymph nodes, and when its complete resection has been carried out, cure is likely in at least four out of five patients, with or without postoperative radiotherapy. Unfortunately many primary gut lymphomas present as emergencies following a perforation or obstruction when the laparotomy is commonly performed by a relatively inexperienced surgeon, late at night. In addition to excising the primary tumor, the surgeon's immediate problems include dealing with a perforation or obstruction in a patient who may be shocked and ill, and he is unlikely to spend much

Table 6. Postoperative Staging of Gastrointestinal Lymphomas

IA:	Single tumor confined to gut
IB:	Multiple tumors confined to gut
IIA:	Tumor with local lymph node involvement
IIB:	Tumor with local extension to adjacent tissues
IIC:	Tumor with perforation and peritonitis
III:	Tumor with widespread lymphadenopathy
IV:	Tumor with disseminated disease in nonlymphoid tissue

Source: From Ref. 20.

time carefully considering the possibility of staging the patient. When the primary tumor arises in the stomach or large bowel, the provisional diagnosis is a carcinoma and again no attempt will be made to stage the tumor as is necessary for a lymphoma. It is therefore usual for primary NHL arising in the gut to be understaged. Most of these tumors are grade II histology. It is not surprising that the results of treating patients with irradiation after surgical resection are in general poor. Crowther believes that postoperative radiotherapy has little effect on patients with advanced disease and is probably unnecessary for the small number of fortunate individuals whose disease is limited to the gut and immediately adjacent lymph nodes.

The possibility of a second-look staging laparotomy is considered in some centers, but this is often contraindicated by the age and general condition of the patient. In some patients with primary lymphoma of the gut, the possible diagnosis is considered before the initial laparotomy, usually because of the radiological appearances and microscopical findings of material removed on endoscopic examination. Surgical removal is still the first essential step in treatment, partly to remove bulk tumor but also to avoid late complications. NHL arising in the wall of the gut often invades all layers, and treatment with radiotherapy or chemotherapy followed by a satisfactory tumor response may be followed by an acute perforation with disastrous results.

The following treatment program for NHL arising in the alimentary canal below the diaphragm is suggested: (1) When the diagnosis is considered preoperatively, total excision of the tumor and its adjacent lymph nodes should be undertaken. At the same operation, if the patient's general condition allows it, the normal staging procedures for a lymphoma should be carried out, including a splenectomy, at least four liver biopsies, and removal of representative lymph nodes from all regions of the abdominal cavity. If histological examination of all this material shows that the tumor is limited strictly to the gut and immediately adjacent lymph nodes, then Crowther's (20) suggestion that no further treatment is indicated should be considered. However, most of these lymphomas are grade II tumors and their unpleasant microscopic appearances will suggest strongly to most clinical oncologists that further treatment is essential. It is suggested that whatever the stage of the disease, the next logical step should be the use of combination chemotherapy, in an attempt to control not only any local macroscopic disease but also micrometastases which may already be present in the liver and in the body elsewhere. Localized radiotherapy may be used after chemotherapy to control bulk disease sites which were demonstrated and recorded by scanning of the abdomen after the original operation. (2) When the diagnosis is not considered preoperatively, total excision of the original tumor with its adjacent lymph nodes may be carried out at operation, but staging procedures will not be undertaken. When the operation is carried out as an emergency, the operation is likely to be even more limited in extent. Under both these circumstances the patient should be staged postoperatively. If investigation suggests that disease is limited to the abdominal cavity, consideration should be given to exact determination of its extent. Gallium 67 and CT scanning of the abdomen may provide valuable information as to its macroscopic extent. After this the possibility of a second-look laparotomy should be considered at which, of course, full staging procedures will be carried out in addition to the removal of any remaining bulk disease. Following successful surgery, treatment will proceed as above. When a second-look laparotomy is inadvisable, a laparoscopy should be considered a much less traumatic procedure. Unfortunately it is more likely to be necessary in the more ill patient, and in particular those patients who presented as emergencies, often after acute perforation of the gut. Intraabdominal adhesions will be commonly encountered, making laparoscopy increasingly dangerous and less likely to provide useful information. When a second-look operation is not possible and when bulk disease is known to have been left behind after an operation, the possibility of irradiation should be considered. However, chemotherapy may be preferable at this stage, as its effect on measurable lymphoma masses as demonstrated by serial scans is likely to influence the choice of further cytotoxic drugs. Radiotherapy to the sites of bulk disease may be considered at a later date.

Extranodal Primary Lymphoma: Other Sites

As already indicated, non-Hodgkin lymphomas may originate in any part of the body. Some sites are rarely affected, but others are involved frequently enough for a reasonable course of action to be planned in advance. Consideration will not be given in this chapter to lymphomas originating in the skin.

Bone: Non-Hodgkin lymphoma originating in bone is considered by some authors to be a clearly identifiable tumor with special characteristics and as such was originally recognized as reticulum cell sarcoma of bone. From the diagnostic, and therefore also the management, point of view the tumor is best regarded initially as a round cell tumor of bone and investigated carefully in order to exclude the other possible causes of this finding (1).

Primary non-Hodgkin lymphoma of bone: Characteristically this tumor shows absent septa, reticulin production, no rosette formation or cystoplasmic glycogen production, and rarely any perivascular cuffing. Typically these lymphomas are composed of diffuse undifferentiated or poorly differentiated non-Hodgkin lymphoma cells with an admixture of mature lymphocytes, with a well-marked reticular framework which can be demonstrated very well with silver impregnation. Differentiation between other bone tumors is particularly difficult when the patient is under the age of 20. Fortunately, many of the investigations which are necessary to establish the correct diagnosis are common to all.

Differential diagnosis: (1) Metastasis from an undifferentiated tumor elsewhere. If the primary tumor is intraabdominal the correct diagnosis may be particularly difficult to establish. (2) Myeloma-A solitary myeloma which may be atypical with scanty or even absent plasma cells may be particularly difficult to identify satisfactorily. (3) Ewing tumor of bone typically shows fibrous septa, no diffuse reticulin, no rosette formation, occasionally perivascular cuffing, and usually there is cytoplasmic glycogen present. (4) Neuroblastoma may sometimes present as a solitary large bone tumor, the primary tumor remaining very small. Microscopical examination typically shows no diffuse reticulin, septa can be present, perivascular cuffing may be found, and some attempt at rosette formation is common. The diagnosis is often confirmed by finding an excess of catecholamines and their degradation products, homovanyllic acid (HVA) and vanillylmandelic acid (VMA) in the urine.

Primary non-Hodgkin lymphoma of bone is frequently found to be part of a generalized lymphoma and the exact site of the primary tumor becomes of academic importance only. The frequency of generalized disease is indicated in a paper by Boston et al. (8) who analyzed 191 patients seen at the Mayo Clinic between 1967 and 1970. Of 179 patients whose full details were obtainable, just over half had an apparently solitary bone lesion at the time of, or up to within 6 months of, diagnosis. It is of course likely that many of these patients with so-called solitary bone tumors would have been shown to have widespread disease if they had been investigated by modern methods. Primary non-Hodgkin lymphoma of bone is a rare disease.

Surgical removal is not indicated in the treatment of this tumor, as radiotherapy offers as good a result. The whole bone must be irradiated in continuity to a tumor dose of 4500 rads/4-5 weeks using megavoltage. Some radiation oncologists then prefer to reduce the treated volume to that of the original tumor bulk to which they then add 1500 rads/10-14 days, attempting to reduce the local relapse rate. The treatment plan should, if possible, provide an unirradiated strip of tissue down the limb, as through-and-through irradiation of the whole limb is usually followed by a constricting circle of fibrous tissue which may impair the peripheral blood supply. The response to irradiation is usually rapid with bone recalcification appearing by the end of treatment.

The 5-year survival rate after radical radiotherapy is about 50% (8,83); this result should be improved in the future with modern investigations which exclude widespread deposits with more certainty. With true localized primary non-Hodgkin lymphoma of bone the value of adjunctive chemotherapy is not known.

Testicle: Most published reports on primary non-Hodgkin lymphoma of the testes include only a small number of patients. Gowing (34) reviewing 2106 cases of testicular tumor referred to the Testicular Tumor Panel and Registry found 140 testicular lymphomas. One hundred and twenty occurred in patients with no previous manifestations of lymphoma. There is a particular tendency for bilateral involvement. Many patients will be found to have distant spread if fully investigated, and their treatment is that of stages III and IV disease, after the testicle has been removed. When the disease is considered to be localized to the testicle, it is customary to irradiate the lymph nodes draining the primary site in a manner identical to that adopted in testicular seminoma. The usual dose given is 3000-4000 rads/4-5 weeks.

Female Reproductive Tract: Primary non-Hodgkin lymphomas arising in the ovary, uterus, or cervix are all rare. Most are undifferentiated or poorly differentiated and the prognosis is poor. The best reported survival rate after treatment with radical surgery and postoperative radiotherapy for NHL of the breast is 64% at 5 years (21). Because of their rarity and, until recently, their lack of adequate investigation, it is difficult to advise authoritatively on their management. When localized and of grade I histology, local radiotherapy may be adequate treatment, but with the more aggressive tumors it is probable that there is a place for adjuvant chemotherapy with or without bulk radiotherapy, after surgical removal.

Thyroid: Although the thyroid may be involved sometimes with any of the lymphomas, the differential diagnosis of NHL from a so-called small-cell carcinoma may be extremely difficult. Retrospectively, it is probable that most tumors of this type are lymphomas. Modern investigations often reveal widespread manifestations typical of lymphoma, which is a reasonable explanation for the frequent rapid spread of these tumors after a satisfactory local response. From the practical point of view patients with a non-Hodgkin lymphoma or an undifferentiated carcinoma of the thyroid should be investigated in the same way.

If the tumor is found to be apparently localized to the thyroid, it is customary to irradiate widely; treatment includes the whole neck and the thoracic inlet down to the tracheal bifurcation. Some oncologists prefer to include the whole mediastinum in the treatment field. The usual dose recommended is 4000 rads/4 weeks, using a megavoltage unit. Adjuvant chemotherapy is of unknown value because of the rarity of these tumors. When the disease is widespread then the patient will normally be treated with cytotoxic drugs.

Stage III, IV, Grade I

When a grade I NHL has become generalized there are four possible approaches. (1) Symptomatic treatment only: If it is accepted that treatment makes little difference to the length of survival with generalized grade I NHL, then it is reasonable to adopt a similar approach to that used with chronic lymphatic leukemia. In an individual case it is very difficult to know that therapy is affecting the outcome, particularly in older people it may be reasonable to adopt an expectant attitude and treat only when necessary. However, with increased knowledge on the part of most patients, it is increasingly difficult to avoid active treatment. (2) Single-agent chemotherapy: Early publications suggested that single agents had become outmoded following the introduction of combination chemotherapy in the management of generalized grade I NHL (37). Collaborators in the British National Lymphoma Investigation found little in the literature to confirm this and since 1974 have compared single-agent with combination chemotherapy. To date, no obvious difference has been discovered; this has been confirmed by other workers (54). Unless a special study is being undertaken, when chemotherapy is considered for generalized grade I NHL, single-agent therapy, either chlorambucil or cyclophosphamide, is as effective and less upsetting than combination chemotherapy. (3) Combination chemotherapy: Most reported series refer to the use of various combinations of cyclophosphamide, vincristine, and corticosteroids. While undoubtedly effective (2,75,76), this approach is not the best one for the average patient with low-grade lymphoma of this type. (4) Radiotherapy: With grade I, stage III NHL there might be a rational place for the use of total nodal irradiation as is used for the treatment of Hodgkin disease (31,35). However, as has been already indicated, subdiaphragmatic NHL is associated with involvement of lymph nodes other than those in the central axis of the body. Both the mesenteric nodes and lymphatic tissue in the gut are frequently involved and this would obviously be untreated by inverted Y-type irradiation. It is more reasonable to consider irradiating the whole abdomen when treating non-Hodgkin lymphoma (32). A logical extension of this was the reintroduction of total-body irradiation for stage III and even more obviously for stage IV disease (43). Since then TBI has been widely used as a method of controlling extensive grade I NHL. It is probable that this method of treatment is at least as effective as combination chemotherapy, and it is extremely well tolerated by patients whose marrow has not been damaged by previous chemotherapy (13,44,73).

The techniques recommended by Johnson (44) include: (1) TBI giving 10 rad daily fractions from either side alternately to a maximum of 100-150 rads midline dose, and (2) a hemibody technique, giving 50 rads daily to either the upper or to the lower half of the body, to a total of 300-600 rads. After one-half is treated, the patient is rested to allow bone marrow recovery and then the other half is treated in a similar way.

These techniques are tolerated by patients remarkably well with little or no systemic side effects. The only common complication is that there is a fall in the platelet count which usually appears 10-14 days after completion of irradiation but spontaneous recovery is the rule. With well-differentiated and follicular lymphomas Johnson has achieved a 5-year survival rate of about 80%.

When assessing the results of all the above methods of treatment, it is important to remember that many patients will survive for many years without treatment, and that it is not uncommon for patients to have no systemic symptoms before the commencement of treatment. When comparing treatment methods with this type of disease, it is important to consider the quality of life that is offered to the patient.

Stage III, IV, Grade II

The clinical picture with generalized lymphoma of this histological type is usually very different from that with grade I tumors. An appreciable number of patients with grade II lymphomas have symptoms either of the B type or associated with anemia or related to the rapidity of the growth of many of these tumors. In addition they have a much poorer prognosis with a median survival of between 6 and 14 months (74). If patients are to be treated successfully there is not much time to be lost. Previous experience and the natural tempo of grade II lymphomas indicate that neither a wait-and-see policy nor single-agent therapy is permissible.

In 1973 the only available treatment methods which appeared to be possible effective were combination chemotherapy and total-body irradiation using the techniques advocated by Johnson (44). A prospective trial was therefore undertaken by the British National Lymphoma Investigation between January 1974 and August of 1978. This study compared a modification of the combination chemotherapy originally described with TBI. The modification included increasing the dose of cyclophosphamide and dividing the dose of adriamycin and giving both on days 1 and 8 (Table 7). Neither form of treatment proved satisfactory as 36% of patients achieved complete remission with cyclophosphamide, adriamycin, vincristine, and prednisone (CHOP) and only 24% of patients with TBI. In addition, 55% of patients treated with CHOP and 72% treated initially with TBI were dead by 58 months. Although there is no statistically significant difference between the groups, in practice TBI proved to be less flexible. When dealing with tumors which have a rapid growth potential, it can be disastrous if relapse occurs while the platelet count is low, as it may be for many weeks after completion of TBI.

On the whole, with grade II non-Hodgkin lymphomas, chemotherapy appears to offer more hope for the future than radiotherapy. Radiotherapy may still offer excellent rapid palliation, and renewed interest is at present being shown in hemicorporeal, large, single-dose irradiation, which may prove useful with a small number of patients.

Table 7. Modified CHOP*

Cyclophosphamide	750 mg/m^2	Days 1 and 8
Hydroxydaunorubicin	25 mg/m^2	Days 1 and 8
Oncovin	1.4 mg/m^2	Days 1 and 8
Prednisone	50 mg/m^2	Days 1-8

* Repeat course every 4-6 weeks, depending upon the blood count, to minimum total of six courses. When the response is (virtually) complete by course 3, courses should be continued so that three courses are given after complete control has been achieved.

Lymphomas in Childhood

In this section, childhood will be accepted as the period of life before the age of 15. The management of childhood lymphomas presents special problems.

Hodgkin Disease

Hodgkin disease in childhood behaves on average much as it does in adult life. It is only in those over 45 years old that the disease behaves in a measurably more malignant fashion.

The special problems encountered are two, and they are interconnected. When the disease can be shown to be localized in extent, then irradiation can be given to the smallest reasonable volume with the least possible effect on growing bone. Most patients with localized disease will require irradiation to the neck and mediastinum. This will be followed in adult life by deformity which is usually tolerable. If TNI is necessary, the deformity becomes increasingly obvious. The need for avoiding unnecessary irradiation of growing bone is obvious and from this it follows that careful localization is even more important than in the adult.

It is recognized that splenectomy, which is such an essential part of a diagnostic laparotomy, may be followed by increased susceptibility to infection when the operation is performed in childhood and this susceptibility is very marked when the spleen is removed under the age of 5. A compromise has to be made. The author's view is that accurate localization is so essential that a diagnostic laparotomy should be carried out in all children over the age of 5, provided the usual indications are present. Fortunately, Hodgkin disease is a rarity below the age of 5. It is then debatable whether a diagnostic laparotomy should be carried out, or the child treated with bulk radiotherapy to a lower than normal dose, followed by combination chemotherapy.

Both irradiation and chemotherapy offer the usual hazards to the gonads. In girls, at least one ovary should be transposed at the diagnostic laparotomy and, with boys, testicular function should be preserved if possible, the possibility of sperm storage should be considered in the older age group.

Non-Hodgkin Lymphoma

In childhood, and often in young adults, non-Hodgkin lymphomas behave in a more malignant fashion. The only exception to this rule is the follicular lymphoma, which is almost never seen in childhood, and the patient with a solitary lymph node presenting high up in the neck, the disease remaining localized after full investigation.

In young people, the disease often behaves as does acute leukemia, spreading to involve the bone marrow and later the cerebrospinal fluid. For this reason it is becoming customary to treat most children with non-Hodgkin lymphomas as if they had acute leukemia (60). Treatment with combination chemotherapy is followed by craniospinal prophylaxis, using intrathecal methotrexate and cranial irradiation. Following this, it is customary to continue with maintenance chemotherapy until treatment has been given for a total of about 2 years.*

* Supported financially by the Cancer Research Campaign and the C.C.C. Trust Fund.

REFERENCES

1. Arthur, J.F., Bennett, M.H., Jelliffe, A.M., Kendall, B.K., Millett, Y.L., and Tucker, A.K.: Small round cell tumors of bone. In Symposium Ossium, edited by A.M. Jelliffe and B. Strickland, Edinburgh and London, Livingstone, 1970, pp. 136-140.

2. Bagley, C.M., De Vita, V.T., Berard, C., and Canellos, G.: Advanced lymphosarcoma: Intensive cyclical chemotherapy with cyclophosphamide, vincristine and prednisone. Ann. Intern. Med. 76:227-234, 1972.

3. Baker, J.W., Morgan, R.L., Peckham, M.J., and Smithers, D.W.: Preservation of ovarian function in patients requiring radiotherapy for para-aortic and pelvic Hodgkin's disease. Lancet 1:1307-1308, 1972.

4. Bennett, M.H. and Millett, Y.L.: Nodular sclerotic lymphosarcoma. A possible new clinicopathological entity. Clin. Radiol. 20:339-343, 1969.

5. Bennett, M.H., Farrer-Brown, G., and Henry, K.: A classification of the non-Hodgkin's lymphomas. Presented at the Workshop on Classifications of non-Hodgkin's Lymphomas, University of Chicago, 1973.

6. Bennett, M.H.: Sclerosis in non-Hodgkin's lymphomata. Br. J. Cancer 31, Supplement II:44-52, 1975.

7. Bonnadonna, G., Castellani, R., Narduzzi, C., Spinelli, P., and Rilke, F.: Pathological staging in adult previously untreated non-Hodgkin's lymphomas. In Recent Advances in Cancer Research. Lymphoid Neoplasias II. Clinical and Therapeutic Aspects, edited by G. Mathe, M. Seligmann, and M. Tubiana, Berlin, Heidelberg, New York, Springer-Verlag, 1978, pp. 41-50.

8. Boston, H.C., Dalhin, D.C., Ivins, J.C., and Cupps, R.E.: Malignant lymphoma (so-called reticulum cell sarcoma) of bone. Cancer 34:1131-1137, 1974.

9. British National Lymphoma Investigation Report: The value of laparotomy and splenectomy in the management of early Hodgkin's disease. Clin. Radiol. 26: 151-157, 1975.

10. British National Lymphoma Investigation Report. Initial treatment of stage IIIA Hodgkin's disease. Comparison of radiotherapy with combined chemotherapy. Lancet 2:991-995, 1976.

11. Britton, K.E. and Brown, N.J.G.: The use of the radioactive renogram in the reticuloses. Br. J. Radiol. 42:34, 1969.

12. Bruun, S., and Engeset, A.: Lymphadenography. A new method for the visualization of enlarged lymph nodes and lymphatic vessels. Acta Radiol. 45: 389-395, 1956.

13. Canellos, G.P., De Vita, V.T., Young, R.C., Chabner, B.A., Schein, P.S., and Johnson, R.E.: Therapy of advanced lymphocytic lymphoma - a preliminary report of a randomized trial between combination chemotherapy (CVP) and intensive radiotherapy. Br. J. Cancer 31, Supplement II:474-480, 1975.

14. Carbone, P.P., Kaplan, H.S., Musshoff, K., Smithers, D.W., and Tubiana, M.: Report of the committee on Hodgkin's disease staging classification. Cancer Res. 31:1860-1861, 1971.

15. Carr, I., Hancock, B.W., Henry, L., and Ward, A.M.: Lymphoreticular Disease, Oxford and London, Blackwell Scientific Publications, 1977, pp. 93-100.

16. Chabner, B.A., Johnson, R.E., Chretien, P.B., Schein, P.S., Young, R.C., Canellos, G.P., Hubbard, S.H., Anderson, T., Rosenhoff, S.H., and De Vita, V.T.: Percutaneous liver biopsy, peritoneoscopy and laparotomy; an assessment of relative merits in the lymphomata. Br. J. Cancer 31, Supplement II: 242-247, 1975.

17. Chapman, R.M., Sutcliffe, S.B., Rees, L.H., Edwards, C.R.W., and Malpas, J.A.: Cyclical combination chemotherapy and gonadal function. Retrospective study in males. Lancet 1:285-289, 1979.

18. Corder, M.P., Elliott, T.E., Maguire, L.C., Leimert, J.T., Panther, S.K., and Lachenbruch, P.A.: Phase II study of cis-dichlorodiammineplatinum (II) in stage IVB Hodgkin's disease. Cancer Treat. Rep. 63:763-766, 1979.

19. Craver, L.F.: Hodgkin's disease. In Practice of Medicine, Vol. 6, edited by F. Tice and E.M. Harvey, Hagerstown, Md., W.F. Prior, 1964, pp. 1017-1063.

20. Crowther, D. and Blackledge, G.: Gastrointestinal lymphomas. Br. J. Radiol. 51:75, 1978.

21. De Cosse, J.J., Berg, J.W., Fracchia, A.A., and Farrow, J.M.: Primary lymphosarcoma of the breast. Cancer 15:1264-1268, 1962.

22. DeVita, V.T., Serpick, A., and Carbone, P.P.: Combination chemotherapy in the treatment of advanced Hodgkin's disease. Ann. Intern. Med. 73:881-895, 1970.

23. Durrie, B.G.M. and Salmon, S.E.: A clinical staging system for multiple myeloma. Correlation of measured myeloma cell mass with presenting clinical features, response to treatment and survival. Cancer 36:842-854, 1975.

24. Easson, E.C. and Russell, M.H.: The cure of Hodgkin's disease. Br. Med. J. 1:1704-1707, 1963.

25. Easson, E.C.: Possibilities for the cure of Hodgkin's disease. Cancer 19: 345-350, 1966.

26. Edland, R.W. and Hansen, H.: Irregular field shaping for 60-Co teletherapy. Radiology 92:1567-1569, 1969.

27. Farrer-Brown, G., Howarth, C., Benneth, M.H., and Henry, K.: Follicular lymphoma. Communication to the 131st Meeting of the Pathological Society of Great Britain and Ireland, 1975.

28. Gazet, J.C.: Laparotomy and splenectomy. In Hodgkin's Disease, edited by Sir David Smithers, Edinburgh and London, Churchill Livingstone, 1973, pp. 190-202.

29. Gilbert, R.: Radiotherapy in Hodgkin's disease (malignant granulomatosis): anatomic and clinical foundations; governing principles; results. Am. J. Roentgenol. 41:198-241, 1939.

30. Glatstein, E., Guernsey, J.M., Rosenberg, S.A., and Kaplan, H.S.: The value of laparotomy and splenectomy in the staging of Hodgkin's disease. Cancer 24:709-718, 1969.

31. Glatstein, E., Fuks, Z., Goffinet, D.R., and Kaplan, H.S.: Non-Hodgkin's lymphomas of stage III extent. Is total lymphoid irradiation appropriate treatment? Cancer 37:2806-2812, 1976.

32. Goffinet, D.R., Glatstein, E., Fuks, Z., and Kaplan, H.S.: Abdominal irradiation in non-Hodgkin's lymphomas. Cancer 37:2797-2805, 1976.

33. Goodman, I.S., Wintrobe, M.M., Dameshek, W., Goodman, M.J., Gilman, A.Z., and McLennan, M.T.: Nitrogen mustard therapy. Use of methyl-bis-(chloroethyl) amine hydrochloride and tris-(chloroethyl) amine hydrochloride for Hodgkin's disease, lymphosarcoma, leukemia and certain allied and miscellaneous disorders. JAMA 132:126-136, 1946.

34. Gowing, N.F.C.: Malignant lymphoma of the testicle. In Pathology of the Testis, edited by R.C.B. Pugh, Oxford, London, and Edinburgh, Blackwell, 1976, pp. 334-355.

35. Hellman, S., Chaffey, J.T., Rosenthal, D.S., Moloney, W.C., Canellos, G.P., and Skarin, A.T.: The place of radiotherapy in the treatment of non-Hodgkin's lymphomas. Cancer 39:843-851, 1977.

36. Henry, K., Bennett, M.H., and Farrer-Brown, G.: Morphological classification of non-Hodgkin's lymphomas. In Recent Results in Cancer Research. Lymphoid Neoplasias I. Classification, Categorization and Natural History, edited by G. Mathe, M. Seligmann, and M. Tubiana, Berlin, Heidelberg, and New York, Springer-Verlag, 1978, pp. 38-65.

37. Hoogstraten, B., Owens, A.H., Lenhard, R.E., Glidewell, O.J., Leone, L.A., Olson, K.B., Harley, J.B., Townsend, S.R., Miller, S.P., and Spurr, C.L.: Combination chemotherapy in lymphosarcoma and reticulum cell sarcoma. Blood 33:370-377, 1969.

38. Hreshchyshyn, M.M., Sheehan, F.R., and Holland, J.F.: Visualization of retroperitoneal lymph nodes. Lymphangiography as an aid in the measurement of tumor growth. Cancer 14:205-209, 1961.

39. Jelliffe, A.M. and Thomson, A.D.: Prognosis in Hodgkin's disease. Br. J. Cancer 9:21-36, 1955.

40. Jelliffe, A.M.: The present place of radiotherapy in the cure of Hodgkin's disease. Clin. Radiol. 16:274-277, 1965.

41. Jelliffe, A.M., Millett, Y.L., Marston, J.A.P., Bennett, M.H., Farrer-Brown, G., Kendall, B., and Keeling, D.H.: Laparotomy and splenectomy as routine investigations in the staging of Hodgkin's disease before treatment. Clin. Radiol. 21:439-445, 1970.

42. Jelliffe, A.M.: Hodgkin's disease: The pendulum swings. Knox lecture, Royal College of Radiologists, 1977. Clin. Radiol. 30:121-137, 1979.

43. Johnson, R.E.: Evaluation of fractionated total body irradiation in patients with leukemia and disseminated lymphomas. Radiology 86:1085, 1966.

44. Johnson, R.E.: Management of generalized malignant lymphomas with systemic radiotherapy. Br. J. Cancer, Supplement II:450-455, 1975.

45. Johnson, R.E., DeVita, V.T., Kun, L.E., Chabner, B.R., Chretien, P.B., Berard, C.W., and Johnson, S.K.: Pattern of involvement with malignant lymphoma and implications for treatment decision making. Br. J. Cancer 31, Supplement II:237-241, 1975.

46. Kaplan, H.S.: The radical radiotherapy of regionally localized Hodgkin's disease. Radiology 78:553-561, 1962.

47. Kaplan, H.S.: Role of intensive radiotherapy in the management of Hodgkin's disease. Cancer 19:346-367, 1966.

48. Kaplan, H.S.: Hodgkin's Disease. Cambridge, Mass., Harvard University Press, 1972.

49. Kaplan, H.S.: Hodgkin's Disease. 2nd edition, Cambridge, Mass., Harvard University Press, 1980.

50. Lacher, M.J. and Durant, J.R.: Combined vinblastine and chlorambucil therapy of Hodgkin's disease. Ann. Intern. Med. 62:468-476, 1965.

51. Lacher, M.J.: Staging laparotomy in patients with Hodgkin's disease. In Hodgkin's Disease, edited by M.J. Lacher, New York, London, Sydney, and Toronto, Wiley, 1976, pp. 117-128.

52. LeBourgeois, J.P., Meigham, M., Lasser, P., Parmentier, C., Pene, F., and Tubiana, M.: Complications of total abdominal and spleen irradiation in patients with lymphomas. In Recent Results in Cancer Research. Lymphoid Neoplasias II. Clinical and Therapeutic Aspect, edited by G. Mathe, M. Seligmann, and M. Tubiana, Berlin, Heidelberg, and New York, Springer-Verlag, 1978, pp. 170-180.

53. Lipton, A. and Lee, B.J.: Prognosis of stage I lymphosarcoma and reticulum cell sarcoma. N. Engl. J. Med. 284:230, 233, 1971.

54. Lister, T.A., Cullen, M.H., Beard, M.E.J., Brearley, R.L., Whitehouse, J.M.A., Wrigley, P.F.M., Stansfield, A.G., Sutcliffe, S.B.J., Malpas, J.S., and Crowther, D.: Comparison of combined and single agent chemotherapy in non-Hodgkin's lymphoma of favorable histological type. Br. Med. J. 1:533-537, 1978.

55. Lukes, R.J. and Butler, J.J.: The pathology and nomenclature of Hodgkin's disease. Cancer Res. 26:1063-1081, 1966.

56. Lukes, R.J. and Collins, R.D.: A functional classification of malignant lymphomas. In The Reticuloendothelial System, edited by J.W. Rebuck, C.W. Berard, and M.R. Abell, Baltimore, Williams and Wilkins, 1975.

57. Lukes, R.J. and Collins, R.D.: New approaches to the classification of the lymphomas. Br. J. Cancer 31, Supplement II:1-28, 1975.

58. McElwain, T.J., Toy, J., Smith, I.E., Peckham, M.J., and Austin, D.E.: A combination of chlorambucil, vinblastine, procarbazine and prednisone for treatment of Hodgkin's disease. Br. J. Cancer 36:276-280, 1977.

59. Millett, Y.L., Bennett, M.H., Jelliffe, A.M., and Farrer-Brown, G.: Nodlar sclerotic lymphosarcoma. A further review. Br. J. Cancer 23:683-692, 1969.

60. Murphy, S.B.: Combined modality therapy of childhood non-Hodgkin's lymphoma. In Recent Results in Cancer Research. Lymphoid Neoplasias II. Clinical and Therapeutic Aspects, edited by G. Mathe, M. Seligmann, and M. Tubiana, Berlin, Heidelberg, and New York, Springer-Verlag, 1977, pp. 207-213.

61. Nice, C.M. and Stenstrom, K.W.: Irradiation therapy in Hodgkin's disease. Radiology 62:641-653, 1954.

62. Nicholson, W.M., Beard, M.E.J., Crowther, D., Stansfield, A.G., Vartan, C.P., Malpas, J.S., Fairley, G.H., and Bodley Scott, R.: Combination chemotherapy in generalized Hodgkin's disease. Br. Med. J. 7-10, 1970.

63. Nisce, L.Z. and D'Angio, G.J.: A new technique for the irradiation of large fields in patients with lymphomas. Radiology 106:641-644, 1973.

64. Peters, M.V.: A study of survivals in Hodgkin's disease treated radiologically. Am. J. Roentgenol. 63:299-311, 1950.

65. Peters, M.V. and Middlemiss, K.C.H.: A study of Hodgkin's disease treated by irradiation. Am. J. Roentgenol. 79:114-121, 1958.

66. Prosnitz, L.R., Hellman, S., Von Essen, C.F., and Kligerman, M.M.: The clinical course of Hodgkin's disease and other malignant lymphomas treated with radical radiotherapy. Am. J. Roentgenol. 105-618, 1969.

67. Rappaport, H.: Tumors of the Hemopoietic System. Armed Forces Institute of Pathology, Washington, D.C., 1966.

68. Ray, G.R., Trueblood, H.W., Enright, L.P., Kaplan, H.S., and Nelson, T.S.: Oophoropexy: A means of preserving ovarian function following pelvic megavoltage radiotherapy for Hodgkin's disease. Radiology 96:175, 1970.

69. Robb Smith, A.H.T.: The classification and natural history of the lymphadenopathies. In Treatment of Cancer and Allied Diseases, Vol. 9, 2nd edition, edited by G.T. Pack, I.M. Ariel, New York, Hoeberg, 1964.

70. Robinson, T., Fischer, J.J., and Vera, R.: Reticulum sarcoma treated by radiotherapy. Radiology 99:669-675, 1971.

71. Rosas-Uribe, A. and Rappaport, H.: Malignant lymphoma histiocytic type with sclerosis (sclerosing reticulum cell sarcoma). Cancer 29:946-953,

72. Rosenberg, S.A., Ribas-Mundo, M., Goffinet, D.R., and Kaplan, H.S.: Staging in adult non-Hodgkin's lymphomas. In Recent Advances in Cancer Research. Lymphoid Neoplasias II. Clinical and Therapeutic Aspects, edited by G. Mathe, M. Seligmann, and M. Tubiana, Berlin, Heidelberg, and New York, Springer-Verlag, 1978, pp. 51-57.

73. Royston, A.Y. and Peckham, M.J.: Total body irradiation in advanced non-Hodgkin's lymphomas. Eur. J. Cancer 13:1241-1249, 1977.

74. Santoro, A. and Bonnadonna, G.: Prolonged disease-free survival in MOPP resistant Hodgkin's disease after treatment with adriamycin, bleomycin, vinblastine, and dicarbazine (ABVD). Cancer Chemother. Pharmacol. 2:101-106, 1979.

75. Schein, P.S., Chabner, B.A., Canellos, G.P., Young, R.C., Berard, C., and DeVita, V.T.: Potentials for prolonged disease-free survival following combination chemotherapy of non-Hodgkin's lymphoma. Blood 43:181, 1974.

76. Skarin, A.T., Pinkus, G.S., Myerowitz, R.L., Bishop, Y.M., and Moloney, W.C.: Combination chemotherapy of advanced lymphocytic lymphoma. Cancer 34:1023-1029, 1974.

77. Smithers, D.W. and Freeman, J.E.: Radiotherapy. In Hodgkin's Disease, edited by Sir David Smithers, Edinburgh and London, Churchill Livingstone, 1973.

78. Stein, R.S., Ultmann, J.E., Byrne, G.E., Moran, E.M., Golomb, H.M., and Oerzel, N.: Bone marrow involvement in non-Hodgkin's lymphoma. Implications for staging and therapy. Cancer 37:629-636, 1976.

79. Sutcliffe, S.B., Wrigley, P.M.F., Stansfield, A.G., and Malpas, J.S.: Adriamycin, Bleomycin, Vinblastine, and Imidazole Carboxamide (ABVD) therapy for advanced Hodgkin's disease resistant to Mustine, Vinblastine, Procarbazine, and Prednisolone (MVPP). Cancer Chemother. Pharmacol. 2:209-215, 1979.

80. Taylor, C.E.: Hodgkin's Disease and the Lymphomas. Montreal, Eden Press, and Lancaster, England, Linesdale House, 1977.

81. Van der Werf-Messing, B.: Reticulum cell sarcoma and lymphosarcoma. Eur. J. Cancer 4:542-557, 1968.

82. Van Dorssen, J.G., Mellink, J.H., and Thomas, P.: Construction of auxiliary diaphragms for megavoltage irradiation of large irregularly shaped fields. Radiol. Clin. Biol. 39:47-53, 1970.

83. Wang, C.C. and Fleischli, D.J.: Primary reticulum cell sarcoma of the bone with emphasis in radiation therapy. Cancer 22:994-998, 1968.

chapter 7

BREAST CANCER

Florence C. H. Chu, M. D.

Breast cancer is the most common malignancy in women, and it is the leading cause of death in women in the United States. The American Cancer Society estimated that there will be 110,900 new breast cancers and 37,000 deaths in the year 1981. One out of thirteen females will develop breast cancer. The high frequency of this disease makes breast cancer of particular importance.

The management of breast cancer requires multidisciplinary team approach. Radiation therapy, an important member of the team, makes valuable contributions to the care of patients with this disease. Radiation therapy has been used for cure, for adjuvant therapy, and for palliation, depending on the clinical situation (63).

In the radiotherapeutic management of breast cancer the following general principles must be considered:

The inherent radiosensitivity of breast carcinoma: Breast carcinoma is moderately sensitive to ionizing radiation. This implies high doses are needed for tumor destruction. The limiting factor for delivering high radiation doses is normal tissue tolerance, as the differential sensitivity between tumor destruction and normal tissue damage is narrow.

Normal tissue tolerance vs. large-volume irradiation: Breast cancer spreads through three mechanisms: local extension, lymphatics, and hematogenous routes. The lymphatics of the breast, briefly described, drain laterally to the axillary nodes and medially to the internal mammary nodes. From these two chains the lymphatics drain to the supraclavicular nodes at the base of the neck. The lymphatics then enter the venous system at the junction of the internal jugular and subclavian veins.

In the treatment of primary breast cancer it is therefore necessary for the breast as well as its regional node areas to be irradiated. Large-volume irradiation reduces normal tissue tolerance. One must apply appropriate treatment techniques to spare the normal tissues as much as possible.

Radiation dose vs. tumor size: It has been shown, both radiobiologically and clinically, that a large tumor mass requires higher radiation dose than a small tumor for sterilization. A large tumor mass contains a large number of cancer cells and most are hypoxic. Hypoxic cells are known to be more resistant to the effects of ionizing radiation than well-oxygenated cells. There are ways to improve the therapeutic ratio. Proper utilization of megavoltage photon irradiation, high-energy electron beam therapy, and interstitial implantation permits the delivery of high tumor doses with sparing of normal tissues. It is also advantageous to fractionate the radiation dose and protract the course of therapy over several weeks.

Normal tissues usually recover from radiation injury faster than neoplastic tissues, and fractionation allows repair of sublethal damage between two treatment fractions. Fractionation further enhances the effectiveness of irradiation because the tumor decreases in size with each treatment. As a result cells at the periphery of the mass receive better blood supply and become well-oxygenated and radiosensitive.

It has been demonstrated by Fletcher (39) and Kim et al. (51) that a dose of 4500-5000 rads delivered in 4 and 5 weeks is very effective in sterilizing subclinical disease. On the other hand, a bulky tumor may need 8000-9000 rads, delivered in 10-12 weeks. This kind of high-dose irradiation may produce unacceptable morbidity in some cases. When feasible, surgery can be used to remove the breast or the bulky tumor prior to radiation therapy to facilitate efficiency of irradiation.

Radiation dose technique vs. aim of treatment: The aim of treatment may be curative, adjunctive, or palliative. In curative therapy the breast and its regional lymph node areas are irradiated, delivering high radiation doses in the order of 6000-7000 rads/7-8 weeks. In adjunctive therapy one is dealing with subclinical disease in the regional lymph node areas and the chest wall. A dose of 4500-5000 rads/4-5 weeks is usually adequate. For palliative treatment it is desirable to give a short course of therapy, delivering moderate amounts of radiation of 4000-4500 rads/3-4 weeks for symptomatic relief.

Radiation modalities: Megavoltage photon beam therapy, high-energy electron beam therapy, and interstitial radiation should be fully utilized depending on the clinical situation. Megavoltage x-ray or ^{60}Co therapy has the advantages of deep penetration, skin sparing, and bone sparing effects. High-energy electron beam irradiation has the advantages of abrupt termination of radiation in the depth and controllable depth of penetration by varying the energy. Interstitial implantation delivers a highly concentrated radiation dose to the tumor volume with sparing of the surrounding normal structures.

The influence of chemotherapy: If chemotherapy is also used one must bear in mind the combined effects of radiation and chemotherapy. If the toxicities of combined treatment are prohibitive, one must compromise chemotherapy dose, radiation dose, or both. Sometimes chemotherapy and radiation therapy should be used sequentially rather than concurrently to avoid undue toxicity.

THE PLACE OF RADIATION THERAPY IN THE MANAGEMENT OF EARLY BREAST CANCER

In the management of early, operable breast cancer, surgery is the primary treatment. The role of radiation therapy has been to supplement and complement surgery, except in the case of curative radiation therapy given to patients who refuse mastectomy. Surgical procedures used range from the most radical to the most conservative. These include radical mastectomy, modified radical mastectomy, extended radical mastectomy, simple (total) mastectomy, and segmental mastectomy, or local excision. Regardless of the type of surgery performed, radiation therapy is employed to treat subclinical residual disease as well as potential areas of regional spread.

Radical Mastectomy and Adjuvant Radiation Therapy

Although controversy exists regarding the choice of surgical procedure, radical mastectomy and modified radical mastectomy are the most widely performed procedures for operable breast cancer. Overall 10-year survival rates of 55-60% have been reported by several large institutions (3,41,45,52,76). Postoperative radiation therapy is often given as an adjuvant to radical mastectomy, particularly in patients with positive axillary nodes. The rationale for giving adjuvant radiation is based on the effectiveness of irradiation in destroying occult lesions which may be present in the operative field and in the regional lymphatic drainage areas. Combined surgery and radiation therapy offer better local and regional tumor control than surgery alone.

In the recent past there have been drastic changes in treatment policies. The value of adjuvant radiation therapy in increasing survival has been seriously doubted. Several studies (38,64,73) have shown that routine postoperative radiation therapy did not increase the patients' survival. In addition, chemotherapy is being widely used as an adjuvant to radical mastectomy since the publications by Bonadonna (9,10) and others (35,36) on the results of their clinical trials. They have found lower relapse rates in patients who received adjuvant chemotherapy as compared with those who did not. Therefore, the number of patients receiving postoperative radiation therapy has decreased significantly. It would be useful to review some of the clinical trials and retrospective studies on adjuvant radiation therapy.

The first clinical trial to determine the value of routine postoperative irradiation therapy was carried out by Paterson and Russell (64) in the early 1950s and involved more than 1400 patients. One group of patients received routine postoperative radiation therapy immediately after the mastectomy and the other group was observed and treated only when local recurrence developed. They used two different radiation techniques during two different periods. First they used a quadrate technique, treating the axilla and the chest wall. During the second period they used a peripheral technique, treating only the peripheral lymph nodes without treating the chest wall. Orthovoltage radiation was used and the tumor dose delivered was about 3500 rads/3 weeks. They demonstrated no statistically significant difference in the survival rates at 5 years between the treated and observed groups. They revealed a lower recurrence rate where postoperative radiation was administered. For example, when the skin flaps were irradiated, the recurrence rate in the area was reduced from 20 to 11%. When the supraclavicular area was irradiated, the recurrence rate in this region was lowered, from 17 to 6%.

Following the Paterson and Russell report, a clinical trial was initiated by the National Surgical Adjuvant Breast Project (NSABP) (38) to evaluate the efficacy of postoperative radiation therapy. Radiation was given to the internal mammary and supraclavicular areas and the average dose was about 4000 rads/4 weeks. The results of the study were reported by Fisher et al. in 1970. There was no significant difference in the 5-year survival rates of patients who received postoperative radiation therapy and those who did not. The incidence of recurrence in the regional nodes was significantly lower in the irradiated than in the control group.

At Memorial Hospital a retrospective study (74) of about 700 patients revealed no significant difference in the overall survival rates between the irradiated and nonirradiated groups. Radiation therapy definitely reduced local and regional recurrences. For example, in patients with positive axillary lymph nodes, the incidence of supraclavicular nodal recurrence at 5 years was 26% without radiation. When patients were treated with orthovoltage irradiation, receiving a tumor dose of 3500 rads/3.5 weeks, the incidence of supraclavicular recurrence was reduced to 13%. When megavoltage radiation was used and the dose delivered was 4000-4500 rads/4 weeks, the recurrence rate was further reduced to 6% (51). These data not only confirm the effectiveness of radiation therapy in reducing recurrence in the irradiated area, but also demonstrate that tumor control is dose dependent.

In another Memorial Hospital retrospective study (25), it was found that when the axillary lymph nodes were positive in the low and midaxilla, the survival rates of the two groups of patients were similar. However, when the axillary nodes were positive in the apex of the axilla, those patients who received postoperative treatment had a higher percentage of survival (39 vs. 22%). This difference of 17% is statistically significant. Many patients with apical axillary involvement received vigorous radiation treatment, not only to the lymph node areas, but also to the entire chest wall. The vigorous treatment may have contributed to the good results accomplished. It is conceivable that adequate postoperative radiation therapy, given to a selected subset of patients, may improve their chances of survival.

Fletcher and Montague (41), in a retrospective analysis of the M. D. Anderson Hospital data, reported beneficial effects of adjuvant radiation therapy on survival. They compared the results of radical mastectomy with those of radical mastectomy followed by irradiation of peripheral lymphatics. In the radical mastectomy group 11.5% had histologically positive axillary nodes, whereas in the irradiated group, 65.7% had positive axillary nodes. The 10-year survival rates for patients who had peripheral lymphatic irradiation was 56% as compared to 54% for patients who were treated by radical mastectomy alone. The authors state: "Since it is a well-established fact that the survival rates correlate well with the percentage of patients with histologically positive axillary nodes, the survival rate would be expected to be much lower for the irradiated patients. Although the data is not from a randomized trial, it does suggest strongly that irradiation of peripheral lymphatics to an adequate dose has been curative in a significant number of patients."

Fletcher (39) also demonstrated that a total dose of 4500-5000 rads/5 weeks is very effective in controlling subclinical disease in the nodal areas. Control is achieved in more than 90% of the cases.

There are two prospective, randomized clinical trials which showed improved survival rates in patients who received adjuvant radiation therapy. One was reported by Host and Brennhovd (46) in 1977 at the Norwegian Radium Hospital, Oslo, Norway. A total of 1090 patients were included in the study. In the first part, orthovoltage x-rays were used, delivering modest doses to the chest wall and regional lymph node areas. In the second part, ^{60}Co was used to irradiate the internal mammary and supraclavicular areas, delivering a higher radiation dose (5000 rads/4 weeks). All patients also had radiation castration.

Postoperative radiation, given either by orthovoltage x-rays or by ^{60}Co radiation, did not influence the survival or the relapse rate in stage I patients. In stage II, orthovoltage radiation therapy reduced the incidence of local and regional recurrences, but did not affect the survival. On the other hand, ^{60}Co irradiation in patients with stage II disease significantly reduced the relapse rate, as well as increased the cumulative survival rate up to 5 years. Although the numbers of patients in the subgroups were small, these authors believe that the prognosis was improved by postoperative radiation therapy in adequate doses, particularly in patients with medially located tumors.

Another clinical trial was conducted by the Stockholm group (32,88,89) to compare the results of preoperative radiation therapy, postoperative radiation therapy, and surgery alone. The radiation dose given was 4500 rads/5 weeks to the breast (preoperatively) or the chest wall (postoperatively), and the internal mammary, axillary, and supraclavicular areas. A total of 960 patients were entered into this study from 1971-1976. The number of patients with recurrent disease is higher in the group treated by surgery only than in any of the groups given radiation therapy. Both radiation groups showed a higher recurrence-free survival than the surgery alone group; the difference, however, is statistically significant only in the preoperative irradiated group.

It is obvious that the question of whether or not adjuvant radiation therapy prolongs the survival of patients is not quite settled. There is no dispute, however, regarding the fact that radiation therapy reduces local and regional recurrences and, therefore, offers better tumor control than surgery alone. Successful treatment should result in satisfactory local tumor control and prolonged survival. Radiation therapy of recurrence may achieve good results; however, it is better to prevent the problem before it occurs. Gross tumor nodules are usually more difficult to sterilize than subclinical lesions. Patients usually suffer from emotional trauma upon discovering tumor nodules on their chest after a mastectomy. There may be symptoms such as pain and ulceration. Finally, it is conceivable that sterilization of occult disease in the local-regional areas by postoperative radiation therapy may eradicate the disease in some patients, even though the chance may be small.

It appears that postoperative radiation therapy is indicated in patients with a high risk of developing local or regional recurrence. Patients with inner quadrant or central lesions should receive postoperative radiation therapy to the internal mammary and supraclavicular areas, even though the axillary nodes are negative. Patients with large primary tumors, greater than 4 or 5 cm in diameter, extensive metastases to the axillary lymph nodes, or histological evidence of lymphatic permeation of the skin by cancer cells should receive postoperative radiation therapy to the chest wall and the lymph node areas. A total dose of 4500-5000 rads/4-5 weeks is recommended.

At the present time it is difficult to make firm recommendations regarding postoperative radiation therapy. We must await further data to clarify the value of adjuvant chemotherapy, the value of adjuvant radiation therapy, and the interactions of the two. In our clinical practice a significant number of patients are referred for radiation therapy of chest wall, parasternal or supraclavicular recurrence after failing adjuvant chemotherapy. It is obvious that some combined approach should be worked out to improve the overall result. Surgery, radiotherapy, and chemotherapy each have advantages and limitations. These methods should not be considered competitive, rather, they should be used to complement one another. Multidisciplinary team approach is essential in order to offer our patients the best possible treatment and the best possible results.

Simple (or Total) Mastectomy and Radiation Therapy

Simple mastectomy followed by radiation therapy was first advocated by McWhirter (54) in the 1950s. Since then there has been a number of clinical trials to compare simple mastectomy with radical or extended radical mastectomy (17, 48,49). One of the most frequently quoted clinical trials is by Kaae and Johansen (48,49) who compared simple mastectomy plus irradiation with "extended radical mastectomy" and found no difference in the results. Kaae and Johansen's results, however, have been criticized for their high recurrence rates and low 10-year survival rates in both groups. Crile (31) advocates simple mastectomy alone because he believes that the axillary lymph nodes are important for immune defense and, therefore, should be left intact.

In 1971 the National Surgical Adjuvant Breast Project started a protocol to compare total mastectomy with other methods of treatment. Patients with clinically negative axillary nodes are randomized into three arms: radical mastectomy, total mastectomy plus radiation therapy, and total mastectomy alone followed by axillary dissection, should the patient develop subsequent positive ipsilateral axillary nodes. Patients with clinically positive axillary nodes are randomly assigned to either radical mastectomy or to total mastectomy plus radiation therapy. Fisher (29,37) reported that findings after a mean follow-up time of 70 months have failed to demonstrate a significant difference in terms of survival between the three clinically negative axilla groups or between the two clinically positive axilla groups. A significant number of patients in the total mastectomy alone group, however, developed axillary involvement and required surgical dissection. Crile's theory cannot be substantiated by Fisher's findings.

The National Institute of Health sponsored a "consensus development" conference on treatment of primary breast cancer which was held in Washington in May, 1979. The conference panel concluded that total mastectomy with axillary node dissection can be considered a satisfactory alternative to the Halsted radical mastectomy and should be recognized as the current treatment standard for stage I and selected stage II breast cancers. However, this conference has stirred up more controversy than it settled, as many surgeons disagree with its conclusions.

When the surgical procedure is simple or total mastectomy with no, or limited axillary dissection, radiation therapy should be given. The radiation fields must include the axilla in addition to the chest wall, internal mammary, and supraclavicular node areas. The dose given should be about 5000 rads/5 weeks with a boost dose of 1000-1500 rads/1 week to the residual axillary node or any high-risk area through a reduced field.

Local Excision and Radiation Therapy

There is another school which advocates local excision and radiation therapy (59,65). The concept for conservative surgery and radiation is based on successful treatment while preserving the breast. Mustakallio (59) reported his experience of treating about 700 patients with stage I disease by this method. Orthovoltage radiation was used and the tumor dose delivered to the breast and lymph node areas was about 2500 rads/3 weeks. He reported a 5-year survival rate of 87% and a 10-year survival rate of 75%. The local recurrence rate was high, about 25%, but Mustakallio stated that recurrent tumors can still be treated effectively without jeopardizing the overall survival.

Another strong proponent for conservative surgery and radiation therapy is Peters (65,66). She treated both stage I and II cases with this method. In an early series of 105 patients (65), the 5 and 10 year survival rates were 75 and 45%, respectively. Later, Peters (66) did a study matching patients according to age, size of tumor, and year treated (2-30 year follow-up). There were 203 patients with T1T2N0M0 lesions treated by excision and radiation therapy and 609 patients treated by radical mastectomy and radiation therapy. Survival without further evidence of carcinoma was identical in the two groups.

Rissanen (71,72), who succeeded Mustakillio at the Helsinki Clinic in Finland, brought their data up to date, and presented a report at the International Radiological Congress in Brazil in late 1977. Some patients had been followed for 20 years. Rissanen compared the 10-year survival rates of local excision and radiation therapy with radical mastectomy according to the size of the tumor. Radical mastectomy gave better results in patients with T2 tumors (64 vs. 49%), while there was no significant difference in survival in the groups with T1 lesions (77 vs. 73%). He further analyzed the 20-year results in a series of 91 patients with T1 lesions, who were less than 51 years of age when the treatment was started, in order to minimize the influence of other causes of death. The results of conservative treatment were as good as those of radical mastectomy. The absolute 20-year survival rate was 78% for radical mastectomy and 73% for local excision. The local recurrence rate was higher in the excision group. Rissanen believes that the results of local excison and radiation therapy can be improved by using megavoltage irradiation, delivering a higher tumor dose. Indeed, since the use of megavoltage therapy in 1969, he has seen a definite reduction in recurrence rates.

At the Guy's Hospital in London, Atkins et al. (5) did a randomized study to compare radical mastectomy and radiation therapy with wide excision and radiation therapy in the treatment of stages I and II breast carcinoma. These investigators also used orthovoltage radiation, delivering a tumor dose in the range of 2500-3000 rads/2-3 weeks. In stage I cases no significant difference was found between survival in the two groups. In stage II cases there was a significantly higher survival rate and a lower recurrence rate in the radical mastectomy group at 10 years.

Since all patients in these studies were treated in the orthovoltage era, it was not possible to deliver a really effective tumoricidal dose comparable to present day standards. It is not surprising to see a high recurrence rate with orthovoltage therapy, delivering a modest tumor dose.

Data are now being accumulated on the results of treatment by modern radiotherapy techniques. Calle and colleagues (15,16) used local excision and cobalt therapy to treat patients with tumors less than 3 cm in diameter. He gives about 5000 rads tumor dose in 5 weeks to the breast and regional lymph areas. An additional dose of 1000-2000 rads/1-2 weeks is given to the tumor site through a small field. In a series of 109 patients treated, the 5-year disease-free survival rate was 87%. There were 80 patients who were followed for more than 10 years. The 10-year disease-free survival rate was 74%. Only 14 patients, or 9% developed local or regional recurrence that required mastectomy.

Prosnitz et al. (69) reported the results, accumulated from four institutions, of conservative surgery and definitive radiation therapy of 150 patients with stages I and II carcinomas of the breast. The radiation dose given was about 4500-5000 rads/5 weeks. The site of excisional biopsy was sometimes given an additional boost of 1000-2000 rads, either by external therapy or by means of implantation of ^{192}Ir.

The results of treatment show that in stage I patients the disease-free survival at 5 years was 91%. The disease-free survival in stage II cases was 60% at 5 years. The local failure rate was 7%. The authors concluded that mastectomy is not a necessary part of the treatment for small breast cancers and that radiation without mastectomy is an acceptable alternative with superior cosmetic and functional results. These authors also commented that adjuvant chemotherapy should be given, particularly in stage II patients in view of their 50% relapse rate.

It appears evident that most patients with tumors less than 3 cm do well with conservative surgery and radiation therapy. No firm recommendation can be made at this time, however, except that this method can be safely offered to patients who have early cancer and wish to preserve the breast. A few clinical trials are being conducted in various parts of the world to compare conservative surgery and radiation therapy with radical surgery.

There is a current National Surgical Adjuvant Breast Project (NSABP) study to compare the efficacies of segmental mastectomy ("lumpectomy," local excision, partial mastectomy) with segmental mastectomy plus radiation therapy and modified total mastectomy (including axillary sampling). This study is having problems accruing patients (29).

The Milan National Cancer Institute group compares radical mastectomy with segmental mastectomy (one-quarter of the breast) plus radiation therapy. Veronesi and colleagues (29, 86, 87) report that with follow-up to 6 years there is no difference between the two groups in recurrence or survival. Veronesi cautioned that it is premature to drwa firm conclusions since a 10-year follow-up is needed to evaluate the results of treatment.

Radiation Therapy Alone

Although radiation therapy is capable of eradicating breast cancer, it is not recommended for use alone for the treatment of early breast cancer. Tumor control probability is less than that of surgery and high doses of radiation may produce unacceptable morbidity.

Let us review some of the experiences of the treatment of operable breast cancer with radiation therapy alone. Baclesse (6,7), a pioneer radiotherapist, treated a large series of breast cancer patients with orthovoltage radiation therapy. He used a protracted, ultrafractionated radiation technique, delivering a tumor dose of 8000-9000 rads over a prolonged period of 3-4 months. The basis for using the ultrafractionated scheme was to avoid a moist skin reaction. Baclesse was able to achieve a 5-year disease-free survival rate of 59% and a 10-year disease-free survival rate of 33% for stage II cases. This was a remarkable accomplishment considering the relatively poor quality of x-rays from orthovoltage machines and the limited radiosensitivity of most breast cancers.

Guttmann (44), in cooperation with Haagensen, treated a series of patients with radiation therapy after a triple biopsy of the breast, the internal mammary lymph nodes, and the apex of the axilla. If the internal mammary nodes were positive or there was fixation of the axilla by tumor, or both, the patients were considered to be inoperable and were referred for definitive radiation therapy. Guttmann used 2 MeV x-ray, delivering a tumor dose of approximately 6000 rads over a period of 6-7 weeks. The 5-year survival rate was 60%, but the 10-year survival rate dropped to 33%. This sharp drop was disappointing, but it should be recognized that these patients had relatively advanced disease with positive internal mammary nodes or apical axillary nodes, or both.

Baclesse's pioneering work is being continued by the radiotherapists at the Foundation Curie. The treatment policy was modified and ^{60}Co therapy was instituted. Tumors equal to or less than 3 cm without palpable axillary nodes are treated with local excision and radiation therapy. Larger tumors, 3-10 cm in diameter, with and without palpable axillary nodes, are treated with radiation therapy alone. The patients are followed closely and if there are signs of residual or recurrent disease, mastectomy with axillary dissection is carried out. Calle (15, 16) recently reported the results of treatment: in a series of 356 patients treated by radiation therapy alone as the primary treatment, 220 cases, or 60%, survived 5 years free of disease. One-half of these patients required mastectomy and the remaining patients have kept their breasts. Calle stated that radiation as the primary modality for treating stages I and II breast cancer is difficult and should not be encouraged for general use. It requires meticulous technique and very close follow-up of patients to determine whether or not surgery should be performed. At times the differentiation between radiation fibrosis and residual or recurrent tumor is not possible. Some patients have been operated on unnecessarily because of doubt concerning the nature of residual masses. Examination of the surgical specimen failed to reveal an active neoplasm.

It is clear that if preservation of the breast is important to the patient, at least the primary tumor should be excised prior to radiation therapy.

RADIATION THERAPY IN THE MANAGEMENT OF LOCALLY ADVANCED BREAST CANCER

Radiation therapy plays a major role in the management of inoperable locally advanced carcinoma. These patients are inoperable because of extensive primary tumor, massive involvement of the regional lymph nodes, or both. The primary tumor is usually larger than 5 cm and is often associated with skin infiltration, edema, or fixation. The axillary lymph nodes may be large, matted, and fixed. Radiation therapy can produce permanent tumor control and significant survival rates in cases which are not too far advanced (6,7,11,14,21,40,43,56,57,78,79,85). Baclasse (6,7) used an orthovoltage, multiple-field, and ultrafractionated technique to treat a large series of patients with radiation therapy alone. Most patients received high doses of radiation, 8000-9000 rads, in an overall period of 3-4 months. In 1959 Baclesse reported on the results of treatment of 310 patients with stages II, III, and IV disease. The overall disease-free survival rates were 32% at 5 years and 15% at 10 years. For stage III cases the 5- and 10-year disease-free survival rates were about 20 and 10%, respectively.

Fletcher and Montague (40), in 1965, reported their experience of treating locally advanced breast carcinoma using Baclesse's long protracted technique. Either 250 kV x-ray or cobalt therapy was used. They achieved, in a series of 288 M. D. Anderson category III cases, a 5-year survival rate of 27% and a 5-year disease-free survival rate of 20%. In a later publication (56) a 10-year survival rate of 10% in a series of 148 patients was reported. The local control rate was 74% (39). These data indicate that radical radiation therapy can eradicate breast cancer in a significant number of patients.

Another large series of advanced cases treated by radiation therapy alone was reported by Strickland (78, 79). There were 385 cases, most of whom had stage III disease. He gave a tumor dose of about 6500-7000 rads in an overall period of 5-6 weeks, using a 5 MeV linear accelerator. The 5-year disease-free survival rate of the T3 cases was 32% (89 of 275). The local recurrence within 5 years was 5%. The 10-year disease-free survival of patients with advanced carcinoma was 21%.

The price paid by the survivors, however, is considerable. Many patients developed soft tissue fibrosis with deformity of the breast, some very severe. These were sometimes associated with repeated bouts of inflammation. There were fractures of the ribs and occasionally the sternum. Other less severe complications included slight lung damage, mild lymphedema, and brachial plexus neuritis.

These tumor control rates and survival rates are impressive for advanced cancer, but the high morbidity warrants some changes in their treatment policy, i.e., patients should be better selected for radical radiation therapy and the radiation dosage or fractionation scheme should be adjusted to minimize the normal tissue injury.

A more recent publication by Bruckman et al. (14) reported a series of 166 patients with stage III carcinoma treated by primary radiation therapy. The 5-year actuarial survival and relapse-free survival rates were 25 and 22%, respectively. The 5-year actuarial probability of local tumor control for the entire group was 64%. These authors point up the efficacies of interstitial radiation and surgical excision of gross tumor, and also the importance of high-dose irradiation. In patients who had either an excisional biopsy or an implant, the 5-year actuarial probability of local control was 77 and 76%, respectively. In contrast, the patients having neither excision or implant, local control was only 41%. In patients receiving a total dose of greater than 6000 rads, the local control was 78% compared to 39% in patients receiving less than 6000 rads.

There has been a recent revival of interstitial implantations. The improved technique using removable afterloading ^{192}Ir has contributed to the increasing use of interstitial irradiation (1). The major advantage of implantation is the ability of delivering a highly concentrated radiation dose to the tumor volume with sparing of the surrounding normal tissues. Interstitial implantation is used mainly for boost treatments. Bruckman et al. (14), Alderman (2), and Pierquin et al. (67) all reported favorable results.

Radiation Therapy Technique

There are various techniques to treat breast cancer. Most are comprised of 3-5 fields. The entire breast, the axilla, the internal mammary nodes, and the supraclavicular areas are irradiated. It is necessary to deliver high radiation doses to these tumor-bearing or potential tumor-bearing areas. Skillful planning and execution of the course of treatment is essential in order to deliver an adequate tumor dose without undue injury to the surrounding normal tissues.

Since the breast requires deep penetration, megavoltage x-rays or telecobalt are utilized. The breast is irradiated with opposing medial and lateral tangential fields to avoid or minimize unnecessary irradiation to the underlying lung. The treatment plan should be individualized in order to achieve a satisfactory dose distribution in each case. Bolus or wedge compensators should be applied, depending on the size and contour of the breast. In patients with advanced carcinoma, the skin of the breast is often involved and, therefore, it is desirable to treat the skin. On the other hand, excessive skin dose causing moist reaction is to be avoided or minimized.

The internal mammary lymph nodes can be incorporated in the medial tangential field, but they are better treated with an anterior field. Most internal mammary nodes lie along the border of the sternum about 2-4 cm from the midline and about 2-3 cm deep from the skin. Some nodes could be more lateral, or more deep. An anterior field provides better coverage of these nodes than a tangential field.

The supraclavicular, infraclavicular, and axillary regions are irradiated through an anterior field with the dose to the axilla supplemented by a small posterior field. In some techniques the lower axilla is incorporated in the lateral tangential field.

A tumor dose of approximately 6000-7000 rads should be delivered in 7-8 weeks. This is accomplished by giving a basic dose of about 5000 rads to the whole breast and lymph node areas. An additional dose of 1000-2000 rads/1-2 weeks is given to the primary tumor and to any residual mass in the lymph node areas through reduced fields, using photon beam, electron beam, or interstitial implantation of radioactive material.

This type of intensive radiation treatment usually produces a brisk skin reaction, even with the use of megavoltage therapy. Care must be taken to keep the amount of reaction to its minimum, while not compromising therapeutic effectiveness. The daily dose should be reduced and the bolus removed, or a rest period given to the patient when skin erythema becomes too brisk.

In those patients whose disease is obviously incurable due to massive local and regional involvement, only palliative radiation treatment can be given. The purpose of such treatment is to reduce the tumor size, to relieve pain, and to heal or prevent ulceration. The dose required for palliative treatment is about 4000-5000 rads delivered in 3-4 weeks.

Inflammatory carcinoma is the most aggressive form of breast cancer. It is characterized clinically by diffuse enlargement of the breast and redness, warmth, and induration of overlying skin. The diagnosis of inflammatory cancer is established by both the clinical appearance and the histological evidence of permeation of dermal lymphatics by cancer cells. Radiation therapy usually achieves good local control when the disease is still confined to the breast and its neighboring areas. The typical behavior of this disease, however, is one of continuous spread to the skin beyond the radiation field and early metastases to distant organs, such as the liver, lung, and brain. Most patients die of widespread metastases within 2 years of initial presentation (74,90). The preliminary results of combined chemotherapy and radiation therapy in the treatment of inflammatory cancer appear encouraging (8).

Toilet Mastectomy and Radiation Therapy

It is sometimes technically difficult to deliver an adequate tumor dose to a bulky tumor or to a breast that is large and pendulous. In such cases toilet mastectomy is performed prior to radiation therapy. Better local control and better survival may be achieved in selected cases treated by toilet mastectomy and radiation therapy than those treated by irradiation alone.

Atkins and Horrigan (4) in 1961 reported on a series of patients with locally advanced cancer treated by either radiation therapy alone or by simple mastectomy and radiation therapy. The radiation dose was 4250 rads/3-4 weeks. In the radiation alone group 17 of 20 patients (85%) had local failure. In the simple mastectomy and irradiation group 2 of 12 patients (17%) had local failure. It is to be noted, however, that the high radiation failure rate is most likely related to the low dose given.

Montague (56) reported higher 5- and 10-year survival rates in patients treated by simple mastectomy plus radical irradiation than in patients treated by protracted irradiation. The 5- and 10-year survival rates for the mastectomy and irradiation group were 44.5 and 22%, respectively. However, Montague states that patients who received a simple mastectomy were those with less advanced lesions.

Urban and Castro (83) reviewed a series of patients treated with palliative radical mastectomy and radiation therapy for locally advanced carcinoma and found that the results achieved were superior to those of radiation therapy alone. Brown et al. (12) in 1964 reported high local and regional control rates, more than 90%, by the treatment method of simple mastectomy and radiation therapy.

Montague (57), in a recent review of the M. D. Anderson experience, reported on the long-term follow-up of the survivors treated with supervoltage radical irradiation to a dose of 8000-9000 rads/10-12 weeks. It became clear that the high dose necessary for eradication of large tumor masses exceeded soft tissue and bone tolerance. Patients have disabling fibrosis, particularly when the treated area involves the shoulder girdle. Severe fibrosis is described in 40% of patients, most often in the breast, although the axilla may also be involved. Necrosis of soft tissue and bones appears in 15% of patients and commonly is delayed as long as 10-15 years. Rib fractures occur in 13% of patients. Twenty percent of the patients treated with ^{60}Co have had recurrences, 80% of which occurred in the breast. These experiences led the M. D. Anderson group to change their direction in the use of irradiation in the treatment of advanced breast cancer. Since the late 1960s most of their patients have been treated by simple mastectomy with axillary dissection, followed by radiation therapy. A tumor dose of 5000 rads is delivered in 5 weeks to the chest wall and lymph node areas. Sites of increased risk, i.e., the mastectomy scar, receive through small fields, an additional 1000-1500 rads tumor dose. Montague reports good local tumor control and minimal incidence of complications with this method of treatment. Local control rate was about 85%. The 10-year survival rate in patients with clinically unfavorable, but resectable, tumors was 31%. In patients with tumors that cannot be resected with clear margins, the 10-year survival rate was 16%.

There is no question that radiation therapy is the primary treatment for locally advanced cancer. No surgery can clear all the local and regional disease. Radiation therapy has produced not only significant survival rates, but also permanent control of tumors in the breast and regional lymph nodes. In suitable cases radiation therapy needs the assistance of surgery to remove a bulky tumor or a bulky breast so that the therapeutic effects are improved.

Both surgery and radiation therapy offer good local tumor control and should be used to complement each other whenever feasible in the management of both early and late breast cancers (58). The removal of bulky radioresistant tumor would facilitate the effectiveness of radiation therapy in sterilizing the residual disease. The application of radiation therapy to treat subclinical lesions that cannot be removed by surgery would certainly improve the surgical results. This is precisely the reason for emphasizing the importance of team work, and the importance of exercising flexibility. Each patient should be evaluated individually to determine the best treatment for her. In the management of early breast cancer, radiation therapy may be used as an adjuvant to surgery. In late cases we should consider using surgery as an adjuvant to radiation therapy.

The overall prognosis of patients with locally advanced breast carcinoma is poor. The fact remains, however, a significant number of patients treated primarily by irradiation survive 5 or more years despite the poor prognosis and advanced stage of the lesions. Since most patients die of distant metastases, the use of adjuvant chemotherapy may improve the results of radiation therapy in locally advanced cancer. The limited experience at Memorial Sloan-Kettering with combined radiation therapy and multiple drug chemotherapy, as well as that reported by Zucali et al. (93), is encouraging. In Bruckman's report of 116 patients, 41 received some form of chemotherapy (14). Both local control and relapse-free survival were improved since receiving chemotherapy with or without an endocrine ablative procedure. These results indicate that primary radiation therapy provides local control in a high proportion of patients with advanced cancer and suggest that chemotherapy may be effective in improving both local control and survival in these patients.

RADIATION THERAPY IN THE MANAGEMENT OF LOCAL AND REGIONAL RECURRENCE

Local or regional recurrence of the disease after initial primary treatment is a common problem in the management of patients with breast cancer. These lesions, if untreated, tend to grow, spread, ulcerate, and produce symptoms. Radiation therapy is a very effective means of controlling this troublesome problem.

Whether breast cancer will recur is influenced by multiple factors, the most important of which are stage of the disease, size and location of the primary tumor, presence or absence at diagnosis of ominous signs such as fixation, skin involvement, or edema, and status of axillary lymph nodes. Basically, the more advanced the local disease at diagnosis, the more often is recurrence encountered after primary treatment. Recurrence rates are also higher in those cancers of aggressive histological type and grade. The quality of the surgery performed and the radiation therapy given influence both the incidence and the patterns of local and regional recurrence.

Most recurrences after a radical mastectomy occur in patients with positive axillary lymph nodes. Dao and Nemoto (33) and Donegan and Perez-Mesa (34) found a direct correlation between the number of involved axillary nodes and local recurrence. The level of axillary nodal involvement also plays a role. Urban and Marjani (84), in their report of 383 patients treated by standard radical mastectomy, found that the local recurrence rate was 2% when the axillary nodes were negative. The recurrence rates in patients with nodal involvement in low axilla, midaxilla, and the apex of the axilla were 8, 19, and 27%, respectively.

The size of the primary tumor has been correlated with the incidence of local recurrence. Conway and Neumann (30) found that 50% of the recurrences developed in patients with tumors 7 cm or more in diameter and only 4% with tumors less than 3 cm in diameter. Spratt (77) found a 33% local recurrence rate in cancers larger than 8 cm in diameter. There was no recurrence in patients with small tumors, i.e., less than 1 cm in diameter. Haagensen (45) noted recurrence rates of 28 and 71% in patients with stages C and D disease, respectively. All these patients were treated by radical mastectomy but did not receive postoperative radiation therapy.

The local and regional recurrences depend also on the type of surgery performed. Cases treated by simple mastectomy and radiation therapy usually show a higher recurrence rate than those treated by radical mastectomy and radiation therapy. This is particularly true for axillary recurrence, which is rare (around 1%), in radical mastectomy cases (25,39,83). Bruce et al. (13) reported a series of 423 stages I and II cases treated by simple mastectomy and radiation therapy. Their 5-year recurrence rates for axillary, chest wall, and supraclavicular areas were 21, 20, and 40%, respectively. Tough (82) in his review of 573 cases treated by simple mastectomy and radiation therapy stated that as far as axillary nodes are concerned, surgery is more effective than radiotherapy in preventing recurrence. It has been demonstrated clearly by many studies (25,38,39,51,73) that postoperative radiation therapy reduces the incidence of recurrence in the irradiated areas.

Recurrence may be local, regional, or both. The term local recurrence is usually applied to lesions appearing in the skin and subcutaneous tissues of the chest wall at the mastectomy site, while regional recurrence means lymph node lesions in the internal mammary chain, the axilla, and the supraclavicular area of the ipsilateral side. In the majority of patients the first manifestation of recurrence is in the chest wall, adjacent to the mastectomy scar. Most recurrences develop during the first 2 years after mastectomy.

Chest wall recurrence may be of the nodular or the inflammatory forms. Nodular recurrence may be solitary or multiple, and in the most advanced cases, confluent nodules may encircle the chest to form cancer en cuirasse.

Inflammatory recurrence is relatively uncommon. Patients with this form of relapse have a grave prognosis and usually die of widespread metastases within a short period of time (74). The lesions appear as a diffuse reddening of the skin, associated with slight induration and an increase in local temperature. Inflammatory cancer, whether primary or recurrent, is a clinical entity, but its diagnosis must be confirmed by skin biopsy which shows cancer cell invasion of the skin lymphatics.

Internal mammary lymph node recurrence usually is manifest as a parasternal nodule, growing through the intercostal space. Most patients who develop internal mammary nodal recurrence are those with inner quadrant or central primary tumors who did not have either internal mammary lymph node dissection or postoperative radiation therapy directed to this chain. Large parasternal masses may cause destruction of the sternum and involvement of the deep mediastinum and other intrathoracic structures.

Supraclavicular and axillary nodes are usually easily palpable. The tumor may extend through the capsule to involve the brachial plexus, producing neuropathy in the upper extremity.

Treatment

Prior to initiating treatment of local or regional recurrence, a biopsy of the lesions must be done to confirm the diagnosis of recurrent mammary carcinoma. Thorough workup should be carried out to determine the extent of the disease, specifically, whether or not the disease is still localized. If there is no clinical evidence of distant metastasis and the local or regional recurrence is of limited extent, one should take an aggressive approach, aiming for permanent or long-term control. If the disease is locally extensive or if distant metastases are present, only palliative therapy can be offered.

Treatment planning of recurrent disease must take into consideration not only the delivering of an adequate radiation dose to the tumor-bearing volume, but also the minimizing of dose to the adjacent normal tissues. We advocate electron beam therapy for chest wall irradiation because of the unique physical characteristics of electrons which permit excellent dose distribution with relatively simple techniques (20,26,27,80).

The chief advantages of high-energy electron therapy include: (1) controllable depth of penetration by varying the energy of electrons; (2) abrupt termination of radiation in depth; (3) minimal differential energy absorption in tissues, such as muscles, lung, air, and bone, gram for gram; and (4) easy beam shaping with the use of tissue equivalent compensators. These can be applied directly to the skin to deliver a homogenous dose to the chest wall and the lymph node areas without unnecessary radiation to the underlying lung. This method is superior to megavoltage x-ray or telecobalt therapy because highly penetrating photon beams require tangential field setups which are sometimes associated with uncertain dose distribution.

Chest Wall Recurrence

For skin and subcutaneous recurrences the radiation field should cover the site of recurrence with a wide margin in order to include other occult lesions which may exist in the neighboring skin. The whole anterior chest wall on the affected side should be treated, even though the recurrent nodule may appear solitary. A tumor dose of 4500-5000 rads is given over a period of 4-5 weeks with a supplementary dose of 500-1000 rads/1 week, given to any residual nodule or nodules.

Whenever possible it is preferable to treat the chest wall lesions with one field. When more than one field is necessary to cover a large cutaneous area or a cutaneous area plus a nodal region, special attention must be paid to the problems of junction points. Converging fields, for example, may create a "hot spot" close to 200%, causing fractures of the ribs (27) or other complications. The use of polystyrene wedges at the interface of adjoining fields may eliminate undesired accumulation of dose in overlapping irradiated regions. Different shapes and thicknesses of polystyrene absorbers are employed to obtain desired depth of penetration. Hot and cold spots can also be minimized by changing the location of the junction area during the course of irradiation.

All treatment plans should be individualized and tailored to suit the patient's particular needs. The procedure and some of the commonly used techniques are described in detail in previous publications (20,26,27). When high-energy electron therapy facilities are unavailable, the chest wall can be treated through tangential fields using telecobalt or megavoltage x-rays. Bolus should be used in order to fully utilize back-scatter and to facilitate accurate dose calculation.

Regional Lymph Node Recurrence

Small parasternal masses from internal mammary lymph node involvement also are best treated with the electron beam. Large parasternal masses, particularly with mediastinal involvement, may require megavoltage photon therapy. Supraclavicular lymph nodes are treated either by megavoltage photon or high-energy electron beam with equally good tumor control dose for dose. Axillary lymph node recurrence is rare after a Halsted-type radical mastectomy, but when it occurs, electron beam therapy is preferred. We recommend a tumor dose of 4500-5000 rads, delivered in a period of about 4-5 weeks, with an additional dose of about 500-1000 rads/1 week given to the residual mass through a reduced field.

Publications in the literature reporting on the fate of patients after the development of local or regional recurrence have shown a general impression that recurrence is soon followed by distant metastasis and most patients die within a short period of time. Spratt (77) reported a 5-year survival rate of 3 and 9% after chest wall recurrence and there were no 10-year survivals. Zimmerman et al. (92) revealed a 10% 5-year survival (7 out of 70 patients) after appearance and treatment of local recurrence.

A study of a series of 215 patients (24), treated at Memorial Hospital has shown somewhat better results. The survival and tumor control by radiation therapy of these 215 patients with limited recurrence in the chest wall and/or lymph node areas were evaluated. These patients all had thorough workup which showed no evidence of distant metastasis prior to the radiation therapy. The survival data showed 21% of the patients survived 5 years and 5% survived 10 or more years following radiation therapy of the recurrent disease. Indeed, some women never developed other problems. Radiation therapy produced a high rate of local response. Complete control was achieved in 67% and partial control in 24%. In those patients with complete control the local remission lasted 2-3 years on an average and the patients were free of local problems during this prolonged period of time. In those patients with partial control most symptoms associated with recurrent disease were alleviated although persistent disease was present. Control of tumor is dose related. Most patients with complete control received about 5000 rads/5 weeks. Bulkier lesions received a higher dose. Among the complete control group there were seven patients who remained free of cancer for periods ranging from 5-15 years. It is entirely possible that some recurrent disease is truly localized and can be eradicated by aggressive therapy. These data indicate that intensive irradiation for patients with limited recurrence is worthwhile. However, local relapse does imply poor prognosis as 80% of patients die within 5 years. This intensive radiation therapy probably should be combined with chemotherapy in an attempt to improve the survival.

For patients with extensive local or regional recurrence, palliative therapy is given to alleviate symptoms or to prevent undesirable complications such as pain, ulceration, or brachial plexus syndrome. Most of these patients have systemic disease and are receiving hormonal or chemotherapeutic treatment. The radiation dose used for adequate palliation should be about 3500-4500 rads, delivered over 3-4 weeks. Effective control of symptomatic lesions can be achieved in a majority of patients. In a study (26) of 630 cases of mostly advanced chest wall recurrence treated by electron beam, there was a control of the local disease in 74% for a mean duration of 13 months. Similarly, in 297 cases of lymph node recurrence, 71% were controlled for a mean duration of 16 months. Symptomatic, ulcerated lesions regressed after therapy and improvement usually lasted to the time of the patient's death.

RADIATION THERAPY IN THE MANAGEMENT OF DISSEMINATED DISEASE

The management of disseminated breast cancer requires hormonal manipulation or chemotherapy and, often, simultaneous or sequential irradiation to relieve localized symptoms. Radiation therapy is very useful in the treatment of a host of problems (19,21). Palliative therapy improves the quality of life and, when metastatic lesions involve vital organs, may actually prolong life.

Breast cancer may metastasize to any part of the body. The most common site of metastasis is the bone. Radiation therapy is very effective in relieving pain. A dose of about 2000-3000 rads/1-2 weeks will relieve pain in 90% of the cases. Recalcification of osteolytic lesions occurs in about 75-80% (42). Pathologic fractures can often be prevented.

Metastasis to external soft tissues or lymph nodes can cause pain, ulceration, and bleeding. A dose of 3500-4500 rads/3-4 weeks will control most of these problems.

Metastatic lesions may produce serious complications of obstruction. Superior vena caval syndrome due to metastatic mediastinal lymph nodes is a genuine emergency requiring prompt institution of radiation therapy. A treatment schedule consisting of three daily doses of 400 rads, followed by daily doses of 200 rads, to a total of about 3600-4000 rads would relieve obstruction in the majority of patients. Prompt therapy is important because delay in treatment may result in thrombus formation which cannot be reversed by radiation therapy.

Other obstructive lesions may occur in the esophagus causing dysphagia; in the bronchus causing atelectasis of the lung; and in the porta hepatis causing jaundice. Occasionally breast carcinoma may metastasize to periureteral tissue, producing obstruction of the ureter, hydronephrosis, and uremia. A dose of 3000-4000 rads delivered over a period of 2-3 weeks would resolve most of the obstruction (28).

Central nervous system involvement is common in breast carcinoma. Whole head irradiation for brain metastasis with a dose of about 3000-4000 rads/2-3 weeks, combined with corticosteroids, would provide good palliation in about 60% of cases (22,60,61,91). Spinal cord compression due to extradural metastasis is also an emergency situation requiring prompt radiation therapy. The most commonly used treatment schedule is three daily doses of 400 rads followed by 200 rads daily to a total of about 3200-4000 rads. Approximately 50% of patients respond to radiation therapy and become ambulatory (50,55,68,70,75). The prognosis is better in patients with minimal neurological dysfunction than in those with severe symptoms and signs, such as paraplegia. In our institution spinal cord compression is treated by radiation therapy alone. Laminectomy is seldom indicated. It has been found by Posner and colleagues (68,70) that laminectomy followed by radiation therapy produces a response rate of 50%, similar to the results of 47% for radiation therapy alone. Further, the surgical procedure is associated with a 10% complication rate. Most patients have metastatic lesions in the spine with partial collapse of the vertebral bodies. The bulk of tumor is anterior to the cord and, therefore, inaccessible to the surgeon.

Lung and liver metastases are common, but these are seldom treated by radiation therapy, as the normal lung and liver tissue do not tolerate radiation well. If radiation therapy is indicated to these sites, the therapy should proceed with caution, in order to avoid pneumonitis or hepatitis.

Breast carcinoma can also metastasize to the eye and orbit. Intraocular lesions usually occur in the choroid membrane, causing elevation and sometimes detachment of the retina. The main symptom is blurred vision. Radiation therapy to the posterior pole of the eye through a small precision field restores vision in the majority of patients (23,62,81). The dose given is about 3500-4000 rads/3 weeks. Metastasis to the orbit usually involves the retrobulbar region, producing proptosis. Good results can also be expected from radiation therapy (47).

Another serious complication of advanced cancer is metastasis to the heart and pericardium. The diagnosis is difficult and often missed because there are no characteristic symptoms and signs. However, when a cancer patient with no previous history of cardiac disease suddenly develops arrhythmia, congestive failure, or pericarditis, and when these symptoms do not respond to conservative treatment, cardiac metastasis should be strongly suspected. Diagnostic procedures such as electrocardiography, echocardiography, angiocardiography, and pericardiocentesis can establish the diagnosis. External beam therapy to the heart, delivering a dose of 3500 rads/4 weeks will relieve the distressing symptoms and avert a life-threatening situation in a significant number of patients (18). Pericardial effusion with tamponade can be treated by pericardial catheterization and instillation of ^{32}P, which provides prompt relief of the tamponade (53).

REFERENCES

1. Afterloading: 20 Years of Experience, 1955-1975. Proceedings of the Second International Symposium on Radiation Therapy, edited by Basil S. Hilaris, New York, Robert C. Gold and Associates, 1975.

2. Alderman, S.J.: Combination teletherapy and iridium implementation in the treatment of locally advanced breast cancer. Cancer 38:1936-1938, 1976.

3. Anglem, T.J. and Leber, R.E.: Operable breast cancer: The case against conservative surgery. Cancer 23:330-333, 1973.

4. Atkins, H.L. and Horrigan, M.D.: Treatment of locally advanced carcinoma of the breast with roentgen therapy and simple mastectomy. Am. J. Roentgenol. 85:860-864, 1961.

5. Atkins, Sir H., Hayward, J. L., Klugman, D. J., and Wayte, A. B.: Treatment of early breast cancer: A report after ten years of clinical trial. Br. Med. J. 2:423-429, 1972.

6. Baclesse, F.: Five-year results in 431 breast cancers treated solely by roentgen rays. Ann. Surg. 161:103-104, 1965.

7. Baclesse, F.: Roentgenotherapy alone in cancer of the breast. Acta Int. Union Against Cancer 15:1023-1026, 1959.

8. Blumenscheim, G.R., Montague, E.D., Eckles, N.E., Hortobaguy, G.N., and Barker, J.L.: Sequential combined modality therapy for inflammatory breast cancer. Breast 2:16-20, 1976.

9. Bonadonna, G., Brusamolino, E., Valagussa, P., Brugnatelli, L., Rossi, A., Brambilla, C., DeLena, M., Tancini, G., Bajetta, E., and Veronesi, U.: Combination chemotherapy as an adjuvant treatment in operable breast cancer. N. Engl. J. Med. 294(8):405-410, 1976.

10. Bonadonna, G., Rossi, A., Valagussa, P., Banfi, A., and Veronesi, U.: The CMF program for operable breast cancer with positive axillary nodes: Updated analysis on the disease-free interval, site of relapse and drug tolerance. Cancer 39:2904-2915, 1977.

11. Bouchard, J.: Advanced cancer of the breast treated primarily with irradiation. Radiology 84:823-842, 1965.

12. Brown, R., Horiot, J.C., Fletcher, G.H., White, E.C., and Ange, D.W.: Simple mastectomy and radiation therapy for locally advanced breast cancers technically suitable for radical mastectomy. Am. J. Roentgenol. 120:67-73 1974.

13. Bruce, J., Carter, D.C., and Fraser, J.: Patterns of recurrent disease in breast cancer. Lancet 1:433-435, 1970.

14. Bruckman, J.E., Harris, J.R., Levene, M.D., Chaffey, J.T., and Hellman, S.: Results of treating stage III carcinoma of the breast by primary radiation therapy. Cancer 43:985-993, 1979.

15. Calle, R.: Primary treatment of breast cancer with radiation therapy: A conservative treatment of operable breast cancer. New York Metropolitan Breast Cancer Group Bulletin, Vol. III, pp. 1-5, No. 1, 1979.

16. Calle, R., Pillerson, J.P., Schlienger, P., and Vilcoq, J.R.: Conservative management of operable breast cancer. Ten years experience at the Foundation Curie. Cancer 42:2045-2053, 1978.

17. Cancer research campaign: Management of early cancer of the breast. Report on an international multicentre trial supported by the cancer research campaign. Br. Med. J. 1:1035-1038, 1976.

18. Cham, W.C., Freiman, A.H., Carstens, H.B., and Chu, F.C.H.: Radiation therapy of cardiac and pericardial metastases. Radiology 114:701-704, 1975.

19. Chu, F.C.H.: Radiotherapy for symptomatic relief. In Breast Cancer Management Early and Late, edited by Basil A. Stoll, London, William Heinemann Medical Books Ltd., pp. 101-108, 1977.

20. Chu, F.C.H.: The role of electron beam therapy in the treatment of breast cancer. In Frontiers of Radiation Therapy, Oncology, edited by J.M. Vaeth, New York, Karger, 1968, pp. 224-237.

21. Chu, F.C.H.: Radiation therapy for locally advanced, recurrent, or disseminated breast cancer. In The Breast, edited by H.S. Gallager, H.P. Leis, R.K. Snyderman, and J.A. Urban, St. Louis, C.V. Mosby, 1978, pp. 343-355.

22. Chu, F.C.H. and Hilaris, B.S.: Value of radiation therapy in the management of intracranial metastases. Cancer 14:577-581, 1961.

23. Chu, F.C.H,, Huh, S.H., Nisce, L.Z., and Simpson, L.D.: Radiation therapy of choroid metastases from breast cancer. Int. J. Radiat. Oncol. Biol. Phys. 2:273-279, 1977.

24. Chu, F.C.H., Lin, F.J., Kim, J.H., Huh, S.H., and Armatis, G.J.: Locally recurrent carcinoma of the breast - results of radiation therapy. Cancer 37:2677-2690, 1976.

25. Chu, F.C.H., Lucas, J.C., Farrow, J.H., and Nickson, J.J.: Does prophylactic radiation therapy given for cancer of the breast predispose to metastasis? Am. J. Roentgenol. 99:987-994, 1967.

26. Chu, F.C.H., Nisce, L.Z., Baker, A.Z., Sattar, A., and Laughlin, J.S.: Electron beam therapy of cancer of the breast. Radiology 89:216-233, 1967.

27. Chu, F.C.H., Nice, L.A., and Laughlin, J.S.: Treatment of breast cancer with high energy electrons produced by 24 MeV betatron. Radiology 81:871-880, 1973.

28. Chu, F.C.H., Solis, M., and Grabstald, H.: Radiation therapy of ureteral metastases from breast cancer. Clin. Bull. 7:105-108, 1977.

29. Consensus Development Conference on Treatment of Primary Breast Cancer: Management of Local Disease, May, 1979, Washington, D.C., Sponsored by NCI's Division of Cancer Treatment and the NIH Office of Medical Applications Research.

30. Conway, H. and Neumann, C.G.: Evaluation of skin grafting in the technique of radical mastectomy in relation to local recurrence of carcinoma. Surg. Gynecol. Obstet. 88:45-49, 1949.

31. Crile, G. Jr.: Results of simple mastectomy without irradiation in the treatment of operative stage I cancer of the breast. Ann. Surg. 168:330-336, 1968.

32. deSchryver, A.: The Stockholm Breast Cancer Trial: Preliminary report of a randomized study concerning the value of preoperative or postoperative radiotherapy in operable disease. Int. J. Radiat. Oncol. Biol. Phys. 1:601-609, 1976.

33. Dao, T.L. and Nemoto, T.: Clinical significance of skin recurrences after radical mastectomy in women with cancer of the breast. Surg. Gynecol. Obstet. 117:447-453, 1973.

34. Donegan, W.L., Perez-Mesa, C.M., and Watson, F.R.: A biostatistical study of locally recurrent breast carcinoma. Surg. Gynecol. Obstet. 122:529-540, 1966.

35. Fisher, B., Carbone, P., Economou, S.G., Relick, R., Glass, A., Lerner, H., Redmond, C., Aelen, M., Katrych, D.L., Wolmark, N., Band, P., Fisher, E.R., and other cooperating investigators: L-phenylalanine mustard (L-PAM) in the management of primary breast cancer: A report of early findings. N. Engl. J. Med. 292:117-122, 1975.

36. Fisher, B., Glass, A., Redmond, C., Fisher, E.R., Barton, B., Such, E., Carbone, P., Economou, S., Foster, R., Frelick, R., Lerner, H., Levitt, M., Margolese, R., MacFarlane, J., Plotkin, D., Shibata, H., Volk, H., and other investigators: L-phenylalanine mustard (L-PAM) in the management of primary breast cancer: An update of earlier findings and a comparison with those utilizing L-PAM plus 5-flurouracil (5-FU). Cancer 39:2883-2903, 1977.

37. Fisher, B., Montague, E., Redmond, C., Barton, B., Borland, D., Fisher, E.R., Deutsch, M., Schwarz, G., Margolese, R., Donegan, W., Volk, H., Lesnick, G., Crux, A.B., Lawrence, W., Nealon, T., Butcher, H., Lawton, R., and other NSABP investigators: Comparison of radical mastectomy with alternative treatments for primary breast cancer. A first report of results from a prospective randomized clinical trial. Cancer 39:2827-2839, 1977.

38. Fisher, B., Slack, N.H., Cavanaugh, P.J., Gardner, B., Ravdin, R.G., and cooperating investigators: Postoperative radiotherapy in the treatment of breast cancer: Results of the NSABP clinical trial. Ann. Surg. 172:711-732, 1970.

39. Fletcher, G.H.: Local results of irradiation in the primary management of localized breast cancer. Cancer 29:545-551, 1972.

40. Fletcher, G.H. and Montague, E.D.: Radical irradiation of advanced breast cancer. Am. J. Roentgenol. 93:573-584, 1965.

41. Fletcher, G.H. and Montague, E.D.: Does adequate irradiation of the internal mammary chain and supraclavicular nodes improve survival rates? Int. J. Radiat. Oncol. Biol. Phys. 4:481-492, 1978.

42. Garmatis, C.J. and Chu, F.C.H.: The effectiveness of radiation therapy in the treatment of bone metastases from breast cancer. Radiology 126:235-237, 1978.

43. Griscom, N.T. and Wang, C.C.: Radiation therapy of inoperable breast carcinoma. Radiology 79:18-23, 1962.

44. Guttmann, R.J.: Effects of radiation on metastatic lymph nodes from various primary carcinomas. Am. J. Roentgenol. 79:79-82, 1958.

45. Haagensen, C.D.: Treatment of curable carcinoma of the breast. Int. J. Radiat. Oncol. Biol. Phys. 2:975-980, 1977.

46. Høst, H. and Brennhovd, I.O.: The effect of postoperative radiotherapy in breast cancer. Int. J. Radiat. Oncol. Biol. Phys. 2:1061-1067, 1977.

47. Huh, S.H., Nisce, L.Z., Simpson, L.D., and Chu, F.C.H.: The value of radiation therapy in the treatment of orbital metastasis. Am. J. Roentgenol. 120:589-594, 1974.

48. Kaae, S. and Johansen, H.: Breast cancer: Five-year results: Two random series of simple mastectomy with postoperative irradiation versus extended radical mastectomy. Am. J. Roentgenol. Radium Ther. Nuclear Med. 87(1): 82-88, 1962.

49. Kaae, S. and Johansen, H.: Simple mastectomy plus postoperative irradiation by the method of McWhirter for mammary carcinoma. Ann. Surg. 170:895, 1969.

50. Kahn, F.R., Glicksman, A.S., Chu, F.C.H., and Nickson, J.J.: Treatment by radiotherapy of spinal cord compression due to extradural metastases. Radiology 489:495-500, 1967.

51. Kim, J.H., Chu, F.C.H., and Hilaris, B.S.: The influence on acute and late reactions in patients with postoperative radiotherapy for carcinoma of the breast. Cancer 35:1583-1586, 1975.

52. Leis, H.P., Jr.: Selective moderate surgical approach for potentially curable breast cancer. In The Breast, edited by H.S. Gallager, H.P. Leis, R.K. Snyderman, and J.A. Urban, St. Louis, C.V. Mosby, 1978, p. 247.

53. Martini, N., Freiman, A.H., Watson, R.C., and Hilaris, B.S.: Malignant pericardial effusion. N.Y.S. J. Med. 76:719-721, 1976.

54. McWhirter, R.: The value of simple mastectomy and radiotherapy in the treatment of cancer of the breast. Br. J. Radiol. 21:599-617, 1948.

55. Millburn, L., Hibbs, G.G., and Hendrickson, F.R.: Treatment of spinal cord compression from metastatic carcinoma - Review of the literature and presentation of a new method of treatment. Cancer 21:447-452, 1968.

56. Montague, E.D.: Radiation therapy for locally advanced carcinoma of the breast. Breast cancer: Early and late. Proceedings of the Annual Clinical Conference on Cancer sponsored by the University of Texas M.D. Anderson Hosp. and Tumor Inst., at Houston, and published by Year Book Medical Publishers, Inc., Chicago, Ill., 1970, pp. 191-198.

57. Montague, E.D.: Radiotherapy as primary modality in treatment of curable breast cancer. In The Breast, edited by H.S. Gallager, H.P. Leis, R.K. Snyderman, and J.A. Urban, St. Louis, C.V. Mosby Co., 1978, pp. 271-283.

58. Montague, E.D.: Radiation management of advanced breast cancer. Int. J. Radiat. Oncol. Biol. Phys. 4:305-307, 1978.

59. Mustakallio, S.: Conservative treatment of breast carcinoma - Review of 25 years follow up. Clin. Radiol. 23:110-116, 1972.

60. Nisce, L.Z., Hilaris, B.S., and Chu, F.C.H.: A review of experience with irradiation of brain metastases. Am. J. Roentgenol. 111:329-333, 1971.

61. Order, S.E., Hellman, S., Von Essen, C.F., and Kligerman, M.M.: Improvement in quality of survival following whole-brain irradiation for brain metastasis. Radiology 91:149-153, 1968.

62. Orenstein, M.D., Anderson, D.P., and Stein, J.J.: Choroid metastasis. Cancer 29:1101-1107, 1972.

63. Paterson, R.: The Treatment of Malignant Disease by Radium and X-rays. London, Arnold, 1948, p. 309.

64. Paterson, R. and Russell, M.H.: Clinical trial in malignant disease, part III: Breast cancer - evaluation of postoperative radiotherapy. J. Fac. Radiol. 10: 175-180, 1959.

65. Peters, M.V.: Wedge resection and irradiation. An effective treatment in early breast cancer. JAMA 200(2):144-145, 1967.

66. Peters, M.V.: Wedge resection with or without radiation in early breast cancer. Int. J. Radiat. Oncol. Biol. Phys. 2:1151-1156, 1977.

67. Pierquin, B., Baillet, F., and Wilson, J.F.: Radiation therapy in the management of primary breast cancer. Am. J. Roentgenol. 127:645-648, 1976.

68. Posner, J.B.: Spinal cord compression. A neurological emergency. Clin. Bull. 1:65-71, 1971.

69. Prosnitz, L.R., Goldenberg, I.S., Packard, R.A., Levene, M.B., Harris, J., Hellman, S., Wallner, P.E., Brady, L.W., Mansfield, C.M., and Kramer, S.: Radiation therapy as initial treatment for early stage cancer of the breast without mastectomy. Cancer 39:917-923, 1977.

70. Raichle, M.E. and Posner, J.B.: The treatment of extra dural spinal cord compression. Neurology 20:391, 1970.

71. Rissanen, P.M.: A comparison of conservative and radical surgery combined with radiotherapy in the treatment of stage I carcinoma of the breast. Br. J. Radiol. 42:423-426, 1969.

72. Rissanen, P.M. and Holsti, P.: Late results of local excision combined with radiotherapy in the treatment of early breast cancer. Twenty-year follow-up. Effect of megavoltage therapy on incidence of local recurrences. Presented at the International Congress of Radiology, Rio de Janeiro, Brazil, October 1977.

73. Robbins, G.F., Lucas, J.C. Jr., Fracchia, A.A., Farrow, J.H., and Chu, F.C.H.: Evaluation of postoperative prophylactic radiation therapy in breast cancer. Surg. Gynecol. Obstet. 122:979-982, 1966.

74. Robbins, G.F., Shah, J., Rosen, P., Chu, F.C.H., and Taylor, J.: Inflammatory carcinoma of the breast. Surg. Clin. N. Am. 54:801-810, 1974.

75. Rubin, P., Mayer, E., and Poulter, C.: Extradural spinal cord compression by tumor. Part II: High daily dose experience without laminectomy. Radiology 93:1248-1260, 1969.

76. Schottenfeld, D., Nash, A., Robbins, G.F., and Beattie, E.J.: Ten-year results of the treatment of primary operable breast carcinoma: A summary of 304 patients evaluated by the T.N.M. system. Cancer 38:1001-1007, 1975.

77. Spratt, J.S.: Locally recurrent cancer after radical mastectomy. Cancer 29: 1051-1053, 1967.

78. Strickland, P.: The management of carcinoma of the breast by radical supervoltage radiation. Br. J. Surg. 60:569-573, 1973.

79. Strickland, P.: Radical radiation therapy for locally advanced disease. In Breast Cancer Management, Early and Late, edited by Basil A. Stoll, London, William Heinemann Medical Books Ltd., 1977, pp. 43-51.

80. Tapley, N. duV., Fletcher, G.H., and Montague, E.D.: Breast: Clinical Application of the Electron Beam. Edited by N. DuV. Tapley, New York, Wiley, 1976, pp. 199-231.

81. Thatcher, N. and Thomas, P.R.M.: Choroidal metastases from breast carcinoma: A survey of 42 patients and the use of radiation therapy. Clin. Radiol. 26:549, 1975.

82. Tough, I.C.K.: The significance of recurrence in breast cancer. Br. J. Surg. 53:897-900, 1966.

83. Urban, J.A. and Castro, El B.: Selecting variations in extent of surgical procedure for breast cancer. Cancer 28:1615-1623, 1971.

84. Urban, J.A. and Marjani, M.A.: Significance of internal mammary lymph node metastases in breast cancer. Am. J. Roentgenol. Rad. Ther. Nuclear Med. 111:130-136, 1971.

85. Vaeth, J.M., Clark, J.C., Green, J.P., Schroeder, A.F., and Lowry, R.O.: Radiotherapeutic management of locally advanced carcinoma of the breast. Cancer 30:107-112, 1972.

86. Veronesi, U.: New trends in the treatment of breast cancer at the Institute of Milan. Am. J. Roentgenol. 128:287-289, 1977.

87. Veronesi, U., Banfi, A., Saccozzi, R., Salvadori, B. , Zucali, R. , Uslenghi, C., Greco, M., Luini, A., Rilke, F., and Sultan, L.: Conservative treatment of breast cancer. A trial process at the Cancer Institute of Milan. Cancer 39:2822-2826, 1977.

88. Wallgren, A.: A controlled study: Preoperative versus postoperative irradiation. Int. J. Radiat. Oncol. Biol. Phys. 2:1167-1169, 1977.

89. Wallgren, A., Arner, O., Bergstrom, J., Blomstedt, B., Granberg, P.O., Karustrom, L., Raf, L., and Silversward, C.: Preoperative radiotherapy in operable mammary cancer: Results in the Stockholm Breast Cancer Trial. Int. J. Radiat. Oncol. Biol. Phys. 6:287-290, 1980.

90. Wang, C.C. and Griscom, N.T.: Inflammatory carcinoma of the breast. Results following orthovoltage and supravoltage radiation therapy. Clin. Radiol. 15:167-174, 1964.

91. Young, D.F., Posner, J.B., Chu, F.C.H., and Nisce, L.Z.: Rapid course radiation therapy of brain metastases: Results and complications. Cancer 34: 1069-1076, 1974.

92. Zimmerman, K.W., Montague, E.D., and Fletcher, G.H.: Frequency, anatomical distribution and management of local recurrences after definitive therapy for breast cancer. Cancer 17:67-74, 1966.

93. Zucali, R., Uslenghi, C., Kenda, R., and Bonadonna, G.: Natural history and survival of inoperable breast cancer treated with radiotherapy and radiotherapy followed by radical mastectomy. Cancer 37:1422-1431, 1976.

chapter 8

COLORECTAL ADENOCARCINOMA

Bernard Roswit, M.D.
George A. Higgins, M.D.

Colorectal carcinoma has come to be the most common major malignant disease in adult men and women in this country, already reaching all of the proportions of a national health calamity. The American Cancer Society has estimated a record of 120,000 new cases for 1981 and 54,900 deaths (4). The incidence is highest in the affluent nations in North America, northwest Europe, and other Anglo-Saxon areas, and low in South America, Africa, and Asia. Diet appears to be the major etiological factor (8,9,75,82). Epidemiological evaluation suggests that there is a strong association of large bowel carcinogenesis and high intake of dietary fat and meat, notably beef, and a deficiency in dietary fiber.

The overall 5-year surgical survival of patients with colorectal cancer is relatively good, when compared with other major visceral cancers. Surgery is still the mainstay of treatment. Nevertheless, survival has not been significantly improved in the last 30 years, despite great improvement in surgical knowledge (34, 41). Adjuvant cancer chemotherapy has been disappointing in the control of the disease in operable patients, despite more than 20 years of investigation by the Veterans Administration Surgical Adjuvant Cancer Chemotherapy Study Group (VASAG) and many other workers.

The surgical failure rate in operable cases remains at about 50% and the overall survival (all cases included) is no better than 30%. When there is gross involvement through the gut wall, the outlook for survival after surgical resection is no better than 35-40%, and should there be lymph nodes involved as well, only 20-25% will survive to the fifth year.

It has been well established that the principal cause of surgical failure is local and regional recurrence because of viable cells beyond the surgical field or dissemination during the surgical procedure. This is particularly true in lesions below the peritoneal reflection and when they have gone through the wall (Dukes B2) and involve nodes (Dukes C) (11,22,25,28,33,34,40,43,56,57,76).

Morson and Bussey, at the St. Marks Hospital in London, reviewed nearly 2000 colorectal operations in 1967 and declared that "surgery has little more to offer in the treatment of rectal cancer. It is hard to see what more can be done by surgical treatment alone. Our experience suggests that radiotherapy is most likely to improve the survival rates of those patients who are at greatest risk of incomplete removal of tumor in the pelvis or deposits in the lymph glands" (41).

It is technically difficult to ensure complete excision of disease in the rigid, narrowing, funnel-shaped lower pelvic compartment (Figs. 1 and 2). Gilbertsen

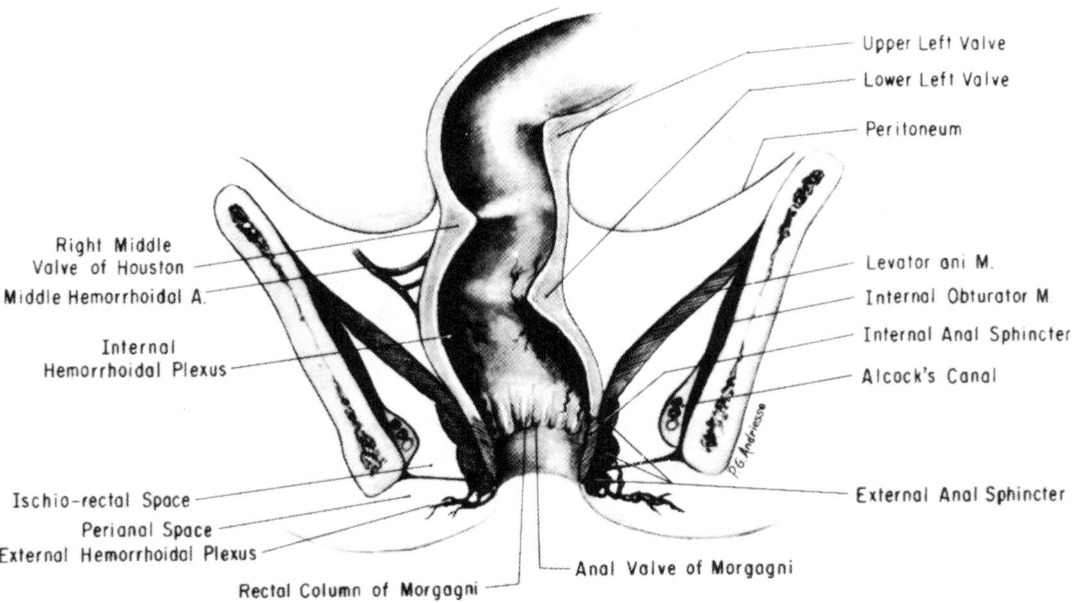

Figure 1. Anatomy of the anorectum. (From Ref. 26.)

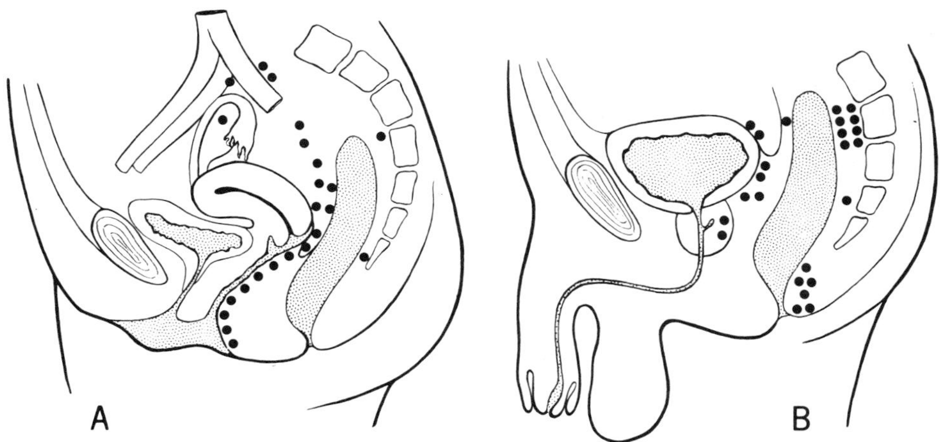

Figure 2. The location of local recurrences in (A) female and (B) male patients having had previous resection for carcinoma of the rectum. (From Ref. 23.)

reported fully 70% local recurrence after curative resections for carcinoma of the rectal ampulla in Dukes C cases (23). Taylor, at the University of Indiana, analyzed autopsy material in 125 patients who died after palliative and curative resections for colorectal cancer, showing that 79 and 72% of patients, respectively had local continuance or recurrence as a principal cause of death by cancer (70).

It seems unlikely that any improvement in surgical techniques can result in a substantial gain in survival. Abdominoperineal resection, first described by Miles in 1908, is being reassessed because operative mortality and morbidity with a permanent colostomy is high, especially in elderly and feeble patients. Nor has chemotherapy given us any real promise of significantly improving the outlook for cure in operable patients.

Clearly, the time has come for a new perspective, a radical change in treatment strategy. There is a wealth of documented retrospective clinical experience over six decades demonstrating the benefits of adjuvant and even primary radiation therapy in rectal and rectosigmoid cancer at every stage of disease (34, 57). The outlook for survival of the operable patient has been improved through preoperative radiation treatment, reducing local recurrence, involvement of lymph nodes, and even distant metastasis. Borderline operable lesions have been converted to operability and some to curability. Our potential in preoperative therapy appears to be greatest for tumors which have the worst outlook for recurrence, notably those invading through the wall and involving lymph nodes or adjacent organs in the lower pelvic compartment. Even some patients with inoperable tumors now appear to have a chance for cure through radical irradiation alone. Postoperative treatment, now being explored in several pilot studies, is already yielding benefits in reduction of recurrence and improved survival. These clinical experiences have excited interest in the possible benefits of "sandwich" therapy (preoperative plus postoperative) now being tested, and the early results look promising.

Of special interest are the reports of high cure rates by intracavitary contact therapy to small rectal cancers near the anal verge in medically inoperable patients (too old, too ill, too feeble). Striking relief from distress and disability can be offered to the majority of patients with locally advanced and even metastatic disease through supervoltage beam therapy.

Of paramount importance is an accurate appraisal and clear statement of the stage of the disease. The original staging established by Dukes is too simplified for accurate assessment of prognosis and survival (6, 13-15). It has been modified by Astler and Coller (6) and still further refined recently by Gunderson (28) (Table 1).

The principal problem at present is how best to utilize radiation treatment to give each patient the maximum opportunity for benefit. Not yet fully established is the optimal tumor dose or the timing and sequence in relation to surgery. To deal with these alternatives is the difficult task in this chapter. It is our objective to develop, at this point in time, clear-cut logistics for the involvement of the radiation oncologist at every stage of this formidable disease.

PREOPERATIVE RADIOTHERAPY

Rationale

All retrospective and controlled studies to date, with one exception, point to significant gains from preoperative irradiation at all dose levels - low, moderate, and high. The rationale is to alter the viability of cancer cells so that they will no longer be capable of local implantation and growth. Treatment failure following surgery for colorectal cancer is most frequently the outcome of recurrence in the perineum or pelvic region, due to local seeding of tumor cells or failure to excise all locally invasive disease. Tumor cells already present in adjacent lymph nodes may be destroyed, thus changing the staging category to a more favorable therapeutic level. Indeed, every study here and abroad has found this to be one of the most consistent rewards of preoperative treatment. The radiosensitivity of adenocarcinoma of the large bowel is a reality.

Table 1. Staging Systems for Colorectal Carcinoma

Dukes	Modified Astler-Coller	TNM+	
A	A	T_1N_0	Nodes negative; lesion limited to mucosa
B	B_1	T_2N_0	Nodes negative; extension of lesion through mucosa but still within bowel wall
	$^*B_2$	T_3N_0	Nodes negative; extension through entire bowel wall (including serosa if present)
C	C_1	T_2N_1	Nodes positive; lesion limited to bowel wall
	$^*C_2$	T_3N_1	Nodes positive; extension of lesion through entire bowel wall (including serosa)

* Modification by Gunderson and Sosin: Separate notation regarding degree of extension through bowel wall: microscopic only (m); gross extension confirmed by microscopy (m&g); adherence to or invasion of surrounding organs or structures (B_3 + C_3).

\+ By definition M_0 or no evidence of metastases.

In the light of the evidence, the reluctance of many members of the surgical community to give serious consideration to preoperative treatment is disheartening. Their anxiety over possible increase in surgical complications has proven invalid. Concern over the perturbation (downgrading) of the surgical stage of disease is unacceptable, in the face of the record of improved survival.

Indications

The indications for preoperative irradiation are best for those adenocarcinomas with the highest risk for local and regional recurrence. These include low-lying lesions arising below the peritoneal reflexion, especially if they are bulky, circumferential, of high-grade histology, and of borderline operability. Patients who are least likely to benefit from preoperative therapy are those with small, freely movable tumors which appear to involve only the mucosa (Dukes A). However, for such patients too old, too feeble, or too ill for the surgery, or who refuse the operation, cure rates comparable to surgical resection are now available through intracavitary contact therapy alone (42,65).

Treatment Plans

There are wide differences in opinion concerning tumor dosage, treatment volume, and sequence with surgery. Preoperative treatment plans have ranged from 500 rads in one fraction to the whole pelvis, followed promptly by resection, to 5000 rads/25 fractions to the primary only, followed by surgery in 4-6 weeks. All have yielded patient benefits. Although there appears to be no clear-cut relationships as yet between dose level and response, it is generally agreed that the higher the dose the greater the cancer kill. The limitation of dose rests principally upon the tolerance limits of the small bowel and the risks of potentiating surgical complications.

With the intent to offer the patient an optimum preoperative treatment plan, one should give serious consideration to a tumor dose of 4000-4500 rads/4-5 weeks to the entire pelvis by means of paired, shaped, opposing anterior and posterior portals, both portals always treated daily (Fig. 3). The treatment field includes the primary tumor and adjacent lymph node drainage area in the pelvis (Fig. 4). Inferiorly the boundaries will be the bottom of the obturator foramen; laterally, 1 cm lateral to the bony margin (iliopectineal line) at its widest point, superiorly to the L5 level. With this regimen, diarrhea will be moderate and manageable, and one may expect impressive regression of tumor in at least one-third of the cases (71). For optimum dose distribution the highest energy available should be employed. In our opinion this plan will offer the highest yield in tumor control and yet will fall short of complications that may trouble the patient and the surgeon. The pelvic operation can then be accomplished with relative safety and greater ease.

One should reduce the preoperative dose to 3500-4000 rads if there is a risk that small bowel loops may be tethered in the beam by adhesions because of previous operation or episodes of pelvic infection. Caution is also advised in the very old, hypertensive, or diabetic, whose radiation bowel tolerance may be limited. Operation should be performed in not less than 3 weeks and not later than 6 weeks.

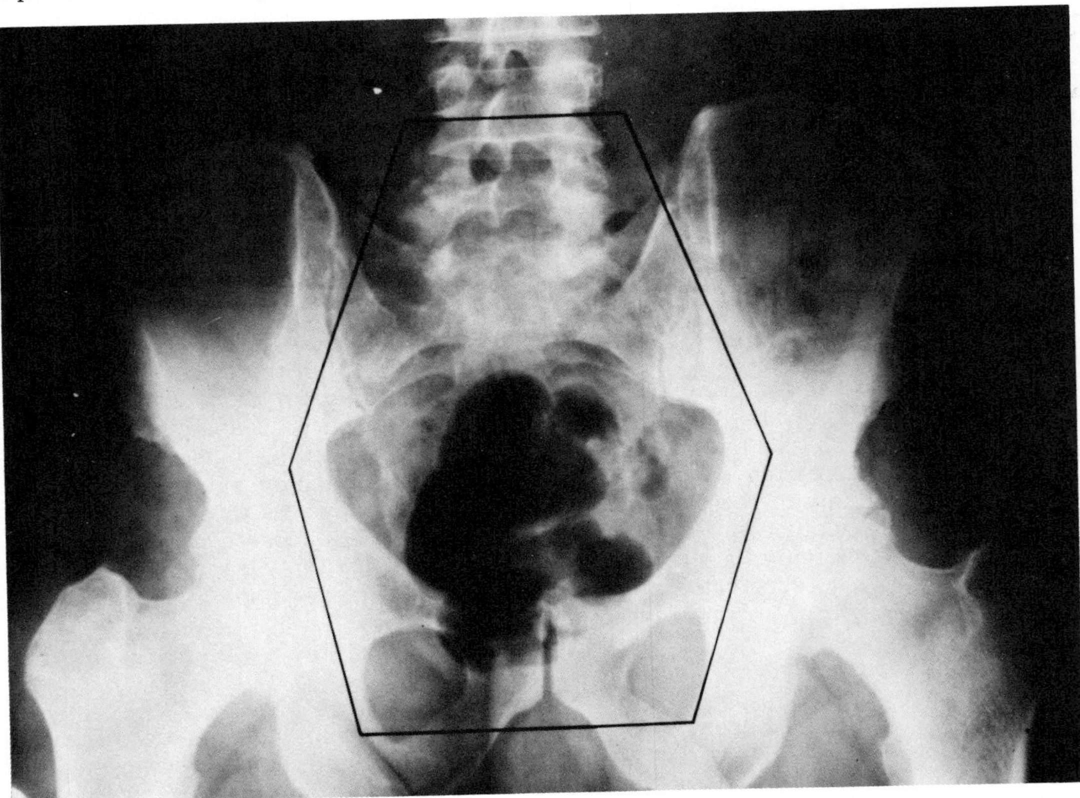

Figure 3. Typical pelvic portal pattern for preoperative or postoperative radiotherapy in patients with rectal or rectosigmoid carcinoma.

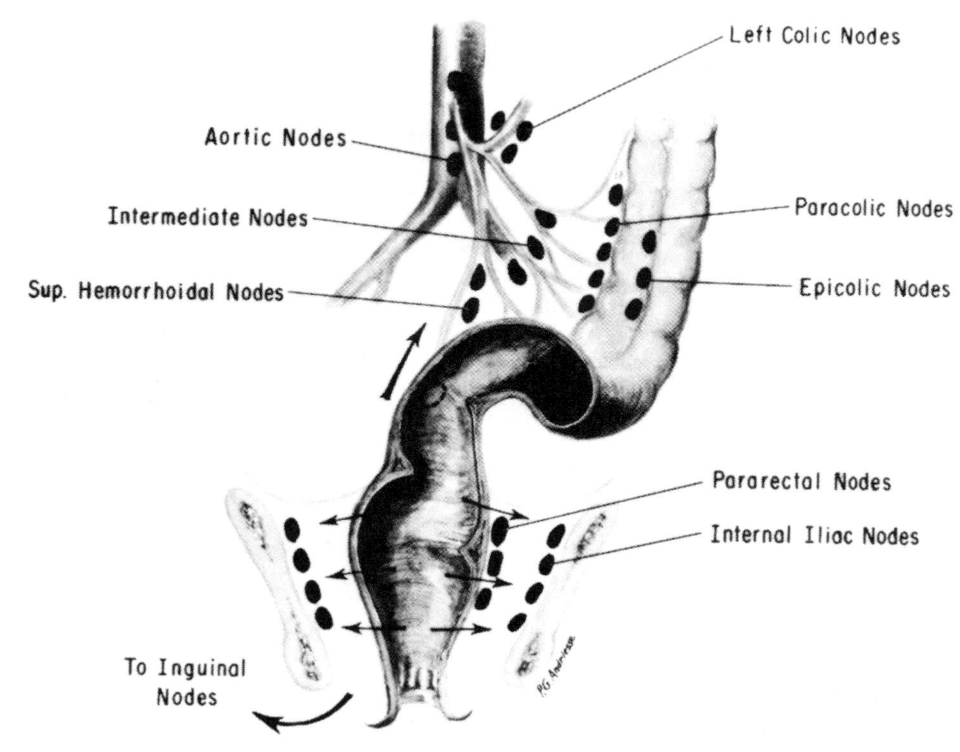

Figure 4. Lymphatic drainage of the anorectum and sigmoid region. (From Ref. 26.)

When surgeons are impatient to delay the surgery, they may be offered the alternative of the 200 rads x 10 program (plus 500 rads pelvic boost) (32, 55), proven by the VASAG in a well-controlled study to offer fruitful benefits, or even on occasion to propose a "rare" tumor dose of only 500 rads within 8 hr of surgery as reported by Rider (48). Other compromise regimens may be considered, such as 400 rads x 5, whose biological equivalent is estimated to be about 3000 rads. An advantage of low-dose regimens is the opportunity to add post-operative radiation for high risk patients, i.e., residual cancer, provided the small bowel has been raised out of the low pelvis during surgery.

As long ago as 1914, Symonds of London reported a favorable result of radium treatment before surgery in a large, apparently inoperable rectal tumor (69). Other favorable historical experiences were subsequently documented by many investigators (34, 57).

Binkley, at the Memorial Hospital in New York, in 1932, employed orthovoltage preoperative radiation in patients with tumors of borderline operability using several large portals and tumor dosage of 800-2000 rads/2 weeks followed in 2 weeks by surgery (7). In 1959, Stearns et al. published a retrospective review of 729 patients so treated vs. 549 comparable patients treated by surgery alone (66). The irradiated patients with lymphatic spread (Dukes C) had a 5-year survival of 37% compared with only 23% by surgery alone. In the 10-year assessment, the combined therapy revealed a 27% survival vs. a 10% figure for surgery alone.

However, in a subsequent prospective and randomized study comparing combined therapy at 2000 rads against surgery alone, these authors reported no difference in survival (67). This is the only negative report. It is appropriate to indicate here that there is considerable doubt about the comparability of the two groups because of serious questions regarding the schema of randomization. Their report covers a mixture of randomized and nonrandomized patients and selection was at the discretion of the surgeons in more than one-half of the patients.

The Binkley experience was a stimulus for a national, large scale, randomized, and controlled preoperative radiation protocol by the Veterans Administration Surgical Adjuvant Group (VASAG) in 1964. This was the first controlled test of adjuvant radiotherapy in colorectal cancer (32,55).

A total of 700 patients in 25 hospitals were included, equally divided between combined therapy and surgery alone. All were males with histologically proven operable adenocarcinoma of the rectum and the rectosigmoid colon. The treatment plan was modeled after the original Memorial regimen except for the fact that supervoltage was then available to only 40% of the VA patients. A tumor dose of 2000 rads/2 weeks, 200 rads daily, was delivered to the entire pelvis through paired opposing AP/PA portals, 20 x 20 cm each, from the anus to the pelvic brim. When the tumor was within 8 cm of the anal verge, a booster dose of 50 rads/day for 10 days was given through a 10 x 10 cm perineal portal.

The operation was nearly always an abdominoperineal resection, carried out within less than a week. However, anterior resections and other procedures were also done without difficulty. The patients were divided into curative and palliative groups and several other groupings, but in all instances pretreatment with radiation showed improved 5-year survival (32,55). Resectability rates were essentially the same in the treated and controlled groups. Preoperative irradiation did not hamper the surgery or induce complications. Patients with abdominoperineal resections (414) who received radiation treatment had a better outcome than the controls when one compares 5-year survival (40.8 vs. 28.4%) and a lowered incidence of positive lymph nodes (24 vs. 38%). Local and regional recurrence were reduced (29 vs. 40%); distant metastases were found at postmortem (180 cases) in only 47% of the treated cases vs. 60% treated by surgery alone. No benefit in survival was recorded in patients with higher lesions who had anterior resections and other procedures.

The VASAG, encouraged by the outcome of this protocol, embarked on a second controlled study in 1976 in male patients planned for AP resections with resectable, potentially curable adenocarcinomas of the rectum. The study employed a higher dose (3150 rads/8 fractions/24 days) using supervoltage only to the entire pelvis plus a narrow extension to the level of L2 to include paraaortic nodes (34). The portals were anterior-posterior opposed. There has been noted a decrease in the percentage of patients with positive lymph nodes in the radiation-treated group. There are not enough cases in the study to assess comparative survival past the third year. In the 3-5 year postoperative interval, there is improved survival in irradiated patients when compared with the controls. There is no impairment of healing or increase in postoperative complications.

Rodriquez-Antunez et al. at the Cleveland Clinic gave 800 rads on each of 3 successive days with surgery 10-15 days later. Of 42 operated patients 58% were alive at 5 years. We would not support these hyperintensive fractions for fear of late small bowel complications (50).

Under the aegis of the European Organization for Research and Treatment of Cancer (EORTC) many institutions in Europe are engaged in a two-arm trial giving 3450 rads/19 days before surgery vs. intravenous 5-FU in a second arm in the first week of radiotherapy (20). Of 232 patients thus far evaluated there is a substantially lower percentage of involved lymph nodes than would be anticipated (23% in one group and 31% in the other). No visible tumor was found in eight patients. However, survival data is not available and a surgery-only arm has not been added.

The Southwest Oncology Group (SWOG) has undertaken a pilot study combining 3000 rads/3 weeks before surgery with 5-FU plus mitomycin C. There were no unusual problems during surgery or in the postoperative period. These workers reported an obvious decrease in the size of most of the lesions, and in 4 of the 28 resected specimens no tumor could be found (34).

Cass et al., at the University of Southern Florida and the Tampa Veterans Medical Center, found 37% of 280 patients developed recurrent disease; of these, 60% were local only (10). They recently initiated a preoperative study using 3500 rads/4 weeks, anticipating a 50-60% decrease in local recurrence and improved survival.

In Leningrad, Simbertsiva et al. at the Petrov Research Institute of Oncology (1975), report on a controlled protocol involving 242 patients receiving surgery only vs. a group getting 3000 rads before surgery, the operation being done only 5-10 days later (64). At 6 years they reported comparative survival rate as 52.5% for the combined treatment and 40% for the controls, ascribing this radiation benefit to significant reduction in local recurrence and remote metastasis. Of particular interest is their observation that the improved survival occurred principally in those patients with unfavorable prognosis. Many of the irradiated tumors showed striking dystrophic cell changes making them less viable.

At the Kiev Diagnostic and Oncologic Institute, Zybina and Nabatich (84) reported on a series of 236 patients receiving 500 rads/day to 3000 rads followed by surgery in 24-48 hr, with no increase in surgical complications. This group, when compared with 246 patients treated by surgery alone revealed a 3-year survival rate in endophytic lesions of 76.1% in the combination treatment group compared with 45% in the surgery-alone group (73).

In 1975, Zybina et al. selected 25 patients with large, far advanced, immobile rectal cancers for intensive preoperative irradiation (3000 rads in six fractions of 500 rads each) plus an additional 1000 rads (500 x 2) just before surgery 6 weeks later. Of these 25 patients, 14 proved operable and 7 are reported to be alive and well in follow-up of more than 3 years (83).

Rider, at the Princess Margaret Hospital in Toronto (1977), acted upon the animal studies of Powers and Tolmach (44), Powers and Palmer (45), and Hoye and Smith (35) who reported that a single preoperative dose of 500 rads enhanced survival, provided that surgery was carried out in less than 8 hr after the irradiation. ^{60}Co irradiation of 500 rads delivered to the whole pelvis (AP/PA portals) a few hours before surgical excision approximately doubled the survival at 5 years (37 vs. 19%) in stage C rectal cancer (48). This was a controlled study in 125 patients. Rider is uncertain whether the mechanism of action is due to direct radiation cell death or to the initiation of some yet occult immunological process.

The British Medical Research Council (1976) has engaged several hospitals in a three-arm trial comparing surgery alone with a single fraction of 500 rads just before surgery and a third arm giving 10 daily fractions for a total of 2000 rads. Treatment was well tolerated but survival data are not available. Those who received 2000 rads had far fewer positive nodes than those in the other two arms (34).

High-Dosage Studies

At the University of Oregon and the VA Medical Center in Portland (1965) Fletcher and colleagues gave 5000-6000 rads/5-8 weeks before surgery to 97 patients with extensive rectal tumors, of whom only 57 were clinically operable (2, 17,19,68). Only the primary tumor itself was treated through AP/PA portals measuring no larger than 10 x 10 cm. For low-lying lesions, wedged posterior and perineal fields were used. Operation was performed 4-7 weeks after treatment. The 5-year survival of those who had curative resections was 53% compared with 38% for comparable historical controls with surgery only. Only four of their treated cases have thus far died of tumor. Twenty-one percent of the resected patients had positive lymph nodes. No viable tumor was found in 19% of the specimens and only in situ carcinoma remained in an additional 10%. It is notable that none have developed pelvic recurrence.

Kligerman and his surgical colleagues in the Yale-New Haven Medical Center in 1977 carried out a well-planned but limited randomized preoperative trial using 4500 rads/4.5-5 weeks to the entire true pelvis and the paraaortic nodes to the level of the second lumbar vertebra (37,38,71). There was no increase in the difficulty of the abdominoperineal resections. Anterior resections were carried out in two cases. No increase in postoperative complications or mortality was encountered. This report was outstanding in the exhaustive and meticulous examination of the surgical specimens. All specimens showed extensive tumor damage and no tumor was found in 4 of the 15 cases irradiated. The only shortcoming was the paucity of cases entered into this trial (15 combined, 16 controls). Nevertheless, the record for survival was 41% in the combined group compared with 25% in those treated by surgery alone.

The Borderline Operable Patient

The patient harboring a borderline, operable colorectal cancer has a chance, through moderate-dose preoperative radiotherapy, of conversion to an operable and resectable setting, with a reasonable hope for cure. Radium was first used for this function more than 50 years ago by Symonds (69). Ruff et al. at the Mayo Clinic described a series of 96 patients (of whom 10 were definitely inoperable) in which radium was used before surgery (63). No residual tumor could be found in the operative specimens in 10 of the 96 patients and 8 of these lived without disease from 4-19 years; fully 43.7% of the total survived 5 years. The 5-year cure rate for those with abdominoperineal resection was 66.7%. Of the 10 inoperable patients, 4 were among the cured.

Urdaneta-Lafee at the Yale-New Haven Medical Center in 1972 converted 13 inoperable rectal cancer patients to operability and 9 to resectability. Of these nine patients, three are alive and well more than 5 years (74).

Fletcher et al., at the University of Oregon and the Portland Veterans Hospital, converted to operability and resectability 10 of 22 patients with inoperable, extensive, and fixed lesions. Three of the resected patients are alive and well at 5 years after preoperative therapy to 4500-5000 rads/5-6 weeks and a 4-6 week delay to surgery (17,68).

More recently (1980) Emani and his associates, at the Tufts-New England Medical Center, treated 44 patients with unresectable colorectal carcinoma with the hope of conversion to operability, resectability, and possible cure (16). Unresectability was determined clinically in 26 cases and with pretreatment laparotomy in 18. The preoperative dose was 4500-5000 rads. Of the 44 cases, 26 were resected (70%) and 18 of the 26 (70%) are alive and well (NED) with a minimal follow-up of 36 months.

POSTOPERATIVE RADIOTHERAPY

Rationale

There is a rapidly growing interest in postoperative irradiation after abdominoperineal resection for patients at highest risk from local and regional recurrence, the principal cause of early death. They include those whose tumor was found penetrating through the entire gut wall, invading adjacent organs or lymph nodes spilled into the operative field, of anaplastic histology or clear indications of gross or microscopic residual tumor. The proponents of the postoperative regimen argue that surgeons are more prone to participate because surgical staging is not perturbed; there is no delay to surgery; early lesions are well cured surgically and need no radiation; and, above all, they need have no anxiety regarding potentiation of surgical morbidity and mortality.

On the other hand, there is a calculated risk of injury to the small bowel, sometimes lethal, with tumorocidal dosage in a postoperative setting, unless there is meticulous treatment planning and delivery to exclude the small bowel. Further, radiotherapy may be unduly delayed because of slow healing of the perineal wound. Nevertheless, there are a number of interesting nonrandomized pilot studies already in progress in major radiation centers. Careful selection of patients (Dukes B2 and C) after curative resections, as well as those with residual disease, is yielding gains in local control and even survival, albeit still with only short-term follow-up (21,29,30,51,73,80,81).

Treatment Plan

For patients with appropriate indications (stage B2 B1,2) therapy should begin 3-6 weeks after abdominoperineal resection, anterior resection, or other surgical procedures. Initial dose levels should be in the range of 4000-4500 rads with daily fractions of 180 rads/5 days per week. This is followed by booster therapy to 6000 rads through carefully shaped and reduced portals excluding the small bowel.

A four-field technique is best employed at the outset to the 4500 rads level using AP/PA and two laterals, with all four fields being treated daily in a 2:1/1:1 ratio. The perineal scar must be included after designation by lead wire or B-B shot. A "chimney" extension to L2 should be avoided because it may substantially increase the rate of intestinal complications. The patient should be treated in the prone position and the bladder distended with fluid. He should void 2 hr prior to treatment and drink a quart of fluid in the next hour. It is important to mention that the "brick" in this portal regimen, unlike that used in cervical and prostate cancer, is well posterior. Recurrent disease is primarily a posterior pelvic problem and the bony presacrum must be included. Perineal failures must be anticipated and cared for in portal planning because they are often the tip of the iceberg, overlying very large pelvic disease revealed only on the CAT scan (Fig. 5). The actual technique in a particular patient must vary with the anatomy of the patient, type of surgery, and the location of the tumor (30). Posterior wedged portals are valuable for posterior cul-de-sac disease or sacral involvement.

For local control of gross residual inoperable tumor, dosage of 6000-7000 rads is needed, but good control of microresidual tumor can be achieved with no more than 6000 rads. After 4500 rads and four portal techniques, the boost can be delivered with reduced posterior and lateral portals (7 x 7 = 10 x 10).

Both Gunderson (30) and Green et al. (27) have described special procedures to spare the small bowel (18). A small bowel film study is imperative before undertaking high-dose postoperative therapy (Fig. 6). The small bowel is often seen fixed in the posterior cul-de-sac, especially in the female patient, and must be excluded from the beam after 4500 rads. If the small bowel cannot be displaced by patient positioning, inflated bladder, etc., then the surgeon may be asked to reoperate to displace it from the treatment volume.

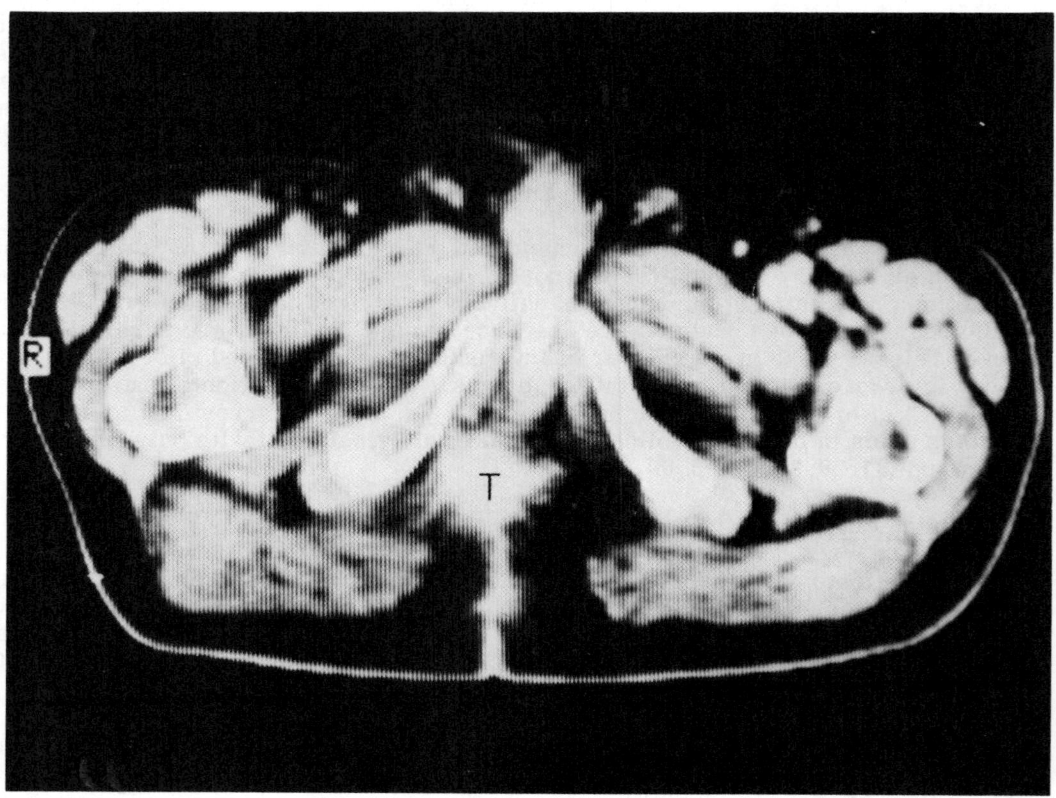

Figure 5. CAT scan of pelvis of a 76-year-old male veteran with obstructed urinary stream and severe perineal pain 9 months after AP resection of stage Dukes C adenocarcinoma of the rectum. Note recurrent tumor (T) at base of penis. Megavoltage therapy completely relieved pain at 2000 rads and effort will be made to control the recurrence.

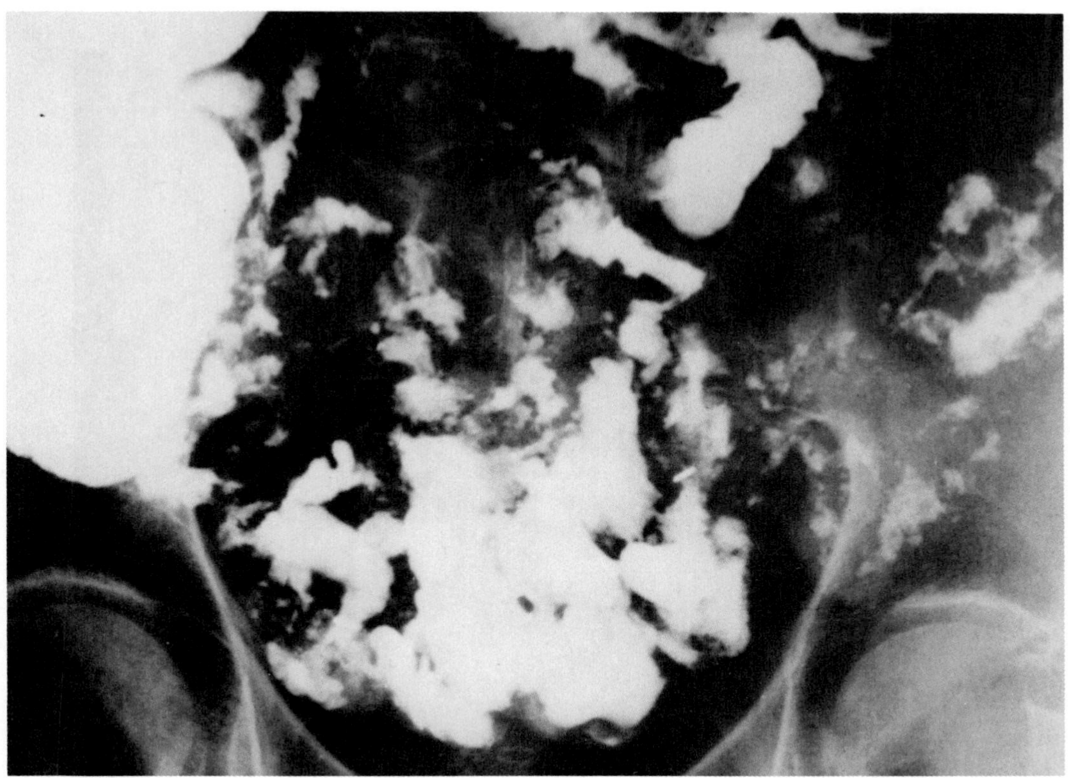

Figure 6. Small bowel study prior to development of high-dose radiotherapy treatment plan in patient with nonresectable rectal carcinoma. The high risk of bowel injury is clearly apparent unless every effort is made to diminish the danger through patient positioning, distended bladder, modified portals, and other protective and preventive measures.

Surgical colleagues must provide a precise description of the involved site and clip it well at surgery (Fig. 7). They should be urged to reperitonealize traumatized tissue surfaces to reduce adhesions and to close the posterior cul-de-sac by any means, such as peritoneal or omental pedicle flaps, or by interposing other pelvic organs such as the uterus or the bladder, or by employing tissue-tolerant obstructive devices such as polyurethane mesh (Fig. 8). Finally, we regard the CAT scan as essential for displaying gross residual or recurrent pelvic tumor (Fig. 5).

Postoperative Studies

At the Albert Einstein Medical Center in New York, Ghossein and his colleagues have treated 57 patients at high risk (B2 and C) and those with residual disease of the rectum and rectosigmoid colon with high-dose postoperative therapy (21). The whole pelvis was treated with up to 4600 rads with a booster of 1000-1500 rads to reduced portals. At 26 months, local recurrence was encountered in only 9% of cases and 74% were still living without disease. In the same period 38 colonic cancer cases at high risk were treated with a moving strip plus a fixed booster portal. At 26 months 70% were alive and well and 16% had a local recurrence.

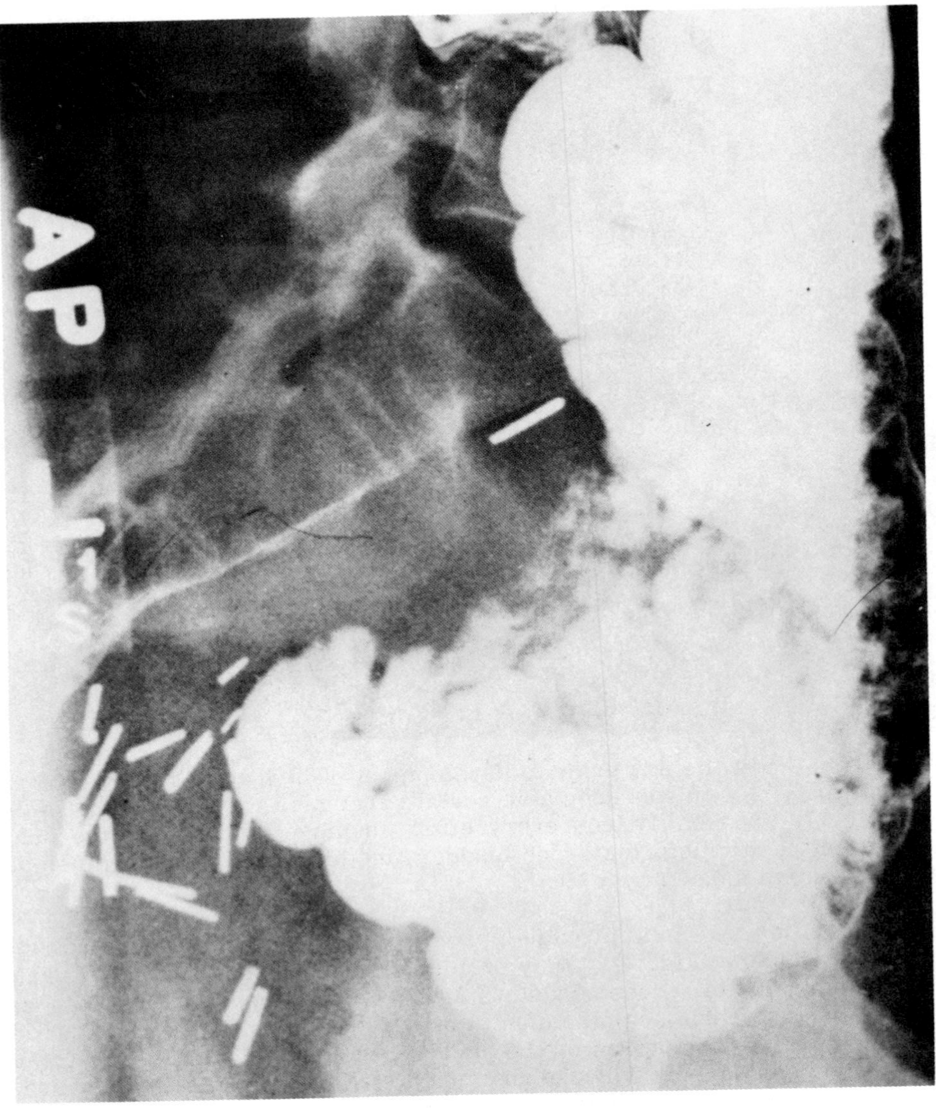

Figure 7. Lateral view of lower abdomen and pelvis with contrast barium in small bowel which occupies the space anterior to sacrum in the pelvis - in the treatment portal. Surgical clips indicate lateral and distal sacral extent of surgical resection. Extreme care is advised to exclude the small bowel from the portal when planning treatment in excess of 4500 rads. (From Ref. 51.)

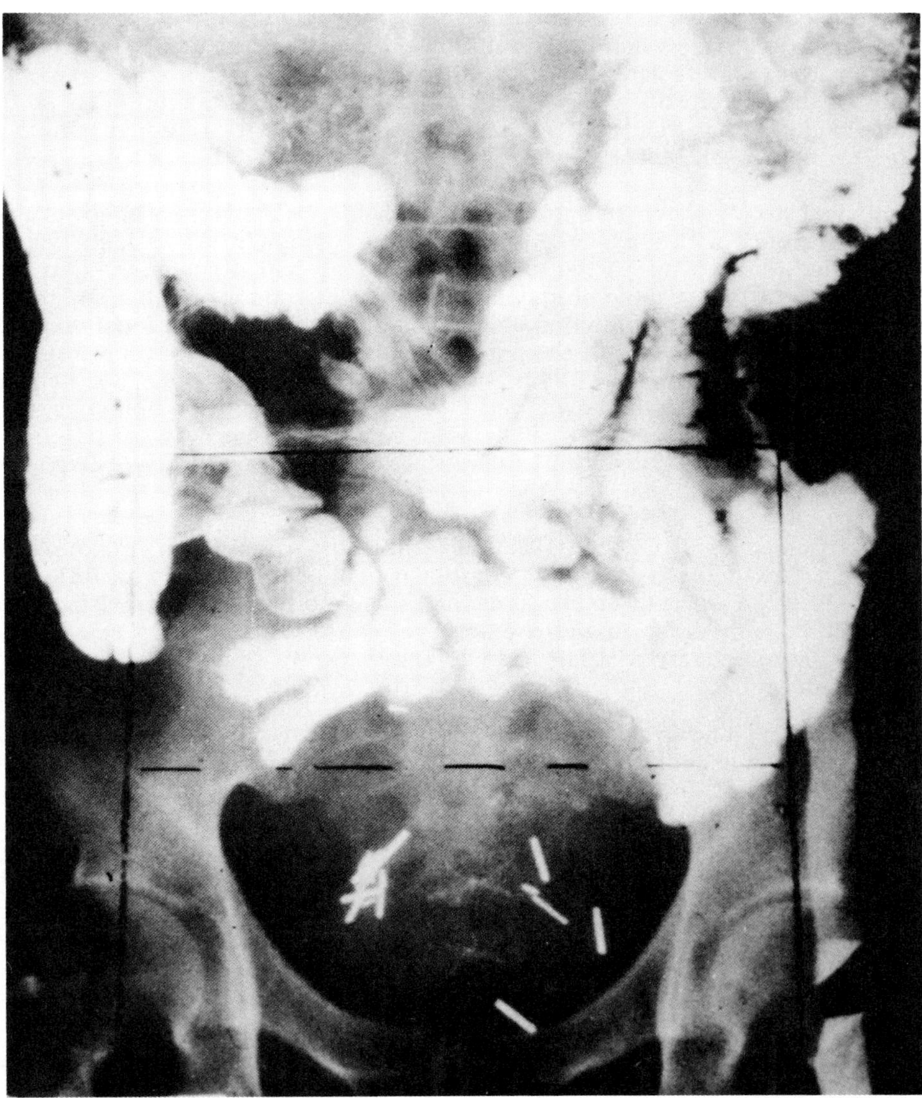

Figure 8. Small bowel barium study after abdominoperineal resection for rectal carcinoma, illustrating how the procedure may obliterate the inferior peritoneum excavation and raise of the pelvic floor. The upper line delineates the superior border of the whole pelvis treatment field. The lower line delineates the superior border of the reduced treatment field used to deliver booster doses to the volume of resection with relative immunity of the small bowel from serious radiation injury. (From Ref. 27.)

Gunderson et al. reported a pilot series of patients after curative resections treated with 4500-5100 rads to the L4 level in 5-6 weeks (29). A pelvic boost was added to high-risk sites when the small bowel proved to be mobile and could be excluded from the treatment portal. A total of 31 of these patients had gross extension outside the bowel wall and/or involved nodes. There was no increase in complications and only one recurrence. Of 29 other cases with residual tumor, only 2 of 29 (6.9%) have been local failures.

Romsdahl and Withers and colleagues at the M.D. Anderson Hospital reported on their experience with high-dose postoperative therapy in 62 patients whose tumors extended through the entire bowel wall and/or had disease in their lymph nodes (80,81). A tumor dose of approximately 5000 rads was delivered to the pelvis over a 6-week period beginning 3-6 weeks after surgery. A local control rate of 92% was achieved and 79% of the patients were free of disease in a follow-up period up to 48 months (median of 34 months). These benefits were not achieved without complications, since seven patients developed radiation enteritis which required eight surgical procedures. These authors warn that only the pelvis should be treated and extreme precautions taken to exclude the small bowel from the maximum dose.

The GI Tumor Study Group (GITSG) has initiated a four-arm randomized trial of treatment after curative surgery combined with chemotherapy as follows: (1) surgery only; (2) 4600 rads in 30-40 days; (3) chemotherapy with 5-FU and methyl CCNU; and (4) both radiation and chemotherapy (34). Preliminary results indicate that survival and reduction of recurrence are better in arms 2 and 4. Recently arm 1 was abandoned.

The RTOG has undertaken a four-arm postoperative protocol to include patients at high risk for recurrence, as follows: (1) no further treatment; (2) 4500-5100 rads in 5-6 weeks; (3) 5-FU plus methyl CCNU; and (4) radiotherapy and chemotherapy, the latter started 4-8 weeks after irradiation (34).

The ECOG has adopted a three-arm protocol for patients after curative resections as follows: (1) chemotherapy; (2) postoperative radiotherapy using 4500-5100 rads; and (3) radiotherapy plus chemotherapy. At this point in time the codes remain unbroken in these on-going protocols (34).

"SANDWICH" RADIOTHERAPY

Rationale

In the light of the benefits of both preoperative and postoperative therapy, why not combine them to best advantage? Preoperative radiotherapy is damaging to cells that may be spread locally or distantly at the time of surgery. For postoperative treatment we can select high-risk patients, based upon operative, pathologic, and microscopic findings. Patients found with metastatic disease or those with surgically curable early lesions can be deleted.

It is our experience that many surgeons balk at high-dose preoperative regimens (4000-4500 rads), and even moderate treatment schedules (3000-3500 rads), because of impatience with the delay as well as concern over the viability of the anastomosis should an anterior resection become feasible during the operation instead of a planned abdominoperineal resection with colostomy. Further, some are disturbed about the perturbation of the surgical staging.

Treatment Plan

Why not, then, employ the single preoperative dose of 500 rads proposed by Rider (47,48,49) or the low dose of 2000-2500 rads tested with success in the VASAG protocol, and follow with more radical postoperative irradiation for carefully selected high-risk patients? The treatment can thus be tailored to the disease, with little delay to surgery, and no compromise of surgical technique.

Sandwich Studies

At the Thomas Jefferson University Hospital in Philadelphia, Mohiuddin et al. have recently presented a report on their initial experience with this alternative (39). A group of 62 patients with rectal carcinoma were given 500 rads on the day of or the day before surgery. In the majority of the cases, an abdominoperineal resection was performed. There were 42 patients with poor prognostic characteristics (stages B2, C1, C2). Twenty-one were given 4500 rads (in 5 weeks) of postoperative pelvic. No further therapy was given to 18 patients with early disease (stages A or B).

In a follow-up of 6-36 months (median, 20 months) none of the 21 patients receiving postoperative treatment have failed in the pelvis, but 2 have developed metastatic disease. Of the 21 who received no postoperative treatment, 2 have recurred in the pelvis, and 2 others have developed metastatic disease. Of patients with stage A or B tumors, one has died with metastasis. It is important to indicate that the majority of failures after radical surgery alone in rectal cancer are encountered within the first year after surgery. We agree with these authors that adjuvant sandwich radiotherapy in the surgical treatment of this disease has considerable potential for improving survival. In the VASAG, we are giving serious consideration to testing this premise in a national, large scale, randomized, and controlled Rectal Protocol-III.

Gunderson and his associates at the Massachusetts General Hospital initiated a similar sandwich project in March 1976 and have reported on 31 patients of whom 15 fulfilled the criteria for the postoperative therapy arm (31). Only two of these failed and neither had a pelvic component of failure. Of the 16 patients with early lesions who received low-dose treatment, only 1 developed later evidence of cancer (an anastomotic recurrence salvaged by further irradiation and surgery).

PRIMARY RADIATION THERAPY

Medically Inoperable Patients

Radiation therapy now offers a chance for cure to rectal cancer patients whose lesions are mobile and clearly operable but for whom surgery is out of the question because of serious medical contraindications or for those who refuse operation. Untreated, these patients will suffer progressive distress and disability and nearly all will die of their disease by the third year.

Rider, at the Princess Margaret Hospital, was among the first to report his experience (1975) with 35 such patients with mobile rectal cancers who would certainly have had an abdominopelvic resection had they been clinically acceptable for the operation. None had a colostomy before or within 3 months of irradiation. The crude 5-year survival was 73% in this group of selected cases (47,49).

Intracavitary Radiotherapy

For patients medically ineligible for surgery, with very small lesions near the anal margin, still another treatment option is available through intracavitary contact radiation. One of the most important and dramatic new approaches to the nonsurgical curative treatment of early rectal cancer has been introduced by Papillon in Lyon, France, employing direct-contact radiation (50 kV) through a long conical rectal applicator (Fig. 9) (42). His results show a 75% 5-year crude survival rate in nearly 200 patients and his 10-year figures are almost as favorable. The death rate from cancer was only 10%. Sischy and his colleagues at the Highland Hospital in Rochester, New York, have adopted and improved this technique, designing special proctoscopes which incorporate a fiberoptic system assuring accurate evaluation and treatment and allowing the taking of color photographs (65).

Candidates for this treatment are carefully selected, with movable lesions no more than 10 cm from the anal verge, up to 5 cm in diameter, well or moderately well-differentiated adenocarcinomas, with a low probability for lymphatic spread. Treatment is delivered on an outpatient basis without anesthesia in 3 min (3000 rads) and repeated every 2 weeks for a total of 9000-12,000 rads. There appears to be little risk of morbidity and the rectum is preserved. This ambulatory treatment is applicable even to the oldest and most fragile patients, as well as to those who refuse surgical treatment with or without colostomy. The infrequent local failure can

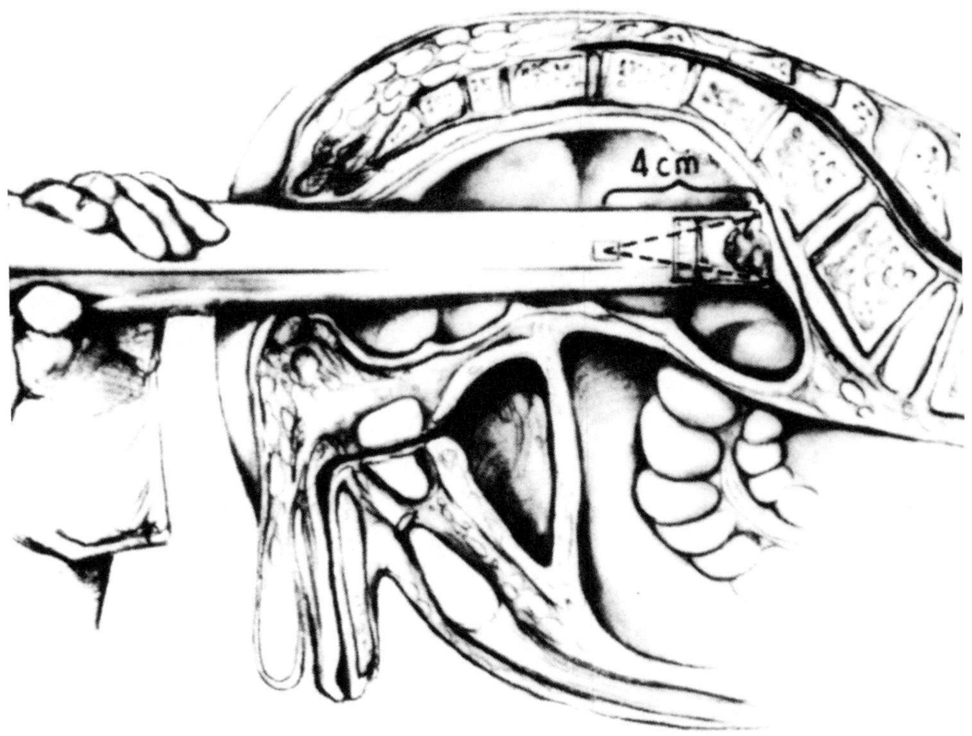

Figure 9. Illustration to show positioning of x-ray tube and special proctoscope over the lesion. (From Ref. 65.)

be salvaged by later surgery. There is prompt and striking shrinkage of the tumor after the first and second applications as well as maintained well-being of all of the patients during and after the treatment course (Fig. 10). Those few lesions which show a grudging response receive booster therapy with iridium implants.

Sischy has now treated 39 patients for cure and 31 for palliation, providing relief from tenesmus, distressful bleeding, and other local symptoms. Some of these palliative cases appear to be cured. Of the 39 patients treated for cure at the Highland Hospital only 2 patients have failed locally. One of these had an anaplastic lesion and underwent an abdominoperineal resection 10 months after treatment and is now alive and well. The other, an obese diabetic, recurred in the pelvis and died from liver metastasis. At autopsy, the rectum proved to be free of disease. There is now an endocavitary therapy program for rectal cancer in our Regional VA Radiotherapy Center to serve veterans in the Northeastern states.

Surgically Incurable Patients

The natural history of untreated colon carcinoma (either unresected or postoperative recurrence) is one of rapid advancement and short survival. The median survival from time of proven incurability is 7 months, with only 10% surviving 18 months. In a group of 95 patients with fixed, technically inoperable rectal carcinoma reported by Rider, 13 had a relative actuarial 5-year survival after radical radiation therapy. Standing virtually alone, Rider asks a provocative question in one of his reports: "Is the Miles operation really necessary for the cure of rectal cancer?" (47). Amalric and his associates in France accepted a mandate to attempt curative radiotherapy in a group of 73 patients with locally advanced disease (3). We are advised that he achieved a 3-year survival of 43%.

PALLIATIVE RADIOTHERAPY

Patients with distressing and disabling symptomology from advanced disease, local, regional, or metastatic, can be relieved in the majority of cases for weeks and months with supervoltage treatment and minimal morbidity. This has been our own experience in nearly 500 such patients since 1952, an experience shared by many others (78). For example, Wang and Schultz treated 111 patients at the Massachusetts General Hospital and reported palliative benefit in 84% of cases, with cessation of intractable bleeding, pain, tenesmus, and perineal discharge. Dosage of the order of 4000-4500 rads is needed for maximum benefit and minimal morbidity (77). Patients with the phantom rectum syndrome should be treated on the basis of symptoms, without waiting for proof of recurrent cancer. The CAT scan can be helpful in the discovery of the extent of involvement as a prelude to therapy (5).

Patients are often in pain when the liver capsule is stretched by bulky metastases. Relief can be promptly provided using dose levels up to 3000 rads in 3-4 weeks (72). Larger dosage to the entire liver invites the risk of radiation hepatopathy with further enlargement of the organ, ascites, jaundice, and even death from liver failure (36). Ramming et al. have recently made a systematic painstaking review of regimens for managing metastatic liver disease (46). Metastatic bone lesions which give much pain and disability or threaten pathologic fractures are effectively treated with daily fractions of 300-3000 rads total. Troublesome lung metastases are treated with daily fractions of 200-2000 rads for the whole lung, but no more, for fear of radiation pneumopathy (62).

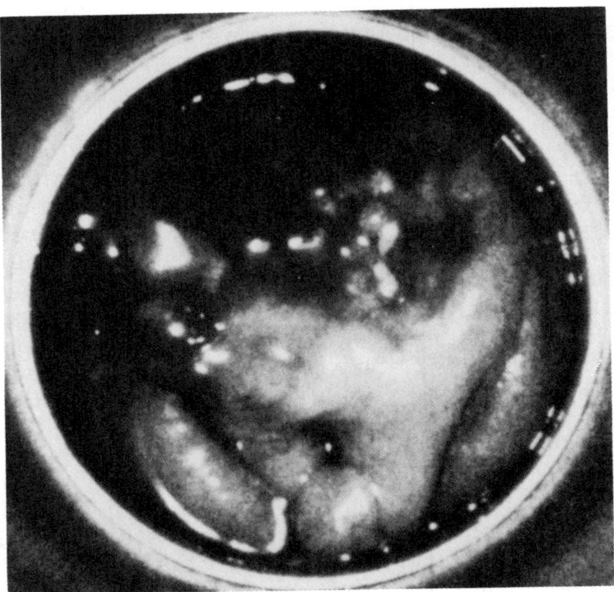

Figure 10. A: Photograph through special proctoscope illustrating a 4 cm polypoid adenocarcinoma on right rectal wall 5 cm from the anal verge in an 80-year-old man too frail for surgery.

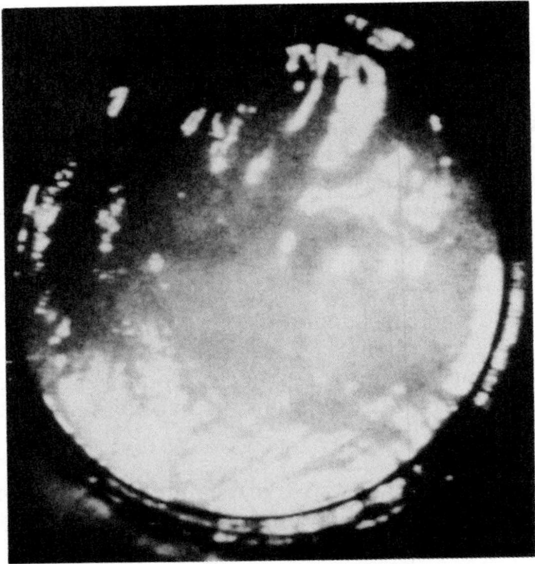

Fig. 10. B: Photograph through special proctoscope illustrating complete disappearance of tumor after 8650 rads in three fractions at 2-week intervals. (From Ref. 65.)

COMBINED THERAPY

Current strategy in cancer management involves integration of all therapeutic modalities in concomitant or sequential regimens. However, radiation oncologists are becoming increasingly apprehensive over the risk of heightened radiation toxicity, particularly in the bowel, when chemical agents are allied with radiation. Danjoux and Catton have recently called attention to such an experience in the RTOG study affiliating high-dose radiotherapy and 5-FU (12). They reported that fully 29% of the patients had late reactions, often serious and sometimes fatal, suffering bowel necrosis, perforation, and fistula about 8 months after treatment. A reduction of radiation dosage, of at least 10% or more, is recommended when planning combined therapy.

COMPLICATIONS

In all of medical and surgical practice there are calculated risks of injury to normal structures, in an uncompromising attack upon a life-threatening disease. Radiation therapy for colorectal cancer is no exception.

In the abdominopelvic compartment our principal concern is for the small intestine, whose tolerance is sharply limited to a dose of no greater than 4500 rads. Indeed, the sensitivity of the small bowel remains the principal barrier to further improvement of cure by primary and/or adjunct radiotherapy for colorectal cancer. This barrier can only be overcome by excluding the small bowel from the high-dose radiation volume by surgical means (interposition of barriers to its cul-de-sac entry such as omentum, bladder, uterus, plastic mesh) (18); improved localization (through small bowel films, ultrasound, CAT scans) (30), optimal positioning (prone with inflated bladder) (30), precisional treatment planning (simulation, customized portals); optimized dose distribution (computerization, in vivo dosimetry) (54); extreme caution (with elderly, diabetic, hypertensive, and previously operated patients); and, above all, great respect for the integrity of the small intestine. Severe radiation enteropathy can give rise to more acute and long-term suffering, disability, and risk of death, than damage to any other abdominopelvic viscera. Surgical repair is hazardous after stricture, ulceration, or perforation. In several other communications we have described the pathogenesis of radiation enteropathy, the clinical presentation, radiographic profile, elements of high risks, surgical management, and guidelines for safer practice (58-62).

The principal factors of high risk include fixed loops after surgery, hyperintensive cumulative dose, high-dose fractions, overlapping portals, single portal daily treatment in a multiportal plan (79), poorly calibrated or uncalibrated dosimeters, and masking of acute distress signals with overmedication. These interlacing factors constitute, in our opinion, a formula fatale.

Treatment of the early acute syndrome (characterized by nausea, vomiting, cramps, and diarrhea) is symptomatic and supportive, including the use of antispasmodics and low-residue nutritional support. If treatment is briefly interrupted (split-course program), there is nearly always prompt recovery of the injured and reactive mucosa. Epithelial regeneration is rapid, and recovery may be complete in 1-2 weeks. Serious large bowel complications will be encountered after dosage in excess of 6000 rads, characterized by tenesmus, cramps, diarrhea, and bleeding, ending in chronic ulceration and stricture, nearly always demanding colostomy.

As a rule, bladder reactions are transient and manageable, rarely ending in ulceration after dosage not exceeding 7000 rads, an unlikely prospect in treating colorectal disease.

FUTURE PROSPECTS

Colorectal cancer has already reached all of the proportions of a major health disaster in this country for men and women in the prime of life. More than 50,000 deaths are predicted for this year (4). Prospects for turning the wheel back must clearly depend upon earlier recognition of the disease and, above all, on a major national preventive effort. Despite a sustained effort by the American Cancer Society, the proportion of patients who present with the earliest, curable lesions remains distressingly small and almost unchanged for many years. Nor can we expect an early and radical change in the American diet despite the fact that dietary factors such as fat, meat, and low fiber content appear to be the principal causative agents.

Nevertheless, we seem to be entering into new areas of investigation which will offer a greater understanding of the pathogenesis of this formidable disease, and improved methods for diagnosis, staging, and treatment (24). Computerized transverse tomography is becoming more available, and will be of enormous help in cancer staging and in better selection of patients for surgery and/or radiation therapy (5). Above all, we must define factors which will assist in selecting patients in whom the risks are greatest, so that therapy may be designed to optimize the benefit-risk ratio. The involved area, including pelvic lymph nodes and contiguous normal organs, can be delineated by CT scanning, far better than by any other method. It is especially helpful when other methods have failed. The transverse image is the only realistic basis for the development of an optimal treatment plan (5,52,53).

Since the liver is the major site for establishment of a beachhead by spreading colorectal cancer, serious consideration is being given to irradiating this sanctuary in a prophylactic effort. Occult hepatic micrometastases may yield to moderate and relatively safe dose levels such as 2000 rads. Clearly, far better multiagent chemotherapy treatment programs need to be developed to control the disseminated disease that kills nearly 30% of all patients despite effective local control. More than 5 dozen experimental trials of chemotherapeutic and immune agents are already in progress.

Is there a rationale for the use of adjuvant radiotherapy for selected extrapelvic colonic adenocarcinomas? Cass et al. at the University of Southern Florida found a significant proportion of local recurrence in 280 patients with tumors originating in the cecum (39%), transverse colon (26%), and descending colon (29%) (10). They urge that adjuvant radiotherapy should be undertaken by treating patients on their side for at least one-half of this treatment. Turner and her group in New York have reported a favorable experience with such patients employing the moving-strip technique (73).*

Intraoperative high-energy electron beam therapy has gained interest, principally in Japan (1). In this country, Gunderson has been effectively employing this system in treating 31 patients, giving 1000 rads in a single dose, the biological equivalent of 3000 rads of fractionated treatment (30).

What may be expected from advances in hyperthermia, chemical potentiators, and high-energy particle beams is still a matter for conjecture, but significant gains may be confidently predicted in this decade.

In the meantime there is a burgeoning effort as never before, in regional, national, and international experimental clinical trials to find newer and better radiation treatment regimens with and without adjuvant chemotherapy. Most believe that progress in this formidable disease will be made in a stepwise fashion and each forward move will be dependent upon the strength and accuracy of the preceding advance. We will be delighted if a revolutionary discovery is introduced which will bring the solution in a single giant step. We are unwilling to wait for that glorious day in idle hopefulness.

REFERENCES

1. Abe, M., Jakahoshi, M., Yahamato, E., Torizuke, K., Tobe, T., and Mori, K.: Techniques, indications and results of intraoperative therapy of advanced cancer. Radiology 116:693-702, 1975.

2. Allen, C.V. and Fletcher, W.A.: A pilot study on preoperative irradiation of rectosigmoid carcinoma. Am. J. Roentgenol. 114:504-508, 1972.

3. Amalric, R., Clement, R., Jin, P., Lipowsky, G., and Spitalier, J.M.: La radiotherapie des cancers in rectum. J. Radiol. Electrol. 54:613-616, 1973.

4. Cancer Facts and Figures, American Cancer Society, New York, 1980.

5. Asbell, S.O. and Schlager, B.A.: The usefulness of CT scanning in the evaluation of patients with primary and recurrent rectosigmoid carcinoma. Int. J. Radiat. Oncol. Biol. Phys. 6 (Suppl. 1):40, 1979.

6. Astler, V.G. and Coller, F.A.: The prognostic significance of direct extension of carcinoma of the colon and rectum. Ann. Surg. 139:846, 1954.

7. Binkley, G.E.: Radiation therapy of rectal cancer. Trans. Am. Proctol. Soc. 33:84, 1932.

8. Burdette, W.J.: Colorectal carcinogenesis. Cancer (Suppl.) 34:872-877, 1974.

9. Burkitt, D.P., Walker, A.R.P., and Painter, N.S.: Dietary fiber and disease. JAMA 229:1068, 1974.

10. Cass, A.W., Million, R.R., and Pfaff, W.W.: Patterns of recurrence following surgery alone for adenocarcinoma of the colon and rectum. Cancer 37: 2861, 1976.

11. Copeland, E.M., Miller, L.D., and Jones, R.S.: Prognostic factors in carcinoma of the colon and rectum. Am. J. Surg. 116:875-881, 1968.

12. Danjoux, C.E. and Catton, G.A.: Delayed complications in colorectal carcinoma treated by combination radiotherapy and 5-Fluorouricil-Eastern Cooperative Oncology Group Pilot Study. Int. J. Radiat. Oncol. Biol. Phys. 5: 441-443, 1979.

13. Dukes, C.E.: The classification of cancer of the rectum. J. Path. Bact. 35: 323-332, 1932.

14. Dukes, C.E., Bussey, H.J.R.: The spread of rectal cancer and its effect on prognosis. Br. J. Cancer 12:309-320, 1958.

15. Dukes, C.E.: Cancer of the rectum. In Monographs on Neoplastic Disease, Baltimore, Williams and Wilkins, 1970.

16. Emani, B., Willet, C., Pileprich, M., and Miller, H.: Preoperative radiotherapy of unresectable colorectal carcinoma. Int. J. Radiat. Oncol. Biol. Phys. 6 (Suppl. 1):39, 1979.

17. Fletcher, W.S., Allen, C.V., and Dunphy, J.E.: Preoperative irradiation for carcinoma of the colon and rectum: A preliminary report. Am. J. Surg. 109:76-83, 1965.

18. Freund, H., Gunderson, L.L., Krause, R., and Fisher, J.E.: Prevention of radiation enteritis after abdominoperineal resection and radiotherapy. Surg. Gynecol. Obstet. 149:206-208, 1979.

19. Galante, M., Dunphy, J.E., and Fletcher, W.S.: Cancer of the colon. Ann. Surg. 165:732-744, 1967.

20. Gerard, A.: Preoperative radiation protocol for cancer of the rectum: Cooperative group for cancer of the gastrointestinal tract (EORTC), Hospital Saint-Pierre, Bruxelles, Belgium, Personal Communication, 1979.

21. Ghossein, N.A., Ager, P.J., Ragins, H., Turner, S.S., DeLuca, F., Alpert, S., and Lowy, S.J.: The treatment of locally advanced carcinoma of the colon and rectum by a surgical procedure and radiotherapy postoperatively. Surg. Gynecol. Obstet. 148:916, 1979.

22. Gilbert, Stuart G.: Symptomatic local tumor failure following abdominoperineal resection. Int. J. Radiat. Oncol. Biol. Phys. 4:801-807, 1978.

23. Gilbertsen, V.A.: Adenocarcinoma of rectum: Incidence and location of recurrent tumor following operation for cure. Ann. Surg. 150:340-348, 1960.

24. Gilbertsen, V.A.: Improving the prognosis for patients with intestinal cancer. Surg. Gynecol. Obstet. 124:1253, 1967.

25. Gilchrist, R.F. and David, V.C.: A consideration of pathological factors influencing five-year survival in radical resection of the large bowel and rectum for carcinoma. Ann. Surg. 126:411-420, 1974.

26. Goligher, J.C.: The surgical anatomy of the colon, rectum and anal canal. In Diseases of the Colon and Anorectum, edited by R. Turell, New York, Saunders, 1959, pp. 21-60.

27. Green, N., Ira, G., and Smith, W.R.: Measures to minimize small intestine injury in the irradiate pelvis. Cancer 35:1633-1640, 1975.

28. Gunderson, L.L. and Sosin, H.: Areas of failure found at reoperation (second or symptomatic look), following "curative surgery" for adenocarcinoma of the rectum. Cancer 34:1278-1292, 1974.

29. Gunderson, L.L. Votava, C., Brown, R.C. and Plenk, H.P.: Colorectal carcinoma: Combined treatment with surgery and postoperative radiation - L.D.S. Hospital Experience (Abstr.). Int. J. Radiat. Oncol. Biol. Phys. (Suppl. 1):64, 1976.

30. Gunderson, L.L.: Combined irradiation and surgery for rectal and sigmoid carcinoma. New roles of radiotherapy in the management of cancer. In Current Problems in Cancer, edited by R. Hickey, 1979.

31. Gunderson, L., Dosoretz, D., Hedberg, S., Rodkey G., Rich, T., Blitzer, P., Shipley, W., and Cohen, A.: Low dose preoperative plus postoperative irradiation for resectable carcinoma of the rectum and rectosigmoid. Int. J. Radiat. Oncol. Biol. Phys. (Suppl. 6):38, 1979.

32. Higgins, G.A., Conn, J.A., Jordan, P.H., Humphrey, E.W., Roswit, B., and Keehn, R.J.: Preoperative radiotherapy for colorectal cancer. Ann. Surg. 181:624-631, 1975.

33. Higgins, G.A.: Surgical considerations in colorectal cancer. Cancer 39:891-895, 1977.

34. Higgins, G.A. and Roswit, B.: The role of radiotherapy in the surgical treatment of large bowel cancer. In Progress in Clinical Cancer, Vol. VII, edited by I.M. Ariel, New York, Grune and Stratton, 1978, pp. 71-81.

35. Hoye, C.H. and Smith, R.R.: The effectiveness of small amounts of pre-op irradiation in preventing the growth of tumor cell dissemination of surgery. Cancer 14:284, 1961.

36. Ingold, J.A., Reed, G.B., Kaplan, H.S., and Bagshaw, M.A.: Radiation hepatitis. Am. J. Roentgenol. 93:200-208, 1965.

37. Kligerman, M.M., Urdaneta, N., Knowlton, A., Vidone, R., Hartman, P.V. and Vera, R.: Preoperative irradiation of the rectosigmoid carcinoma including its regional lymph nodes. Am. J. Roentgenol. 114:498-503, 1972.

38. Kligerman, M.M.: Irradiation of the primary lesions of the rectum and rectosigmoid. JAMA 231:1381-1384, 1975.

39. Mohiuddin, M., Dobelbower, R.R., Kramer, S., and Marks, G.: Selective sandwich and adjuvant radiotherapy for rectal cancer. Int. J. Radiat. Oncol. Biol. Phys. (Suppl. 1):37, 1979.

40. Moosa, A.R., Ree, P.C., Marks, J.E., Lerien, B., Platz, C.E. and Skinner, D.B.: Factors influencing local recurrence for cancer of the rectum and rectosigmoid. Br. J. Surg. 62:727-730, 1975.

41. Morson, B.C. and Bussey, H.J.R.: Surgical pathology of rectal cancer in relation to adjuvant radiotherapy. Br. J. Radiol. 40:161-165, 1967.

42. Papillon, J.: Intracavitary irradiation of early rectal cancer for cure: A series of 186 cases. Cancer 36:696-701, 1975.

43. Polk, H.C. and Spratt, J.S.: Recurrent colorectal carcinoma: Detection, treatment and other consideration. Surgery 69:9-23, 1971.

44. Powers, W.E. and Tolmach, L.J.: Preoperative radiation therapy: Biological basis and experimental investigation. Nature 201:272-273, 1964.

45. Powers, W.E. and Palmer, I.A.: Biologic basis of preoperative radiation treatment. Am. J. Roentgenol. 102:176-192, 1968.

46. Ramming, K.P., et al.: Management of hepatic metastases. Semin. Oncol. 4:71, 1977.

47. Rider, W.D.: Is the Miles operation really necessary for the treatment of rectal cancer? J. Can. Assoc. Radiol. 26:167-175, 1975.

48. Rider, W.D., Palmer, J.A., Mahoney, L.H., and Robertson, C.T.: Preoperative irradiation in operable cancer of the rectum: Report of the Toronto Trial. Can. J. Surg. 20:335-338, 1977.

49. Rider, W.D., Hawkins, N.V., Cummings, B.J., Harwood, A.H., and Thomas, G.M.: Radiation therapy for cure of adenocarcinoma of the rectum. Int. J. Radiat. Oncol. Biol. Phys. 5(Suppl. 1):62-63, 1979.

50. Rodriguez-Antunez, A., Chernak, E.S., Jelden, G.L., and Hunter, T.W.: Preoperative irradiation of carcinoma of the rectum. Radiology 108:689-690, 1973.

51. Romsdahl, M.M. and Withers, R.: Radiotherapy combined with curative surgery: Its use as therapy for carcinoma of the sigmoid colon and rectum. Arch. Surg. 113:446-453, 1978.

52. Roswit, B., Unger, S.M., Stein, J., Malsky, S.J., and Reid, C.B.: Transverse laminography: Applications in radiation therapy. Am. J. Roentgenol. 81:130-139, 1959.

53. Roswit, B. and Unger, S.M.: Tumor localization with transverse tomography: Diagnostic and therapeutic applications. Radiology 74:705-720, 1960.

54. Roswit, B., Malsky, S.J., and Reid, C.B.: In vivo radiation dosimetry: Review of a 12-year experience. Radiology 97:413, 1970.

55. Roswit, B., Higgins, G.A., and Keehn, R.J.: Preoperative irradiation for carcinoma of the rectum and recto-sigmoid colon. Report of a national randomized study. Cancer 35:1597, 1975.

56. Roswit, B. and Higgins, G.: The present outlook for the patient with colorectal cancer - a new perspective. Int. J. Radiat. Oncol. Biol. Phys. 6 (Suppl. 1);40, 1979.

57. Roswit, B.: The role of radiation therapy in the surgical management of colorectal carcinoma. In Management of the Patient with Cancer, edited by T.F. Nealon, New York, Saunders, 1976, pp. 574-584.

58. Roswit, B., Malsky, S.J., and Reid, C.B.: Severe radiation injuries of the stomach, small intestine, colon and rectum. Am. J. Roentgenol. 114:460, 1972.

59. Roswit, B., Malsky, S.J., and Reid, C.B.: Radiation tolerance of the gastrointestinal tract. In Frontiers in Radiation Therapy Oncology, Vol. 6, edited by J. Vaeth, Basil, Karger, 1972, pp. 160-181.

60. Roswit, B.: Complications of radiation therapy. The alimentary tract. Semin. Roentgenol. 9:51-63, 1974.

61. Roswit, B.: Radiation injury of the colon and rectum. In Radiographic Atlas of Colon Disease, edited by E.I. Greenbaum, Chicago, Year Book Medical Publishers, 1980.

62. Roswit, B. and White, D.C.: Severe radiation injuries of the lung. Am. J. Roentgenol. 129:127-136, 1977.

63. Ruff, C.C., Dockerty, M.B., Frickie, R.E., and Waugh, J.M.: Preoperative radiation therapy for adenocarcinoma of rectum and rectosigmoid. Surg. Gynecol. Obstet. 112:715-723, 1961.

64. Simbertsiva, L.P., Sneshko, L.I., and Smirnov, N.M.: Results of intensive combined therapy for carcinoma of the rectum. Vopr. Onkol. 21:7-12, 1975.

65. Sischy, B., Remington, J.H., and Sobel, S.H.: Treatment of rectal carcinomas by means of endocavitary irradiation. Cancer 42:1073-1076, 1978.

66. Stearns, M.W., Jr., Deddish, M.R., and Quan, S.H.: Preoperative roentgen therapy for cancer of the rectum. Surg. Gynecol. Obstet. 109:225, 1959.

67. Stearns, M.W., Deddish, M.R., Quan, S.H., and Leaming, R.H.: Preoperative roentgen therapy for cancer of the rectum and rectosigmoid. Surg. Gynecol. Obstet. 138:584-586, 1974.

68. Stevens, K.R., Jr., Allen, C.U., and Fletcher, W.S.: Preoperative radiotherapy for adenocarcinoma of the rectosigmoid. Cancer 37:2866-2874, 1976.

69. Symonds, C.W.: Cancer of the rectum: Excision after application of radium. Proc. Soc. Med. (London), 1913-1914, (Clin. Sec. 7, 152).

70. Taylor, F.W.: Cancer of the colon and rectum. A study of routes of metastases and death. Surgery 52:305-308, 1962.

71. Tepper, M., Vidone, R.A., Hayes, M.A., Lindenmuth, W.W., and Kligerman, M.M.: Preoperative irradiation in rectal cancer: Initial comparison of clinical tolerance, surgical and pathologic findings. Am. J. Roentgenol. 102: 587-595, 1968.

72. Turek-Maischeider, M. and Kazem, I.: Palliative irradiation for liver metastasis. JAMA 232:625, 1975.

73. Turner, S.S., Vieira, E.F., Ager, P.J., and Ghossein, N.A.: Effective postoperative radiotherapy for locally advanced colorectal cancer. Int. J. Radiat. Oncol. Biol. Phys. 2 (Suppl. 1):64, 1976.

74. Urdaneta-Lafee, N., Kligerman, M.M., and Knowlton, A.H.: Evaluation of palliative irradiation in rectal carcinoma. Radiology 104:673-677, 1972.

75. Walker, A.R.P. and Burkett, D.P.: Colon cancer: Epidemiology. Semin. Oncol. 3:341-350, 1976.

76. Walz, B.J., Lindstrom, E.R., Butcher, H.R., Jr., and Baglan, R.J.: Natural history of patients after abdominoperineal resection: Implications for radiation therapy. Cancer 39:2437-2442, 1977.

77. Wang, C.C. and Schulz, M.D.: The role of radiation therapy in the management of carcinoma of the sigmoid, rectosigmoid, and rectum. Radiology 79: 1-5, 1962.

78. Whiteley, H.W., Jr., Stearns, M.W., Jr., Leaming, R.H., and Deddish, M.R.: Palliative radiation therapy in patients with cancer of the colon and rectum. Cancer 25:343-346, 1970.

79. Wilson, C.S. and Hall, E.J.: On advisability of treating all fields at each radiotherapy session. Radiology 98:419-424, 1971.

80. Withers, H.R. and Romsdahl, M.M.: Postoperative radiotherapy for adenocarcinoma of the rectum and rectosigmoid. Int. J. Radiat. Oncol. Biol. Phys. 2:1069-1074, 1977.

81. Withers, H.R., Romsdahl, H., Barkley, H.T., Saxton, J., Jr., McBride, C., and McMurtrey, M.: Postoperative radiotherapy for rectal cancer. In Adjuvant Therapy of Cancer, II, edited by S.E. Jones and S.E. Salmon, New York, Grune and Stratton, 1979.

82. Wynder, E.L. and Reddy, B.S.: Metabolic epidemiology of colorectal cancer. Cancer (Suppl.) 34:801-806, 1974.

83. Zybina, M.A., Chernichenko, V.A., Lure-Pokrovskaia, T.A., Arungazycva, V.V., and Zaichuck, A.L.: Combined therapy for rectal cancer. Vopr. Oncol. 21:59-65, 1975.

84. Zybina, M.A. and Nabatich, N.N. Results of combination treatment for rectal cancer. Vestn. Khir. 114:67-69, 1975.

SUGGESTED READING

1. Compilation of Cancer Therapy Protocol Summaries, 4th edition, Washington, D.C., U.S. Department of Health, Education and Welfare, Public Health Service, National Institutes of Health, April, 1980.

2. Enker, W.E. (Ed.): Carcinoma of Colon and Rectum. Chicago and London, Year Book Medical Publishers, 1979.

3. Glenn, F. and McSherry, C.K.: Carcinoma of the distal large bowel: 32-year review of 1026 cases. Ann. Surg. 163:838-849, 1966.

4. Kinsie, J.J.: Radiation therapy in the treatment of large bowel cancer. In Carcinoma of Colon and Rectum, edited by W.E. Enker, Chicago and London, Year Book Medical Publishers, 1979, pp. 187-199.

5. Moss, W.T., Brand, W.N., and Baltifara, H.: Radiation Oncology - Rationale, Technique, Results. 4th edition, St. Louis, C.V. Mosby, 1973, pp. 335-342.

6. Votava, C.H.: Carcinoma of the rectum and colon. Chapter 10: Textbook of Radiotherapy, 2nd edition, edited by G. Fletcher, Philadelphia, Lea and Febiger, 1973, pp. 611-619.

7. Votava, C.H. and Gunderson, L.L.: Carcinoma of the rectum and colon. In Textbook of Radiotherapy, 3rd edition, edited by G. Fletcher, Philadelphia, Lea and Febiger, 1980, pp. 704-716.

chapter 9

GYNECOLOGIC CANCER

SECTION I. CARCINOMA OF THE UTERUS, VAGINA, AND VULVA

Margaret Snelling, M.B., B.S.

CERVIX

Cancer of the cervix is one of the most common tumors treated in any radiotherapy department. In many developing countries it provides one-third of the female patients and, as with carcinoma of the breast, there are about 500 new patients per 1 million population each year. In more than 90% of cases the growth is a squamous cell carcinoma arising close to the squamous endometrial junction. It is a venereal disease in that the origin of squamous cell carcinoma is almost without exception related to sexual intercourse. It is now well known that the high-risk population for this disease includes those who commence intercourse at a very early age (59), those who marry early, those who remarry after a broken marriage, and those with multiple partners. The incidence of precursors of carcinoma is high in prostitutes and a high incidence of infection with herpes virus is also recognized (1,17,25,40,51).

For many years carcinoma of the cervix was considered as a disease occurring commonly at 45-55 years - soon before the menopause - in multipara and thought to be associated with chronic irritation, untreated birth injuries, chronic infection, and with a standard of hygiene. The disease was thought to be more common in the lower social and economic groups. Recently the change in social attitudes, the more permissive outlook associated with use of birth control, and the more common termination of pregnancy for social reasons has produced a rise in the incidence of squamous cell carcinoma in the younger members of the more affluent and better educated classes (4,9). Research has shown the incidence of carcinoma in situ and preinvasive carcinoma to be greatest in the groups mentioned (5,61). While in many patients the epithelium reverts to normal without treatment, in some the condition proceeds after a latent interval, which may last many years, to frank invasive carcinoma.

The relation of carcinoma to early intercourse is recognized, although not completely understood, and it is suggested that this is due to a particularly sensitive condition of the cervical epithelium which occurs in adolescence and at the first pregnancy and that the development of the carcinoma depends upon the addition of a cocarcinogen after a latent period. The role of circumcision, the importance of smegma as an irritant, the possibility of the addition of DNA from the sperm, the existence of racial immunity and of the importance of the Mosaic law which regulates intercourse in the Jewish race, have all been investigated but are still unproven. The relationship of early and frequent intercourse and the importance of multiple partners still remain our most important indications of risk to this disease and such a concept can explain much, including the relationship of the disease to certain racial and religious customs which determine the age of first intercourse, the age of marriage, the frequency of intercourse, and a number of partners.

There is no doubt that public education, which must include the education of children and adolescents, is a high priority, and that the public health services including the birth control, antenatal, and postnatal services, must be involved in this education and in the screening of high-risk populations.

In addition to cervical smears on these occasions and follow-up smears in patients whose previous ones are abnormal, routine smears should be carried out every 3 years during the active sexual periods of the lives of every woman (11,18, 36,50,63). In view of the expense, it is thought that a more frequent investigation in the symptomless is not necessary except for those in the high-risk group and those whose first smear showed a possible precancerous change.

Squamous cell carcinomas vary greatly in differentiation and activity and therefore in malignancy (70). While some reported series show the results to be worse in those rapidly growing undifferentiated tumors which appear to the clinician to have the worst prognosis, this is not always confirmed. The cells vary in size, as well as in mitotic activity (54). It is the large-celled tumors that have been shown to be more dangerous than the smaller celled (29).

Adenocarcinoma of the Cervix

An adenocarcinoma arising from the endometrium in the endocervical canal must be considered as a different clinical entity since its clinical behavior and its response to radiotherapy differ from those of squamous cell carcinoma and since it poses special problems to the radiotherapist because of its higher radioresistance.

The tumor extends up the endocervical canal and infiltrates deeply the cervical muscle producing a barrel-shaped tumor without extension to the vaginal epithelium. With a lateral extension of the tumor into the base of the parametria it is very difficult to irradiate it adequately with vaginal and intrauterine sources. This and a degree of radioresistance have been used in the past to suggest a combination of radiotherapy and surgery as the best chance of cure. It used to be believed that lymphatic glandular spread occurred early in adenocarcinoma, but this is probably associated with a late appearance of symptoms in endocervical disease since the tumor is less liable to trauma or infection at intercourse than is an exocervical carcinoma.

The differential diagnosis of carcinoma of the cervix includes melanoma, hypernephroma, other müllerian tumors, mixed carcinoma-sarcoma, and myosarcoma usually arising in a fibroid. The prognosis of all these tumors tends to be poor. The use of surgery combined with irradiation is usually preferred to radiation therapy alone.

Body of the Uterus

This is an adenocarcinoma arising in the endometrial lining of the uterus and its behavior and therefore its treatment differs from carcinoma of the cervix. Its development is related to the production of hormones in the body and especially to estrogens. It appears at a later age than does carcinoma of the cervix, i.e., after the menopause. It is associated with relative sterility and with a typical physique: a short, obese woman with small hands and feet and with a tendency to diabetes, hypertension, and often with a history of other gynecological disorders, such as fibromyomata and ovarian cysts.

This adenocarcinoma varies in malignancy but is usually lower than that of carcinoma of the cervix. Because of the relative scarcity of lymphatic vessels in the uterus, spread to the lymphatic glands occurs at a later stage and often only after there has been deep myometrial invasion or the cervix is invaded by direct extension. Spread to the vagina occurs by implantation of cells or via the lymphatic plexus.

As the tumor increases in size, deep extension takes place into the myometrium and from here the tumor may spread to the peritoneal surface and to the pelvic or abdominal glands. The ovaries may become involved by tumor extending along the fallopian tubes or via lymphatic vessels.

PRINCIPLES GOVERNING THE MANAGEMENT OF CARCINOMA OF THE UTERUS

The management of all uterine tumors, whether squamous cell carcinoma of the cervix, adenocarcinoma of the cervix, adenocarcinoma of the fundus, or the rarer tumors mentioned, involves radiation therapy (49, 73) or surgery (66), alone or in combination. The many variations of the clinical problems they present are so great that individualization of treatment is essential. Each patient must be assessed and considered separately by an experienced team which includes a surgeon and a radiotherapist specializing in gynecological malignant disease and provided with a fully equipped radiotherapy department with a strong infrastructure. The aim (10) is to achieve the complete cure of the patient with no more than easily tolerated morbidity of the irradiated normal tissues or to palliate the symptoms of advanced disease which should be so controlled as to allow the patients a number of months or even years of comparatively normal, even though restricted, life.

Over 90% of early cases and well over one-half of all the cases of squamous cell carcinoma treated should live many years without evidence of disease as should more than two-thirds of the cases of carcinoma of the endometrium. Cure is obtained by the removal or destruction of the primary growth together with its direct and lymphatic extensions. While bloodstream metastases may eventually occur, there is no evidence of the early spread of micrometastases such as occurs in carcinoma of the breast. Death from carcinoma of the uterus is associated, almost invariably, with residual pelvic or lower abdominal disease.

Where surgery and radiotherapy fail, the contribution of chemotherapy is, at present, disappointing. Although hormone therapy using progesterones may cause occasional remarkable regression in well-differentiated adenocarcinoma, these additional disciplines are ineffective in the control of other tumors of the uterus. These tumors depend essentially upon an accurate assessment of the disease followed, as soon as possible, by accurate and intensive radical surgery and/or high-dose radiotherapy.

FIRST ASSESSMENT OF A NEW PATIENT WITH CARCINOMA OF THE CERVIX

Each patient presents a new and different problem requiring careful assessment and individualized treatment for a complicated condition that often involves a number of different organs (Table 1). After a full investigation, treatment is prescribed, but it must be expected that in many cases this will be replanned and altered as it proceeds (65). Continuation of the treatment to the best solution possible requires continual observations, reassessments, and often replanning as the tumor regresses (23).

Table 1. Comparative Staging of Cervical Carcinoma

UICC	Cervix	FIGO
T1S	Carcinoma in situ	0
T1	Confined to cervix	0
T1(a)	Microinvasive	I(a)
T1(b)	All other stage 1 cases	I(b)
T2	Extends beyond cervix but not to the pelvic wall	II
T2(a)	No parametrial involvement	II(a)
T2(b)	Parametrial involvement	II(b)
T3	Extends to pelvic wall/lower vagina/hydronephrosis or nonfunctioning kidney	III
T3(a)	No extension to pelvic wall	III(a)
T3(b)	Extension to the pelvic wall and/or hydronephrosis or nonfunctioning kidney	III(b)
T4	Extends beyond true pelvis or involves the bladder or rectum	IV
T4(a)	Extends to adjacent organs	IV(a)
T4(b)	Metastases	IV(b)

Time is never wasted when taking a detailed careful history from the patient. In addition to the important development of a doctor-patient relationship which must last for many years, there are the advantages gained from knowledge of the patient's mentality and attitude to the disease. The patient's account of her symptoms gives an accurate picture of the nature and of the extent of the disease on which her prognosis and treatment depend. While a complete examination and thorough investigation must follow, the first estimation of the patient's general health may at once indicate advanced metastatic disease or suggest the presence of some quite different pathology requiring prior attention. The general examination includes a check for any previous condition of the abdomen which may interfere with treatment such as surgery causing adhesions (laparotomy for appendicitis, or cesarean section) or inflammation (colitis, diverticulitis).

An examination under anesthesia is essential in the determination of the treatment policy, although it is best left as the last item in the investigations, after the history has been studied and a local and general examination has been followed by full laboratory investigations.

Examination under Anesthesia

An examination under anesthesia by a gynecological surgeon and radiotherapist is essential before the treatment is planned. It allows the accurate staging of the condition, extent of tumor, treatment volumes, and a decision on management by radiotherapy and/or surgery.

The aims of the examination, which is often carried out after the radiological and laboratory tests, are:

1. To assess the tumor volume, including any extension to neighboring organs.

2. To decide the treatment volume, whether treated by surgery or radiotherapy.

3. To discover any additional abnormality or pathology in the region.

4. Where radiotherapy is to be used, a careful assessment of the pelvic anatomy is necessary, including the relationship between uterus, vagina, and the size of the introitus and of the cavities which will contain the intracavitary sources.

The whole of the region is examined carefully, starting with inspection and palpation of the clitoris, labia, urethra, and introitus where deposits are not infrequently missed. The tumors in the vagina and cervix are measured and biopsies taken. The uterus is dilated, the length measured, and a fractional currettage performed. Dilatation to no. 6 Hegar is often sufficient. Splitting a tight cervix by unnecessary dilatation above no. 8 should be avoided. A bimanual vaginal and rectal complete the information concerning the primary neoplasm and its spread to the fornices, parametria, and pelvic wall. Sometimes proctoscopic and sigmoidoscopic examinations are indicated if there are bowel symptoms.

A cystoscopy should be carried out in every case to search for evidence of bladder infiltration, which is unlikely in the absence of palpable infiltration in the anterior fornix. The ureters should be visualized. The intravenous injection of indigocarmine is sometimes useful as a first quick check on renal function. Examination by a urogenital surgeon and the passage of a ureteric catheter are sometimes necessary.

Radiological Examination

This should follow the first clinical assessment and is performed to ascertain the involvement by the carcinoma of the urinary tract when this is suspected. It can be used to evaluate lymph nodes (Fig. 1), the blood supply of the tumor, and the involved organs. Ultrasound and CT scans can give amazing detail of the anatomical extent of the tumor.

SYMPTOMATOLOGY OF CARCINOMA OF THE CERVIX AS AN INDICATION OF THE PATIENT'S DISEASE

The symptoms of carcinoma of the cervix are well known but a good history often reveals a great deal of clinical information.

In general a menopausal woman complains of painless bleeding on intercourse caused by local trauma and followed by menorrhagia and a gradual development of intermenstrual bleeding without obvious cause. Later, as ulceration and infection occur, there is persistent vaginal discharge. Pain is rare, but dyspareunia may indicate rapid infiltration by a highly malignant tumor. A low abdominal pain suggests cervical obstruction with a collection of blood or pus in the uterus. Extensive disease or infection can cause a sacral or lumbosacral backache. Pain referred to the buttocks and backs of the thighs is caused by involvement of the common iliac nodes. This involvement can cause pain in the loin associated with hydronephrosis and reduced renal function. Metastases in the lumbar sacral spine causes sciatica and at a higher level, pain in the front of the thigh. Inguinal pain on the outer aspect of the thigh may also be caused by deposits in the upper lumbar spine but is more often due to disease in the pelvis, groins, near the psoas muscle at the pelvic brim, or above. The pressure of invaded pelvic nodes on the internal and external iliac veins causes edema and results in thrombosis and development of a collateral circulation. This collateral circulation may be inadequate when there is involvement of all the pelvic nodes thus causing increasing edema of the leg and thigh followed by edema of the buttock. When both sides of the pelvis are involved, there will be edema of both legs, the vulva, and mons. Extension of the disease to the lumbar nodes may result in obstruction of the vena cava with edema of the lower trunk, development of a collateral circulation through the portal system, hemorrhoids, and/or a circulation through the superficial abdominal veins.

Urinary Symptoms

Dysuria and frequency of micturition are infrequent with early cervical disease. When these symptoms are severe they suggest a tumor on the anterior lip of the cervix and anterior fornix spreading through the vesicovaginal septum to the trigone of the bladder. Dysuria associated with retention or incontinence may be caused by extension down the anterior vaginal wall with involvement of the urethra.

Bowel Symptoms

Apart from constipation relieved by laxatives, bowel symptoms are rare and unimportant in early disease. An advanced tumor arising from the posterior lip of the cervix or in the posterior fornix may extend to the rectum causing bleeding, discharge, pain, hemorrhoids, and eventually symptoms and signs of obstruction in rectum or sigmoid.

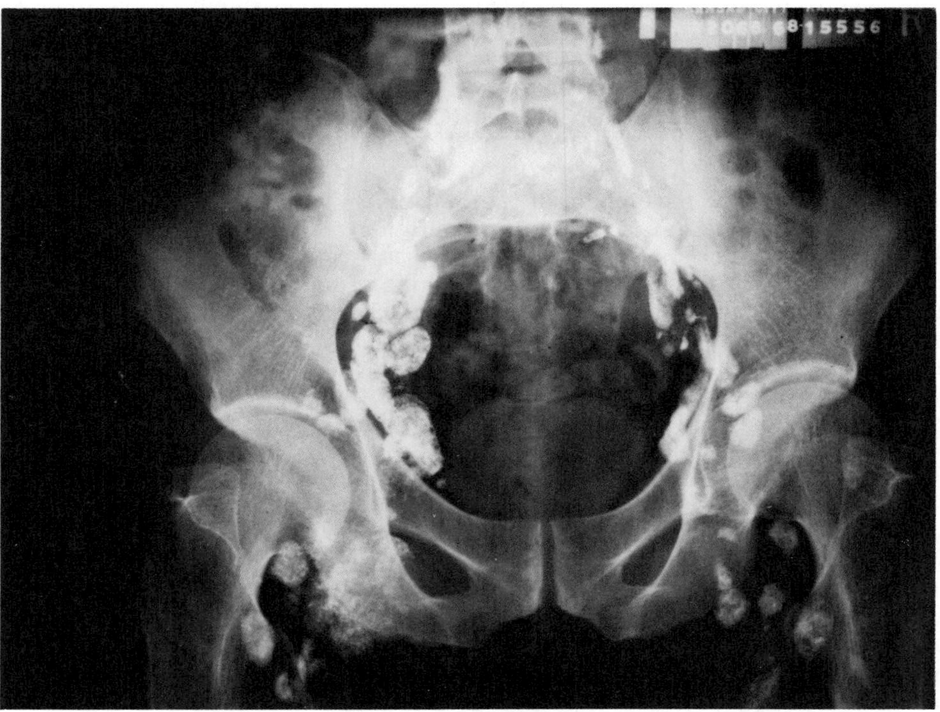

Figure 1. Patient with carcinoma of the cervix and positive lymphangiomas. A: Pelvic nodes.

TREATMENT OF EARLY CASES OF CARCINOMA OF THE CERVIX

Basic Intracavitary Techniques

Whatever technique is used, intracavitary irradiation must be planned and carried out as carefully as external irradiation.

The Paris System of Intracavitary Therapy

A large number of pioneer radiotherapists learned their art at the Foundation Curie in Paris or at the Radiumhemmet in Stockholm, before the Second World War. In the Parisian system the treatment continued for 120 hr with 33.3 mg of ^{226}Ra in the uterine tube and two 13.3 mg in corks of a vaginal colpostat. The colpostats were separated by a spring. Later developments at the Institute Gustave Roussy have included a manual afterloading system using ^{192}Ir and a conventional dose rate remote loader, the Curietron, used in many European centers. Fixation of the vaginal sources is now ensured by a plastic vaginal mold made individually for each patient.

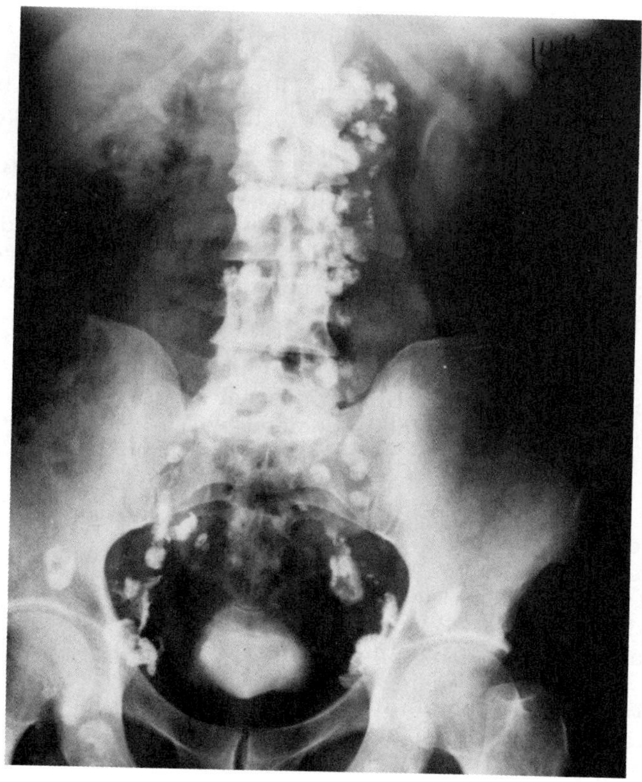

Figure 1. B: Paraaortic nodes.

Stockholm System

In this system devised at the Radiumhemmet, the proportion of the sources in uterus and vagina differ from that used in Paris. There is 50 mg of radium in the uterine tube and 65-80 mg arranged in a flat or curved vaginal box closely apposed to the cervix and occupying the whole width of the vagina.

The dosimetry and the total dose in the paracervical are similar to that delivered in the Paris system but there is a higher dose rate and treatment is given in three fractions of 22 hr delivered at intervals of 1 and 2 weeks. These sources are held in position by packing.

The prolongation of the treatment and the fractionation is favored by many radiotherapists since it allows observation of the response to treatment for appropriate alterations in dosimetry when deemed necessary.

The Manchester System

The Manchester system is in use in centers throughout the world. It was devised at the Christie Hospital and Holt Radium Institute, Manchester, England, and was based on the Paris system with treatment given in two fractionations (insertions) lasting approximately 3 days, with an overall time of 10 days, during which a total dose of up to 8000 rads is delivered to point A. This point is located in the paracervical triangle described as being 2 cm above the vaginal fornix and 2 cm lateral to a point in the uterine tube which is itself 2 cm above the uterine os. When isodose curves are constructed this is the site where the tumor dose falls off quickly. Point A may be impossible to define clinically when there is cervical displacement, destruction of the cervix, or a very bulky tumor. The radiotherapist may have to redefine point A's position in these cases. It is useful, however, as a point of importance to radiotherapists where tumor passes laterally into the parametrium and of importance to surgeons as it is here in the paracervical triangle that the uterine artery and ureter cross. Providing the system and its isodose curves are understood and the loading and position of the sources are known, a knowledge of the dose at point A gives to a radiotherapist and his physicist very complete information concerning the treatment given to a patient.

The Manchester system provides three uterine sources of different lengths which are combined with a choice of three different sizes of vaginal ovoids, each with appropriate sources. The choice is decided by the length of the uterus and the width of the vagina. The dose rate and total dose at point A are the same for all treatments.

This technique provides a rule of thumb method for the treatment of cancer of the cervix and gives a reasonable average treatment with a minimum of complications to all patients. In centers where there is no possibility of individualization of treatment, for instance, in a busy center in a developing area, it offers a well established and reliable method of treatment easy to teach and carry out.

The disadvantages are a certain inflexibility when dealing with abnormal situations and the absence of any rigid attachment between the vaginal and uterine sources, which may cause movement during treatment. There is a real disadvantage in that the uterus is not fixed in anteversion, and the success of the treatment and the avoidance of complications depends upon the position of the sources and firmness of the packing. Measurement or calculations of the rectal dose and radiographs to check the position of the sources during the course are essential.

Common Clinical Problems in Intracavitary Therapy

All radiotherapists are faced with problems involving the positioning of the sources because the dosimetry in the tumor and normal tissue may be affected by pathology and anatomic abnormalities in the pelvic organs.

A narrow vagina in a nulliparous patient may make it impossible to insert sources in the lateral fornices to provide an adequate contribution to irradiation of the cervix and parametrium. The longer central uterine source may be used so that it extends into the vagina, or the usual two fornical vaginal sources may be rotated and placed in tandem. This may be satisfactory for a small tumor in a small cervix, but the dose will drop at the periphery of a large carcinoma on the surface of the cervix as well as at the outer and upper part of an endocervical tumor. An attempt to raise the dose will risk increasing the dose dangerously in the bladder or rectum. The addition of metallic shielding in the vaginal sources to decrease the rectal and bladder dose may improve the overall dosimetry. This shielding is more easily accomplished if sources of ^{137}Cs or, better still, ^{192}Ir, are used. When this is not possible, the contribution from external irradiation should be increased; failing this, surgery should be considered.

A retroversion of the uterus may raise the rectal dose. A mobile retroversion can usually be corrected before the insertion of the sources but may revert to its original position after they have been inserted. In all cases the rectal and bladder dose can be measured directly after insertion of the sources. Check x-rays taken, preferably either orthogonal or stereoscopic shift, and examine as soon as possible. When the treatment is lengthy, further x-rays may be advisable at intervals of 24-36 hr. If a mobile retroversion cannot be controlled, a rigid applicator with fixation of vaginal and uterine sources should be considered.

Fixed anteversion and sometimes anteflexion of the uterus may cause difficulty and may even prevent the insertion of the uterine source in advanced disease and thus raise the dose in the bladder and reduce the dosage that can be given to the tumor. In other cases a mobile, acutely anteverted uterus or a small senile uterus may cause too high a dose to the trigone.

A bulky tumor may distort the vaginal or uterine cavity, or the uterus may be drawn to or pushed away from the tumor. Under these conditions a combination of external and intracavitary treatment should be used with external therapy 5 days a week for 5 weeks to a dose of 4500-5000 rads and intracavitary therapy fractionated weekly over 3 or 5 weeks. As the condition starts to improve after 2 or 3 weeks and the vaginal tumor disappears, a better dosimetry can be achieved. Treatment continues over 5-7 weeks.

A very capacious vagina with a cystocele and rectocele may by its size and laxity prevent the correct positioning and fixation of the sources by packing. Again, the use of a fixed metallic applicator governing the position of all three sources may be necessary. The use of an applicator attached to a belt outside the body is advocated but the individual mold prepared for each patient at the Institut Gustave Roussy, for manual or conventional dose rate remote loading, effectively controls the vaginal sources.

Precancerous Conditions, Carcinoma In Situ, Noninvasive Carcinoma

There is no place for radiotherapy in these cases. There are neither pathological nor radiobiological reasons for it to be effective. It has the disadvantage of producing a menopause in a young woman. There is a possibility of complications from irradiation of the bowel (16,65) and of the late appearance of malignant disease in the normal pelvic tissues irradiated. The patient should be kept under close observation with repeated smears and treated, when necessary, by conization (which may be repeated). There are a wide spectra of the preinvasive conditions, some of which can be managed by laser cauterization. Eventually, and often after childbirth has been achieved, simple hysterectomy may be indicated.

T1N0M0: Early Stage I Cancer of Cervix (Less Than 1 cm in Diameter)

The prognosis is good; involvement of lymph nodes is unlikely. The choice of treatment lies between surgery (35) or radiotherapy alone (8,32), or by the two in combination (43,56,60).

Surgery

A Wertheim radical hysterectomy may be thought wise, but where the tumor is of very low malignancy, an extended hysterectomy without glandular dissection may be performed. If no irradiation is to be given, an ample cuff of vagina must be removed.

Preoperative Radiotherapy

When there is a long history with delay in diagnosis, where the tissues have been widely opened by local surgery, and where histology shows a high degree of malignancy, preoperative intracavitary irradiation is followed by Wertheim hysterectomy. A dose of 5500 rads (^{226}Ra) is given in two insertions in an overall time of 10 days, completed 2 days before surgery, in which the classical operation is modified and only one-third of the vagina removed.

Radiation Therapy Alone

In an elderly patient with a tumor less than 1 cm across and where the malignancy is of a low grade, treatment may be by intracavitary irradiation alone (32). A dose of 6000 rads (^{226}Ra), is given to point A in two applications over a time of 10 days.

T1M0M0: Stage 1 Cases More Than 1 cm Diameter

Treatment should be by a combination of intracavitary and external irradiation (42), except where there is a radioresistant low-grade carcinoma or adenocarcinoma of the endocervical canal when a radical hysterectomy may be performed after preliminary intracavitary irradiation. Several protocols have been suggested for this combined radiotherapy-surgery treatment. As a result of preliminary studies, some clinicians believe that adenocarcinoma of the cervix or the barrel cervix are not as radioresistant as previously thought and recommend that there should be no treatment distinction between squamous cell and adenocarcinoma.

Intracavitary Irradiation Followed by External Therapy to Sides of Pelvis: Center Protected

This is a preliminary treatment with intracavitary sources in which a dose at point A of 6000 rads is given in two treatments with an overall time of 12 days. This is followed by a carefully planned supervoltage irradiation of the lateral structures in the pelvis using opposing fields with the central 5 cm shielded (Fig. 2). In 5 weeks the dose at point A is raised by not more than 1000 rads; the pelvic wall receives 5000 rads. Treatment is given on 5 days each week and all fields are treated each time.

External Irradiation to the Whole Pelvis Combined with Intracavitary Therapy

External supervoltage irradiation is given to the whole pelvis and lower abdomen extending up to the lower border of the fourth lumbar vertebra, that is, it covers the common iliac nodes. There is a recognized hazard from irradiation of the bowel (16), with especial danger to the sigmoid colon, terminal ileum, and the small intestine included in the treatment volume (69). There is evidence to suggest that

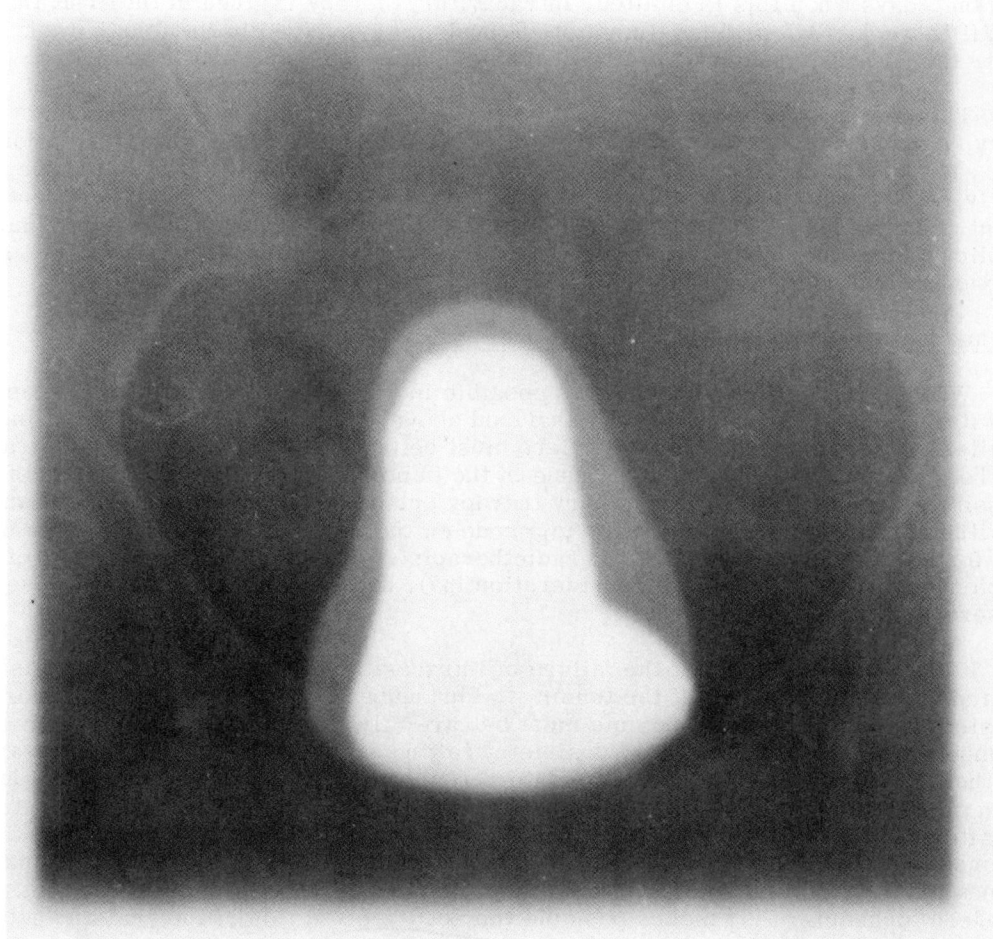

Figure 2. Midline block after intracavitary irradiation.

a dose of 4600 rads in 5 weeks is well tolerated but should be given only in the absence of any history of bowel pathology or previous abdominal surgery.

Intracavitary radiotherapy may be combined with full pelvic irradiation, which may be given either concurrently or as the first stage in the treatment.

When the external irradiation is completed and full benefit from it has been obtained, the insertion of radioactive intracavitary sources is performed. This method has radiobiological advantages, although to perform the insertion in the presence of a reaction and when there is considerable shrinking of the vagina may present some difficulty.

The author prefers the concurrent treatment by intracavitary and external irradiation. The treatment lasts 5.5 weeks and involves a dose to point A of the equivalent of 2750 rads in three fractions (insertions), complemented by 4600 rads to the whole pelvis and lower abdomen, in 20 treatments in 4.5 weeks.

External treatment is given on 4 days each week when intracavitary therapy is given and on 5 days when this is omitted. Intracavitary therapy is given in the first, third, and fifth week. A fourth treatment of 750 rads may be given in the fourth week or after the end of the planned treatment if this appears to be clinically indicated.

This method of management facilitates the individualization of treatment by varying dose and dosimetry according to the response of the tumor to irradiation (8). The early administration of the first insertion has the advantage of producing early relief from bleeding. Where the vaginal tumor is large, a localized treatment at this stage of 1000 rads surface dose to the neoplasm with an intravaginal applicator causes regression in the next week, and this allows an easy second insertion of a uterine tube and the usual vaginal sources.

T2 and T3 with Probable Invasion of Nodes

When curative radical therapy is possible in view of the extent of the disease and its histology, treatment is as described above, i.e., by a combination of intracavitary and external irradiation. Care must be taken not to overstep the tolerance of the bowel or of the connective tissue in the tumor bed (65). However, it is often possible to increase the intracavitary therapy by another fraction or to apply a small additional dose by external therapy to a node on the pelvic wall (35). This is a matter for the clinical judgment of the radiotherapist. Dose/time and dosimetry of each case requires individual consideration (37), and each patient must be closely observed during the treatment.

It has been realized that the failure of intracavitary therapy is frequently associated with the large size of the tumor, the inadequacy of the dose, and the poor dosimetry. The treatment volume must be carefully examined by stereoscopic or orthogonal x-rays and computer dosimetry to find areas of over- and underdosage in the tumor volume. The use of miniature sources made possible by the introduction of radium equivalents and the modern applicators devised during the evolution of afterloading techniques have improved dosimetry and immobilization of the sources during conventional dose rate treatments. The use of high dose rate machines allows virtually complete immobilization throughout the whole treatment. Modern technology also makes possible the accurate addition of internal and external therapy.

While the results obtained by the irradiation of squamous cell carcinoma have improved, there are still many failures in the treatment of the more resistant adenocarcinoma in the barrel cervix. Here success may be achieved by the addition of a simple panhysterectomy to heavy preoperative irradiation with a combination of external and internal therapy advocated by Fletcher et al. (27,28). In a case where the tumor receives a dose of 5000 mg hr, associated with 5000 + rads external therapy, an interval of 5-6 weeks is necessary before reassessment and, where operable, very restricted surgery, with no attempt at a clearance of more than the primary tumor.

Salvage of Advanced Disease by Surgery

Bladder and Rectal Involvement

In cases where the bladder is involved, the possibility of an anterior exenteration following preliminary irradiation should be considered, and similarly the possibility of a posterior exenteration in the case of disease involving the rectum from the cervix. A decision depends on the estimation of the patient's probable survival and the presence of disease in the abdominal nodes and liver. With the improvement in the palliation obtained by irradiation using modern technology a complete exenteration is rarely performed. The combination of a colostomy and ureteric transplant into an ileal bladder often gives significant palliation which may last some years and may, without more treatment, often relieve pain, vaginal bleeding, and discharge.

Ureteric Obstruction

For hydronephrosis and renal failure due to ureteric obstruction by nodes in the abdomen or at the pelvic brim, by the primary tumor at the side of the cervix or at the trigone, ureteric transplantation is indicated. This is providing that there is good reason to expect the patient to profit from a life prolonged for a year or more and that there is sufficient length of one (preferably both) ureter. A pericutaneous ureterostomy or a transposition can be made to an ileal bladder on the abdominal wall. The simpler transposition to the large bowel will give relief, but should be avoided where it is anticipated that at a later stage a colostomy may be necessary. Palliative radiotherapy may then be possible.

Ureteric transposition should be performed for dysuria, frequency and incontinence due to vesicovaginal fistula, caused by tumor or following irradiation. The improvements in urogenital surgery have been so great in recent years that this operation should be advised in many late cases, providing recovery of renal function is expected and the prognosis is suitable. It has relieved distressing symptoms and returned many patients to a happy familial and social life for periods varying from many months to a few years. Ureteral stents are effective in relieving obstructions.

In the author's opinion, drainage through the renal pelvis for ureteric obstruction too high for transplantation of the ureters is, however, contraindicated, since the tumor at this level is not controllable and the patient will almost certainly spend her last weeks with uncontrollable leakage of urine through the loin.

Irradiation of Lumbar Nodes

The value of the irradiation of the lumbar nodes above the lower level of L4 is still under assessment. Many radiotherapists consider that once they are involved, the disease has already metastasized beyond the hope of cure. In order to investigate this point, trials are in progress at the Royal Marsden Hospital and also in other hospitals under the auspices of the European Organization for Research and Treatment of Cancer (EORTC).

Treatment of Recurrent Disease

Once full curative treatment by radiotherapy has failed, further external irradiation is rarely useful. Although a local vaginal or uterine source may help in the control of bleeding, this irradiation must be very localized and given only after full consideration of any previous treatment and prognosis. In general, the beneficial effect lasts only a few months and such treatment is often combined with colostomy or ureteric transposition. When conventional dose rate treatment is used, the discomfort of the insertion and the packing often outweighs any advantage gained. With high dose rate remote loading therapy given under anesthesia or sedation, the patient receives considerable short-term benefits without associated discomfort.

In general the results of chemotherapy are poor although a combination including adriamycin, vincristine, cyclophosphamide, and 5-FU may be of some value in the treatment of very aggressive squamous cell carcinoma.

Treatment of Bowel Complications
Due to Disease or Following Treatment

Rectal Symptoms

When the rectum is involved by the growth, the possibility of a primary adenocarcinoma in the bowel spreading forward to involve the cervix must be remembered. Where rectal symptoms follow irradiation (16) with local erythema, edema, ulceration, and stenosis, it is usually due to heavy irradiation from the vaginal applicators in the fornices. Care is necessary to differentiate these findings from extension of the neoplasm. This is especially necessary in modern therapy as the rectal reaction, once so common, has become very rare in many centers. The author, using high dose rate remote loading, has not seen a rectal reaction for 5 years.

The importance of controlling the position of both uterine and vaginal sources by direct measurement, radiographic checks, careful dosimetry, and by avoiding later displacement of the sources has been mentioned. With the modern increase in the use of external irradiation, its effect on large and small intestines are now receiving urgent consideration (65). Irradiation of the rectosigmoid junction causes pain, bleeding, discharge, and diarrhea, and may result in perforation or obstruction.

Because of the increased long-term cures resulting from the treatment of carcinoma of the cervix by large volume external irradiation, slight bowel complications may occur in more than 20% of patients treated. Although this may be accepted in view of the seriousness of the disease, severe damage cause considerable disability and results ultimately in the death of the patient with the most severe damage. Perhaps ± 10% changes similar to Crohn disease occur in the terminal ileum and ascending colon and throughout the irradiated portion of the small intestine. Excision is indicated but is often impossible because of the length of the bowel involved in postirradiation fibrosis. Treatment is largely prophylactic, by avoiding irradiation of the bowel in patients with a history of bowel disease or abdominal surgery of any kind. In such cases it is better to confine irradiation to the true pelvis and to use intracavitary irradiation to achieve the maximum effect on the tumor. External irradiation to the whole pelvis and lower abdomen should not exceed the equivalent in 5 weeks of 4500-5000 rads (linear accelerator 10 MV or 4000-4500 ^{60}Co.

ADENOCARCINOMA OF THE ENDOMETRIUM

The natural history of this disease differs in many ways from squamous cell carcinoma. It is an adenocarcinoma arising from the endometrial glandular epithelium, varying in malignancy from a slow-growing differentiated form to a rapidly advancing, very undifferentiated form. Mixed tumors with squamous cell or sarcomatous elements occur and are associated with a bad prognosis. Sarcomata may arise in uterine and cervical fibroids.

The tumor appears usually after the menopause and often with a history of increasing menorrhagia and hyperplasia of the endometrium. There may be a history of relative sterility, or dysfunction of the endocrine glands, or other gynecological disorders.

Spread is first by direct extension in the body of the uterus down to the cervix and up through the fallopian tubes. It also spreads deep into the muscle. When the growth is of low malignancy and localized to the fundus, the prognosis is good since the lymphatic supply there is poor. Once the cervix is involved, spread occurs laterally to the parametrium and out through lymphatics to the internal and external iliac nodes and up to the common iliac and aortic nodes. This tumor differs from cervical tumors again in that spread may occur to vagina and vulva by means of cells, by lymphatic spread with typical secondary tumors at the level of the cervix, behind the urethra in the lower vagina, and in the labia at the introitus.

Lymphatic spread differs also from that of cervical tumors. The growths in the upper part of the uterus may spread along the round ligament to the medial group of inguinal nodes which are more often involved in this disease than in carcinoma of the cervix, in which the inguinal spread comes from lower vaginal or vulval disease.

Highly malignant anaplastic tumors in the fundus infiltrate deeply into the myometrium. When the outer third is involved, invasion of the aortic nodes is to be expected either via the common iliac nodes or directly along the ovarian lymphatics to aortic nodes at the level of the renal vessels. Spread to the liver and pulmonary metastases occur eventually.

Prognosis depends upon the extent of the tumor (Table 2), the histology, and the grade of malignancy. It is excellent where a low-grade tumor is limited to the fundus or the superficial layer, but it has long been realized that once the cervical canal is involved the cure rate drops to one-half. Similarly, enlargement of the uterus due to invasion, usually by high-grade tumor, is a bad prognostic sign.

Treatment

The most important element in the curative treatment of carcinoma of the endometrium is a hysterectomy which includes uterus and adnexa with adjacent parametria and pelvic fascia. A cuff of vagina covering the cervix is removed. A Wertheim radical hysterectomy is performed in a woman fit for such surgery where nodal involvement has been proven.

When the tumor is of low-grade malignancy and is confined to the upper part of the cavity without deep infiltration, surgery alone is sufficient providing it is performed with due precautions against the spilling of tumor cells in the wound. Because of postoperative residual disease in the vaginal vault, recurrence here is not uncommon. It has been reported in a number of series as occurring in 14% of cases treated by hysterectomy. Postoperative irradiation is therefore recommended following hysterectomy in cases of low malignancy when only a small length of vagina has been removed, when full precautions have not been taken at operation to avoid local recurrence, and when the details of the pathologic condition and surgery are unknown.

Under these conditions a cylinder with a central linear source is used with a diameter of up to 3 cm - large enough to slightly distend the vagina. When the diameter exceeds 3 cm it must be remembered that the dose in the rectum will rise. A surface dose of 6000 rads is given to the mucosa in two applications separated by

Table 2. Comparative Staging

UICC	Corpus Uteri	FIGO
TIS	Carcinoma in situ	O
T1	Confined to the corpus	I
T1(a)	Length of uterine cavity 8 cm or less	I(a)
T1(b)	Length of uterine cavity greater than 8 cm	I(b)
T2	Involvement of corpus and cervix	II
T3	Extension outside of uterus but not outside of true pelvis	III
T4	Extension outside of true pelvis or involves the bladder or rectum	IV
T4(a)	Extension to adjacent organs	IV(a)
T4(b)	Metastases	IV(b)

an interval of 1 week. Dilators must be used later to prevent vaginal adhesions and to avoid stenosis.

When the disease is of high malignancy, the cervical canal is involved, or the condition has not been accurately staged in preliminary investigations at another hospital, it is wise to give preoperative irradiation. This should be done if sources can be inserted into the uterus and vaginal fornices and so provide an adequate dosimetry. A dose equivalent to 5500 rads should be given in two applications of ^{226}Ra or radium equivalent sources in an overall period of 10 days, followed after 2-3 weeks, or alternatively, 6-8 weeks, by extended hysterectomy. An advantage of preoperative intracavitary irradiation is the fact that the removal of the vagina is limited to the part immediately related to the cervix and the patient is left with an almost full-length functional vagina. It is important to remember that where surgery follows soon after such irradiation with ^{226}Ra, the dose to point A should not exceed the equivalent of 5500 rads in two applications with an overall time of 10 days. After such irradiation, which because of the surgery to follow is deliberately below the lethal tumor dose in the endometrium, the surgery must be carried out with every precaution not to interfere with the blood supply of the bladder base and ureters, or fistulae will result.

Heyman reported the result of the treatment of inoperable carcinoma of the endometrium at the Radiumhemmet, by the now classical technique of packing the uterine cavity with radium capsules. This system gave a greatly improved dosimetry when treating a grossly enlarged uterus with an irregular cavity full of tumor. Today, with general improvement in the health of the population and with modern operative techniques and anesthesia, the incidence of inoperability is well below 10%. Also, cases are usually diagnosed at an earlier stage. Hysterectomy should be performed and should be preceded by intracavitary irradiation as already described. Since the uterus is to be removed, there is no need for a lethal dose in the cavity as long as enough treatment is given to reduce the activity of the tumor in the cervix and potential or real tumor in the vagina receives a lethal dose. The author prefers, therefore, in these cases, not to use Heyman capsules, the preparation and insertion of which involves considerable radiation exposure in the radium and operating rooms. In order to improve radiation protection, the author prefers to use the ingenious manual afterloading system devised by Simon, or to use a simple Manchester system consisting of a uterine tube with a heavy load at the upper end and vaginal ovoids, or some simpler arrangement. Fig. 3 shows modified Simon intrauterine applicators and Fletcher vaginal ovoids that can be used in treating endometrial cancer. Manual afterloading or remote loading techniques should be used whenever possible.

Where radical curative therapy is desired, a dose of 6000 rads should be given to a line 1 cm deep to the surface of the endometrium. Two applications can be given, each lasting 2-3 days and with an overall time of 10 days. This isodose line should be brought down to include the cervix and upper vagina, and the surgery performed after either an interval of 1-2 weeks or postponed for at least 6 weeks until the radiation reaction has developed and subsided.

Treatment of Involved Nodes

When enlarged nodes are shown to be involved by pathological examination or lymphography, or believed to exist because of the deep infiltration of the tumor into the myometrium, they may be irradiated postoperatively. Supervoltage treatment

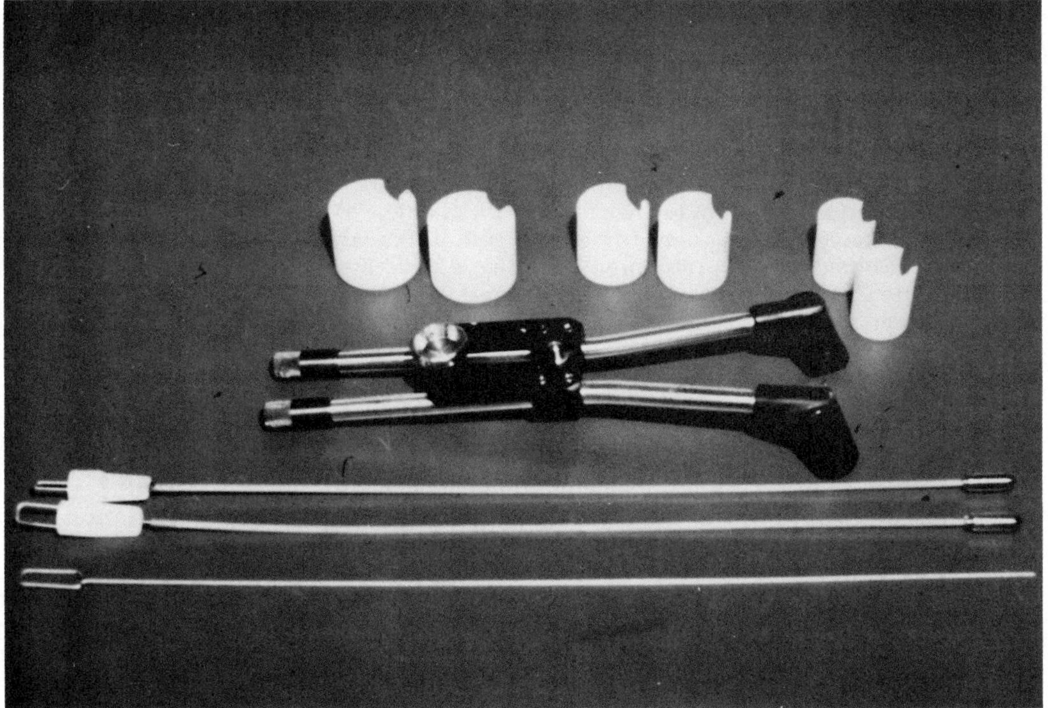

Figure 3. Modified Simon applicators used for the Heyman packing technique. The Fletcher ovoids are used for the intravaginal sources.

may be given using inverted Y opposing fields. A dose of not more than the equivalent of 4000 rads is given in daily treatment in not less than 5.5 weeks.

Salvage of Advanced Inoperable Carcinoma of the Endometrium

Where highly malignant anaplastic tumor fills and invades the whole uterus, the outlook is very bad. Only a short survival is to be expected. Pelvic symptoms of pain, bleeding, and discharge are invariably present. Chemotherapy is of little value in these large avascular tumors, but when the tumor is a well-differentiated carcinoma there may be a remarkable response to very large doses of progesterone therapy and such treatment is well worth a trial. In other cases a preoperative combination of intracavitary with external irradiation may make surgery possible. This can be done with a dose of approximately 4500 rads given over 5 weeks to the whole pelvis, and is combined with fractionated intracavitary therapy, with the reassessment of the possibility of a simple hysterectomy after a further 6 weeks.

CARCINOMA OF THE VAGINA

Primary squamous cell carcinoma of the vagina is rare. When it occurs it is still most commonly found in older women.

Most vaginal tumors are caused by the extension of a squamous cell carcinoma of the cervix, or of an adenocarcinoma of the endometrium, choriocarcinoma, or melanoma. In children, primary adenocarcinoma may be found.

Treatment is by conventional radiotherapy and depends upon the size and accessibility of the tumor. Treatment of the vaginal tumor is by vaginal applicator or by implantation using ^{226}Ra, ^{60}Co, ^{137}Cs, or ^{192}Ir, sources, and is carefully planned to include the whole tumor within the treatment volume. With careful fractionation this volume shrinks with successive treatments.

If the tumor is small, a dose of 6000 rads may be given with a vaginal applicator in two fractions in an overall time of 10-12 days. With a larger tumor and where pelvic nodes are thought to be involved, intracavitary and external therapy must be combined and the treatment prolonged over 5 or 6 weeks. In such treatments the use of intracavitary therapy makes it possible to raise to the required dose in the vaginal mucosa and tumor without subjecting the patient to extensive desquamation of the vulva.

CARCINOMA OF THE VULVA

Primary squamous cell tumors of the vulva are best treated by vulvectomy since the area is often the site of premalignant changes. Where a small basal cell carcinoma or cylindroma occurs in otherwise normal skin, local irradiation may be used, preferably by implantation, but reactions in this site cause considerable pain and healing may be slow. Additionally bleomycin or methotrexate (depending on the grade of the tumors) may be used with radiotherapy for extensive squamous cell tumors. Even a large secondary from an adenocarcinoma of the endometrium should be treated by implantation or by external irradiation, providing the primary tumor can be controlled for a considerable period.

ADVANCES IN RECENT YEARS IN INTRACAVITARY TREATMENT OF CARCINOMA OF THE UTERUS

Since the beginning of the century we have acquired a vast amount of experience in intracavitary therapy using radium sources. This includes the dosimetry of traditional arrangements of the sources, the radiobiology of the tumor and the effects of irradiation on tumors of different types and extent, on the endometrium and vaginal epithelium, and on the radiosensitive bowel and bladder mucosa.

Intracavitary brachytherapy and the interstitial implantation of accessible tumors have maintained their importance throughout the years because we have found that with the accurate positioning of small radioactive sources in a relatively small tumor it is possible to irradiate the whole tumor to a high dose while avoiding areas of over- or underdosage. Although the development of supervoltage external therapy with its high penetration has advanced the treatment of deepseated extensive disease, often, this still requires the addition of brachytherapy with sealed intracavitary sources to raise the dose to a lethal level without producing associated necrosis of the tumor bed or neighboring tissues. It has been agreed internationally that such intracavitary therapy should be available to all women suffering from carcinoma of the cervix or endometrium and that such treatment should be given in a radiotherapy department where associated ^{60}Co teletherapy or treatment with supervoltage x-rays can be added.

Hazards Associated with Use of ^{226}Ra Sources: Change to Radium Substitutes

Since the 1940s there has been increasing general awareness of the hazards associated with the use of ^{226}Ra to the doctors, physicists, and nurses caring for these patients, as well as occasionally to the other patients on the wards, their relatives, and visitors. These matters have been discussed at length in national and international meetings and at conferences sponsored by the World Health Organization and by the International Atomic Energy Authority.

A congress, where these hazards could be discussed, was sponsored in New York by the Department of Health and Mount Sinai Hospital in 1972. In 1973 there was created in Geneva an International Working Party which has discussed and reported on the treatment of cancer of the cervix in developing areas by radium substitutes and afterloading techniques. It has since met in Rio de Janeiro, in Hyderabad (where it participated in a seminar on the same subjects organized by WHO), Yugoslavia, Egypt, and in Istanbul. The next meeting of this international group, sponsored by WHO is planned to take place in Venezuela in 1982. Detailed reports on all the matters discussed in this section will be found in the accounts of these meetings and also in the report of the seminar held in Cambridge in 1978, by WHO, concerning optimization of radiotherapy in developing areas.

While discussions commenced with consideration of the hazards of ^{226}Ra and the advantages of a direct change to ^{60}Co, ^{137}Cs or ^{192}Ir, they later covered the use of miniature sources available, consequent development of manual afterloading techniques, the design of applicators, the improvement in dosimetry, and the introduction of remote loading equipment with conventional dosimetry. In the last meetings, much emphasis has been placed on high dose rate remote loading and radiobiological considerations of different dose rates. The next meeting of the International Working Party will be combined with an international conference of the members with radiotherapists and surgeons from the Middle East and Balkan countries. This conference will also be sponsored by WHO, and will be concerned mainly with the difficulties experienced by radiotherapists in developing areas in the disposal of their radium stocks and their replacement by substitutes.

The most important of the hazards associated with the use of ^{226}Ra is from the production during its disintegration of the radioactive gas radon and alpha particle emitters. If alpha emitters are absorbed into the body as a result of a leaking source, they remain active during a very long physical and biological half-life. In spite of these well-known hazards there is a natural reluctance on the part of many radiotherapists (and of their departments of health and hospitals) to discard sources with such a long life and constant dose rate. However, although ^{226}Ra can be safely handled in a modern development with adequate protective devices, only containers of modern design should be used, and these must be regularly checked. In addition to these special hazards, there is the hazard to hospital personnel and staff from external irradiation of hands and bodies by gamma rays emitted by the sources. These hazards occur in the radium room, where applicators are prepared and sources are stored, in the operating room where they are inserted into the patient, in the x-ray department where the positions of the sources is radiographically checked, and in the wards where nurses and other patients are exposed to irradiation.

Radiotherapists are placed in a position where the number of patients is increasing (especially in developing areas where an increasing proportion of patients with uterine cancer are referred for treatment) and where they have a duty to reduce irradiation to the staff.

The substitutes used in the treatment of cancer are ^{60}Co, ^{139}Cs, and ^{192}Ir. All sources fulfill the chemical and physical safety requirements for the use of isotopes in radiotherapy departments. The choice of the isotope to be used is related largely to the energy of the gamma ray, the specific activity, the half-life, and the expense. The energy must be above the level of that associated with a higher differential absorption in the bone. It is generally accepted by radiobiologists that the action of all these isotopes on the tissues is similar and related to the dose absorbed. More investigation is awaited on the dosimetry close to these sources. A report on this and other aspects of brachytherapy sources will be published by a Working Party of the British Institute of Radiology.

It is generally agreed that the perfect isotope for brachytherapy does not exist. Radium 226 itself has the disadvantage of too high an energy for the small volumes treated. This high energy also involves considerable expense in the provision of thick lead shields for transportation throughout the hospital; a protection that is not only expensive but also very heavy and cumbersome to use. In addition, the relatively low activity of radium sources and the need for thick-walled containers because of gas protection and particle emission result in clumsy containers unsuitable for any but very simple afterloading procedures.

Cobalt 60 (1.17 and 1.33 MeV Gamma Energies, 5.2 Years Half-Life)

These sources are relatively inexpensive but have an energy too high for intracavitary and implantation dosimetry, while protection is very expensive. Its short life requires frequent replacement of sources and regular recalculation of dose rates. For these reasons, it is not suitable for direct placement or for manual afterloading, but ^{60}Co is used for high dose rate remote loading.

Cesium 137 (0. 664 MeV Gamma Energy, 30 Years Half-Life)

Cesium is the isotope of choice in manual afterloading techniques. Although its energy is higher than the ideal, the necessary protection is cheaper and lighter than with radium and cobalt. Sources incorporated in stable, low-solubility glass or ceramic and sealed in stainless sealed containers can reproduce the dosimetry of the radium tubes to which the radiotherapist is accustomed. For instance, in the Simon source, the ceramic source incorporating the ^{137}Ce is sealed in a steel needle of 1 mm external diameter. A length of 10 mm is equivalent to 15 mg ^{226}Ra. (Sources, of course, must be permanently sealed in metallic containers.)

In the Amersham Manchester applicator, flexible source trains of sealed sources are loaded in metallic flexible applicators of 3.2 mm external diameter; the loading is varied according to the user's need (Fig. 4). The life of such applicators is determined by the life of the holder and about 10 years. As well as being important in afterloading techniques, ^{137}Ce is used widely in the place of ^{226}Ra in tubes and needles for surface applicators and for implantation.

Iridium 192 (0. 13-1. 06 MeV Gamma Energy, 74.2 Day Half-Life)

Iridium has many of the characteristics of the ideal isotope for gynecological cancer. It has a suitable energy for the dosimetry required but without specific bone absorption. Protection is simpler, less heavy, and less expensive. It has a high specific activity and is used by many for afterloading interstitial implants and gynecological applicators. It is relatively inexpensive but unfortunately, in spite of these advantages, the half-life is very short. Departments using this isotope must be geared to the work with a regular arrangement for the replacement of sources and with efficient bookkeeping, calibration, and dosimetry. It is the isotope of choice for afterloading implantation techniques, but most centers prefer

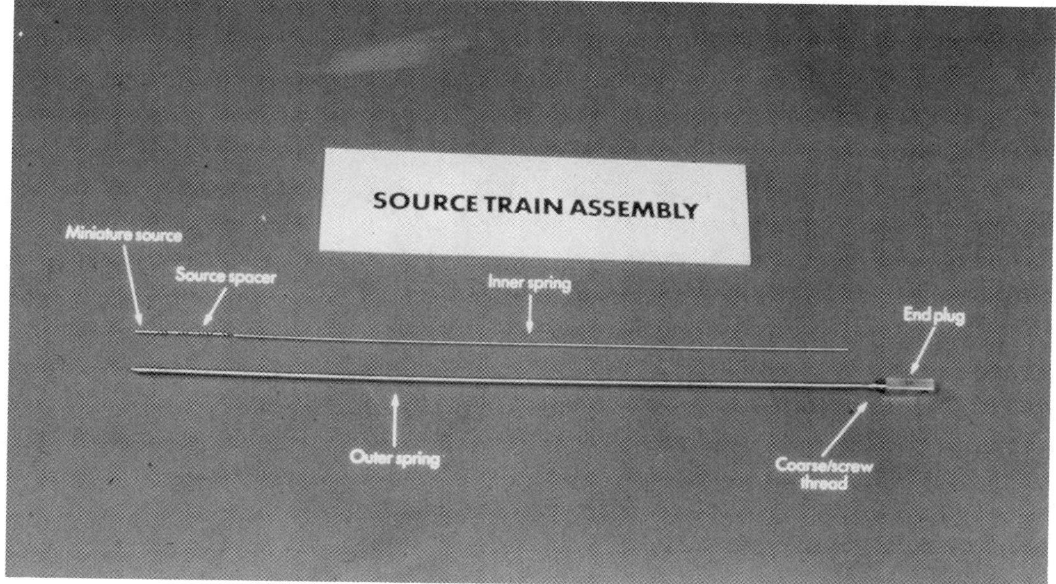

Figure 4. Amersham Manchester applicator.

cesium for the manual afterloading of gynecological applicators. Although the specific activity is sufficient for iridium to be used for high dose rate remote loading, the frequent change of curie-sized sources would provide departmental difficulties much greater than those experienced with ^{60}Co sources.

The Change From ^{226}Ra to Substitutes: Manual Afterloading

The first step in many departments was a change from radium to an alternate source using sources of the same strength and dimensions giving very nearly the same dosimetry. After a few years the introduction of miniature sources made possible by the high specific activity of cobalt, cesium, and iridium stimulated the rapid development of afterloading techniques. The rapid progress of this work was due very largely to the work of Henschke (33) in New York and later of Pierquin (53) in Paris, who brought Henschke's technique back to Europe and founded the European Group of Curietherapists.

The introduction of the principles of manual afterloading in these centers led to the development of many applicators, among them in the United States, the Henschke applicator and sources developed at the Memorial Hospital and later at Howard University, the Fletcher-Suit applicator from Houston (Fig. 5), the Charyulu applicator from Miami, and the Simon applicator from New York. In Paris, Pierquin, first at the Institut Gustave Roussy and later at the Hospital Henri Mondor, developed afterloading iridium applicators. He and Chassagne developed the

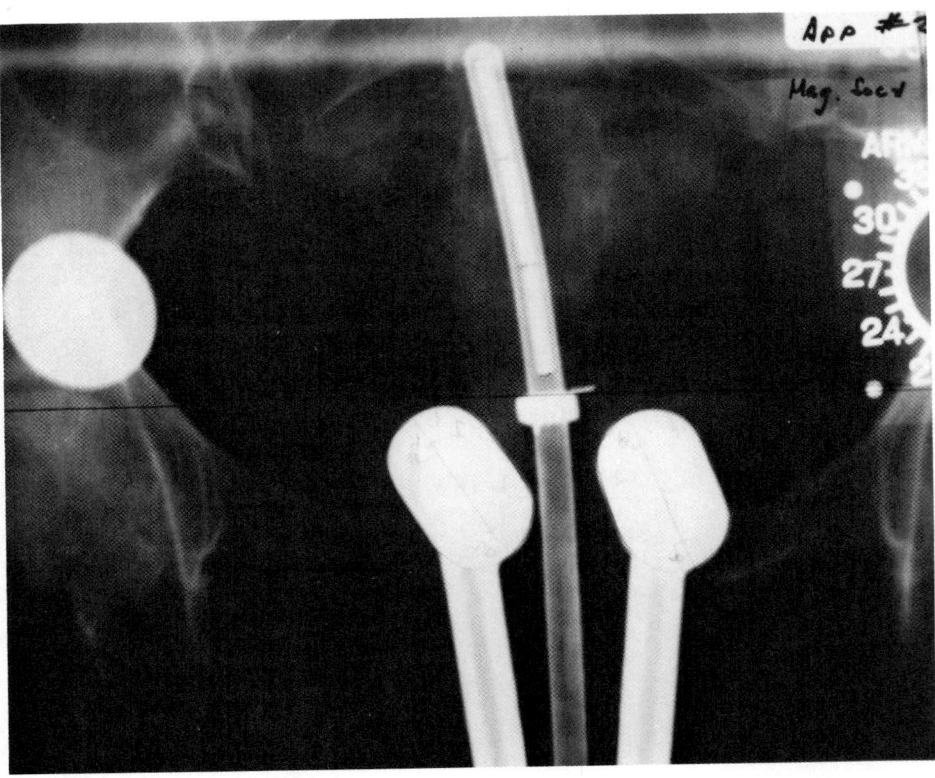

Figure 5. Fletcher-Suit tandem and ovoid in the uterus and vagina.

use of vaginal molds and manual afterloading at the Institut Gustave Roussy. The conventional dose rate remote loading Curietron was developed at the Gustave Roussy and is now used in many hospitals. In the United Kingdom, Haybittle produced at Cambridge a manual afterloading version of the Manchester system and The Radiochemical Center at Amersham has now marketed a disposable plastic set of Manchester tubes and ovoids together with source trains of ^{137}Ce appropriate for reproducing the Manchester dosimetry in patients of different sizes (Fig. 6).

In addition to these applicators and sources, many radiotherapy centers throughout the world have adapted the applicators to which they were accustomed for afterloading techniques using ^{137}Ce. The design of the applicators themselves has received considerable attention; especially with the aim of improving the dosimetry by fixing the position of the sources and avoiding movement during the treatment. Increased comfort to the patient occurs by improving the construction of the applicator, restricting its weight, and using disposable or easily sterilizable applicators.

Remote Loading

The appreciation of the advantages of manual afterloading led to the development of remote loading. This technique avoids all irradiation of staff, the patient being alone in her room for conventional dose rate therapy or in a heavily protected treatment room when high dose rate therapy is used.

Conventional Dose Rate Therapy

The advantages of remote loading were demonstrated by Henschke at the Memorial Hospital in New York, and later the Curietron in Paris was produced by G.E.R. in collaboration with the Institut Gustave Roussy. This machine, using ^{137}Ce sources, reproduces the Paris treatment without alteration in dose, dose rate, or dosimetry. Cesium sources were introduced and removed mechanically and the same holders fixed in a plastic vaginal mold made individually for each patient.

The Cervitron was introduced in the Radiumhemmet and also in Geneva and reproduced a Stockholm-type treatment. In this machine, active and inactive ^{137}Cs sources were arranged as prescribed by the radiotherapist to produce the required isodose curves for each source; thé spheres were then transferred pneumatically to the preplaced catheters.

The Cervitron is no longer constructed but the principles of construction are found again in the Selektron used at present for 50 rads/min medium dose rate therapy. Soon there will be introduced a high dose rate treatment machine.

High Dose Rate Remote Loading

The Cathetron is a British machine made by T.E.M., to specifications agreed on by a national committee of radiotherapists, physicists, radiobiologists, and engineers. It was designed so that radiotherapists might continue the Manchester-type treatments already used in many of our hospitals without any change in the general management of cases of different histologies and stages by intracavitary therapy combined where necessary with external supervoltage irradiation, or with surgery. The Cathetron has been in use in an increasing number of hospitals in industrialized and developing countries since 1966 and many 5- and 10-year results of its cure rates are available.

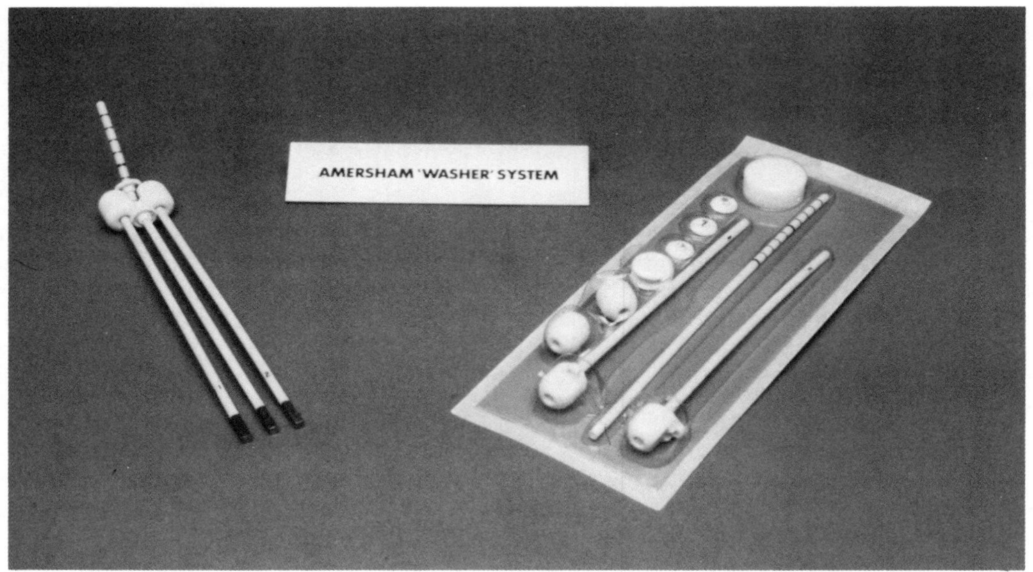

Figure 6. A: The Amersham modified Manchester applicators.

About 50 of these machines are now in use throughout the world. A report on the use of these and of other high dose rate equipment manufactured in Japan and elsewhere was produced after a meeting of the High Dose Rate Users held at the Middlesex Hospital, London, in 1978. These proceedings are to be published by the British Institute of Radiology. A reluctance has been felt by many radiotherapists to change to high dose rate treatment because of the anticipated danger of late complications in the normal tissues. None such have been reported and at the meetings referred to there was general agreement that the use of high dose rate treatment in the doses and fractionation reported should be accepted as of equal value to the traditional low-dose therapy. Details of the Cathetron and its use have been included in this volume because its value has been proven over recent years, especially in the very busy clinics with heavy work loads that are found in developing areas.

The Cathetron (Fig. 7) consists of a heavily protected source-safe which contains nine sources of ^{60}Co varying in strength from 1-10 Ci of which up to three can be used at one time. The safe is so designed that sources totaling 50 Ci of ^{60}Co will give a leakage radiation of no more than 2 mR/hr at 5 cm from the surface of the container. Since, however, 25 Ci or more may be used during the treatment of a patient, the machine must be positioned in a heavily protected room (inclusing floor and ceiling). The patient is watched by television or by a mirror system and by cardiac monitors during the treatment, which may be carried out under anesthesia or under sedation.

Each patient remains 20-25 min in the suite and each treatment lasts 2-5 min. Many radiotherapists who use the Cathetron on only one or two sessions each week have placed the machine in a cobalt treatment room and continue to use that machine on the other days of the week, but in developing areas where the intake of carcinoma of the uterus exceeds several thousands of patients each year and the

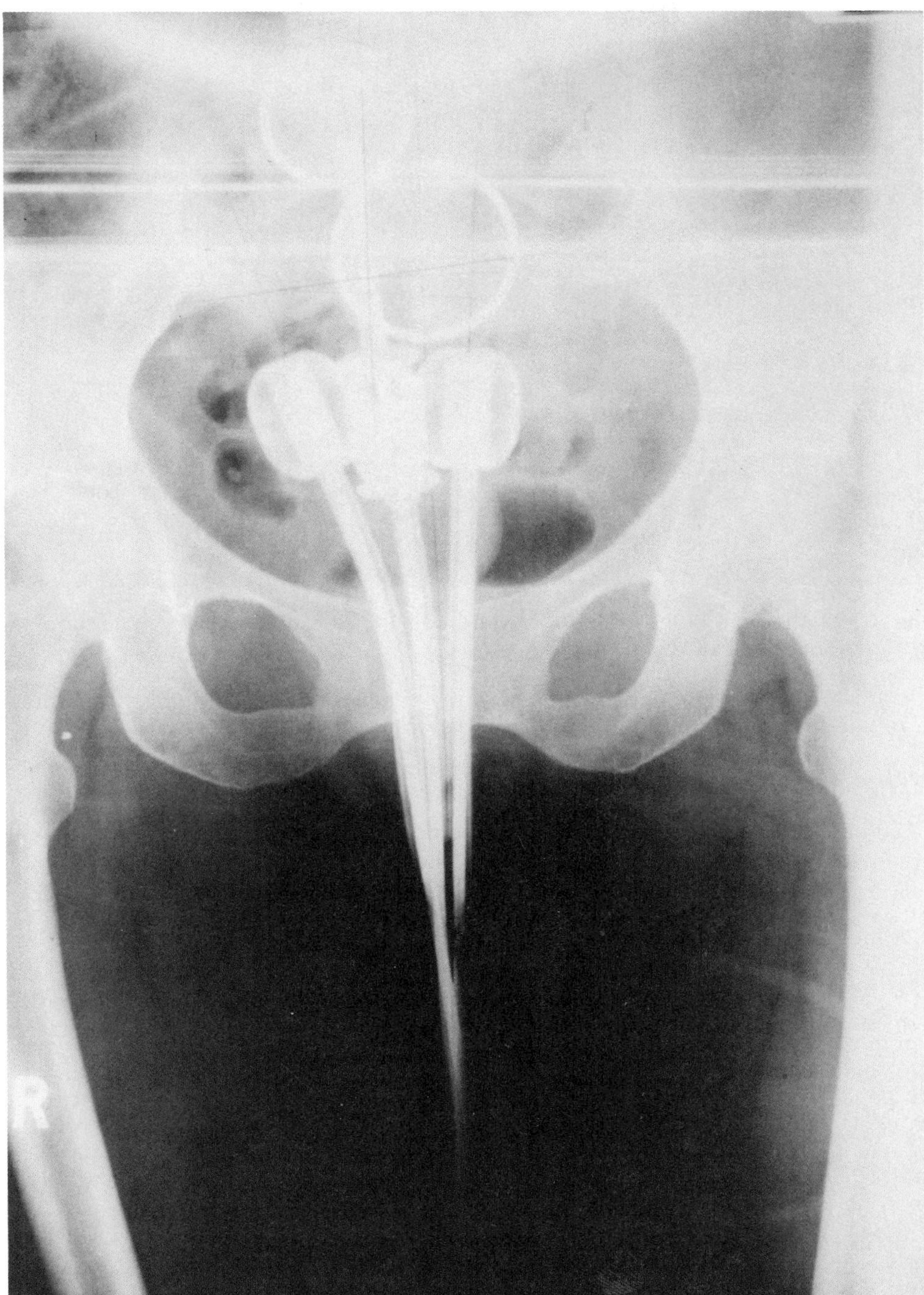

Figure 6. B: Amersham applicators in place.

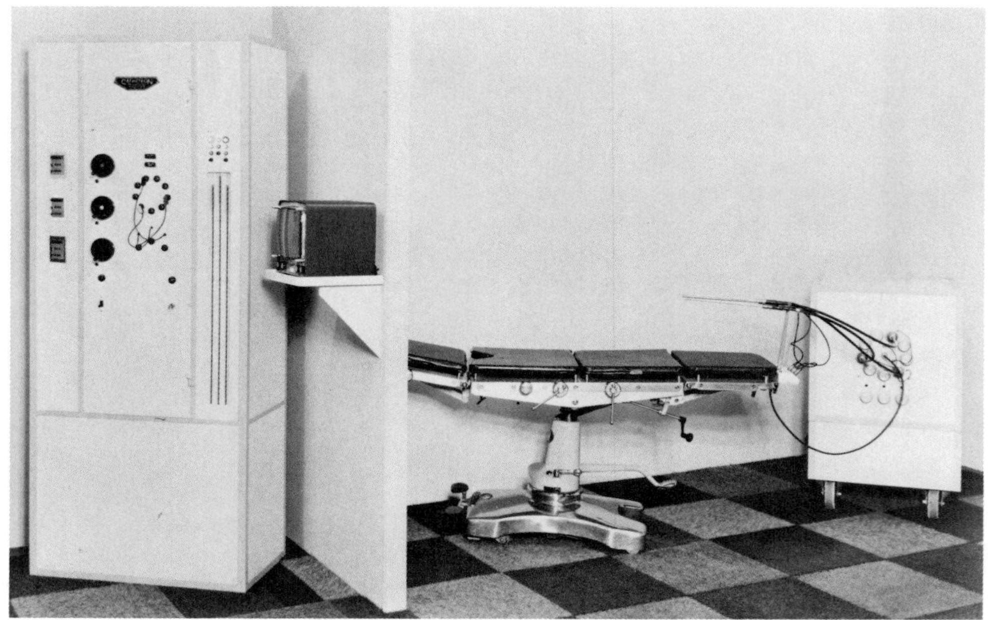

Figure 7. Cathetron. The console is outside the treatment room. The safe and guide tubes are seen in the room.

weekly load is 30, 50, or more intracavitary treatments, a separate treatment suite is used and 12 or more treatments are carried out daily.

Sources

The radiotherapist is provided with the dosimetry to which he is accustomed. The standard arrangement of one intrauterine and two vaginal sources is usually employed, although where necessary a single intrauterine or intravaginal source is used or two or more parallel sources positioned and kept parallel in a plastic Stockholm box.

At the Middlesex Hospital the Manchester dosimetry is used with five sources with a choice of three different uterine lengths (4-7 cm). There are two sources for vaginal ovoids. Three other sources are designed for the preoperative treatment of cancer of the endometrium, where a wider spread of the isodose at the fundus is needed. A ninth source is possible although it was found convenient to keep one socket empty to make checks in position with an empty container. With this equipment a therapist can complete a schedule of 10 or more cases in 3 hr. The therapist has eight or nine sources of different lengths and strengths available from which he can choose. This gives a much wider selection than has been available when using conventional radium sources.

The Treatment

During the treatment, the sources are positioned in metallic catheters inserted with the patient in the lithotomy position on the treatment table. The sources are fixed in place by clamps attached to a rail fixed to the table (Fig. 8). Output source tubes from the safe connect the safe to the catheters and the sources move automatically along these when the start button on the console is pressed. The source

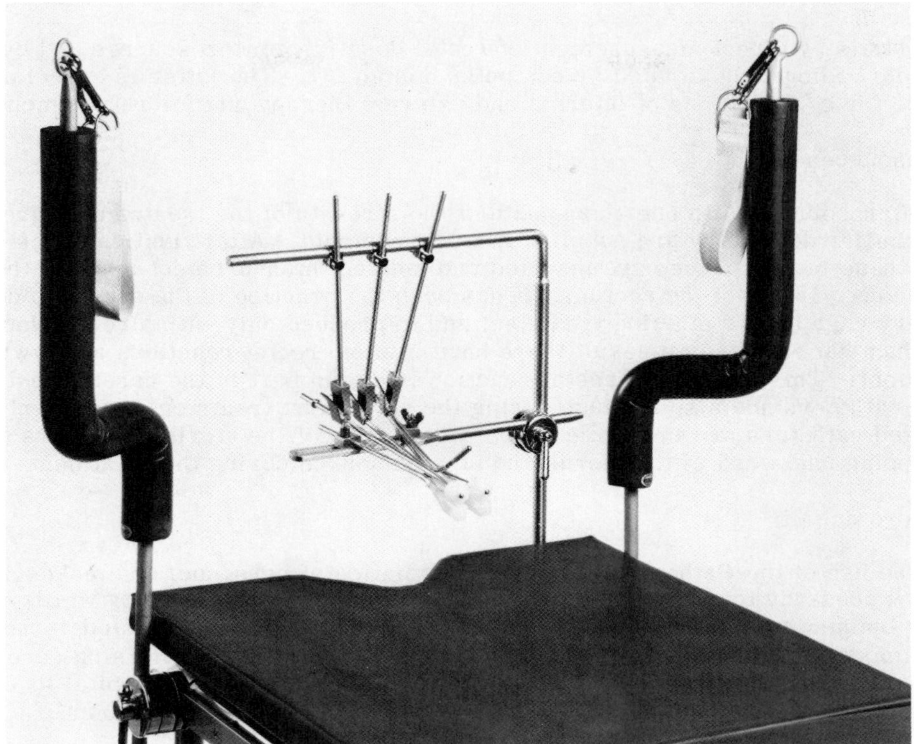

Figure 8. Intracavitary sources of the Cathetron fixed to the treatment table.

moves always to the tip of the catheter, 168 cm from the center of the safe (the output tubes plus the catheter total 134 cm). Since the uterine and vaginal sources are clamped in position and so fixed, additional packing is not necessary to maintain their position, although a rectal retractor or packing may be useful to prevent the ovoids from coming into close contact with the rectum. Should there be any movement of the patient, the sources must be withdrawn and checks made in their position before resuming treatment. At the end of the treatment the sources are automatically withdrawn to the safety of the source container. (The source drive mechanisms are fitted with a gravity return mechanism which, in the event of a main power failure, automatically returns the sources to the source container.)

The remote control (Fig. 7) is positioned outside the treatment room in a safe area and provides a facility for the precise control of the exposure times of each source assembly and a remote indirect indication of its exact position in the catheter. Three predetermined digital countdown and countup timers are fitted, one for each of the three source assemblies being used. Mechanical and electrical interlocks are fitted to the Cathetron, and unless all these are correctly made the channel indicator lamps on the control panel will not light. Because of the very high dose rate the whole treatment takes only 2-5 min. Only when the indicator lamp shows all interlocks are made, and time has been set on the treatment timers, and the start button pressed will the radioactive sources move from the source-safe through the output source tubes into the catheters. Here they take up accurate predetermined positions. Precise mechanically linked indications of the exact position of all three sources are given on the control panel, from the time they leave the container until they reach their final position.

Dosimetry

This is by direct measurement of rectal dose from microsources and by stereoscopic radiographs studied by computer dosimetry. The latter is especially desirable for combinations of internal and external therapy and for retreatments.

Microsources

Microsources with one-thousandth of the strength of the treatment sources and with similar dosimetry are supplied in a storage safe. After fixation of the catheters, these microsources are inserted and a direct measurement made of the dose in the lower 10 cm of the rectum. It has been the practice of the author to do this in every case before starting treatment and to proceed only with a rectal dose of less than 400 rads. As a result there have been no rectal reactions at all with this treatment. This absence of rectal reaction is due in part to the careful positioning of the catheters and also because during the very short treatment the patient and the fixed catheters are immobile. The anteversion of the uterine catheters allows no slipping backward of the uterus and uterine source during the treatment.

Radioprotection

The use of the Cathetron avoids all irradiation of personnel and makes it no longer necessary to nurse these patients in special radiation therapy wards with highly trained nurses and strict precautions. The patients are treated in hostel accommodation, with a freeing of ward beds for others needing nursing care. It is obvious that there are considerable financial advantages for the hospital to offset the initial expense of the machine, the sources, and the treatment room.

In the radiotherapy department there is a large administrative advantage in limiting these treatments to one or more short periods each week when the trained personnel, therapists, physicists, and technicians, can meet together to carry out the treatments and be free to carry out other activities during the remainder of the week.

The patients are themselves freed from the fear and from the discomfort or real pain associated with conventional dose rate therapy and from the involved catheterization and packing. The palliative treatment of recurrent disease, often impossible because of local tenderness, now presents no difficulties, while in all patients the incidence of cystitis and vaginitis almost disappears.

Cost

Although there are many financial savings in staff and ward costs associated with a change to high dose rate remote loading, there is considerable initial expense in the purchase of the machine and in the acquiring or building of a protected suitable treatment room. Provision must also be made for replacement of the sources every 4 or 5 years.

High dose rate remote therapy should be carried out in large hospitals with regional responsibilities to which patients from a large area are referred for therapy. It is of special value in developing areas where, using several teams, 100 or more treatments can be carried out on outpatients each week throughout the year. In some of these, associated external therapy is reduced to a single treatment each week.

In hospitals where less than 10 intracavitary treatments are carried out, the use of manual afterloading with ^{137}Ce or ^{192}Ir sources is sufficient for radioprotection. Where there are only occasional treatments, the replacement of permanently loaded applicators by cesium should suffice.

Total Dose and Fractionation

Compared with ^{226}Ra therapy the total dose is dropped to 66%, while the fractionation is doubled because of the very short treatment times. Thus, with cancer of the cervix the dose with radium was 3000 rads to point A in one treatment of 36 hr. The author now gives three doses of 750 rads at weekly intervals and sometimes a fourth treatment of 500 rads (this is associated with 4500 rads in 4.5 weeks external therapy).

With carcinoma of the endometrium the author used to give 6000 rads to the myometrium in two treatments of 36 hr with an interval of 1 week. She now gives four weekly treatments of 1000 rads. She has found that vaginal extensions of disease are destroyed by two or three doses to the surface of 1000 rads given at weekly intervals. Each of the treatments described are delivered in 2-5 min.

SECTION II. CARCINOMA OF THE OVARY

H. E. Lambert, M. B., B. S.

Carcinoma of the ovary is now the most common cause of death from gynecological cancer in Europe and the United States. The incidence is 15:100,000 women per annum (68) and is rising, with most cases occurring after the age of 40 years with a peak incidence in the seventh decade. The high incidence together with its poor prognosis, 5-year survival of 28%, has led to increased efforts over the last few years to find better methods of treatment. Unfortunately, approximately two-thirds of patients present to the physician when their disease has already spread beyond the pelvis (stages III and IV). This is due to the insidious nature of the signs and symptoms of carcinoma of the ovary which are nonspecific, for example, indigestion, abdominal distention, abdominal pain, anorexia, and weight loss. Later an abdominal mass may be noticed or abnormal menstrual or postmenopausal bleeding. As the disease is asymptomatic in the early stages, patients will continue to present with advanced disease until an adequate screening program has been evolved. In this regard tumor markers such as serum enzymes are being tested and may lead to a biochemical test in the future (55). The marked difference in the 5-year survival in stage I, i.e., disease confined to the ovaries, 60-70%, compared to less than 5% for advanced disease, makes this problem of early diagnosis paramount.

ETIOLOGY

The cause of cases of ovarian cancer are not known. The common epithelial tumors have been found to be more frequently present in single women and women of low fertility suggesting that some factor is lowering fertility and increasing the risk of cancer in these women (39). Cancer of the breast is also more common in such women. No association between the use of oral contraceptives and ovarian cancer has been found, and they may even play a protective role if the effect of continuous ovulation on the ovarian epithelium induces neoplasia. Other possible factors that have been considered are asbestosis and cosmetic talc (44).

PATHOLOGY

Tumors of the ovary are cystic or solid and may be benign, of borderline malignancy, or frank carcinomas. There have been many different classifications of ovarian tumors but the classification used by the World Health Organization is becoming more widely accepted. A modified version is shown on Table 3. More than 85% of malignant ovarian carcinomas are epithelial in origin; the main types being serous, mucinous, and endometrioid (48). The others will mainly be undifferentiated or unclassified.

Malkasian and his coauthors (48) found that low-grade tumors tend to be more often associated with earlier stage disease but that grading is of prognostic significance since, taken stage for stage, patients with poorly differentiated tumors fare worse than those with well-differentiated tumors. The histological cell type is not prognostically significant except that more of the mucinous and endometrioid lesions are lower stage and lower grade than the serous cystadenocarcinomas.

Table 3. Histological Classification of Ovarian Tumors

I. Common epithelial tumors
   - A. Serous tumors
   - B. Mucinous tumors
   - C. Endometrioid tumors
   - D. Clear cell (mesonephroid)
   - E. Brenner tumors
   - F. Mixed epithelial tumors
   - G. Undifferentiated carcinomas
   - H. Unclassified carcinomas

   May be:
   Benign
   Of borderline malignancy
   Malignant

II. Sex cord stromal tumors
   - A. Granulosa stroma cell tumors
   - B. Androblastoma; Sertoli Leydig cell tumors
   - C. Gynandroblastomas
   - D. Unclassified

III. Lipid cell tumors

IV. Germ cell tumors
   - A. Dysgerminoma
   - B. Endodermal sinus tumor (yolk sac tumor)
   - C. Embryonal cell tumor
   - D. Polyembryoma
   - E. Choriocarcinoma
   - F. Terratomas
   - G. Mixed forms

V. Gonadoblastoma

VI. Soft tissue tumors not specific to the ovary

VII. Unclassified tumors

VIII. Secondary (metastatic tumors)

STAGING

A summary of the staging of ovarian cancer as defined by the UICC (1978) and FIGO is shown in Table 4. Readers should consult the UICC Classification of Malignant Tumors for complete details (67).

Accurate assessment of the extent of disease is crucial to the management of each individual and should be performed before any treatment is instituted.

Investigations needed are as follows:

Full clinical examination
Full blood count
Blood chemistry; in particular, urea, electrolytes, and liver function tests
Chest x-ray
Abdominal x-ray
Barium enema
Lymphangiogram
Ultrasonography and/or computerized axial tomography
Cytology of pleural and ascitic fluid if present
Laparoscopy and/or laparotomy

Where disease appears to be confined to the abdomen, laparoscopy and/or laparotomy are essential both in order to confirm the diagnosis by biopsy and to assess the extent of the disease.

Ovarian cancer spreads by the following routes:

Direct
Transcoelomic
Lymphatic
Hematogenous

Table 4. Comparative Staging of Ovarian Carcinoma

UICC	Ovary	FIGO
T1	Limited to ovaries	I
T1a	One ovary; no ascites	Ia
T1b	Both ovaries; no ascites	Ib
T1c	One or both ovaries; with ascites	Ic
T2	With pelvic extension	II
T2a	Uterus and/or tubes; no ascites	IIa
T2b	Other pelvic tissues; no ascites	IIb
T2c	Other pelvic tissues; with ascites	IIc
T3	Extension to small bowel/omentum in true pelvis or intraperitoneal metastases/retroperitoneal nodes	III
M1	Distant organs	IV

Direct spread occurs once the tumor has breached the capsule of the ovary and involves the pelvic peritoneum and pelvic organs. Later spread will involve bowel and omentum.

Transcoelomic spread is the main route. Cells shed from the surface of the tumor can seed throughout the peritoneal cavity, including the diaphragmatic area. Peritoneal fluid, free particles, and cells flow upward through the paracolic gutters and are drained by lymphatic channels on the undersurface of the diaphragm into the subpleural lymph nodes. Blockage of these channels by malignancy will produce ascites. As pointed out by Bush (13) ascites can also be caused, as in benign lesions, by an inability of the lymphatic channels to drain excess fluid. The importance of this subdiaphragmatic lymphatic system in the spread of ovarian cancer has been stressed by, among others, Bagley et al. (6) and Rosenoff et al. (58). The latter found an incidence of 44% of diaphragmatic metastasis in 16 patients who at laparotomy had been staged as I or II, when peritonescopy was subsequently performed to visualize the undersurface of the diaphragm.

The main lymphatic drainage from the ovaries is into the retroperitoneal nodes. Occasionally spread occurs via the broad ligament to the external iliac and hypogastric nodes and rarely via the round ligament to the inguinal nodes. While lymphangiogram will detect gross lymph node involvement, microscopic deposits will not be demonstrated and, therefore, biopsy of the retroperitoneal nodes should be carried out as part of the surgical staging procedure. Unrealized paraaortic node involvement may account for some of the failure to cure apparent stage I or II carcinoma of the ovary.

Hematological spread is usually late and is mainly to the liver and lung. Bone metastasis is rare.

It is therefore essential that a full surgical staging procedure should include:

Cytological examination of peritoneal fluid or in the absence of ascites, peritoneal washings.

Careful exploration of the abdomen including the subdiaphragmatic area and the paracolic gutters.

Biopsy of any suspicious area. Day and Smith (20) advocate a radical approach with multiple blind biopsies of the subdiaphragmatic areas, paracolic gutters, and pelvic peritoneum to rule out occult metastases.

Biopsy of retroperitoneal nodes.

TREATMENT

Surgery

Surgery is the primary treatment in carcinoma of the ovary. The operation performed is a total hysterectomy, bilateral salpingo-oophorectomy, and omentectomy. At the same time the staging procedures described previously should be carried out. Omentectomy is necessary because histological evidence of spread may well be found even if the omentum looks macroscopically normal, and in addition its removal facilitates subsequent laparoscopy. If the omentum cannot be removed, biopsies should be taken. Patients with stage II and early stage III, in whom, for technical reasons hysterectomy and bilateral salpingo-oophorectomy cannot be carried out, fare worse than those in whom the operation is complete. This is probably related to the depth of cancer invasion into neighboring tissues (14). Where there is extensive spread of carcinoma of the ovary, reduction of tumor mass should be as radical as possible, as residual masses larger than 2 cm are associated with a very poor prognosis (20).

In stage I (confined to ovaries) with a well-differentiated tumor and intact capsule, radical surgery alone is the treatment of choice. In all other cases of stage I and for the other stages, additional treatment, radiotherapy, or chemotherapy is advocated, because as even in early stage I there is probably residual disease (30). When initial surgery is incomplete, subsequent therapy may allow complete removal of residual tumor at a second-look operation.

Surgery, i.e., laparoscopy and laparotomy, is the most accurate method of assessing response to treatment. Peritoneal washings can be obtained for cytological evidence of persistent disease, minute deposits not detected by ultrasonic or computerized tomographic scanning can be directly visualized, and biopsies can be taken from any suspicious lesions or from areas likely to be involved, e.g., pelvic peritoneum or under the diaphragm. The aim of the therapy, complete remission, cannot be verified unless these procedures have been carried out.

Radiotherapy

The role of radiotherapy in the management of stages I and II ovarian carcinoma remains controversial and will continue to be so until appropriate clinical trials have been carried out. Inadequate pretreatment staging may explain the relatively disappointing results in early stage disease where postoperative radiotherapy to the pelvis alone has been given, as this cannot be effective when there is already disease outside the pelvis. However, where the extent of the disease has been adequately delineated, there is sometimes a case for limiting the treatment volume to the pelvis in order to reduce the morbidity associated with radiation. More extensive fields to give prophylactic irradiation to the paraaortic nodes, the medial parts of the diaphragm and the subpleural diaphragmatic lymph nodes has been advocated (30), while others include the whole abdomen as well as the pelvis. Dembo et al. (21) found that postoperative abdominopelvic irradiation gave better results, in terms of survival and control of abdominal disease, in stage IB, II and stage III with minimal abdominal spread, than pelvic irradiation or pelvic irradiation and chlorambucil.

In stage III carcinoma of the ovary, irradiation to the whole abdomen and pelvis can be employed where there is minimal residual disease after surgery, but results are poor if deposits are larger than 2 cm. Chemotherapy is therefore the preferred treatment in these latter cases. Radiotherapy may be used in stage IV for palliation.

Technique

Radiotherapy to the pelvis alone is given using megavoltage radiation with three to four fields. The field size is usually 15 x 15 cm. A dose of 5000 rads, tumor dose, in 25 fractions in 5 weeks is sufficient for minimal disease, but larger doses, up to 6000 rads, may be needed for larger masses in which case the top-up dose to 6000 rads should be given to a reduced volume. All fields should be treated daily.

Radiotherapy to the pelvis and abdomen involves treating an area which extends from the top of the diaphragm to the bottom of the obturator foramen. It can be carried out using stationary open fields or moving-strip techniques. A prospective comparison of these two techniques carried out by Fazekas and Maier (26) failed to show any significant difference in length of survival or local tumor control for either of these methods and the complication rate was also similar. Radiotherapy using the open-field method consists of two large fields, anterior and posterior, using megavoltage. Doses vary. Fazekas and Maier (26) gave 4000 rads midplane (40 fractions/56 days), with kidney shielding (estimated dose 2500-2700 rads) but no liver shielding. Fuks (31) gave 5500 rads/27 fractions/37 days to the lower abdomen and 4000 rads/20 fractions/33 days to the upper abdomen, but shielding to the liver and diaphragm limited the dose to these organs to 2000 rads. Earlier studies (34) had shown an 18% incidence of symptomatic radiation hepatitis where 3000 rads or more was delivered to the whole liver. We follow the policy outline by Order et al. (78) using delayed split abdominal irradiation to give 3000 rads to the abdomen with opposed fields with kidney shielding and to top up the true pelvis to 4000 rads. A maximum dose rate of 600 rads midplane in 4 fractions per week to the upper abdomen and 800 rads midplane to the lower abdomen is given and then increased to 1000 rads weekly for the reduced volume to the true pelvis.

The moving-strip technique has been described in detail by Dembo et al. (22). Using a 22 MeV betatron this technique is started with 10 fractions of 225 rads treating five times weekly to a 15 x 15 cm field to the pelvis using opposed anterior-posterior portals. This is immediately followed by downward moving-strip abdominopelvic irradiation, using either ^{60}Co or a 25 MV photon beam, from 1 cm above the domes of the diaphragm in expiration to below the obturator foramen. The field length is divided into 2.5 cm strips. Starting with a 5 cm length, the field size is slowly increased to a maximum length of 10 cm. The prescribed dose is 2250 rads midplane in 10 fractions making the total pelvic dose 4500 rads in 20 fractions. Posterior renal shielding is used throughout but no liver shielding is used.

Radioactive Isotopes

The intraperitoneal use of radioactive isotopes is limited to stages I and II carcinoma of the ovary. Radioactive colloidal chromic phosphorus ^{32}P has been used postoperatively and appears to be safe (3). The use of colloidal gold (^{198}Au) has been compared with pelvic irradiation (41) and while there was no difference in survival, stage I patients treated by intraperitoneal ^{198}Au had a lower recurrence rate but a greater number of fatal complications. Colloidal gold is not available in the United States.

Toxic Effects of Radiation

The consequences of treating large volumes of tissue cannot be ignored. These will include: bone marrow depression occurring during therapy with a fall in white blood cell and platelet count and later in the level of hemoglobin, but rarely of much significance; and gastrointestinal toxicity, nausea, vomiting, and diarrhea, occurring to some extent in all patients especially if total abdominal irradiation is carried out. Late gastrointestinal complications also occur. Fuks (31) reported that 24 out of 167 patients (14%) developed severe bowel stenosis or hemorrhage requiring surgical intervention. Radiation damage to the liver and kidneys can be prevented by limiting the dose to below 2500 rads.

Chemotherapy

Chemotherapy is playing an increasingly important role in the treatment of carcinoma of the ovary. It is the treatment of choice in stage IV, in stage III where debulking is initially impossible, and where tumor deposits larger than 2 cm remain in the abdominal cavity after surgery. Chemotherapy is also used as an adjunct to surgery in earlier stages as an alternative to postoperative radiotherapy (62).

Single Agents

The alkylating drugs have been the most commonly used agents, in particular, cyclophosphamide, melphalan, chlorambucil, and thiotepa. Objective responses as reported in the literature vary between 35-65% initially, with 5-15% of all patients still responding after 2 years (74).

Unfortunately, the criteria used for assessing responses were usually based on clinical findings only, and it is difficult to interpret the true response rate in most of the published studies. Hopefully, with the use of more sophisticated scanning techniques to detect subclinical tumor masses and the use of laparoscopy and laparotomy to obtain pathological confirmation of response, future assessments of drug efficacy will be more valuable.

Alkylating agents are usually given continuously or in pulsed courses, by mouth, by the intravenous route, and directly into the peritoneal or pleural cavities, the latter route for the local control of ascites or pleural effusion. There is no evidence that ascites are better controlled by giving the drugs intraperitoneally compared to systemic administration nor are large abdominal masses affected.

Drugs, other than alkylating agents, which have been used with some success in the treatment of ovarian carcinoma, include the antimetabolites, 5-FU and methotrexate; the antitumor antibiotic, adriamycin, and hexamethylmelamine which is derived from an alkylating agent triethylene-melamine. This latter drug has been found to have activity where resistance has developed to alkylating agents (38). Young (75) reports on prospective studies at the M. D. Anderson Hospital comparing objective responses of at least 3 months' duration in patients with stages III and IV ovarian cancer to melphalan, 5-FU, adriamycin, and hexamethylmelamine. This showed an equal response rate of approximately 30% for melphalan, adriamycin, and hexamethylmelamine and a much lower rate of 17% for 5-FU. Progestogens have been used with little success in ovarian cancer, but there are a few reported cases of long survival following its use (47); some response could be expected in endometrioid tumors.

Over the last few years great interest has been taken in the drug cis-platinum (cis-dichlorodiammineplatinum) (21). Work at The Royal Marsden Hospital showed a 26.5% response rate with a median duration of 6 months in patients with advanced adenocarcinoma of the ovary who had become resistant to conventional chemotherapy (71). This activity in patients resistant to alkylating agents has been confirmed by Young et al. (76) who obtained a 29% response rate in 24 patients. Cis-platinum has been used to a much lesser extent in previously untreated patients. One such report (12) showed a response rate of 35% in 17 cases.

In the future, cell culture techniques or xenografts may be valuable in determining the optimum chemotherapeutic agent in each patient with ovarian cancer.

Combination Chemotherapy

Combination chemotherapy has the theoretical advantage that it allows ovarian cancer to be treated by several drugs which have been shown to have activity when used singly. Drugs which are phase specific and cycle specific and which have differing toxicities are combined. The use of several cytotoxic agents together may require lowering the dose of each to less than would be given as a single agent to ensure patient tolerance. Unfortunately, if only one of the drugs being used is actually active in an individual patient, then that patient may receive a suboptimal dose.

In the management of advanced ovarian cancer, the place of combination chemotherapy is at present unresolved. Many studies have been carried out after single alkylating agents or radiotherapy have failed, usually with a poor response. Only a few prospective trials have taken place and pathological confirmation of response has not always been obtained. Chemotherapy, like radiotherapy, is more effective where residual disease is minimal (less than 2 cm), and Young (77) in a comparative study of melphalan with a four-drug combination [hexamethylmelamine, cyclophosphamide, methotrexate, and 5-FU (Hex-CAF)] found that the combined drugs gave a significantly increased response rate, especially in these cases of minimal residual disease. At the Mayo Clinic, cyclophosphamide plus adriamycin was found to be no better than cyclophosphamide alone in advanced ovarian cancer, but the combination was better than the single agent in patients with minimal residual disease after surgery. Complete excision of disease prior to chemotherapy had an even better prognosis (24). Other work has failed to show any improvement in survival by the addition of other drugs to an alkylating agent, e.g., melphalan (7). Of interest is the work by Ozols et al. (52) who found using a modified system of Broders' grades I-IV based on cytological detail that Hexa-CAF improved survival compared to single alkylating drugs in patients with grades II and III lesions, but there was no advantage over the single agent in grades I or IV.

Cis-platinum is now being investigated in various combinations in patients with advanced ovarian cancer who have not had previous chemotherapy. In one such study carried out at The Royal Marsden Hospital (72) in 58 patients, none of whom had had radical surgery, cis-platinum and chlorambucil combination was compared with cis-platinum, chlorambucil, and adriamycin. Complete clinical responses were seen in 32 and 41% of the patients. Second-look operations were performed in 12 of the responders to carry out debulking and to assess response, and in 6 of these patients there was no histological evidence of residual carcinoma. Whether cis-platinum alone will give as good results as when used in the various combinations now being assessed in several centers still remains to be determined.

Toxicity

All cytotoxic drugs have important immediate toxic effects. For example:

1. Bone marrow depression occurs with the use of almost all the drugs.

2. Alopecia is marked with cyclophosphamide and adriamycin.

3. Gastrointestinal toxicity such as nausea and vomiting is particularly severe with hexamethylmelamine and cis-platinum and stomatitis with methotrexate and 5-FU.

4. Renal tubular damage occurs with cis-platinum unless it is given with adequate hydration, and hemorrhagic cystitis can complicate the administration of cyclophosphamide.

5. Neurological toxicity, particularly peripheral neuropathy, occurs for example with hexamethylmelamine and cis-platinum.

6. Liver damage is produced by methotrexate, adriamycin can cause cardiac failure, and bleomycin can cause pulmonary fibrosis.

7. A long-term complication is the increased risk of acute leukemia occurring especially if radiotherapy has also been given or chemotherapy has been administered for more than 2 years. The incidence in one series of patients reported was 0.3% (57).

Chemotherapy Plus Radiotherapy

The two modalities have been frequently combined in the treatment of ovarian cancer but no advantage has as yet been shown.

Immunotherapy

The use of nonspecific immunotherapy with BCG (bacille Calmette-Guerin) or Corynbacterium parvum, in addition to chemotherapy is now being studied. One such randomized trial is being carried out by the Southwest Oncology Group (2) where BCG with adriamycin and cyclophosphamide is being compared to the two cytotoxic agents alone, in advanced ovarian carcinoma. Preliminary results suggest an advantage to the addition of passive immunotherapy as does another study (19) when C. parvum is the agent used, but it will be some time before the value of immunotherapy, if any, is proven.

Conclusion

Of the three main modalities of treatment of cancer of the ovary, surgery, radiotherapy, and chemotherapy, surgery remains the most important because of its role both in staging and debulking. If these two functions can be successfully carried out, then adjuvant therapy (radiotherapy or chemotherapy), essential in all but the very earliest stage of the disease, has an increased chance of improving the survival of the patient.

The type of adjuvant treatment to be used in each stage remains controversial with a choice of radiotherapy or chemotherapy in the earlier stages (IB, II, and minimal stage III) but with chemotherapy accepted as the treatment of choice for the advanced cases (stages III and IV). Over the next few years, results from properly conducted randomized trials with pathological confirmation of remissions will become known and will help in the choice of optimal treatment. We must, however, not lose sight of the fact that about three-quarters of cases of cancer of the ovary present late and research effort must continue to be directed towards early diagnosis as well as to new treatment modalities in advanced cases.

OTHER OVARIAN TUMORS

These constitute approximately 10% of all ovarian tumors.

SEX CORD STROMAL TUMORS

The most common sex cord stromal tumors are the granulosa and theca cell tumors, but the latter are almost never malignant. Granulosa cell tumors frequently produce excess estrogen but can be hormonally inert. They occur at all ages with 40% in postmenopausal women. The treatment is primarily surgery, abdominal hysterectomy plus bilateral salpingo-oophorectomy, although conservative surgery is indicated in stage IA in women who wish to have children. Granulosa cell tumors are characterized by a tendency to recur many years after surgery, and this makes it difficult to assess the efficacy of postoperative radiotherapy or chemotherapy (64). However, irradiation is indicated in advanced cases where there is spread beyond the ovary to the pelvis or abdomen. Chemotherapy is indicated in cases where radiotherapy has failed. In cases of late recurrence a second operation should be considered.

GERM CELL TUMORS

Dysgerminoma which accounts for 2-5% of primary malignant ovarian tumors occurs in young women usually before the age of 30 years. It is a very radiosensitive tumor and behaves similarly to seminoma in men, spreading mainly by the lymphatic route to paraaortic, mediastinal, and supraclavicular nodes. Occasionally mixed tumors occur with elements of choriocarcinoma, endodermal sinus tumor, or terratoma, and these tumors have a much poorer prognosis. Treatment is surgery, oophorectomy in stage IA cases in young women wishing to have children, and hysterectomy plus bilateral salpingo-oophorectomy followed by postoperative radiotherapy in more advanced cases. The dose of radiation recommended is 2000-2500 rads/2-3 weeks to the pelvis and paraaortic nodes unless the nodes are grossly involved, when 3000-4000 rads are needed. The mediastinal and supraclavicular nodes are also treated if there is evidence of paraaortic involvement (44). When spread has occurred to the peritoneal cavity radiation should be given to the whole abdomen. In a review of 33 cases of pure dysgerminoma from the Christie Hospital, Manchester (45), a 5-year survival rate of 85% was obtained. Excepting for cases of unilateral stage I disease, postoperative radiotherapy to the whole abdomen, 3000 rads/20 fractions/28 days was recommended. If malignant elements other than dysgerminoma are present, chemotherapy is required.

Malignant germ cell neoplasms such as malignant terratomas and endodermal sinus tumors are very rare. They usually occur in children. Following surgery to remove as much tumor as possible, chemotherapy is the treatment of choice as these tumors are not radiosensitive. In a study at the M. D. Anderson Hospital, a combination of vincristine, cyclophosphamide, and actinomycin D was given to all stages in a variety of germ cell tumors following debulking, the latter two drugs for 2 years. In 21 girls there were only 5 deaths, 4 with stage IV disease (15). This combination with surgery is therefore the treatment of choice at the present time for this group of tumors although new combinations with cis-platinum are being tried.

REFERENCES

1. Adam, Ervin, Kaufman, Raymond H., Melnick, Joseph L., Levey, Allan H., and Rawls, William E.: Seroepidemiologic studies of herpesvirus type 2 and carcinoma of the cervix IV. Dysplasia and carcinoma in situ. Am. J. Epidemiol. 98:77-87, 1973.

2. Alberts, D.S., Moon, T.E., Stephens, R.A., Wilson, H., Noburu, O., Hilgers, R.D., O'Toole, R., and Thigpen, J.T.: Randomized study of chemoimmunotherapy for advanced ovarian carcinoma: A preliminary report of a Southwest Oncology Group study. Cancer Treat. Rep. 63:325-331, 1979.

3. Alderman, S.J., Dillon, T.F., Krummerman, M.S., Phillips, B.P., and Chung, A.F.: Postoperative use of radioactive phosphorus in Stage I ovarian carcinoma. Obstet. Gynecol. 49:659-662, 1977.

4. Alexander, E.R.: Possible etiologies of cancer of the cervix other than herpesvirus. Cancer Res. 33:1485-1496, 1973.

5. Ashley, David J.B.: The biological status of carcinoma in-situ of the uterine cervix. J. Obstet. Gynec. Brit. Comm. 73:372-381, 1966.

6. Bagley, C.M., Jr., Young, R.C., Schein, P.S., Chabner, B.A., DeVita, V.T.: Ovarian carcinoma metastatic to the diaphragm - frequently undiagnosed at laparotomy. A preliminary report. Am. J. Obstet. Gynecol. 116: 397-400, 1973.

7. Blom, J., Park, R., and Blessing, J.: Treatment of women with disseminated and recurrent ovarian carcinoma with single and multi-chemotherapeutic agent. Proc. Am. Assoc. Cancer Res. 19:338, 1978.

8. Blomfield, G.W., Cherry, Cora P., and Glucksmann, A.: Biological factors influencing the radiotherapeutic results in carcinoma of the cervix. Br. J. Radiol. 38:24-254, 1965.

9. Boyd, J.T. and Doll, R.: A study of the aetiology of carcinoma of the cervix uteri. Br. J. Cancer 18:420-434, 1964.

10. Brady, Luther W.: Future prospects of radiotherapy in gynecologic oncology. Cancer 38:553-564, 1976.

11. Brindle, Georfrey, Wakefield, John, and Yule, Robert: Cervical smears: Are the right women being examined? Br. Med. J. 1:1196-1197, 1976.

12. Bruckner, H.W., Cohen, C.J., Deppe, G., et al.: Chemotherapy of gynecological tumors with platinum II. J. Clin. Hemol. Oncol. 7:619-632, 1977.

13. Bush, R.S.: The Management of Malignant Disease, Series 2. Malignancies of the Ovary, Uterus and Cervix. Edward Arnold, 1979, p. 35, Chicago.

14. Bush, R.S., Allt, W.E.C., Beat, F.A., Bear, H., Pringle, J.F., and Sturgeon, J.: Treatment of epithelial carcinoma of the ovary: Operation, irradiation and chemotherapy. Am. J. Obstet. Gynecol. 127:692-704, 1977.

15. Cangir, A., Smith, J., and van Eys, J.: Improved prognosis in children with ovarian cancers following modified VAC (vincristine sulfate, dactinomycin, and cyclophosphamide). Chemother. Cancer 42:1234-1238, 1978.

16. Cochrane, J.P.S. and Yarnold, J.R.: Management of radiation injuries to the bowel associated with treatment of uterine carcinoma by radiotherapy: Pre liminary communication. J.R. Soc. Med. 72:195-197, 1979.

17. Coppleson, Malcolm: Epidemiology and etiology. Br. J. Hosp. Med. 8:961-980, 1969.

18. Cramer, Daniel W.: The role of cervical cytology in the declining morbidity and mortality of cervical cancer. Cancer 34:2018-2027, 1974.

19. Creasman, W.T., Gall, S.A., Blessing, J.A., Schmidt, H.J., Abu-Ghazaleh, S., Whisnant, J.K., and DiSala, P.J.: Chemoimmunotherapy in the

management of primary stage III ovarian cancer: A gynecologic oncology group study. Cancer Treat. Rep. 63:319-323, 1979.

20. Day, T.G. and Smith, J.P.: Diagnosis and staging of ovarian carcinoma. Sem. Oncol. 3:217-222, 1975.

21. Dembo, A.J., Bush, R.S., Beale, F.A., Bear, H.A., et al.: The Princess Margaret Hospital Study of ovarian cancer: Stages I, II and asymptomatic III presentations. Cancer Treat. Rep. 63:249-254, 1979.

22. Dembo, A.J., Van Dyk, J., Japp, B., Bean, H.A., Beale, R.A., Pringle, J.F., and Bush, R.S.: Whole abdominal irradiation by a moving strip technique for patients with ovarian cancer. Int. J. Radiat. Oncol. Biol. Phys. 5: 1933-1942, 1979.

23. Easley, James D. and Fletcher, Gilbert H.: Analysis of the treatment of stage I and stage II carcinomas of the uterine cervix. Am. J. Roentgenol. 111: 243-248, 1971.

24. Edmonson, J.H., Fleming, T.R., Decker, D.G., Malkasian, G.D., Jorgensen, E.O., Jefferies, J.A., Webb, M.J., and Kvols, L.K.: Different chemotherapeutic sensitivities and host factors affecting prognosis in advanced ovarian carcinoma versus minimal residual disease. Cancer Treat. Rep. 63: 241-247, 1979.

25. Epidemiology and natural history of carcinoma of the cervix. Report of task force. Can. Med. Assoc. J. 114:1003-1012, 1976.

26. Fazekas, J.T. and Maier, J.G.: Irradiation of ovarian carcinomas. A prospective comparison of the open field and moving strip techniques. Am. J. Roentgenol. 120:118-123, 1974.

27. Fletcher, Gilbert H. and Rutledge, Felix N.: Extended field technique in the management of the cancer of the uterine cervix. Am. J. Roentgenol. 114:116-122, 1972.

28. Fletcher, Gilbert H.: Cancer of the uterine cervix. Am. J. Roentgenol. 111: 225-242, 1971.

29. Friedell, Gilbert H. and Graham, John B.: Regional lymph node involvement in small carcinoma of the cervix. Surg. Gynecol. Obstet. 108:513-516, 1959.

30. Fuks, Z.: External radiotherapy of ovarian cancer: Standard approaches and new frontiers. Sem. Oncol. 2:253-266, 1975.

31. Fuks, Z.: The role of radiation therapy in the management of ovarian carcinoma. Israel J. Med. Sci. 13:815-828, 1977.

32. Hamberger, Arthur D., Fletcher, Gilbert H., and Wharton, J. Taylor: Results of treatment of early stage I carcinoma of the uterine cervix with intracavitary radium alone. Cancer 41:980-985, 1978.

33. Henschke, U.K., Hilaris, B.S. and Mahan, G.D.: Afterloading in interstitial and intracavitary radiation therapy. Am. J. Roentgenol. Rad. Ther. Nucl. Med. 90:386-389, 1963.

34. Hintz, B.L., Fuks, Z., Kempson, R., Eltringham, J.R., Zaloudek, C., Williamson, T.J., Bagshaw, M.A.: Results of postoperative megavoltage radiotherapy of malignant surface epithelial tumors of the ovary. Radiology 114: 695-700, 1975.

35. Hsu, Chien-Tien, Cheng, Yung-Sheng, and Su, Shi-Chiuy: Prognosis of uterine cervical cancer with extensive lymph node metastases (special emphasis on the value of pelvic lymphadenopathy in the surgical treatment of uterine cervical cancer. Am. J. Obstet. Gynecol. 114:954-962, 1972.

36. Hulka, Barba S.: Cytologic and histologic outcome following an atypical cervical smear. Am. J. Obstet. Gynecol. 101:190-199, 1968.

37. Jampolis, Samuel, Andras, E. James, and Fletcher, Gilbert H.: Analysis of sites and causes of failures of irradiation in invasive squamous cell carcinoma of the intact uterine cervix. Radiology 115:681-685, 1975.

38. Johnson, B.L., Fisher, R.I., Bender, R.A., De Vita, V.T., Chabner, B.A. and Young, R.C.: Hexamethylmelamine in alkylating agent-resistant ovarian carcinoma. Cancer 42:2157-2161, 1978.

39. Joly, D.J., Lilienfeld, A.J., Diamond, E.L., and Bross, I.D.: An epidemiologic study of the relationship of reproductive experience to cancer of the ovary. Am. J. Epidemiol. 99:190, 1974.

40. Josey, William E., Nahmias, Andre J., Naib, and Zuher, M.: Genital infection with type 2 herpesvirus hominis. Am. J. Obstet. Gynecol. 101:718-728, 1962.

41. Kolstad, P., Davy, M., and Hoeg, K.: Individualized treatment of ovarian cancer. Am. J. Obstet. Gynecol. 128:617, 1977.

42. Lagasse, L.D., Smith, M.L., Moore, J.G., Morton, D.G., Jacobs, M., Johnson, G.H., and Watring, W.G.: The effect of radiation therapy on pelvic lymph node involvement in stage I carcinoma of the cervix. Am. J. Obstet. Gynecol. 119:328-334, 1974.

43. Localio, S. Arthur, Stone, Alex, and Friedman, Milton: Surg. Gynecol. Obstet. 129:1163-1172, 1969.

44. Longo, D.L. and Young, R.C.: Cosmetic talc and ovarian cancer. Lancet 2: 349-351, 1979.

45. Lucraft, H.H.: A review of thirty-three cases of ovarian dysgerminoma emphasizing the role of radiotherapy. Clin. Radiol. 30:585-589, 1979.

46. Maier, J.G.: Radiotherapy Treatment of Ovarian Cancer in Gynecologic Oncology, edited by L. McGowan, New York, Appleton-Century-Crofts, 1978, p. 338.

47. Malkasian, G.D., Decker, D.G., Jorgensen, E.O., and Webb, M.J.: 6-Dehydro-6, 17α-dimethylprogesterone (NSC-123018) for the treatment of metastatic and recurrent ovarian carcinoma. Cancer Treat. Rep. 57:241-242, 1973.

48. Malkasian, G.D., Decker, D.G., and Webb, M.J.: Histology of epithelial tumors of the ovary. Clinical usefulness and prognostic significance of the histological classifications and grading. Sem. Oncol. 2:191-202, 1975.

49. Maruyama, Yosh, Van Nagell, J.R., Wrede, D.E., Coffey, II, C., Utley, J.F., and Avila, J.: Approaches to optimization of dose in radiation therapy of cervix carcinoma. Radiology 120:389-393, 1976.

50. Miller, A.B., Lindsay, J., and Hill, G.B.: Mortality from cancer of the uterus in Canada and its relationship to screening for cancer of the cervix. Int. J. Cancer 17:602-612, 1976.

51. Naib, Zuher M., Nathmias, Andre J., and Josey, William E.: Cytology and histopathology of cervical herpes simplex infection. Cancer 19:1026-1031, 1966.

52. Ozols, R.F., Gaivin, A.J., Coste, J., Simon, R.M., and Young, R.C.: Histological grade in advanced ovarian cancer. Cancer Treat. Rep. 63:255-263, 1979.

53. Pierquin, B., Baillet, F., and Wilson, J.F.: Radiation therapy in the management of primary breast cancer. Am. J. Roentgenol. Rad. Ther. Nucl. Med. 127:645-648, 1976.

54. Piver, M. Steven and Chung, Whan S.: Prognostic significance of cervical lesion size and pelvic node metastases in cervical carcinoma. Obstet. Gynecol. 46:507-510, 1975.

55. Piver, M.S., Barlow, J.J., and Bhattacharya, M.: Treatment and immunodiagnosis of advanced ovarian adenocarcinoma. Cancer Treat. Rep. 63:265-267, 1979.

56. Rampone, John F., Klem, Valborg, and Kolstad, Per.: Combined treatment of stage 1B carcinoma of the cervix. Obstet. Gynecol. 41:163-167, 1973.

57. Reimer, R.R., Hoover, R., Fraumeni, J.F. and Young, R.C. Acute leukemia after alkylating cytotherapy in ovarian cancer. N. Engl. J. Med. 297:117, 1977.

58. Rosenoff, S.H., DeVita, V.T., Hubbard, S., and Young, R.C.: Peritoneoscopy in the staging and follow-up of ovarian cancer. Sem. Oncol. 2:223-228, 1975.

59. Rotkin, I.D.: Adolescent coitus and cervical cancer: Associations of related events with increased risk. Cancer Res. 27:603-617, 1967.

60. Rutledge, Felix N., Fletcher, Gilbert H., and MacDonald, Eleanor J.: Pelvic lymphadenectomy as an adjunct to radiation therapy in treatment for cancer of the cervix. Am. J. Roentgenol. 93:607-614, 1965.

61. Savage, Edward W.: Microinvasive carcinoma of the cervix. Am. J. Obstet. Gynecol. 113:708-717, 1972.

62. Smith, J.P., Rutledge, F.N., and Declas, L.: Results of chemotherapy as an adjunct to surgery in patients with localized ovarian cancer. Sem. Oncol. 2: 277-282, 1975.

63. Spriggs, A.I. and Husain, O.A.N.: Cervical smears. Br. Med. J. 1:1516-1518, 1977.

64. Stage, A.H. and Grafton, W.D.: Thecomas and granulosa - theca cell tumors of the ovary. An analysis of 51 tumors. Obstet. Gynecol. 50:21-27, 1977.

65. Strockbine, M.F., Hancock, J.E., and Fletcher, G.H.: Complications in 831 patients with squamous cell carcinoma of the intact uterine cervix treated with 3,000 rads or more whole pelvis irradiation. Am. J. Roentgenol. 108:293-304, 1970.

66. Symmonds, Richard E.: Some surgical aspects of gynecological cancer. Cancer 36:649-660, 1975.

67. TNM Classification of Malignant Tumors, edited by the Committee on TNM Classification of the International Union Against Cancer, Geneva. G. deBuren & Co., 1968.

68. U.I.C.C. Clinical Oncology. A Manual for Students and Doctors, edited by Committee on Professional Education of UICC, 2nd edition, Springer-Verlag, Berlin, 1978, p. 198.

69. Wellwood, J.M. and Jackson, B.T.: The intestinal complications of radiotherapy. Br. J. Surg. 60:814-818, 1973.

70. Wentz, W. Budd and Reagan, James W.: Survival in cervical cancer with respect to cell type. Cancer 12:384-388, 1959.

71. Wiltshaw, E. and Kroner, T.: Phase II study of cis-dichlorodiammineplatinum (II) (NSC-119875) in advanced adenocarcinoma of the ovary. Cancer Treat. Rep. 60:55-60, 1976.

72. Wiltshaw, E., Subramarian, S., Alexopoulos, C., and Barker, G.H.: Cancer of the ovary: A summary of experience with cis-dichlorodiammineplatinum (II) of the Royal Marsden Hospital. Cancer Treat. Rep. 63:1545-1548, 1979.

73. Winterton, W.R. and Windeyer, B.W.: A comparison of results of surgery and radiotherapy in carcinoma of the cervix uteri. Br. Med. J. 1:195-196, 1941.

74. Young, R.C.: Chemotherapy of ovarian cancer past and present. Sem. Oncol. 2:267-276, 1975.

75. Young, R.C.: The EORTC Cancer Chemotherapy Annual I. edited by H.M. Pinedo, 1979, p. 344.

76. Young, R.C., Von Hoff, D.D., Gormley, P., Makuch, R., Cassidy, J., Howser, D., and Bull, J.M.: Cis-dichlorodiammineplatinum (II) for the treatment of advanced ovarian cancer. Cancer Treat. Rep. 63:1539-1544, 1979.

77. Young, R.C., Chobner, B.A., Hubbard, S.P., Fisher, R.I., Bender, R.A., Anderson, T., Simon, R.M., Canellos, G.P., and DeVita, V.T.: Advanced ovarian adenocarcinoma: A prospective trial of melphalan (L-PAM) versus combination chemotherapy. N. Engl. J. Med. 299:1261-1266, 1978.

78. Order, S.E., Rosenshein, N., Klein, J.L., Leibel, S., Torres, J.P.Y., and Ettinger, D.: The integration of new therapies and radiation in the management of ovarian cancer. Cancer 48:590-596, 1981.

chapter 10

BLADDER CANCER

Brigit van der Werf-Messing, M.D.

The evolution of bladder cancer in most cases appears to proceed in an orderly fashion starting in the bladder mucosa. The tumor extends gradually over the surface and into the depth of the bladder wall. Spread occurs to the regional nodes and subsequently to the juxtaregional nodes. Usually the malignancy metastasizes to other organs at a later stage. No spontaneous regression can be expected, the inevitable death from untreated malignancy can be anticipated within 3 years.

Treatment is virtually always required as death due to an untreated bladder cancer is nearly always a protracted and painful event. Bladder death, in which the primary growth dominates the symptoms, is characterized by abundant hemorrhage and nearly unbearable bladder spasm. In case of pelvic death, extension of the primary into the pelvic organs, usually in combination with involvement of regional nodes, causes excruciating pain by involving the sacral plexus. Occasionally uremia, as a sequela of compression of the ureters by the growth, terminates life without distressing bladder and pelvic symptoms. Surgery has been resorted to in an attempt to cure or at least to alleviate symptoms. As cure rates were not satisfactory and as radical surgical approaches are mutilating, radiotherapy became involved in the management of bladder cancer in the beginning of this century.

The benefit of radiotherapy is based on the relatively greater destructive effect of ionizing irradiation on the malignancy than on healthy tissue. This therapeutic margin is small in bladder cancers because they are only moderately radiosensitive, hence requiring a large radiation dose which approaches the tolerance of the normal tissues of the bladder and the adjacent intestinal and pelvic structures. Curative and palliative radiotherapeutic techniques have been developed and applied, over the years, dependent on extent of disease and facilities available. The main radiotherapeutic methods are: intracavitary and interstitial application of radioactive sources, external orthovoltage and later supervoltage irradiation, combined external and interstitial irradiation, combined modality treatments such as external irradiation and surgery, and combinations of irradiation, surgery, and systemic chemotherapy. Since bladder cancer usually tends to remain localized and to spread mainly by local invasion and by gradual involvement of regional and juxtaregional nodes, the main goal of the radiotherapeutic attack has been the bladder itself or the bladder with the adjacent or all regional lymph nodes. Occasionally the juxtaregional nodes are included in the first curative goal of radiotherapy.

In order to assess the value of the various types of radiotherapy in terms of survival rates and in order to compare these with results of other treatment modalities, clinical pretreatment classification of the malignancy is essential. The use of the internationally accepted TNM classification of the Union Internationale Contre le Cancer (UICC) (38,39) and the American Joint Committee (AJC) (Fig. 1) will increase the reliability of such comparisons.

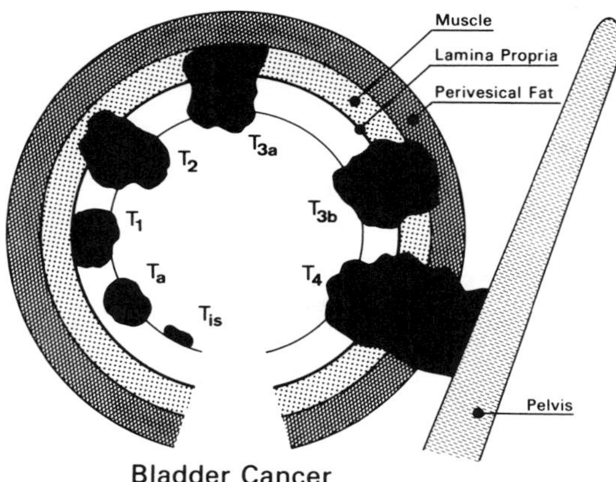

Figure 1. TNM classification of bladder cancer (UICC). A: T classification (of the primary growth) (from Ref. 39).

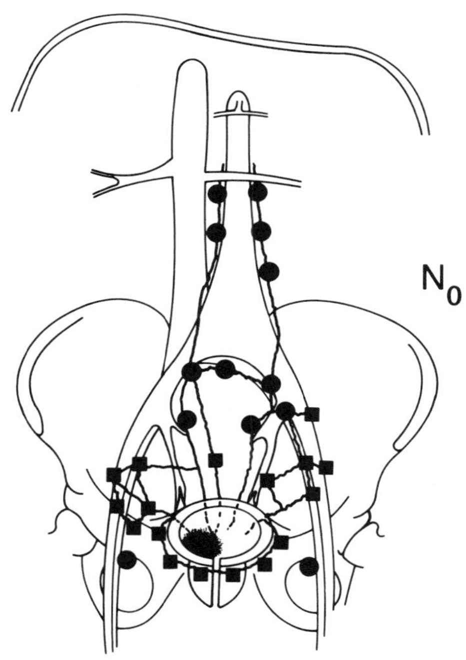

Figure 1. B. N_0. N categories of the TNM-AJC classification (Ref. 38). ■, regional nodes; ▲, involved nodes; ●, juxtaregional nodes; p, primary.

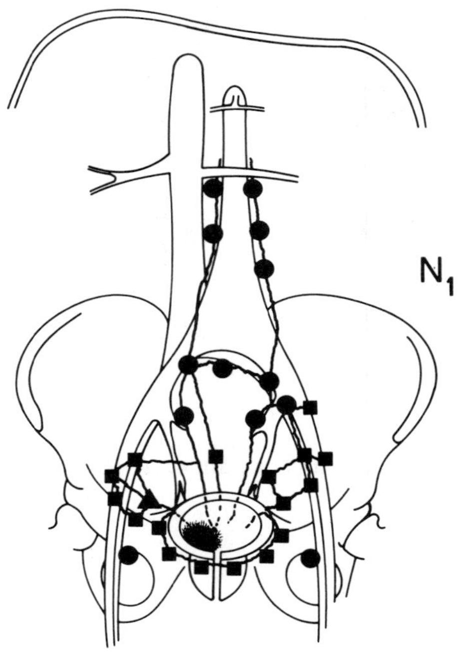

Figure 1. C: N_1.

In the past urologists usually reported their treatment results according to the surgical-pathological classification of Jewett (19) (Fig. 2) as clinical staging often appeared to be unreliable when compared with the surgical and pathological findings. However, for the purpose of comparative evaluation of surgical and nonsurgical treatment modalities the clinical TNM classification is conditio sine qua non!

INTRACAVITARY IRRADIATION WITH SOLID OR LIQUID RADIOACTIVE SOURCES

In 1949 Friedman and Lewis (14) introduced the Walter Reed technique. A 25 mg radium source or a ^{60}Co pellet was introduced into the bladder via cystostomy; the bladder was kept distended by a balloon. The 5-year survival rates appeared promising at that time (15). However, this technique was abandoned until Pedersen and Herting (27) in 1972 reported results of bladder cancer treatment by an intravesical 20 mg radium source, applied transurethrally and placed centrally in a distended balloon. During a 120 hr application a dose of 3500 rads was delivered to the mucosa. At about 12 mm depth the dose decreased to 1750 rads and at about 20 mm approximately to 800 rads. A second application was given after a 2-week interval. All applications were combined with surgical intervention: transurethral resection, segmental resection, or coagulation of the bulk of the growth.

In 1955 Muller (24) reported treatment of bladder cancer by filling an intravesically placed balloon with a ^{60}Co solution. The surface dose was about 10,000 rads with a few millimeters half-depth value penetration. Ninety-six patients were

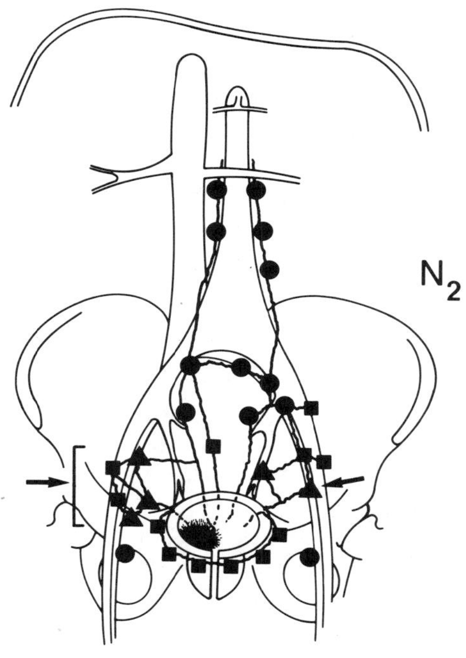

Figure 1. D: N_2.

treated in this manner; 60% of the papilloma and 30% of the carcinoma patients remained tumor free up to 3.5 years. In view of the high half-life time of ^{60}Co, the danger of contamination was considerable. To avoid this disadvantage shortlived γ -ray emitting radioisotopes were tried, such as radioactive ^{24}Na and ^{82}Br with half-life times of 15 hr and 36 hr, respectively.

Most clinicians agree that if adequate tumoricidal doses are delivered by intracavitary application of γ -ray emitters the complication rate is high, e.g., vesicoureteric reflux with risk of metastatic implants in renal pelvis, impaired healing after subsequent diathermy for recurrences, bleeding, and fibrosis resulting in a contracted bladder.

Free instillations of β -ray emitting radioisotopes such as colloidal ^{198}Au had disappointing results. Due to the shallow penetration of the β -rays, clearing of the bladder neoplasm usually could not be obtained and this technique has been abandoned. The more penetrating β -ray emitters such as radioactive ^{90}Y and ^{76}As could theoretically deal with infiltrating growths and yet avoid the complications of the still deeper penetrating γ -ray emitters. However, subsequent bladder bleeding caused by radiation-induced mucosal teleangiectasia necessitated cystectomy in the majority of cases. In 1975 Durrant and Laing (7) published the results of treating patients with diffuse or multiple bladder cancers of the T1 category by transurethrally instillating 80 ml solution of 100 mCi ^{90}Y in the bladder. This solution delivered 1500 rads to the bladder surface during a 2 hr application.

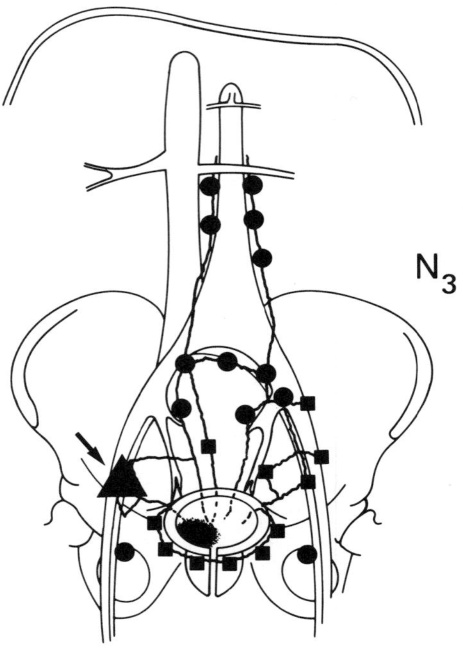

Figure 1. E: N_3.

The treatment was repeated within 46 weeks. Sixty percent of 32 patients were alive after 3 years, however, 28 required further surgical treatment in order to control the disease. The complications such as hematuria and frequency were acceptable.

Intravesical application of radioactive sources is generally not considered to be a satisfactory therapeutic approach in the management of bladder cancer because the complication rate seems prohibitively high if tumor-lethal doses are delivered. Most clinicians have resorted to other types of radiation therapy (Table 1).

INTERSTITIAL IRRADIATION

By suprapubic or transurethral route radioactive material can be implanted into a bladder neoplasm. A high dose of ionizing irradiation can thus be delivered to the malignancy, while sparing the adjacent structures. For curative treatment, interstitial therapy is usually restricted to solitary malignancies in categories T1, T2, or T3, covering an area with a diameter not exceeding 3-5 cm. Because the irradiation dose falls off steeply beyond the implanted area, regional lymph nodes cannot be expected to be sterilized by this method. Good local palliation can be achieved even in cases of more advanced malignancies. In 1910 for the first time in history Pasteau et al. (26) inserted a radium source, transurethrally, into a bladder cancer.

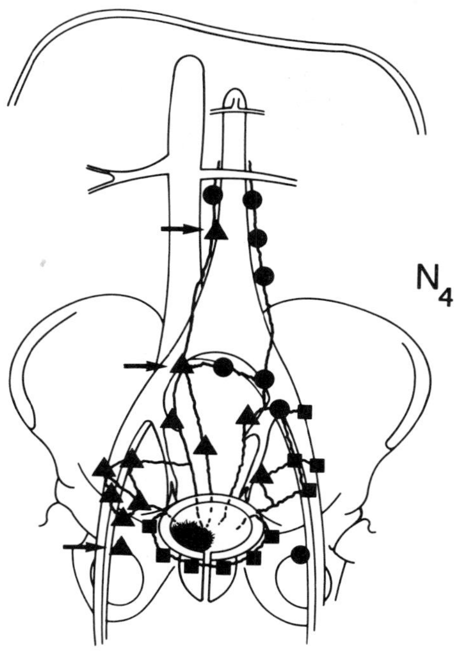

Figure 1. F: N_4.

In 1951 Darget (5) published his suprapubic radium needle implantation technique. Because he left the bladder and abdominal wall open until removal of the radium about a week later, this method appeared to be unattractive to other clinicians. In 1960 Bloom (2) presented his results of treating categories T1, T2, and T3 bladder cancers, with a diameter up to 4 cm, by suprapubic implantation of radioactive ^{182}Ta wires. Accurate dosimetry and readjusting the tantalum wires in case of unsatisfactory implantation permitted a high grade of accuracy in dose delivery. The operative wound could be closed immediately. At the calculated time the tantalum wires were removed transurethrally.

Similar advantages apply to suprapubic radium implantation (Fig. 3), results of which were reported by Van der Werf-Messing (42,46). By this method, application time can be calculated so as to deliver a dose biologically equivalent to 6500-7000 rads in 168 hr. In order to prevent scar implants, postimplant external irradiation was added (1500 rads skin dose in three sessions). After 1962 this scar irradiation was replaced by preoperative external irradiation to the true pelvis (three times 350 rads in order to reduce both the incidence of scar implants and of iatrogenic metastases). The method completely eliminated scar implants and reduced, mainly in the T3 category, the incidence of distant metastases.

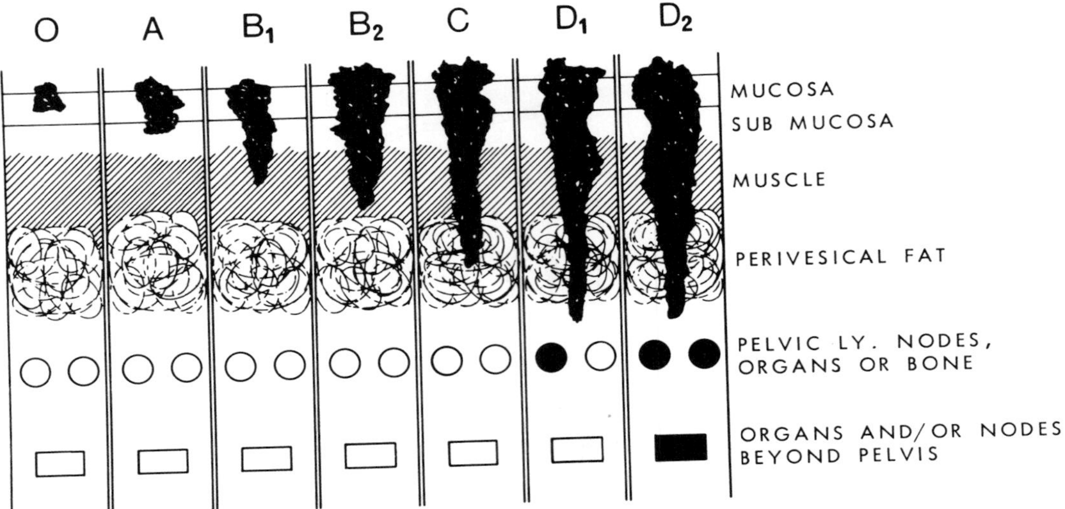

Figure 2. Jewett's classification of bladder cancer. (From Ref. 19.)

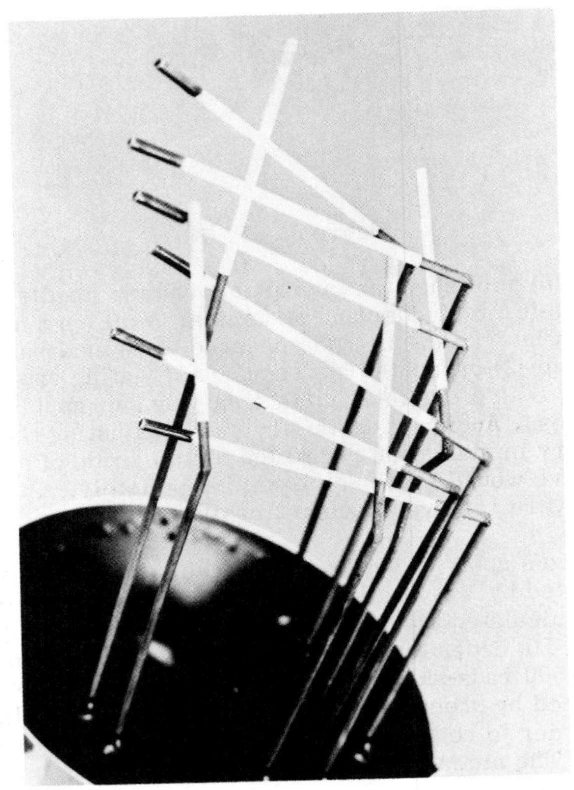

Figure 3. Three-dimensional reconstruction of a radium implant. (From Rotterdam Radiotherapy Institute, Ref. 46.)

Table 1. Survival after Intracavitary Irradiation with Solid or Liquid Radioactive Sources

Study	Technique		Cancer in Situ	Survival by T Category			
				T1	T2	T3	T4
Ref. 15	Walter Reed technique: Central source of radium 25 mg or ^{60}Co pellet, in inflated balloon. Inserted via cystostomy	5-year survival	- -	7/9	4/4	7/18	1/2
Ref. 27	Two applications of radium 20 mg in distended balloon, inserted transurethrally at 2 weeks interval (combined with surgery)	5-year survival	(26)* 55%	(54) 45%	(28) 33%	(36) 25%	(21) 5%
Ref. 7	80 cc 100 mCi ^{90}Y solution, two applications of 2 hr within 4-6 weeks	3-year survival	- -	(32) 60%	- -	- -	- -

* Within brackets is number of treated patients.

Pierquin et al. (28) reported preliminary results of suprapubic ^{192}Ir wire implanation in 28 T1 and T2 growths up to 3 cm in diameter. The flexibility of the material is a practical advantage and dose distribution can be calculated correctly as in case of radium and tantalum implanation. Suprapubic implants of radioactive ^{198}Au grains and ^{222}Rn seeds have been practiced by Munro (25) and by Dix et al. (6). Since the radioactive material is implanted permanently, no adjustments can be made for unsatisfactory dose distribution. Complications after interstitial radiotherapy are: necrosis, calculi formation, vesicoureteric reflux, and chronic cystitis. The incidence of these complications, usually minor, can be reduced by careful preimplant treatment of urinary infections.

Survival rates rank among the highest reported in the literature. However, selection has been introduced, because in each T category this technique is only applicable to solitary growths of limited size. Since the high dose of ionizing irradiation is mainly restricted to the implanted area, theoretically no cure can be expected in case of lymph node involvement beyond the closest proximity to the primary. It is not inconceivable that additional external irradiation, even with limited doses, can eradicate microscopic lymph node deposits. In case of local failure, a full course of external irradiation or cystectomy can still rescue the patient (Table 2).

EXTERNAL IRRADIATION

External irradiation of bladder cancer by means of orthovoltage machines was considered not to be an effective curative method of treatment, though palliation could be achieved. As the penetrating power of the photon beam of ionizing irradiation was relatively poor, a radiation dose high enough to eradicate the bladder cancer could only be achieved by meticulous application of complicated radiation techniques. Even then, the unavoidable high dose to the healthy surrounding tissues, with threat of severe complications, prevented radiotherapists from employing this method as the first choice in a curative approach. Ingenious ways to circumvent the limits of external orthovoltage irradiation such as contact irradiation during 2 or 3 cystotomies (Goin and Hoffman, quoted by Smithers, 37) or during a period of bladder marsupialization (17) have not been accepted by other clinicians.

With the introduction of supervoltage facilities, ionizing irradiation with greater penetrating power and skin-sparing effect could be produced. This permitted the delivery of a high tumoricidal dose in the bladder, and yet the healthy surrounding tissuss and organs could be relatively spared. In order to reduce the bulk of the growth which has to be eradicated by irradiation, it is considered advantageous to remove as much as possible of its exophytic part by transurethral resection.

By various techniques of external supervoltage irradiation, the volume to be irradiated with a cancericidal dose can be adapted to the depth of penetration of the growth. In cases of low T category (T1mT2) (Figs. 4 and 5), most radiotherapists limit the curative attack to the bladder with a small margin of surrounding normal tissue; in cases of growths in categories T3 and T4 the field of irradiation can be extended so as to include regional (Fig. 6) and even juxtaregional nodes (Fig. 7). In 1976 Rider and Evans (33), based on a retrospective analysis, drew the conclusion that in the T3 category elective irradiation of the juxtaregional nodes (3500 rads in 16 fractions, over 3 weeks) does not improve prognosis. Apparently in cases of juxtaregional node involvement, subclinical metastases elsewhere determine survival. The problem is still not solved whether extended-field irradiation, i.e., an additional burden to the usually elderly patient, is justified.

Table 2. Survival after Interstitial Irradiation

Study	Technique	5-Year Survival by T Category		
		Mucosal	Muscular	Perivesical
Ref. 2	Suprapubic ^{182}Ta wire implant	(44)* 70%	(30) 40%	(74) 58%
Ref. 25	Suprapubic ^{198}Au grain implant	(79) 70%	(46) 39%	(26) 0%
Ref. 6	Suprapubic ^{198}Au grain or radon seed implant		T1 T2 T3 (350) 45%	
Refs. 42,46	Suprapubic radium needle implant (total)	T1 (164) 75%	T2 (313) 55%	T3 (129) 25%
	idem with preoperative external irradiation (3 x 350 rads)	(100) 75%	(202) 55%	(43) 35%

* Within brackets is number of treated patients.

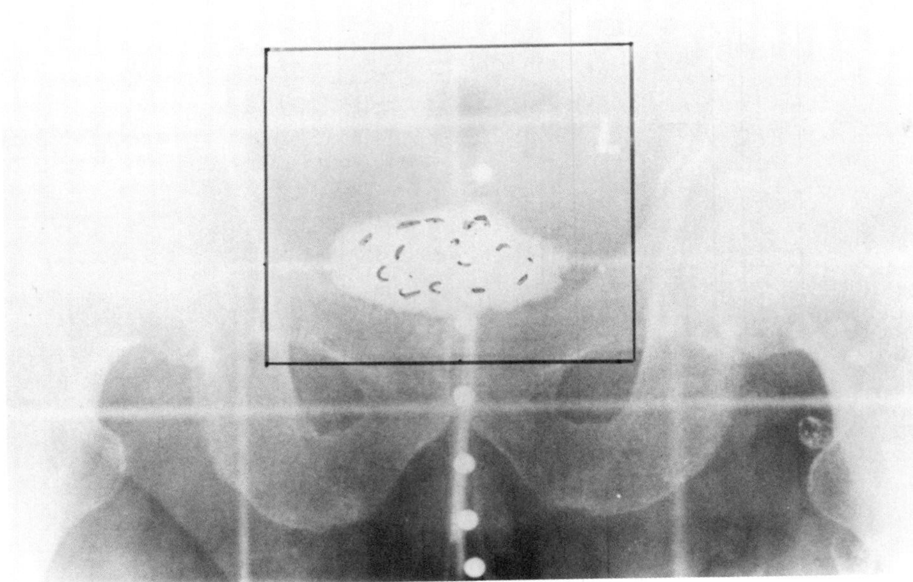

Figure 4. Carcinoma of the bladder category T1 and T2. Standard fields for external irradiation. A: Anteroposterior view of the irradiated field.

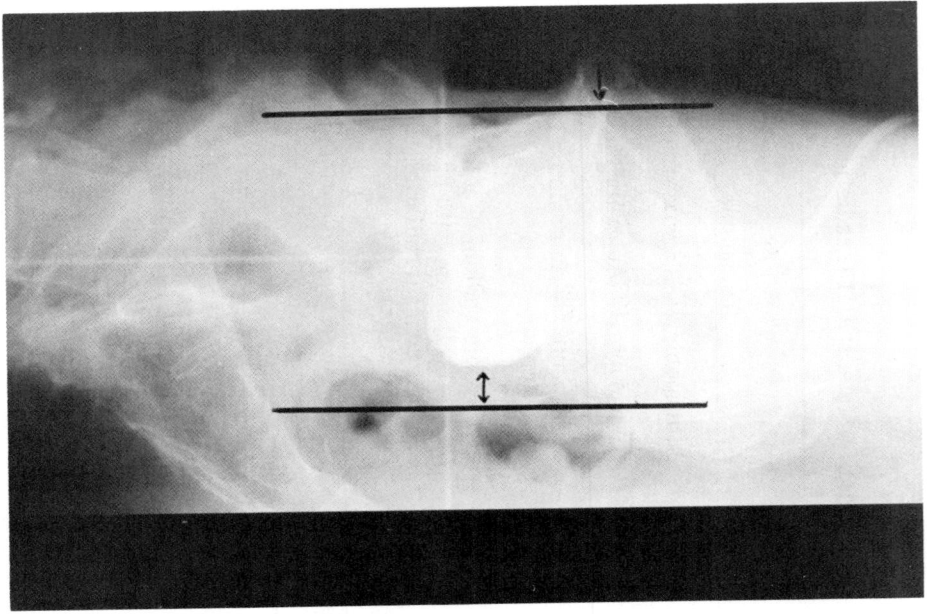

Figure 4. B: Lateral view of the irradiated field.

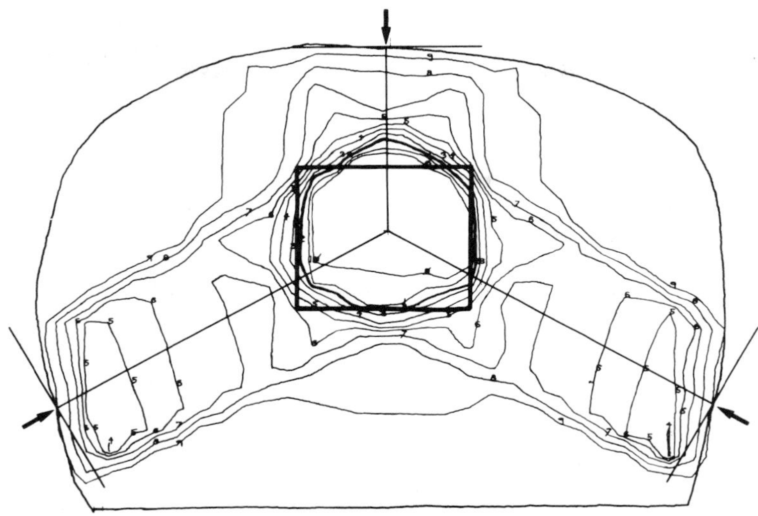

Figure 5. Dose distribution in case of irradiation of a T1 or T2 bladder cancer (Fig. 4) by three irradiation fields.

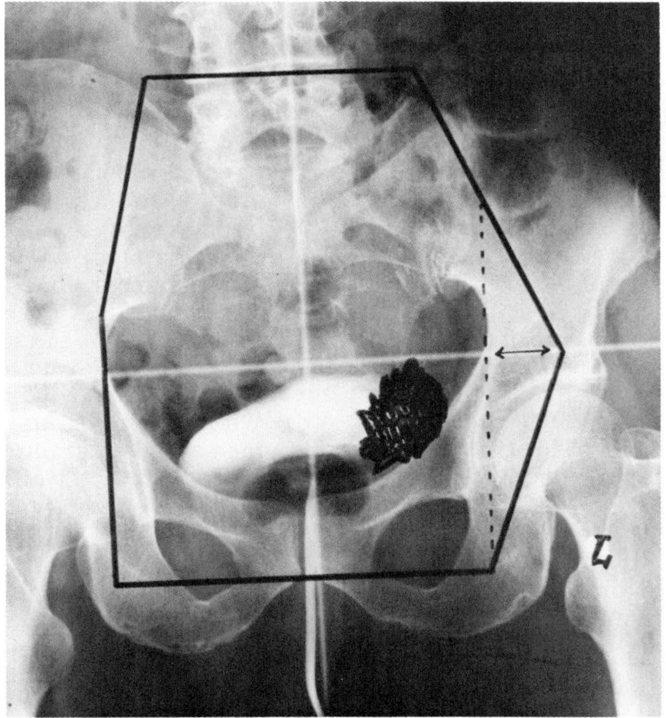

Figure 6. T3 bladder cancer extending toward the left pelvic wall. Irradiation field covering the true pelvis, the regional and the common iliac nodes.

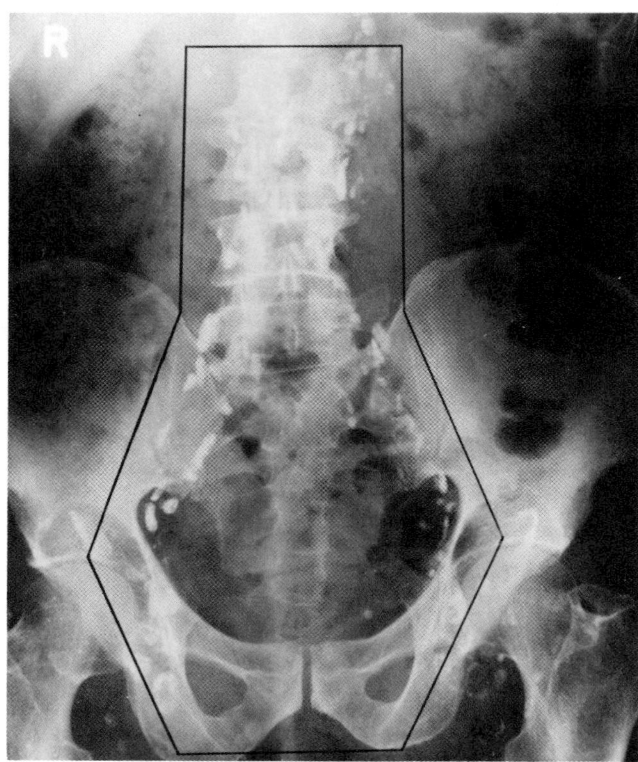

Figure 7. T3 or T4 bladder cancer. The irradiation field includes the majority of the juxtaregional nodes. (From Ref. 33.)

Most authors agree that by daily irradiation a dose of 6000-7000 rads in 6-7 weeks, or its biological equivalent, has to be delivered to the tumor-bearing area if cure is the aim. Usually, the last 1000-2000 rads are given via smaller fields to the primary only. With higher doses, cure rate increases, however; the concomitant higher rate of severe complications limits the upper dose level. Three and five year survival rates, roughly comparable with surgical cure rates, range from 30-50% in the T1 category, are about 40% in the T2, 20% in the T3, and 5% in the T4 category. Reported results vary because of many differing and elusive prognostic factors such as selection of cases, accuracy of staging, and inclusion of palliative treatments in the reported series, etc. With increasing histological grade of malignancy, prognosis becomes worse, but since a higher grade of malignancy is correlated with greater depth of penetration of the growth, most clinicians assume that in each T category the histological grade is of no or only minor prognostic importance (19,46) (Table 3).

Relief of symptoms, caused by metastases, even prevention of disasters such as pathological fractures, spinal cord compression, or suffocation, can usually be achieved by palliative supervoltage irradiation. A short course of irradiation to the bladder (about 5 x 400 rads or its equivalent) can stop hemorrhage without causing inconvenience to a patient in whom curative treatment is not indicated because of poor general condition or metastatic spread of the malignancy.

The immediate reactions to external irradiation are frequency, strangury, dysuria, diarrhea, and tenesmus. These reactions are most severe after 3-4 weeks and can be reduced by treating concomitant urinary infection. In a double-blind, placebo-controlled study, Edsmyr et al. (11) demonstrated that administration of the antiinflammatory drug Orgotein during irradiation significantly ameliorates and prevents irradiation side effects. Late complications after curative external irradiation are: chronic cystitis, progressive fibrosis leading eventually to a crippling contracted bladder which might necessitate ureteric diversion, bleeding from teleangiectasis varying from incidental slight blood loss to intractable hemorrhage, and bowel complications such as chronic proctitis, rectal bleeding, fistula formation, and intestinal obstruction. The risk of late bladder and rectal complications increases with increasing radiation dose (22). The complication rate can be reduced by limiting the number of transurethral resections, by permitting the bladder to heal after previous surgical intervention, and by effectively treating urinary infection.

Various authors have tried to improve the prognosis after external supervoltage irradiation of bladder cancer, in terms both of increased cure rate and decreased morbidity. Scanlon and Furlow (35) demonstrated that split-dose radiotherapy, i.e., introducing a period of rest of about 3-4 weeks after the first half of the radiation course, does not decrease the destructive effect on the cancer but reduces the rate of immediate radiation reactions and of late complications. Some radiation oncologists have investigated the possibility of enhancing the curative radiation effect by irradiating under hyperbaric oxygen conditions. The rationale of this approach was to reduce the radioresistance of hypoxic tumor cells while not enhancing the damage to well-oxygenated normal cells. In spite of some promising reports (3,29), the majority of investigators have abandoned this method as being cumbersome and not convincingly superior to conventional radiation therapy (4). Edsmyr (10) reported the results of another attempt to improve the therapeutic ratio by low dose fractionation. In a prospective trial patients were randomized either to conventional radiotherapy, consisting of 200 rads tumor dose daily, to a total dose of 6400 rads with a 2-week split period after 3200 rads; or to three times daily 100 rads tumor dose, to a total of 8400 rads with a 2-week split in the middle of the course. The preliminary results indicate that after low dose fractionation there is possible an increased cure rate in the categories T3 and T4. Edsmyr suggests that the beneficial effect on the malignancy could be explained by the fact that the relative radioresistance caused by anoxic conditions of cancer cells is of minor importance if low doses like 50-125 rads are given, whereas the intracellular repair of the healthy tissues will take place during the few hours' interval between these radiation sessions. The combination of these two factors can theoretically contribute to an increased therapeutic margin. Results of neutron irradiation of bladder cancer are only scantily reported. Though theoretically more effective (high relative biological effectiveness and low oxygen enhancement ratio) than megavoltage photons and electrons, the complication rate seems to be discouraging. However, pi-meson radiotherapy for the local bladder malignancy appears to be promising (21).

COMBINED MODALITY TREATMENT: PREOPERATIVE RADIOTHERAPY AND SURGERY

In an endeavor to improve prognosis, urologists and radiotherapists have investigated the results of treatment by the combination of radiotherapy and surgery in the various T categories of bladder cancer (Table 4). A preoperative course of external supervoltage irradiation is delivered either to the bladder with a small margin of healthy tissue, or to the bladder with regional and even juxtaregional

Table 3. Survival after External Megavoltage Irradiation

Study	Type of External Irradiation	5-Year Survival by T Category		
Ref. 34	Four field technique or rotation technique including bladder and regional lymph nodes (in deeply invading cancer): 6000 rad to pelvis + 1000 rad booster to bladder/6-8 weeks, 200 rad/day	B1 + B2	(76)*	32%
		C	(46)	25%
		D1	(54)	3%
Ref. 33	3500 rad/16 x/3 weeks to pelvis + lymph nodes including L2 + bladder 1500 rad/5 x/5 days	T1	(142)	58%
		T2	(120)	50%
		T3	(162)	17%
		T4	(74)	26%
Ref. 35	5000-5500 rads in two equally divided courses (3-4 weeks rest) (two or three fields, 10 x 10 cm or 8 x 8 cm)	T4	(47)	19%
Ref. 13	Fractional:			
	200 rad		(28)	18%
	250 rad	T2	(25)	20%
	300 rad		(24)	29%
Ref. 9	Treated by ^{60}Co unit 6 MeV acc. between 1957-1964	T2	(86)	34%
			(125)	25%
		T3	(89)	7%
		T4		

Ref.	Treatment	Dose	Stage		No.	Survival
Ref. 22	Four portals, 20 daily fractions, all portals treated daily T1T2: Fields covering bladder only	Trial 6250 rad	T1 + T2		(44)	80%
		Trial 5500 rad	T1 + T2	2-Year Survival	(46)	61%
	T3: Fields covering whole pelvic cavity	Trial 4250 rad	T3		(45)	38%
		Trial 5000 rad			(40)	55%
Ref. 16	5000 rad/5 weeks via four portals to pelvis + 2000 rad/2 weeks small-field rotation to bladder or 7000 rad/7 weeks rotation to bladder (less invasive cancer)		A		(33)	35%
			B1		(68)	42%
			B2		(123)	35%
			C		(95)	20%
			D1		(65)	8%
Ref. 46	Palliative and curative treatment unsuitable for interstitial radium implant, because of tumor or bad condition; 6000 rad/6 weeks or 6500 rad/6.5 weeks, 200 rad/day		T1		(86)	20%
			T2		(119)	15%
			T3		(290)	10%
			T4		(396)	5%
			M1		(124)	0%

* Within brackets is number of treated patients.

Table 4. Survival after Preoperative Irradiation and Cystectomy

Study	Type of Treatment	Type of Growth T Category	5-Year Survival		
Ref. 1	Prospective cooperative randomized study:				
	1. 4500 rad/4-5 weeks, 4-6 weeks later cystectomy	T2, T3		(12)*	40%
	2. 5-6000 rad/5-6 weeks		3-Year Survival	(10)	40%
	3. Cystectomy			(12)	40%
Ref. 36	Nonrandomized study:				
	1. 5000 rad/4-6 weeks, field size 7 x 7 cm, 4-6 weeks later cystectomy	O, A, B1		(13)	69%
		B2, C		(11)	27%
	2. Cystectomy only	O, A, B1		(19)	53%
		B2, C		(7)	0%
Refs. 48,49,50	1. 4000 rad/4-6 weeks to true pelvis; 1-3 mon later cystectomy	O, A, B1		(44)	36%
		B2, C		(65)	30%
	2. Cystectomy only (historical control group)	O, A, B1		(51)	43%
		B2, C		(89)	20%
	3. 2000 rad/1 week; after 1 week radical cystectomy	T3		(52)	39%
Ref. 31	Cooperative prospective randomized study:				
	1. 4500 rad/28-32 days varying technique, 4-8 weeks later cystectomy	B2, C	Tumor in cyst. spec.	(39)	±29%
			No tumor in cyst. spec. (P0)	(19)	51%
		B1, B2, C		(99)	40%
	2. Cystectomy	B2, C		(72)	25%
		B1, B2, C		(129)	27%

Ref. 41	Prospective cooperative randomized study:			
	1. 4000 rad/4 weeks followed by cystectomy after 4 weeks	All T3	(98)	33%
		60 years	(43)	±40%
	(including juxtaregional nodes level L5)	P0, Pis, P1, P2	(36)	±50%
		P3, P4	(41)	±25%
	2. External irradiation only	All T3	(91)	21%
	4000 + 2000 rad/5 weekly fractions of 200 rad	60 years	(34)	±25%
Ref. 23	5000 rad/5 weeks after 6 weeks simple cystectomy	T3	±(69)	30%
	7000 rad/7 weeks	T3	(137)	±20%
	Randomized study: 5000 rad/5 weeks + simple cystectomy	T3	(35)	46%
	7000 rad/7 weeks	T3	(32)	16%
Ref. 46	4000 rad/4 weeks, portal:	All cases T3	(141)	50%
	until 1972: true pelvis			
	after 1972: including juxtare-	T3 → P3	(43)	20%
	gional nodes level L5	T3 → P0 P1 P2	(96)	60%
	± immediately followed by	T3 → P2	(30)	45%
	cystectomy	T3 → P1, Pis	(24)	75%
		T3 → P0	(42)	60%
		T3 → PX	(2)	

* Within brackets is number of treated patients.

lymph nodes. Varying from center to center, cystectomy, with or without lymph node dissection, is performed subsequently 1 week to 3 months after finishing radiation therapy. The applied radiation dose in the treated volume has varied from 2000 rads in five fractions to approximately 4000-6000 rads in 4-10 weeks.

The rationale of preoperative irradiation is based upon the following considerations: (1) The growth in the bladder, especially its depth of infiltration, might be reduced, thus facilitating the surgical procedure. (2) Lymph nodes in the irradiated area being less massively invaded than the bladder and hence requiring smaller tumor-lethal irradiation doses, might be sterilized; reducing the risk of incomplete surgical clearing or even eliminating the need of lymphadenectomy, by devitalizing or reducing the number of tumor cells, both in the primary and in the lymph node deposits. (3) The risk of iatrogenic dissemination during the surgical procedure might be decreased.

After previous reports in 1963 and 1968, Whitmore et al. (50) presented the following 5-year survival data for patients with a T3 growth, treated in various periods (noncontrolled study): cystectomy only, 20% (89 cases); preoperative irradiation 4000 rads/4-6 weeks to the true pelvis followed 1-3 weeks later by radical cystectomy, 30% (65 cases); 2000 rads in 1 week followed 1 week later by radical cystectomy, 39% (52 cases). In case of less deeply infiltrating growths (categories T1, T2) no beneficial effect of preoperative irradiation could be observed. There was no increased mortality or complication rate due to preoperative irradiation, though slightly more urinary infections were noted.

In a prospective cooperative controlled clinical trial patients with bladder cancer categories T2 and T3 were treated by irradiation only (4000-6000 rads in 5-6 weeks), by cystectomy only, or by preoperative irradiation followed by cystectomy. The irradiation field was not defined in this trial. Cystectomy followed 4-6 weeks after finishing radiotherapy. Blackard et al. (1) reported the preliminary results: 3-year survival in all groups, each consisting of about 12 patients, was about 40%.

Veenema et al. (40) observed tumor regression in 65 out of 150 preoperatively irradiated patients (dose: 3000-4000 rads in 3-4 weeks). Prognostic improvement due to preoperative irradiation could not be ascertained. Scott et al. (36) suggested improvement of prognosis in all stages due to preoperative irradiation: 5000 rads were given in 4-6 weeks through a 7 x 7 cm portal. Cystectomy followed 4-6 weeks later.

In a prospective cooperative trial (31) patients were randomized into either cystectomy or cystectomy preceded by irradiation (4500 rads/28-32 days, 1000 rads/week, the choice of the field size was left to the radiotherapist). Cystectomy followed after 4-8 weeks. Five-year survival was 40% for 99 patients preoperatively irradiated, 27% for 129 patients treated by cystectomy only. In 34% of 98 patients no tumor was found in the cystectomy specimen after preoperative irradiation; however, 10% of patients without preoperative irradiation had also no evidence of malignancy in the cystectomy specimen. The 5-year survival rate for all patients with tumor in the cystectomy specimen was about 25% as compared with about 50% for patients without residual growth.

At the Rotterdam Radiotherapy Institute (43-45,47) patients with a bladder cancer category T3 received preoperative megavoltage irradiation 4000 rads/4 weeks; the irradiation fields covered the true pelvis and since 1972 also the juxtaregional nodes (Fig. 6). Simple cystectomy followed as soon as possible after finishing irradiation. In 96 out of 141 patients (68%), T reduction, i.e., a reduction of the depth of infiltration of the malignancy could be demonstrated in the cystectomy specimen [T3 corresponding with P(0), P(is), P(1), P(2)] , 42 of these 96 appeared to be microscopically free of malignancy (T3 corresponding with P0). In case of such T reduction the 5 year uncorrected survival rate was significantly better than in case of no T reduction (60% and 20%, respectively). Histological grade appeared not to be related to T reduction and hence not to prognosis. Survival after large-field preoperative irradiation was slightly worse than after small-field (true pelvis only) irradiation, this was mainly due to high first year mortality of patients older than 65 years; apparently the therapeutic burden is too large for older patients.

In 1966 Wallace and Bloom (41) started a randomized controlled trial for patients with carcinoma of the bladder T3 category without demonstrable metastases, age not exceeding 70 years. The two trial arms were:

1. 4000 rads external irradiation to the pelvic cavity including lymph nodes at the level of L5, followed in 4 weeks by cystectomy and lymphadenectomy.

2. 4000 rads to the pelvic cavity as in case of treatment 1, followed by 2000 rads to the bladder including the perivesical tissue. The 5 year survival of 98 patients in the preoperative irradiation plus cystectomy group was 33%, for 91 patients irradiated only, 21%. If only patients under 60 years were considered, the difference became even more marked: about 40% 5-year survival in the preoperative irradiation plus cystectomy group as compared with about 25% in the irradiation-only group. Pathological down-staging due to preoperative irradiation was noted in 47% of the patients. The 5-year survival of 36 patients with pathological down-staging was about 50% as compared with about 20% of 41 patients with no pathological down-staging.

In 1977 Miller (23) showed in a controlled prospective trial that preoperative irradiation (5000 rads/5 weeks) followed by simple cystectomy resulted in 46% 5-year survival (35 cases treated), whereas only 16% (32 cases treated) were alive after irradiation, giving 7000 rads/7 weeks. All authors agree that preoperative irradiation can reduce the extent of infiltration of the bladder cancer. As in the T3 category, clinical overstaging seems negligible (46) and T reduction cannot be the result of clinical overstaging. According to most authors, preoperative irradiation does not increase operative mortality (about 10%) nor the rate of serious complications. In earlier studies improvement of prognosis due to preoperative irradiation could only be suggested but not proved; however, since 1973 evidence for its beneficial prognostic influence has accumulated. Though cooperative controlled clinical trials should give aproper answer as to the value of preoperative irradiation, they have often the inherent disadvantages of different institutions contributing to the trial and even of varying investigators in one center. This can result in the possibility of different techniques of staging, different extent of transurethral resection, and different irradiation techniques. These factors could introduce a flaw in the assessment of T reduction as for instance in the study of Prout et al. (31), or in the assessment of prognosis as in the study of Blackard et al. (1).

There is nearly a consensus of opinion that deeply infiltrating growths [T3 (UICC) or B2 and C (Jewett)] benefit most from preoperative irradiation. Probably this beneficial influence is due to sterilizing regional and juxtaregional lymph nodes in those cases with T reduction, as response of the primary to irradiation will also reflect response of involved lymph nodes. This theory is supported by the trial of Wallace and Bloom (41) which showed a correlation between lymph node involvement and T reduction in the cystectomy specimen; 8% lymph node involvement in case of T reduction as compared with 37% in case of no T reduction. Moreover, in the Rotterdam and in Miller's series, no lymph node dissection was performed, yet results were identical to those after lymphadenectomy as reported from other centers. In support of this theory is the finding at Rotterdam that of 43 patients without T reduction (P3), 40% died with clinical lymph node metastases, whereas this was noted in only 7 out of 96 patients with T reduction, the other causes of death being comparable in both groups.

COMBINED MODALITY TREATMENT: SYSTEMIC CHEMOTHERAPY, PREOPERATIVE IRRADIATION, AND CYSTECTOMY

Several investigators suggested that systemic chemotherapy, especially 5-FU, in addition to preoperative irradiation and cystectomy might improve prognosis. Kaufman (20) reported cystectomy specimens free of malignancy in 15 out of 25 cases, stage A and B1, and in 7 out of 17 cases, stage B2 and C, after treatment with 5-FU and preoperative irradiation (3500 rads/3.5 weeks). However, this percentage of tumor destruction is not higher than after preoperative irradiation to a slightly higher dose level.

In a cooperative prospective study (30) bladder cancer patients were randomized into either preoperative irradiation followed by open surgery or into direct open surgery. Each group was again randomized into additional 5-FU treatment or into no chemotherapy. The complication rate appeared not to be increased by additional 5-FU; however, neither tumor regression nor prognosis was favorably influenced by additional 5-FU. Similar conclusions were drawn by Edland et al. (8). In his nonrandomized study of 36 patients 18 were treated with supervoltage irradiation (6000-7000 rads) plus 5-FU, 18 by supervoltage irradiation only. After irradiation, in 21 cases tumor regression of more than 75% was noted, 39% showed total response, additional 5-FU had no significant influence on tumor regression. Since chemotherapy may have a destructive effect on clinical and subclinical metastatic deposits in nodes and other organs beyond the irradiated area, theoretically it should improve prognosis; however, affirmative convincing evidence has not yet been produced.

THE VALUE OF RADIOTHERAPY IN THE MANAGEMENT OF BLADDER CANCER

Comparison of the results of surgical treatment of bladder cancer with those of radiotherapeutic approaches is difficult and full of fallacies: urologists often report survival rates according to surgical-pathological staging; tumor and host factors play an important role in the selection for both minor surgery, such as transurethral resection, and major surgery, such as cystectomy; pure palliation is generally not attempted by surgical procedures.

In assessing the value of the various radiotherapeutic treatment modalities, several aspects have to be considered: the risks and the burden of the treatment, the morbidity including early and late complications, the survival rate, the quality of life after cure, and the possibilities of salvage after failure of the first treatment of choice. Comparison of survival rates in the various treatment groups can be misleading if staging is not comparable, if the histological border between benign and malignant growths is not clearly defined, if tumor factors such as multiplicity and surface extension of the growth are not taken into account, if host factors such as general condition, age, concomitant disease, etc., have influenced the decision as to the applied therapy, i.e., trial results usually apply only to selected groups characterized by identified criteria and referral policy to certain centers often implies selection of the patients. The complication rate tends to decrease with increased experience of the treating clinicians. Yet, the possible early and late complications and the chance of impairment of quality of life inherent to the various radiotherapeutic approaches have to be balanced against the expected cure rate, the individual conditions of the patient, and against his life expectancy apart from the bladder malignancy.

In case of papillomas, radiotherapy is not indicated; surgery with or without intracavitary application of chemicals (Epodyl, or thiotepa) is still the treatment of choice. Hyperthermia as applied by Hall (18) turned out to be disappointing, as it could not prevent recurrences elsewhere in the bladder. Patients with carcinoma in situ, T (is), and with papillary carcinoma, T(A) growths, as a rule do not benefit substantially from any type of radiotherapy. Transurethral resection (TUR) is still the initial method of choice; probably topical (mitomycin, Epodyl, thiotepa) or systemic (adriamycin) administration of chemotherapeutic agents can reduce the recurrence rate and hence prevent eventual cystectomy. The benefit of oral administration of vitamin A (13-cis-retinoic-acid) is being investigated (32). Cytogenic analysis of chromosomal markers might be helpful in identifying patients with high risk of recurrence, who might benefit from elective chemotherapy (12).

In the T1 category, localized bladder malignancies with a diameter not exceeding 4-5 cm and not controllable by transurethral resection only appear to have the best cure rate after interstitial implantation of radioactive material (about 70% 5-year survival). Recurrence rate is less than 10% as compared with TUR only (up to 70% within 1 year). The operative mortality is low (about 2%). Morbidity is negligible, return to normal active life without mutilation or complaints is the rule; however, the general condition of the patient has to be compatible with suprapubic intervention. In case of local recurrence or recurrence elsewhere in the bladder, cure can still be provided by an external course of irradiation or by surgical procedures.

In cases of multiple or diffuse T1 growths not controllable by TUR, intracavitary application of radioactive sources or a full course of external irradiation offer about the same prognosis, the risk of crippling bladder fibrosis is larger with intracavitary treatment. After both types of irradiation, cystectomy is possible in cases of recurrence or in cases of serious complications, however, extensive fibrosis beyond the bladder might render salvage cystectomy hazardous.

Malignancies of the T2 category covering an area with a maximum diameter of 5 cm benefit most from interstitial radiotherapy, preferably preceded by a short course of external irradiation (40-55% 5-year survival). Similar to the T1 category, the patient, fit for suprapubic intervention, will risk negligible morbidity and mortality. Again, in the case of local recurrence, salvage is still possible by a full course of external irradiation or cystectomy. In multiple T2 growths or T2 growths covering a large area, a full course of external irradiation and preoperative irradiation followed by cystectomy offer about the same prognosis (5-year survival, 40-50%); cystectomy patients are usually selected according to good general condition and age (generally accepted upper limit + 70 years). Operative mortality usually does not exceed 5-10%. The complication rate seems acceptable in view of the possible cure rate. A full course of external irradiation is less mutilating to the patient; therefore, a strict selection as to general condition and age of the patient is not required. The immediate and late complication rate can be reduced to a minimum with modern techniques. In case of local recurrence salvage cystectomy is still feasible if the general condition of the patient permits it, though, due to irradiation fibrosis, this procedure might be difficult and associated with delayed healing.

T3 growths restricted to a limited area in the bladder can be treated with interstitial irradiation. Since the incidence of metastatic regional lymph nodes in the T3 category approaches 40-50% and these nodes are usually not adequately attacked by interstitial technique, cure rate cannot be expected to exceed 50%. Cystectomy, preceded by external irradiation (about 4000 rads/4 weeks) in patients eligible for major surgery, will probably provide a better prognosis; however, at the price of mutilation. Combinations of 4000 rads (or its equivalent) of external irradiation with a reduced interstitial irradiation dose might lead to higher cure rate and still avoid cystectomy. This approach is being investigated now at the Rotterdam Radiotherapy Institute. More extensive T3 growths are best treated by preoperative irradiation followed by cystectomy. Again, patients have to be selected according to good general condition and age. The unavoidable operative mortality (up to 10%) and the inherent mutilation are the price to pay for 40-50% chance of cure. The alternative is a full course of external irradiation which still offers 10-30% cure to all patients with a T3 growth, where tumor and/or host conditions do not permit either interstitial therapy or major surgery. Studies to identify markers which indicate T reduction after preoperative irradiation prior to cystectomy might be helpful in the selection of patients for the mutilating cystectomy: as prognosis is very poor (10% 5-year survival) in case of no T reduction, cystectomy might be replaced by a full course of external irradiation in those patients. On the other hand, postoperative elective chemotherapy [adriamycin, 5-FU, methotrexate, cis-dichlorodiamine platinum (II) (DDP), as single agents or in combination] for patients with no demonstrable radiation-induced T reduction, might improve prognosis by killing subclinical metastases in and beyond the irradiation field. However, this more vigorous therapy might surpass the general resistance of the usually elderly patients and hence have an adverse effect.

Patients with a bladder cancer fixed to the pelvic wall or penetrating into other organs (T4 category) are usually unsuitable for curative surgery and only a 5% chance of cure can be offered by a full course of external supervoltage irradiation. In the majority of cases, this irradiation at least prevents a painful bladder or pelvic death. Also in this group selected patients in good general condition might benefit from elective adjuvant chemotherapy.

In all patients with distant metastases (M1) or with a poor condition not compatible with demanding treatment, a short course of irradiation can prevent, abolish, or relieve serious bladder and metastases symptoms. The real value of systemic chemotherapy in case of metastases has still to be assessed. Response rates in small series of selected patients, as reported by various authors, vary between 19-90%.

In an endeavor to broaden the scope of radiotherapy in the treatment of bladder cancer, with the goal of identifying for each individual patient, according to host and tumor factors, the most beneficial type of radiotherapy, with or without combinations of other treatment modalities, imaginative feasibility pilot studies have to be done meticulously. In these studies unconventional fractionation schemes, new combinations, and modifications of existing radiotherapeutic approaches (external and interstitial), and various combinations with surgery, chemotherapy, radiosensitizers, immunotherapy, and perhaps hyperthermia can be tested. In order to assess critically the value of new treatment designs, the feasibility studies have to be followed by prospective randomized studies. Strict rules regarding clinical staging, microscopic classification, treatment details, and patient selection are mandatory for obtaining unequivocal answers to the many questions which remain.

REFERENCES

1. Blackard, C.E., Byar, D.P., and the Veterans Administration Cooperative Urological Research Group: Results of a clinical trial of surgery and radiation in stages II and III carcinoma of the bladder. J. Urol. 108:875, 1972.

2. Bloom, H.J.G.: Treatment by interstitial irradiation using tantalum 182 wire. Br. J. Radiol. 33:471, 1960.

3. Brenk, H.A. van den: Hyperbaric oxygen in radiation therapy. Am. J. Roentgenol. 102:8, 1968.

4. Cade, I.S. and McEwen, J.B.: Clinical trials of radiotherapy in hyperbaric oxygen at Portsmouth. Clin. Radiol. 29:333, 1978.

5. Darger, R.: Tumeurs malignes de la vessie, traitement par la radium-therapie a vessie ouverte, Paris, Marson & Cie, 1951.

6. Dix, V.W., Shanks, W., Tresidder, G.C.: Carcinoma of the bladder; treatment by diathermy snare excision and interstitial irradiation. Br. J. Urol. 42:213, 1970.

7. Durrant, KR. and Laing, A.H.: Treatment of multiple superficial papillary tumor of the bladder by intracavitary yttrium-90. J. Urol. 113:480, 1975.

8. Edland, R.W., Wear, J.B., and Ansfield, F.J.: Advanced cancer of the urinary bladder. Am. J. Roentgenol. 108:124, 1970.

9. Edsmyr, F., Moberger, G., and Wadstrom, L.: Carcinoma of the bladder. Cystectomy after supervoltage therapy. Scand. J. Urol. Nephrol. 5:215, 1971.

10. Edsmyr, F.: Radiotherapy in the management of bladder cancer. In The Biology and Clinical Management of Bladder Cancer, edited by E.H. Cooper and R.E. Williams, Oxford, Blackwell, 1975, p. 229.

11. Edsmyr, F., Huber, W., and Menander, KB.: Orgotein efficacy in ameliorating side effects due to radiation therapy. Curr. Therap. Res. 19:198, 1976.

12. Falor, W.H. and Ward, R.M.: Prognosis in early carcinoma of the bladder based on chromosomal analysis. J. Urol. 199:44, 1978.

13. Finney, R.: The treatment of carcinoma of the bladder by external irradiation. Clin. Radiol. 22:225, 1971.

14. Friedman, M. and Lewis, L.G.: A new technic for the radium treatment of carcinoma of the bladder. Radiology 53:342, 1949.

15. Friedman, M. and Lewis, L.G.: Irradiation of carcinoma of the bladder by a central intracavitary radium or cobalt 60 source (The Walter Reed Technique). Am. J. Roentgenol. 79:6, 1958.

16. Goffinet, D.R., Schneider, M.J., Glatstein, E.J., Ludwig, H., Ray, G.R., Dunnick, N.R., and Bagshaw, M.A., et al.: Bladder cancer: Results of radiation therapy in 384 patients. Radiology 117:149, 1975.

17. Goin, Lowell S. and Hoffman, Eugene F.: A new approach to the treatment of certain bladder carcinomas. Radiology 34:205, 1940.

18. Hall, R.R.: Personal communications, 1976 and 1978.

19. Jewett, H.J.: Cancer of the bladder. Diagnosis and staging. Cancer 32:1072, 1973.

20. Kaufman, J.J.: Treatment of carcinoma of the bladder with combined radiotherapy, chemotherapy and surgery. Arch. Surg. 99:447, 1969.

21. Kligerman, M.M.: Pi-meson radiotherapy of human bladder carcinoma. In: Current Cancer Research on Cancer of the Urinary Tract, International Cancer Research Data Bank, Washington, D.C., U.S. Dept. of Health, Education and Welfare. July 21, 1978, p. 21.

22. Morrison, R.: The results of treatment of cancer of the bladder. A clinical contribution to radiobiology. Clin. Radiol. 26:67, 1975.

23. Miller, L.S.: Bladder cancer. Superiority of preoperative irradiation and cystectomy in clinical stages B2 and C. Cancer 39:973, 1977.

24. Muller, J.H.: Radiotherapy of bladder cancer by means of rubber balloons filled in situ with solutions of a radioactive isotope (Co-60). Cancer 8:1035, 1955.

25. Munro, A.I.: The results of using radioactive gold grains in the treatment of bladder growths. Br. J. Urol. 36:541, 1964.

26. Pasteau, O., Wickham, L, Degrais, L.: Cancer de la prostate et radium. 2. Conf. Intern. pour l'etude du cancer. Paris, Masson and Cie, 1910, p. 707.

27. Pedersen, M. and Herting, S.E.: Intracavitary radium treatment of malignant tumors of the urinary bladder. Acta Radiol. 11:369, 1972.

28. Pierquin, B., Chassagne, D.J., Chahbazian, C.M., and Wilson, J.F.: Urinary bladder. In Brachytherapy, St. Louis, Warren H. Green, 1978, p. 198.

29. Plenk, H.P.: Hyperbaric radiation therapy. Preliminary results of a randomized study of cancer of the urinary bladder and review of the "oxygen experience." Am. J. Roentgenol. 114:152, 1972.

30. Prout, G.R., Slack, N.H., and Bross, I.D.J.: Irradiation and 5-fluorouracil as adjuvants in the management of invasive bladder carcinoma. A cooperative group report after 4 years. J. Urol. 104:116, 1970.

31. Prout, G.R., Slack, N.H., and Bross, I.D.J. Preoperative irradiation and cystectomy for bladder carcinoma. IV: Results in a selected population. 7th National Cancer Conference Proceedings, Los Angeles, September 27-29, 1972. Philadelphia, Lipincott, 1972, p. 783.

32. Prout, G.R.: Retinoid chemoprevention trial begins against bladder cancer. JAMA 240:609, 1978.

33. Rider, W.D. and Evans, D.H.: Radiotherapy in the treatment of recurrent bladder cancer. Br. J. Urol. 48:595, 1976.

34. Sagerman, R.H., Bagshaw, M.A., and Kaplan, H.S.: Linear accelerator supervoltage radiation therapy; carcinoma of the bladder. Am. J. Roentgenol. 93:122, 1965.

35. Scanlon, P.W. and Furlow, W.L.: Split-dose radiotherapy for bladder carcinoma. Radiology 97:141, 1970.

36. Scott, R., Koff, W.J., Hudgkins, Ph. T., and McCullough, D.: Preoperative irradiation in the surgical treatment of transitional cell cancer of the bladder: Preliminary report based on 12 years of experience. J. Urol. 109: 405, 1973.

37. Smithers, W.: Cancer of the bladder. In The X-ray Treatment of Accessible Cancer, London, Arnold & Co., 1946, p. 108.

38. Union Internationale Contre le Cancer (U.I.C.C.): T.N.M. Classification of Malignant Tumors, 2nd edition, Geneva, 1974, p. 79.

39. Union Internationale Contre le Cancer (U.I.C.C.): T.N.M. Classification of Malignant Tumors, 3rd edition, Geneva, 1978, p. 113.

40. Veenema, R.J., Guttmann, R., Uson, A.C., Senyazyn, J., and Romas, N.A. et al.: Improved clinical definition of bladder carcinoma by preoperative external radiotherapy. Transactions of the American Association of Genitourinary Surgeons 64:69, 1972.

41. Wallace, D. and Bloom, H.J.G.: Personal communications, 1966, 1971, and 1976.

42. Werf-Messing, B. van der: Carcinoma of the bladder treated by suprapubic radium implants. The value of additional external irradiation. Eur. J. Cancer 5:277, 1969.

43. Werf-Messing, B. van der: Carcinoma of the bladder treated by preoperative irradiation followed by cystectomy. Eur. J. Cancer 7:467, 1971.

44. Werf-Messing, B. van der: Carcinoma of the bladder treated by preoperative irradiation followed by cystectomy. The second report. Cancer 32:1, 1973.

45. Werf-Messing, B. van der: Carcinoma of the bladder T3NXMO treated by preoperative irradiation followed by cystectomy. Third report of the Rotterdam Radiotherapy Institute. Cancer 36:718, 1975.

46. Werf-Messing, B. van der: Cancer of the urinary bladder treated by interstitial radium implant. Int. J. Radiat. Oncol. Biol. Phys. 4:373, 1978.

47. Werf-Messing, B. van der: Carcinoma of the urinary bladder category T3NX, O-4M0 treated by preoperative irradiation followed by cystectomy in Rotterdam. Int. J. Radiat. Oncol. (to be published).

48. Whitmore, W.F., Phillips, R.F., Grabstald, H., Bronstein, E.L., Mackenzie, A.R., and Hustu, O.: Experience with preoperative irradiation followed by radical cystectomy for the treatment of bladder cancer. Am. J. Roentgenol. 90:1016, 1963.

49. Whitmore, W.F.: Integrated therapy for bladder cancer. In: Cancer Therapy by Integrated Radiation and Operation, edited by B.F. Rush, Jr. and R.H. Greenlaw, Springfield, Thomas, 1968, p. 111.

50. Whitmore, W.F., Betaca, M.A., Hilaris, B.S., Reddy, G.N., Unsl, A., Ghoniem, M.A., Grabstald, N., and Chu, F.: A comparative study of two preoperative radiation regimens with cystectomy for bladder cancer. Cancer 40:1077, 1977.

chapter 11

CARCINOMA OF THE PROSTATE

Eashwer K. Reddy, M.D.
Carl M. Mansfield, M.D.

The prostate gland is an organ composed of glandular and muscular tissue that surrounds the proximal portion of the male urethra. The longest axis of the prostate, which is almost vertical in the erect posture, measures 2.5-3.0 cm; the transverse diameter at the base is 4.0-4.5 cm; and the thickness, 2.0-2.5 cm. Its weight is normally 20-25 g but in old age it may be several times larger. The anterior surface is directly posterior to the pubic symphysis and separated from it by the pudendal plexus of veins and adipose tissue. The posterior surface is separated from the anterior wall of the lower portion of the rectum by a double layer of fascia (Denonvillier). Laterally the prostate is bounded by the levator ani and the prostatic venous plexus.

The prostate gland is rich in lymphatics which form a network on the posterior surface of the gland. About six to eight collecting channels on each side of the prostatic drain to nodes along the internal, external, and common iliacs and obturator nodes (Fig. 1).

Venules from the parenchyma of the gland drain into the prostatic plexus which consists of a mass of thin-walled veins lying between the prostatic fascia and fibrous capsule of the gland. It receives the deep dorsal vein of the penis and the veins of the base of the bladder and, after communicating with the rectal plexus of veins, drains across the pelvic floor into the internal iliac vein. The internal iliac veins communicate freely with veins draining the vertebral column and coxal bone. (Since none of these veins have valves, it is believed that prostate carcinoma often metastasizes through these veins to the coccygeal bones and the lower part of the vertebral column.)

Carcinoma of the prostate is the second most common malignant disease in men in the United States. It causes about 7-8% of all tumor deaths in men over 50 years of age. The United States has the highest incidence of prostatic cancer (21). The American Cancer Society estimated that in 1981 there would be 70,000 new cases and 22,700 deaths from carcinoma of the prostate in the United States (14).

The disease is rare before age 35. The age-specific incidence rates show a steady increase, both in clinical and latent cases, beyond age 50, until the eighth decade. After age 80, clinical cases become less common. Latent cases, however, become increasingly common after 80 years of age; most men over the age of 90 have latent disease. Autopsy findings in men over 50 years, who died from other causes, revealed a 30% incidence of carcinomas that were indistinguishable histologically from active clinical cancer. These are latent or retarded cases; their growth rate is very slow. The microscope in this instance gives us no guide

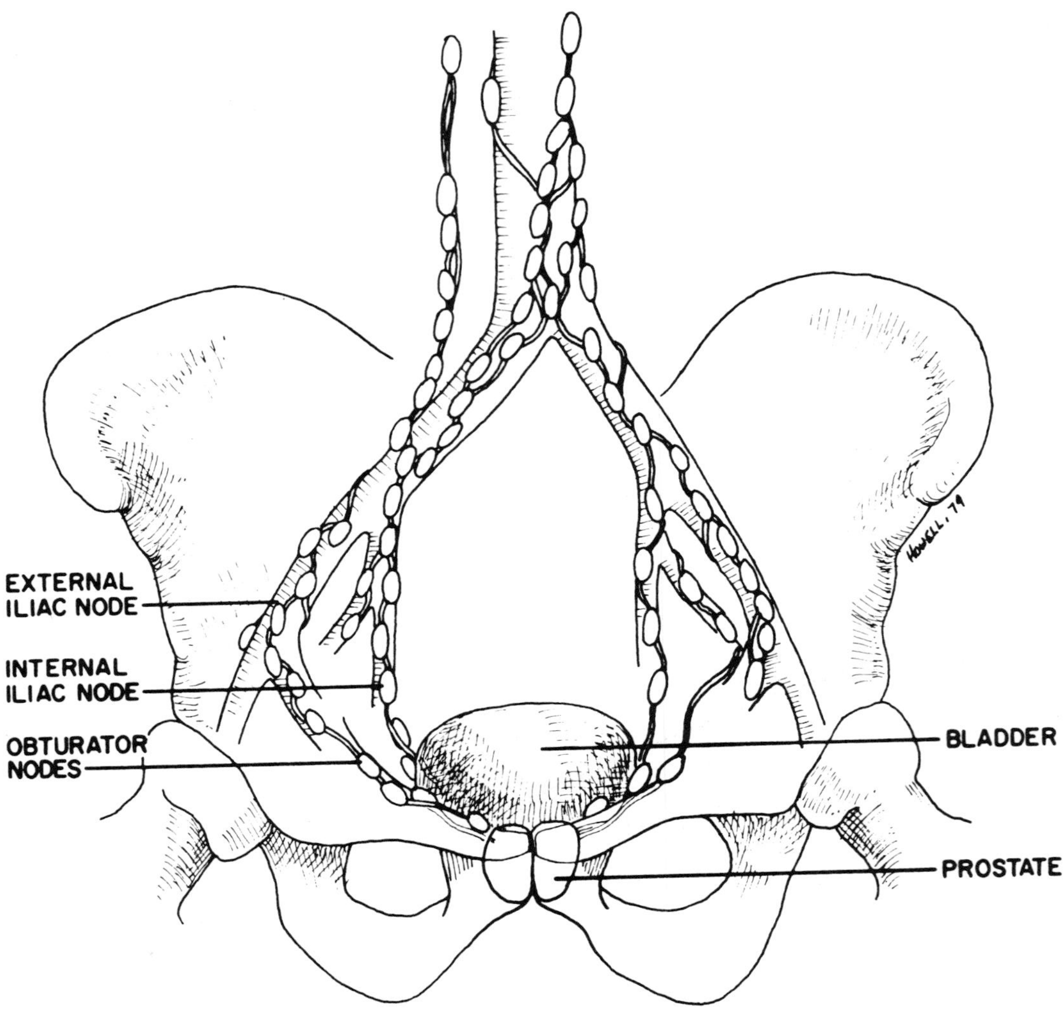

Figure 1. Lymphatic drainage of prostate. A: Anterior view.

to the biological behavior of the tumor (29). These two types of prostatic cancers are morphologically indistinguishable, yet differ in their biological behavior. It is a common observation that the younger the age the more aggressive the disease. There seems to be a factor or factors in the elderly which retards the growth of prostatic cancer or makes it more indolent.

About 50% of cases can be diagnosed by an inexpensive digital rectal examination. Any nodule in the prostate in a man over 50 years of age should be considered malignant until proven otherwise. It is often easy to detect these nodules on digital examination since most malignant tumors of the prostate arise in the peripheral zone of the gland. By the time the tumor causes symptoms, it is locally advanced, usually extending to paraprostatic tissue and/or to regional lymph nodes.

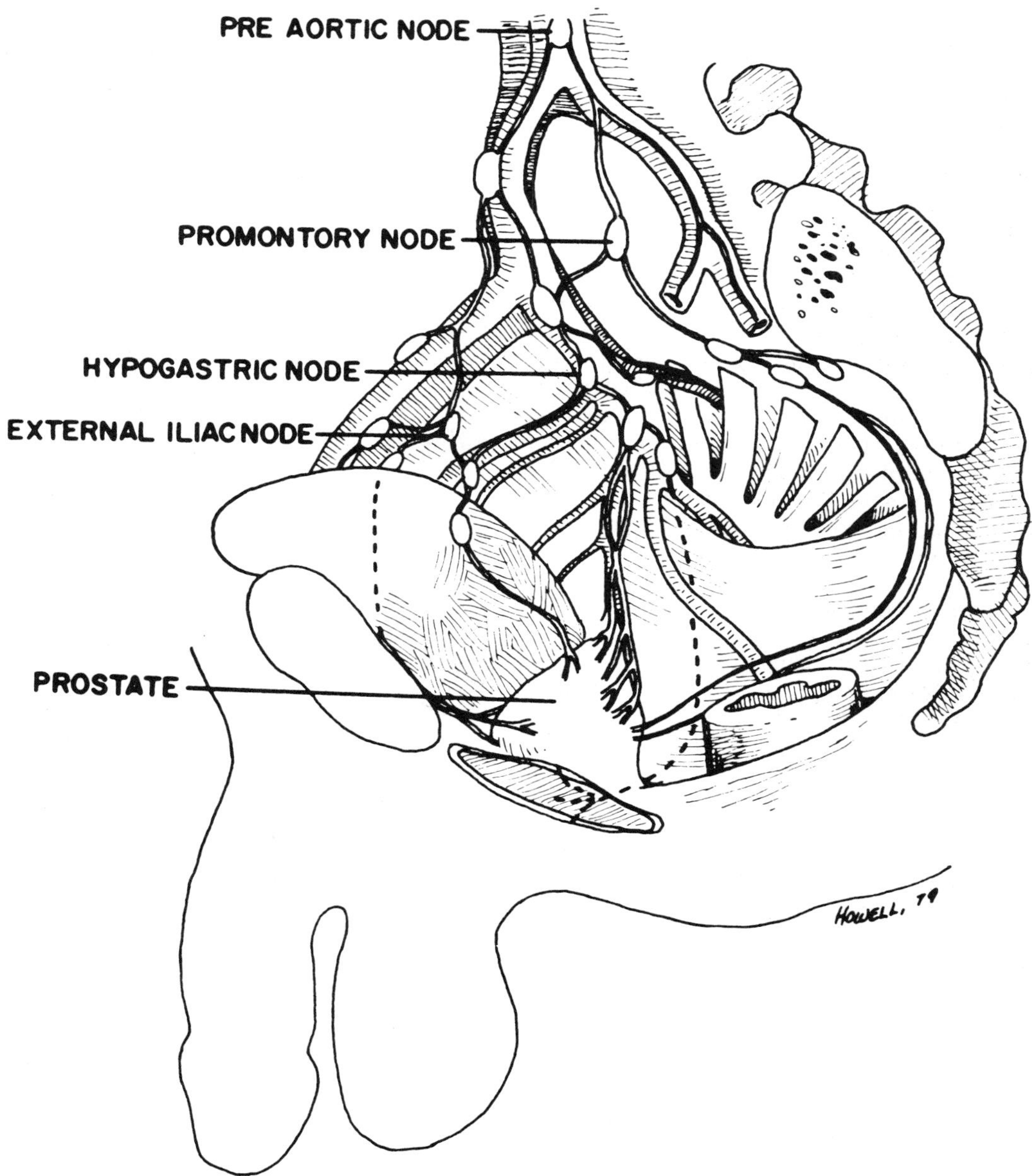

Figure 1. B: Lateral view.

The routine workup should include the following procedures:

1. History and physical examination
2. Routine laboratory work (SMA 12, CBC, urinalysis)
3. Biopsy (perineal, transrectal, or transurethral resection)
4. Serum and prostatic acid phosphatase
5. Lymphangiography
6. Bone scan
7. Computerized axial tomography

Human serum acid phosphatase activity is composed of a mixture of acid phosphatase isoenzymes present in different organs. It has been reported that elevated serum acid phosphatase levels are found in 24-40% of patients with primary carcinoma of the prostate and in 47-85% of patients with metastatic tumor (36,70,80). The serum acid phosphatase levels have been used in the diagnosis and monitoring of therapy for prostatic carcinoma for more than four decades. Unfortunately, it was not possible to single out the prostatic fraction of this enzyme. Using radioimmunoassay, immunofluorescence, and counterimmunoelectrophoresis techniques, it is now possible to separate prostatic acid phosphatase isoenzyme (16,93).

Gutman (37) and associates in 1936 first showed increased acid phosphatase activity in prostatic tumor at metastatic sites and hypothesized that tumor cells produce acid phosphatase similar to normal prostatic tissue. Much effort has also been directed toward direct identification of tumor cells in bone marrow aspirate. The incidence of bone marrow metastasis ranged from 7.5-56% (3,10,18,25,62, 94). Nelson (67) and associates, after reviewing 556 bone marrow aspiration biopsy specimens on 449 patients in a 10-year period, found positive cytology in 7.6% of specimens. Because of this low yield of positive cytology the authors concluded that bone marrow aspiration biopsy was of little help in evaluating patients with carcinoma of the prostate.

Based on the work of Gutman in 1936, Chau et al. (17) noted the potential values of acid phosphatase determination in bone marrow aspirates for early detection of metastatic prostatic carcinoma. Since then several reports (11,22,35,50, 72,87,92) have appeared in the literature supporting the value of bone marrow acid phosphatase for early detection of metastatic carcinoma of the prostate. Although the above reports support the value of this procedure, others (24,26,32,52,73) questioned its value because of a large number of false positive results (74).

The bipedal lymphangiogram (LAG) is of limited value, since the hypogastric and obturator nodes do not routinely fill. Hilaris et al. (40) report that the lymphangiogram is accurate in determining the presence or absence of lymph node metastases in about 70-75% of patients. The high incidence (30-45%) of false negative interpretations (11,40,77) makes lymphangiography too insensitive a diagnostic tool for the determination of lymph node involvement. Transabdominal percutaneous needle biopsy, under fluoroscopic guidance, of suspicious nodes on LAG may help in staging disease (89,103). CT scanning can be helpful in evaluating paraaortic and pelvic nodes. At present it seems that staging laparotomy and pelvic lymphadenectomy are the most accurate methods to assess involvement of the obturator, hypogastric, and external and common iliac nodes. Lymphatic dissemination may occur early in clinical disease. The incidence of lymph node metastases ranges from 27-50% (Table 1). The incidence increases with size and grade of tumor (11, 26,60) and invasion of seminal vesicle (5,47).

The bone scan should be done routinely. Seminal vesiculography (1,31), prostatography (75), and ultrasonography (43,81) with a probe in the rectum can be helpful in delineating the local extent of disease. It is also possible to use computed tomography to help evaluate the extent of disease in the pelvis (84).

In 1956 Whitmore (95) proposed a staging system, separating prostatic malignancy into four stages (96), A, B, C, and D, so that the results of different treatments could be better compared. Other systems are UICC, tumor, nodes, metastases TNM, and Jewett's (48) classification (Table 2).

Table 1. Incidence of Lymphnode Metastases According to Stage by Histological Examination

Author (Ref.)	No. of Patients	Stage A	Stage B	Stage C	Total
Flocks et al., 1959 (26)	411		2/29 (7%)	144/382 (38%)	146/382 (35%)
Arduino and Glucksman, 1962 (5)	44		14/44 (32%)		
McLaughlin et al., 1976 (60)	60		9/36 (25%)	12/24 (50%)	21/60 (35%)
Ray et al., 1976 (77)	50		5/25 (20%)	13/25 (52%)	18/50 (36%)
Hilaris et al., 1977 (40)	208		37/128 (29%)	47/80 (59%)	84/208 (40%)
Bruce et al., 1977 (40)	30	0/3 (0%)	5/19 (26%)	6/8 (75%)	11/30 (36%)
Bagshaw et al., 1977 (8)	60	0/1	7/33 (21%)	20/33 (60%)	27/60 (40%)
Wilson et al., 1978 (101)	87	0/12 (0%)	14/56 (25%)	10/19 (52%)	24/87 (27%)
Golimbu et al., 1978 (33)	30	?/10	?/15	?/5	15/30 (50%)
Herr, 1979 (39)	71		11/41 (26%)	16/30 (53%)	27/71 (38%)
Paulson and Research Group, 1979 (70)	129	8/32 (25%)	30/52 (30%)	21/45 (46%)	59/129 (45%)

Table 2. Carcinoma of the Prostate: Staging

AJCCS (102) (TNM)	Description	Whitmore (95)	Jewett (48)
T0	No tumor palpable; includes incidental findings of cancer in a biopsy of operative specimen	A	A1 (Focal) A2 (Diffuse)
T1	Tumor intracapsular surrounded by normal gland		
T2	Tumor confined to gland, deforming contour, and invading capsule, but lateral sulci and seminal vesicles are not involved	B	B1 one lobe (1.5 cm or less) B2 1.5 cm (invading one or both lobes)
T3	Tumor extends beyond capsule with or without involvement of lateral sulci and/or seminal vesicles	C	C
T4	Tumor fixed or involving neighboring structures		
N0	No involvement of regional lymph nodes		
N1	Involvement of a single regional lymph node		
N2	Involvement of multiple regional lymph nodes		
N3	Free space between primary tumor and fixed pelvic mass		
N4	Involvement of juxtaregional nodes		
M0	No distant metastases		
M1	Distant metastases present	D	D

Prostatic cancer is almost exclusively adenocarcinoma. Adenocarcinoma arises in the peripheral subcapsular zone of the prostate gland. The majority of them are multicentric and diffuse. Transitional cell carcinomas do arise in the larger prostatic ducts (85).

Grading of biopsy specimens of the primary tumor and metastases was suggested by Mostofi (64): grade 1: slight anaplasia; grade 2: moderate anaplasia; and grade 3: marked anaplasia. In cancer showing multiple histologic patterns, the area of greatest anaplasia is considered as the tumor grade. Grading of the tumor is also essential as a prognosticator: patients with high-grade tumors having a poorer outlook (40,54).

TREATMENT

More than 50% of patients present with metastatic disease. Less than 10% (47) of the cases are candidates for curative radical prostatectomy as first advocated by Young (102) in 1904. For the remaining 35-40% of patients, who present with locally extensive disease and/or regional lymph node involvement, radiation therapy plays an important role. The use of ionizing radiation, both external and interstitial, in the definitive treatment of adenocarcinoma of the prostate has greatly increased during the last decade.

Pasteau and Degrais (69) in 1909 used intraurethral radium source to treat the carcinoma of prostate. Barringer (9) in 1915 treated prostatic carcinoma by inserting radium needles into the prostate gland. In 1922 Deming (22) reported the results of radiotherapy in 100 cases with favorable results in 75%. The ability of ionizing radiation to sterilize prostatic carcinoma was further supported when Barringer (10) in 1942 reported four patients treated by interstitial implantation, using radium needles, and gold seeds by suprapubic or perineal route. All four lived for 6-9 years without evidence of disease locally, two had no cancer at necropsy 6 and 7 years after treatment. During the period of 1930-1946 the results of external beam therapy using kilovoltage radiation has been reported by several therapists (6,46,54,86,100). Due to the inherent quality of kilovoltage radiation the tumoricidal dose could not be delivered without undue damage to skin and subcutaneous tissues. Because of these side effects and the impressive results reported by Huggins et al. (44) in 1941 using hormone therapy, treatment by x-ray therapy was rarely used.

External Therapy

Interest in external radiation therapy was renewed with the introduction of supervoltage equipment. Bagshaw and Kaplan (7) reported to the Tenth International Congress of Radiology in 1962 their preliminary observations on the use of radiation therapy as a definitive treatment modality in carcinoma of the prostate. The first published report appeared in the literature in 1964 when Budhraja and Anderson (12) presented the results of treating 36 patients using megavoltage radiation therapy.

Most stage A tumors probably never produce clinical symptoms. It has not been determined whether a transition from stage A to stage B or C lesions is a function of time or some change in the biologic behavior of the cancer cells. Whitmore (97) reports that patients with stage A disease who received no therapy or conservative therapy had a survival which was nearly that of the population at large. Stage A disease has been divided into A1 (focal) and A2 (multifocal and diffuse disease). This better reflects prognosis and is more meaningful since the clinical behavior of stage A2 disease is more aggressive (48, 49) and definitive therapy is warranted. The majority of the patients with stage A disease have negative nodes. Therefore, only local radiation therapy to the prostate is necessary.

In stage B disease more than 30% of patients will have involvement of pelvic lymph nodes; this is higher in stage C disease (50-60%). The incidence is even higher in anaplastic tumors. Therefore, in addition to treating the prostate, it is essential to treat the whole pelvis to include pelvic lymph nodes. The treatment of stage D disease is for symptomatic relief of bone pain, bleeding, or obstruction from local disease.

Megavoltage therapy units are essential in order to deliver a tumoricidal dose to the pelvic lymph nodes and prostate without injury to skin and subcutaneous tissues. It is essential to use multiple-field and treatment planning techniques to minimize the dose to vital structures such as the rectum. In most instances, treatment, delivered by means of two opposed fields only, may risk unacceptable morbidity. An isocentric treatment planning technique with the patient in the supine position is a very commonly used setup. The position of the prostate gland, rectum, and bladder can be obtained by AP and lateral diagnostic film. The localization of the structures can be improved by the instillation of appropriate contrast media into the rectum and bladder. The whole pelvis field extends from the bifurcation of aorta (L4-5 junction) to the lower border of the ischial tuberosity. The lateral borders are 1.5 cm lateral to the ileopectineal line on the AP film to include the external and internal iliac lymph nodes (Fig. 2A). On the lateral film the length of the field remains the same as on the AP film. The posterior border should be drawn to adequately include the promanteric and presacral lymph nodes. The posterior half of the rectum should be blocked. Anteriorly the field extends to the pubic symphysis (Fig. 2B). To define the prostate booster volume, the length of the field can be obtained from the lateral film by identifying the bladder base which can be easily recognized on the lateral film taken with contrast in the bladder. An adequate margin of 2 cm should be allowed.

In stage A disease, the inclusion of seminal vesicles in the booster volume may not be necessary in every case because the incidence of microscopic invasion is rare. The seminal vesicles should be included in stage B and C disease because if one considers stage B disease alone microscopic invasion ranges from 2-24% (5, 8, 13, 101). The lower border of the booster volume is the same as the whole pelvic field (Fig. 2A). The lateral borders are through the middle of the obturator foraminae, the anterior border is through the middle of the pubic symphysis, and the posterior border is through the anterior wall of the rectum (Fig. 2A and B).

Treatment planning and the isodose distribution is essential to visualize and verify the dose distribution throughout the treatment volume. Different combined isodose distributions for whole pelvic radiation and prostate boost are shown in Fig. 3 and for prostate only shown in Fig. 4. Three hundred and sixty degree rotation is a common technique for treatment of the prostate only; other treatment techniques such as two lateral arcs, one anterior arc, or four-fields box technique can reduce the dose to the rectum. The computerized axial tomography (CAT) scan of the pelvis is very helpful in the localization of the tumor and normal structures (Fig. 5).

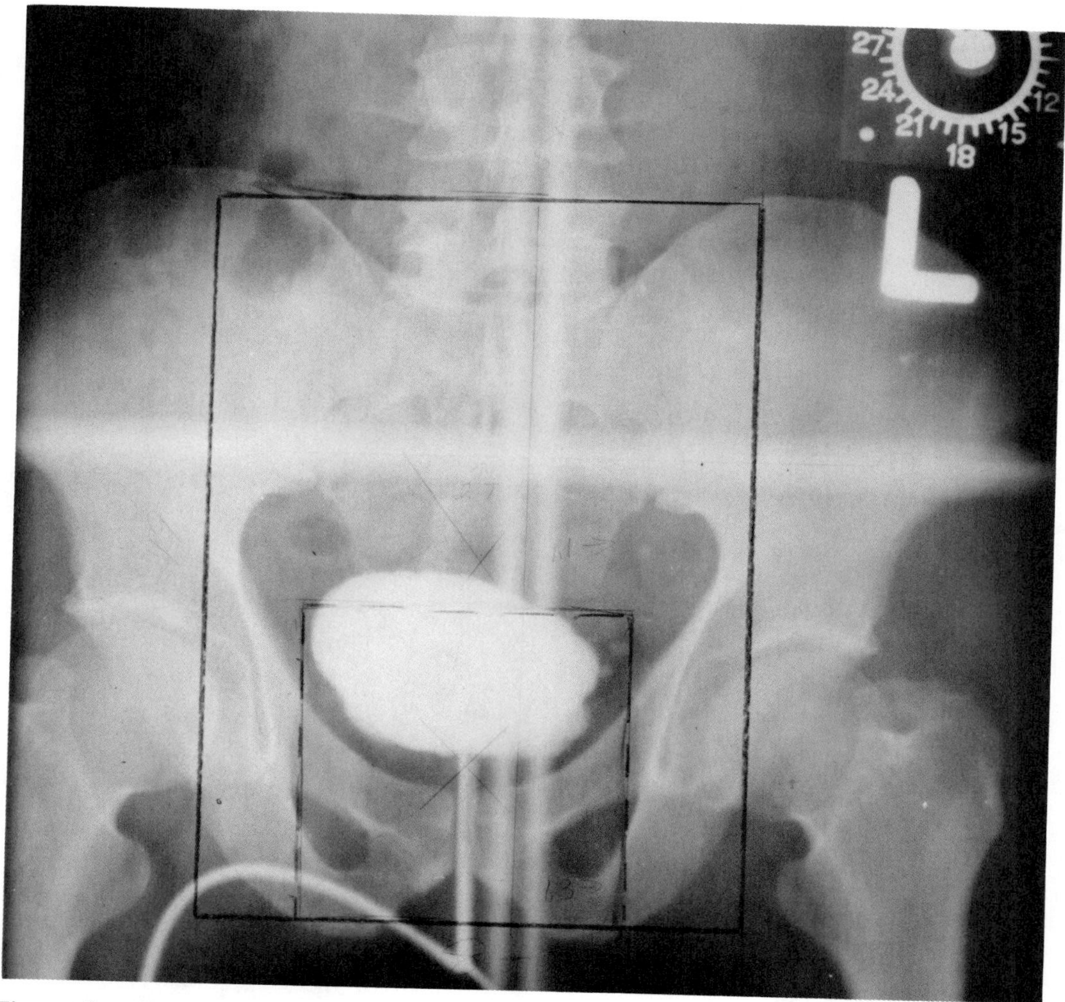

Figure 2. Simulation for whole pelvic and prostate boost volume. A: Anterior view.

A minimum dose should be delivered that is equivalent to 4500-5000 rads to node-bearing areas (whole pelvis) in 4.5-5 weeks at a rate of 180-200 rads/fraction/5 days per week. A booster dose of 1500-2000 rads to the prostate can be delivered immediately after completion of whole pelvic radiation to give a total dose to the prostate of 6000-7000 rads/6-7 weeks. It is advisable to treat all fields every day in order to minimize morbidity and to obtain homogeneous dose distribution within the treatment volume. With higher-energy machines (15 MV and above) using a four-field box technique, it may be possible to treat two fields per day.

The value of radiation therapy in the prophylactic treatment of the paraaortic nodes is still not known (27, 54). At present it appears to be of little value because if paraaortic nodes are negative, prophylactic irradiation is unnecessary, and if the nodes are positive, it is unlikely that the addition of prophylactic radiation will improve survival. However, when nodes are proven positive the general policy has been to irradiate these nodes. This should be continued until evidence shows conclusively that this approach is of no value. When the paraaortic nodes are irradiated,

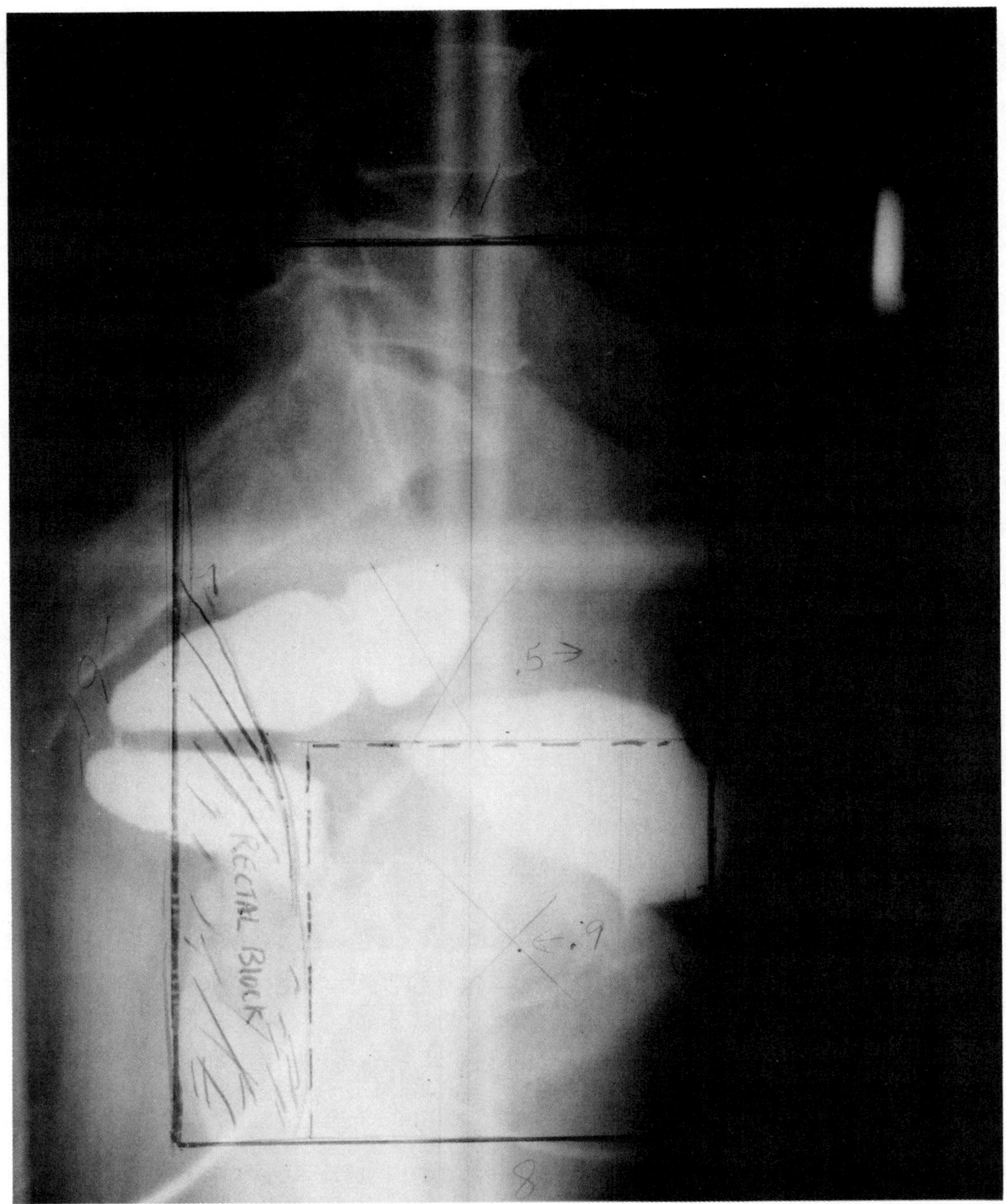

Figure 2. B: Lateral view.

the gap between the pelvic and paraaortic fields should be carefully calculated in order to avoid either overlap or an anatomic miss. Another approach is to abut the fields and shift the junctions every 1000 rads. The superior margin of the paraaortic field should be at the level of T12. The paraaortic nodes can be treated by a multiple-field technique; however, 3000 rads can be given through anterior and posterior fields and an additional 1500-2500 rads given through multiple-field technique depending upon the individual case.

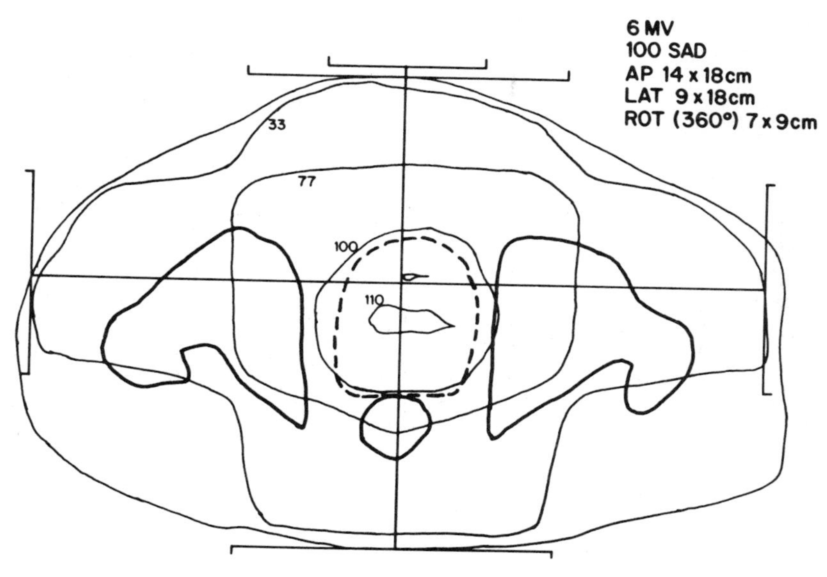

Figure 3. Composite isodose distribution for whole pelvic and prostate boost. A: Four-field whole pelvic fields followed by 360° rotation to prostate boost.

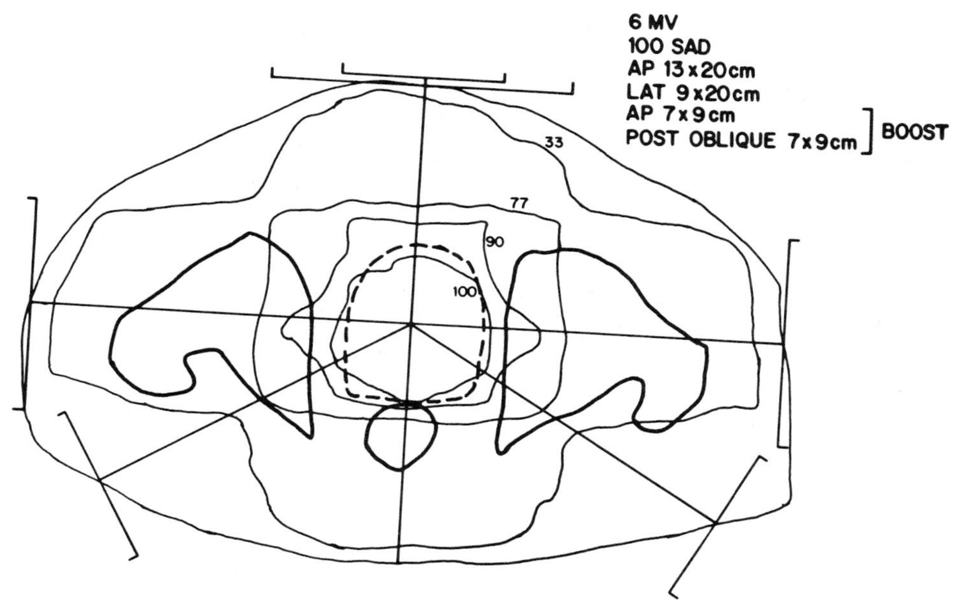

Figure 3. B: Four-field whole pelvic fields followed by three-field (anterior and posterior oblique) technique to prostate boost.

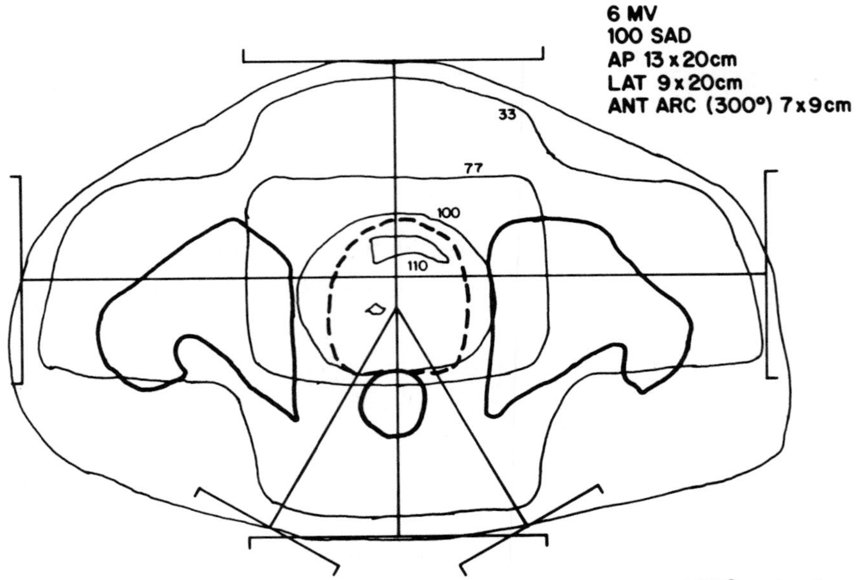

Figure 3. C: Four-field whole pelvic fields followed by single 300° anterior arc rotation to prostate boost.

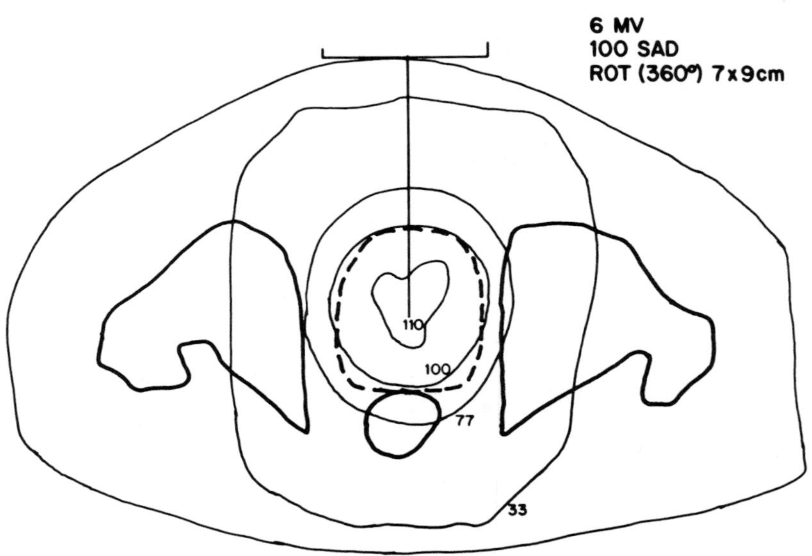

Figure 4. Computerized isodose distribution in the treatment of prostate only. A: 360° rotational field.

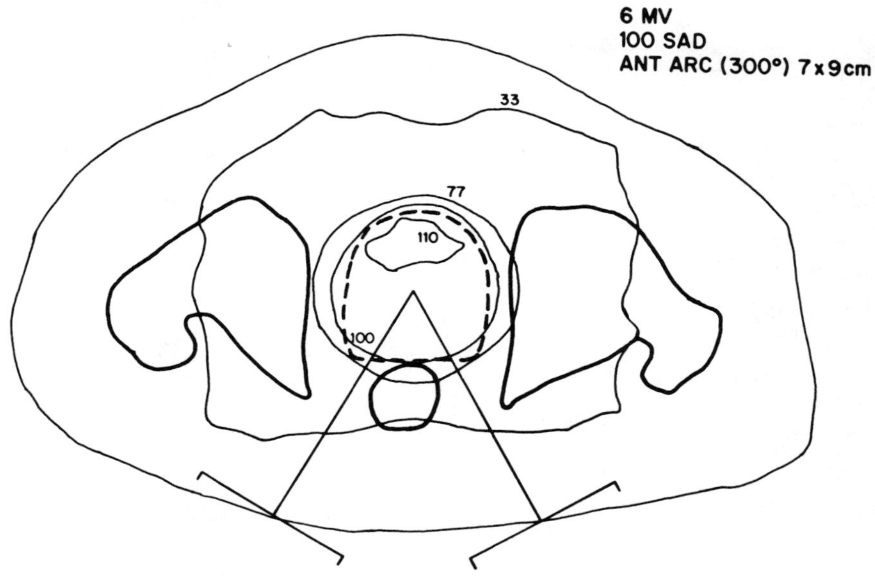

Figure 4. B: 300° anterior arc rotation.

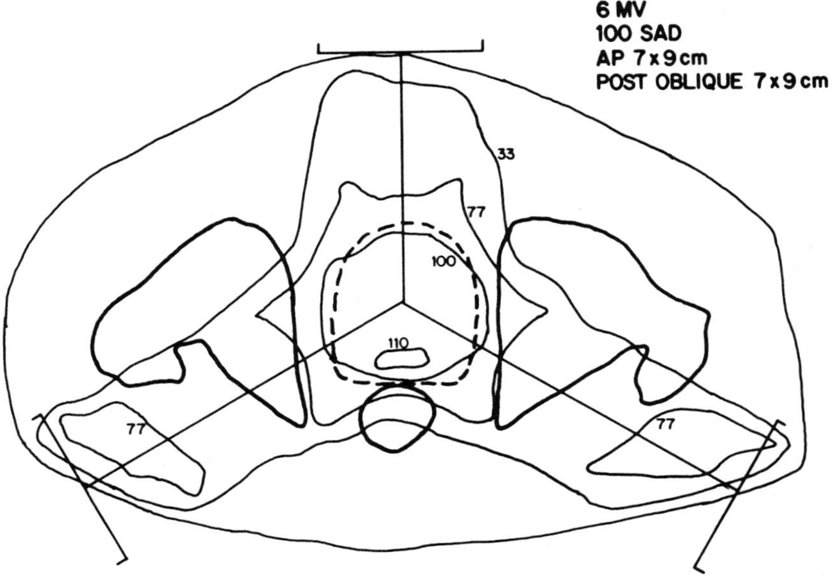

Figure 4. C: Fixed three-field technique (anterior and posterior oblique).

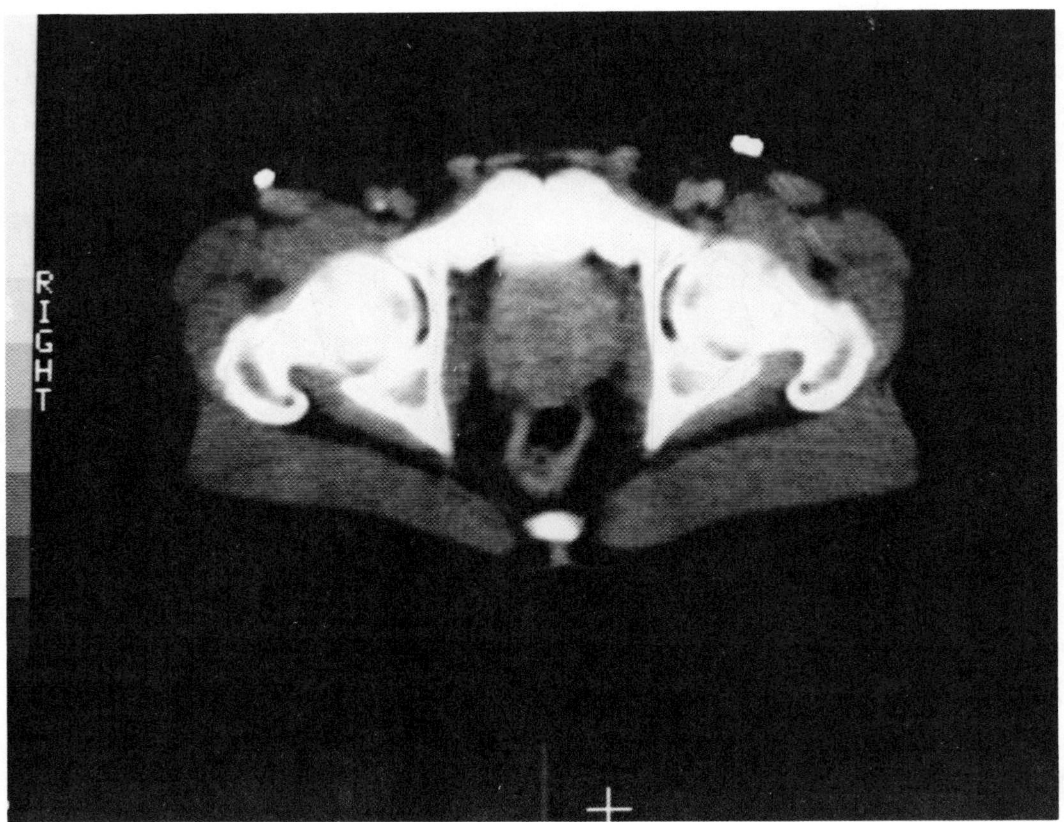

Figure 5. A: CT scan of pelvis through the center of prostate booster volume, with isodose distribution.

Interstitial Therapy

In 1952, Flocks et al. (27) injected a colloidal solution of radioactive gold (^{198}Au) directly into the gland or into the tumor bed after subtotal resection. Each of the above procedures resulted in undue side effects to the patients and exposure to the personnel. In 1970, Whitmore and associates (98) used a new radioisotope, ^{125}I as a substitute for gold (^{198}Au). Since then they have used this isotope (^{125}I) in about 256 prostatic carcinoma patients with minimal complications.

Iodine 125 has practical and theoretical advantages as a radiation source for interstitial therapy because of its half-life of 60 days and a peak energy of 31 kV. The intensity of the gamma radiation is reduced to half by 2 cm of soft tissue, and 8-10 cm of tissue will reduce the activity to 3%. Kim and Hilaris (53) showed that ^{125}I has greater therapeutic ratio when compared to ^{222}Rn and ^{198}Au. This may be due to protracted radiation resulting from the long half-life of this isotope. This type of radiation may be advantageous in the treatment of slow-growing neoplasia with a relatively long doubling time. The ^{125}I seed is dark brown in color, measures about 4.5 mm in length by 0.75 mm in diameter. The iodine is absorbed in two portions of an ion exchange resin, separated by a gold marker (Fig. 6). The marker helps in localization of seeds in the x-rays after the implant. In order to determine the optimal activity (millicuries) of ^{125}I required for the implant, the average dimension method is utilized as described by Henchke and Cevc (38) and Anderson (4).

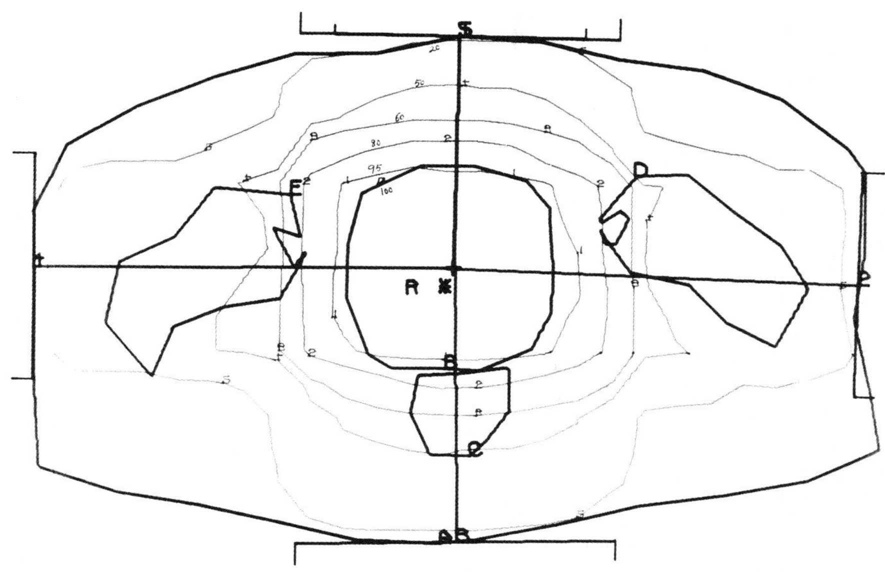

Figure 5. B.

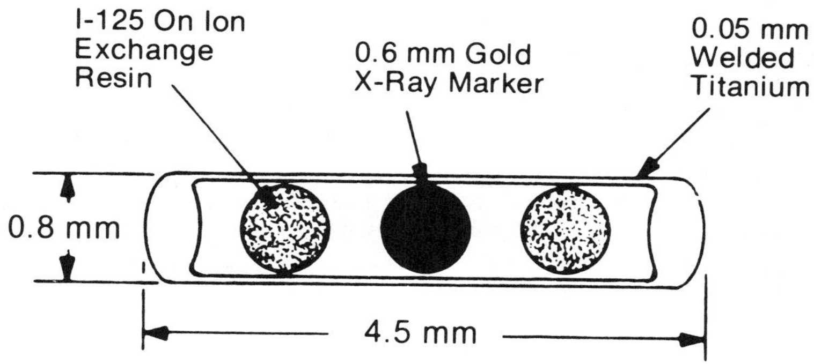

Figure 6. ^{125}I seed.

A = da x K

A = total activity in millicuries required

da = dimension average

K = constant of proportionality, e.g., "5" for ^{125}I

The total millicuries, obtained by average dimension method, divided by the average activity of the ^{125}I seeds available, yields the actual number of seeds required.

All the patients with a diagnosis of localized carcinoma (A, B, C) of prostate and who are in reasonably good health with an estimated life expectancy of 5 or more years are eligible for this combined surgical and radiotherapeutic procedure.

The only exceptions are bulky stage C lesions with tumor extension to the pelvic wall or bladder base, because it is difficult to get a uniform distribution of the isotope. Patients presenting with obstructive symptoms pose a special problem since they require transurethral resection to relieve the obstruction and also to prevent total obstruction from prostate swelling following radioisotope implant. A minimal or conservative transurethral resection (TUR) is advised in these patients, because total TUR will leave no tissue to hold the implant and requires a wait of 3-5 weeks to permit healing and resolution of infection before the implantation can be carried out. There is also evidence that the TUR encourages metastatic spread of the disease (61). The procedure is performed in conjunction with pelvic exploration and lymphadenectomy.

After a bilateral pelvic lymphadenectomy and prostatic exposure, implantation of the entire gland can be carried out by using 15 cm long, hollow, 17 gauge stainless steel needles. The needles are placed starting from base to apex, avoiding the median plane to prevent the insertion of needles into the urethra. They are inserted in a more or less anterior-posterior direction parallel to one another and approximately 1 cm apart. By keeping the index finger inside the rectum and feeling the prostate during insertion of the needles, it is possible to sense the tips of the needles so that they will not perforate the rectal wall (Fig. 7). Prior to actual loading of the needles with ^{125}I seeds, it is important to withdraw the tip at least by 0.5 cm. This is done because each seed measures 4.5 mm in length, and implantation of the seed very close to the rectal wall could result in rectal wall perforation. Bleeding and oozing occurs during insertion of needles because of penetration of the prostatic venous plexus. Occasionally penetration of bladder and urethra by a needle can occur, but this has not created a recognized problem in Whitmore's (99) experience. When the insertion of needles is completed, a manual or semiautomatic applicator (Fig. 8), which uses the magazines holding 14 seeds in each, is utilized to deposit the seeds at 0.5-1 cm intervals as each needle is successively withdrawn. When the patient has recovered from surgery, on the fourth or fifth postoperative day localization films of the implant are done. From these, a computer generated isodose distribution is plotted (Fig. 9). The adequacy of computed dose distribution is based primarily on the following two parameters: (1) matched peripheral dose (MPD) or minimum effective dose of 10,000 or 18,000 and (2) average dose of about 25,000 rads. If this is achieved, it can be expected that this will result in 90% local control rate (41).

COMPLICATIONS

With pelvic lymphadenectomy and ^{125}I implant of prostate, the intraoperative complication was 6%. Twenty-three percent had postoperative complications. About 50% of the patients developed voiding symptoms, but the majority of them had subsidence of symptoms in 1 year (28).

When external radiation therapy is used the most common side effects are transient dysuria and diarrhea that can be managed with conservative treatment such as oral fluids, low-residue diet, and antidiarrheal drugs. Dysuria can be minimized by treating with a full bladder in order to elevate the dome of the bladder out of the irradiated volume during boost volume treatment. A waiting period of 3-4 weeks before initiation of external radiation therapy after transurethral resection could prevent dysuria and stricture of urethra. If patients have an infected necrotic tumor with dysuria, it is best to clear up the infection as much as possible since the combination of irradiation and cystitis can cause increased dysuria and potential long-term fibrosis and bladder contracture. If dysuria is persistent during therapy, urinalysis, cultures, and sensitivity are essential to detect and treat

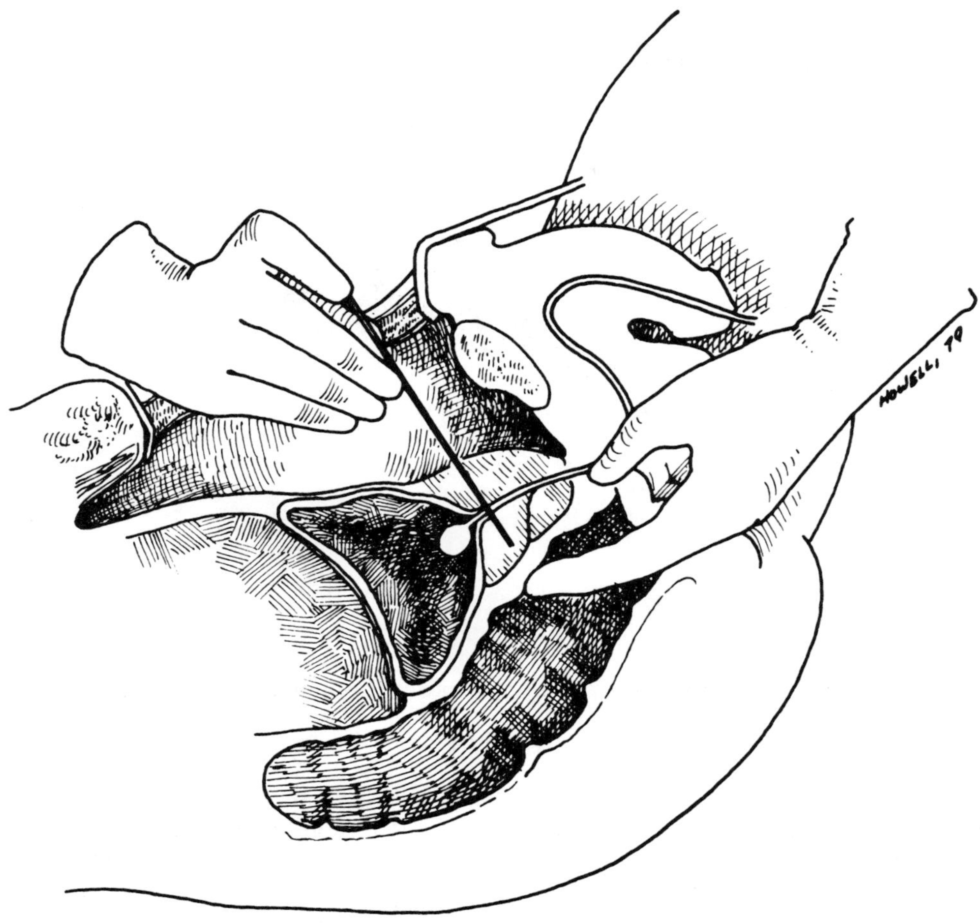

Figure 7. Demonstration of insertion of hollow stainless steel needles into prostate, index finger in the rectum to guide the needle bimanually to prevent the perforation of rectum.

any infection. Proctitis, rectal stricture, and bowel obstruction are possible late complications. The latter is more common if the patient had prior pelvic surgery. Proctitis can be treated by stool softeners and/or Cortifoam applications (corticosteroid foam).

Sexual impotency following treatment of carcinoma of the prostate may not only relate to the specific treatment but also to the definition of the condition, the patient's veracity, persistence of the questioner, posttreatment interval, as well as various social and psychological factors. The reported frequency of impotency following external radiation varies between 23-84% (55,63,78,83) and 7-12% following interstitial radiation (28,45). It can be expected that about 60% of patients can maintain sexual potency following curative radiotherapy in contrast to none being potent following radical prostatectomy.

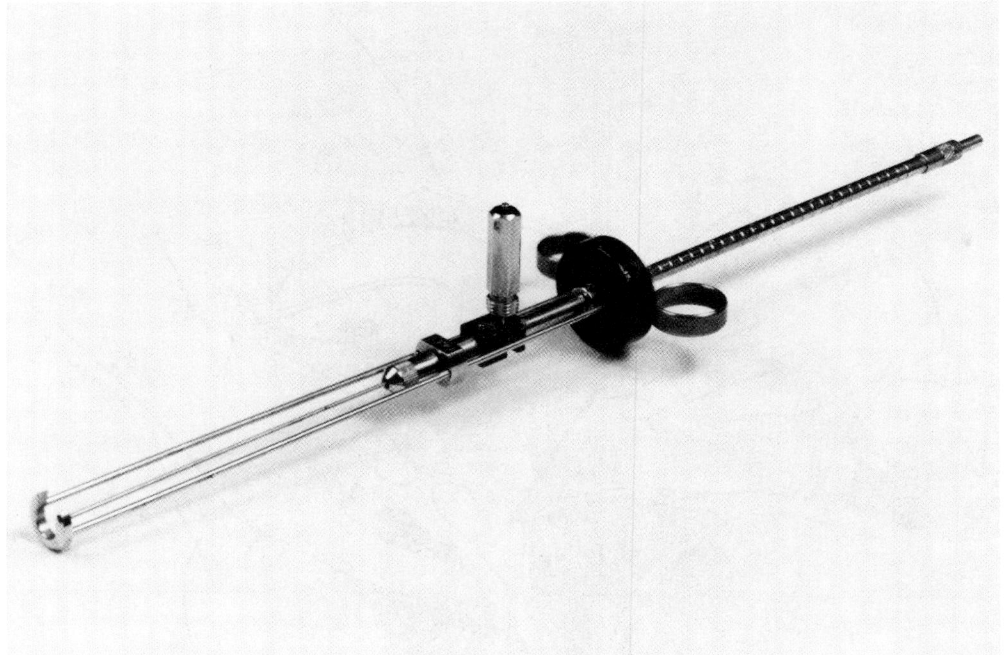

Figure 8. Semiautomatic ^{125}I seed applicator; the magazine holds 14 seeds.

RESULTS

About 30% of the patients will show change in size and/or firmness of prostate at the time of completion of radiation therapy. At 6 months posttreatment, objective response will be found in 80% of the patients (78). In Hulick's (45) experience, based on review of 147 cases, clinical regression of the tumor was seen in 85% of patients at the completion of therapy. A progressive decrease in the size of the irradiated prostate was noted for longer than 1 year in a majority of the patients. Regression of adenocarcinoma of the prostate following implantation by ^{125}I seeds is slow. Only 50% of implanted prostates had regressed completely at 20 months; 90% had regressed at 30 months (42).

Megavoltage radiation therapy has made it feasible to deliver tumoricidal doses without significant damage to normal tissues. In 1964 Budhraja and Anderson (12) reported a group of 53 patients, 36 of whom were treated by megavoltage radiation with concomitant hormone therapy. The 3- and 5-year survival rates were 60 and 25%, respectively. Ray and Bagshaw (78) reported a 71% 5-year actuarial survival for disease limited to the prostate (DLP) and a 41% survival in those with prostatic involvement; subsequently, many reports have appeared in the literature supporting the use of megavoltage radiotherapy for adenocarcinoma of the prostate (Table 2). Bilateral pelvic lymphadenectomy and ^{125}I implant of the prostate have been reported to achieve a 73% overall 5 year survival rate, and 92% of the patients who had negative nodes survived for 5 years or more compared to 46% of those with positive nodes (40).

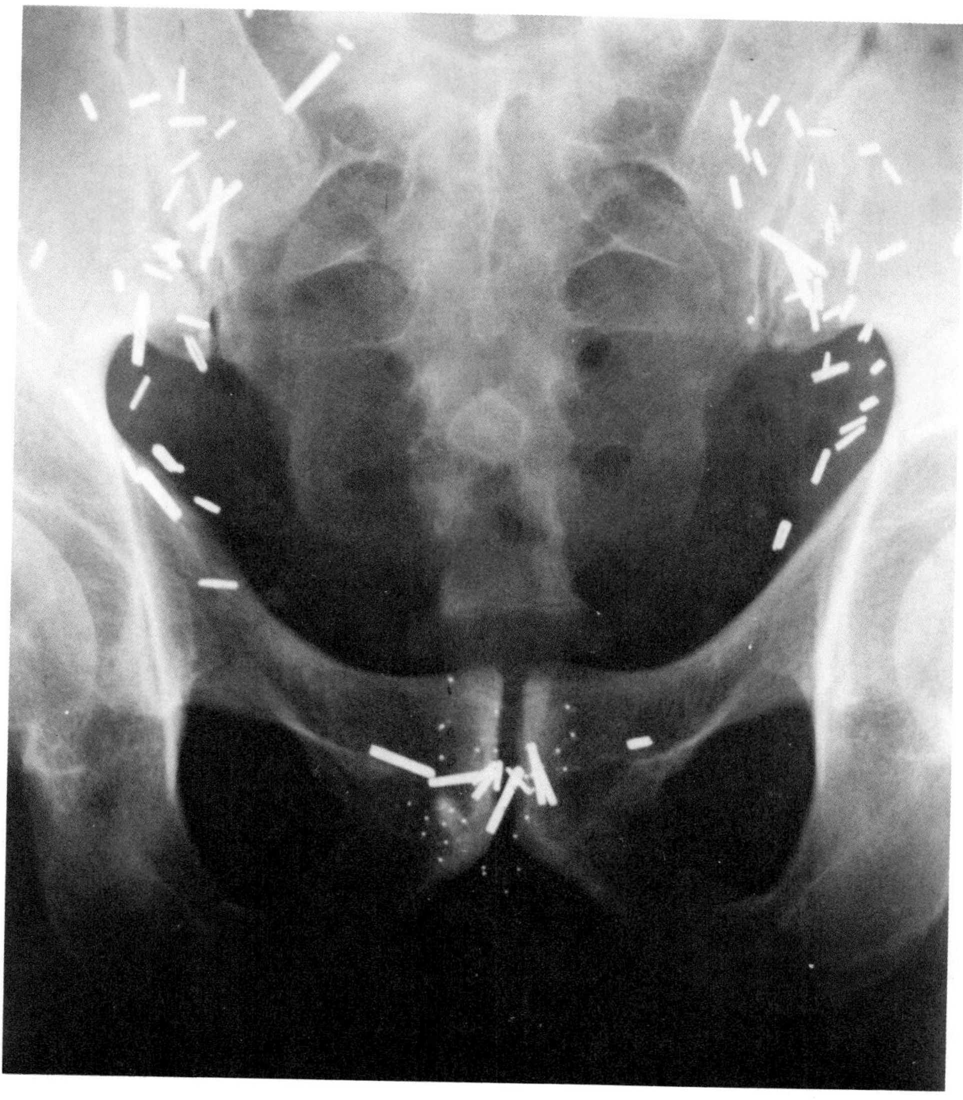

Figure 9. Localization of ^{125}I implant of prostate with isodose distribution. A: Anterior view.

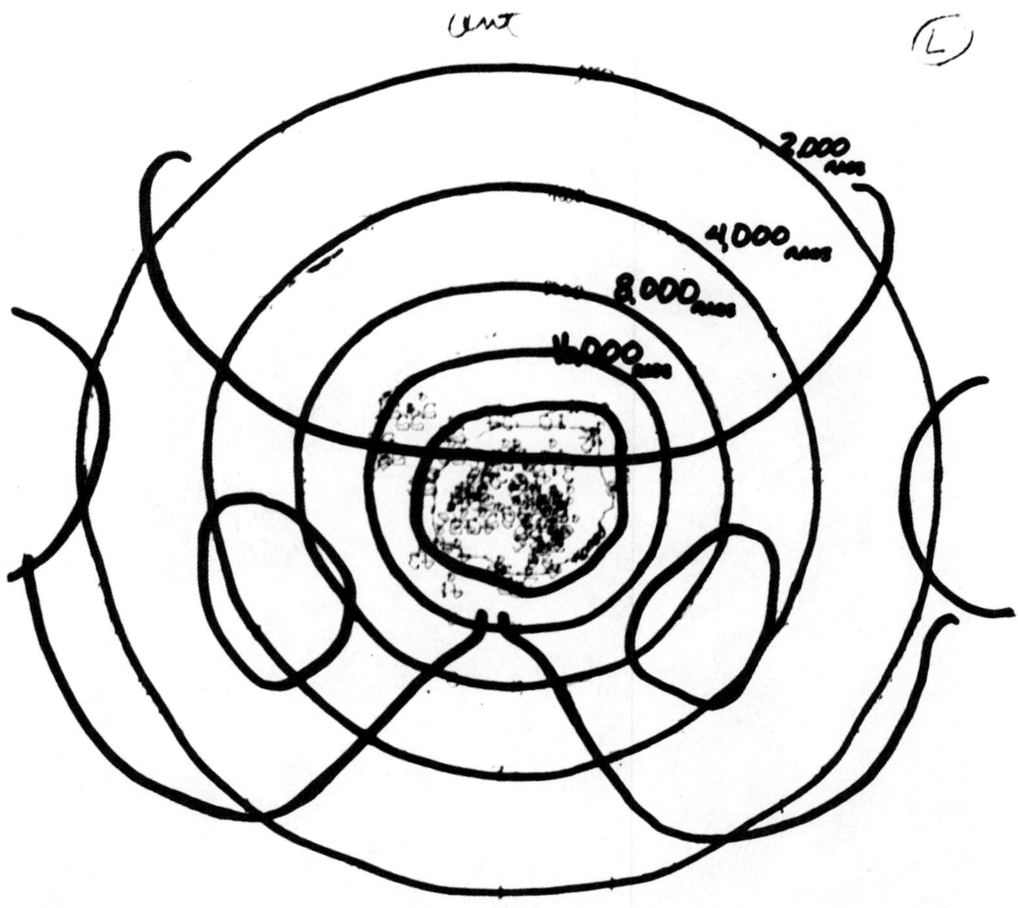

Figure 9. B: With isodose distribution.

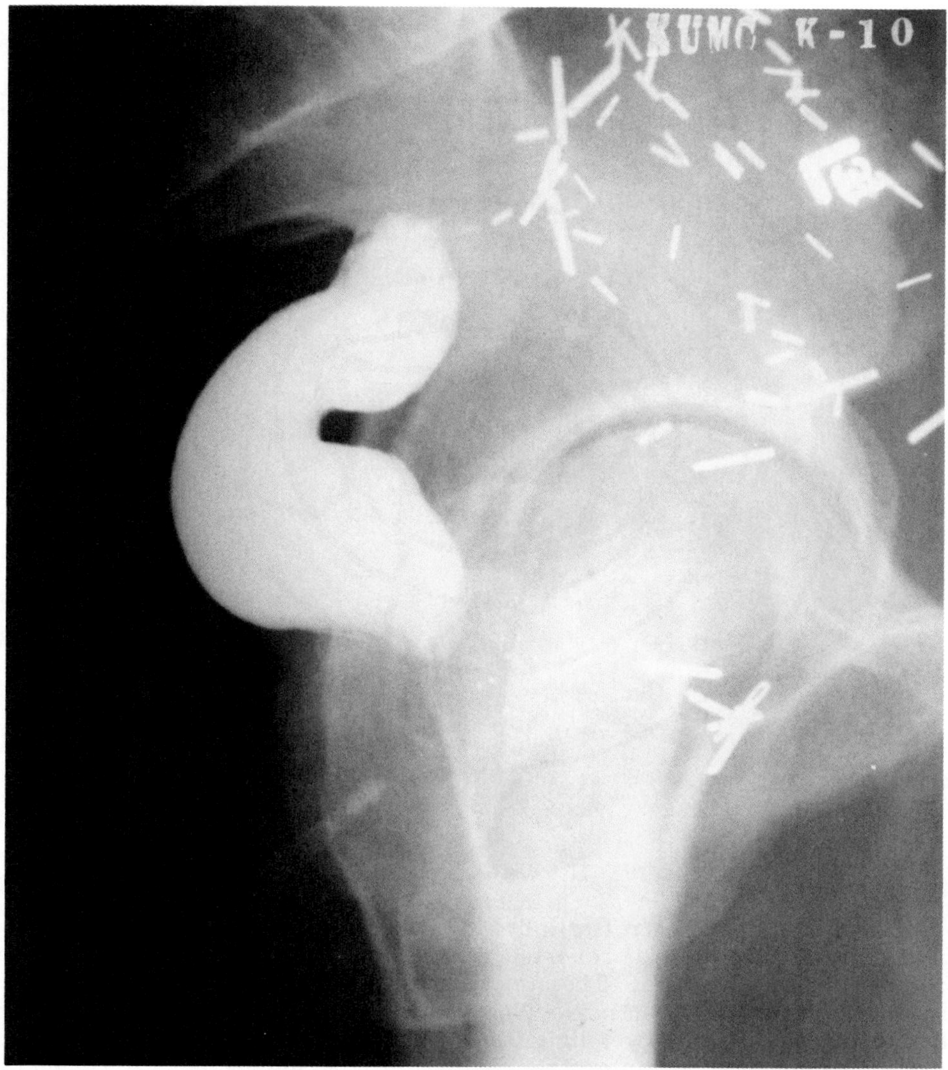

Figure 9. C: Lateral view.

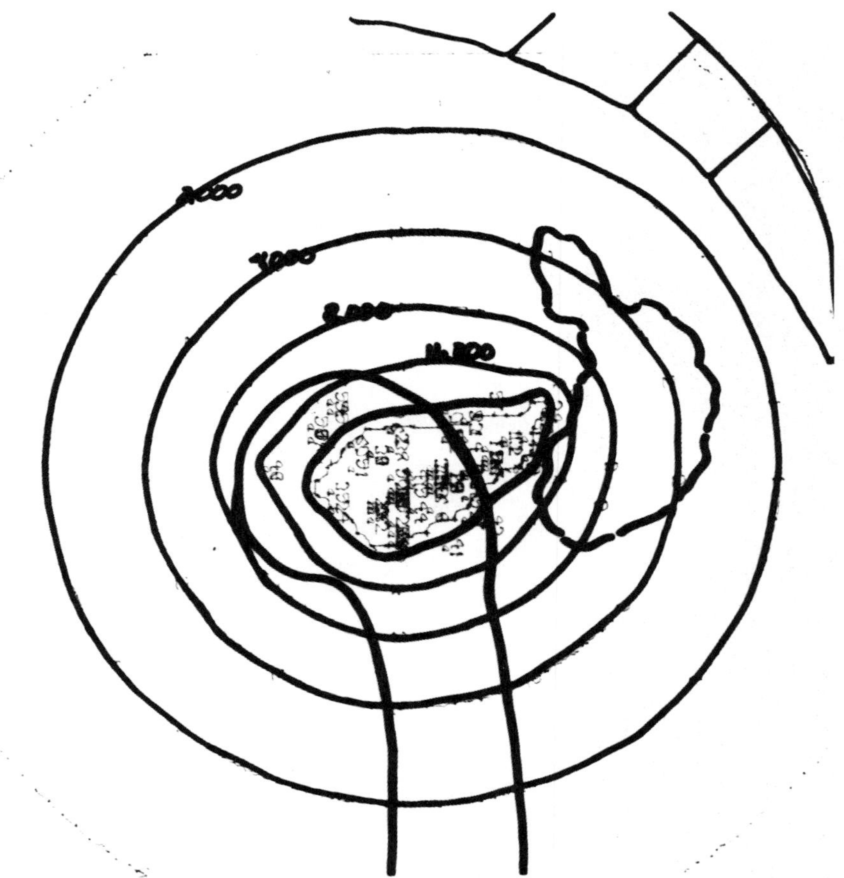

Figure 9. D: With isodose distribution.

The reported local control rate by external radiotherapy ranges from 62-88% (Table 3). Hilaris et al. (41) reported a 90% local control rate with ^{125}I interstitial implants of the prostate. The majority of the local control rates reported have been based on clinical evaluations. This criterion which includes the absence of clinical symptoms or tumor on digital examination of the rectum may not be a very accurate gauge of tumor control. This has been emphasized by recent reports (19,20,51,65) showing persistent carcinoma in biopsies of a clinically normal prostate at varied intervals. Cox and Tizerina (19) in 1974 reported on 68 biopsies on 30 patients 3-30 months after irradiation of the prostate. A striking correlation has been noted between the interval from irradiation to biopsy and the residual histologic evidence of malignancy. During the first 9 months after irradiation 26 of 43 biopsies were positive. From 12-30 months postirradiation, 20 of 25 biopsies were negative. In 1977 Cox and Stoffel (20) reported on 139 biopsies. There were 49 positive and 90 negative. Positive biopsy rate correlated only with the interval after irradiation - 60% at 6 months, 37% at 1 year, 30% at 18 months, and approximately 19% after 2.5 years. The authors concluded that these biopsies provide interesting data about the regression rate of prostatic adenocarcinoma, but they have no significance for the individual patient. A possible explanation for the conversion of positive biopsies to negative is that the histological presence of tumor in the prostate after irradiation does not necessarily indicate persistence of

Table 3. Results of External Radiation Therapy

Author (Ref.)	No. of Pts.	Stage A	B	C	Dose Rad/Week (to prostate)	Follow-up (months)	Local Control	Survival
Budraja and Anderson, 1964 (12)	56				5000/5	1-60		
Odell et al., 1971 (68)	68				4000-6800/5-7	16-120		
Carlton et al., 1972 (15)	106				6000-7500	12-96		
Grossman, 1974 (34)	58				7200/11	12-24		
Ray and Bagshaw, 1975 (78)	430		230	200	7000-7500/7-8	18-92	88%	71%-B 41%-C (Actuarial)
Perez et al., 1977 (71)	112		15	97	7000/7	12-60	82%	60%-B 42%-C
Neglia et al., 1977 (66)	154		4	150	6500-7000/7-8	24	86%	100%-B 68%-C (58% NED)
Van der Werf-Messing, 1978 (91)	110				7000	12		65% ALL (Actuarial)
Hulick, 1978 (45)	147	9	68	70	6500-7000	24-84	62%	77%-A 61%-B 56% 49%-C
Taylor et al., 1979 (88)	257		36	221	6500-7000/7-8			59%-B 58%-C
Reddy et al. (79)	72	6	31	35	6000-7000	6-60		100%-A 87%-B 79% 68%-C

biological activity. An extended follow-up of a significant number of patients by serial prostatic biopsy and correlation of the findings with progression or development of metastatic disease will help to clarify this issue. The histological appearance in 7 of 10 patients with persistent tumor in a study by Lytton and associates (56) would tend to support this contention in that the appearance of the tumor in the postirradiation biopsies was different from that seen before radiation. The principal changes were vacuolation of the cell cytoplasm with pyknosis and disorganization of nuclei. At present, however, it is not possible for pathologists to make firm conclusions as to a cell's biological activity based on morphological appearance.

METASTASES

The most common metastatic site is bone. The primary management is hormonal manipulation such as orchiectomy and stilbesterol therapy. Symptomatic bony metastases can be effectively treated with external beam therapy. About 3000 rads/2 weeks will result in symptomatic relief of pain in the majority of the patients. In widespread bony metastases radioactive chromic ^{32}P had been used in the past (23,59.90), but because of the possible side effect of bone marrow depression, this method is not in common use. A recent study of systemic radioisotope therapy in disseminated bony metastases using ^{89}Sr (90) seems to be promising as the authors have reported 80% response rate with practically no side effects. In our series, 10 of 13 patients showed a good response (unpublished data).

The incidence of gynecomastia is about 70% in patients receiving estrogen therapy (2,57). This condition can be associated with severe mammary pain. Mastectomies have been required in some patients to alleviate the intense disabling pain. A dose of 1200-1500 rads at 300-500 rads/fraction on alternate days confined to the nipple and areola using orthovoltage equipment or electron beam, prior to hormone therapy, is very effective in preventing gynecomastia (30). Higher dose given after breast enlargement has developed is less likely to reverse the process.

REFERENCES

1. Aledia, F.T.: Vasoseminal vesiculography: A diagnostic aid in early metastatic carcinoma of the prostate. J. Urol. 110:242-244, 1973.

2. Alfthan, O. and Kuttunen, K.: The effect of roentgen ray treatment of gynecomastia in patients with prostatic carcinoma treated with estrogen hormones: A preliminary communication. J. Urol. 94:604-606, 1965.

3. Alyea, E.P. and Rundles, R.W.: Bone marrow studies in carcinoma of the prostate. J. Urol. 62:332-339, 1949.

4. Anderson, L.L.: Dosimetry for interstitial radiation therapy. In Hilaris Handbook of Interstitial Brachytherapy. Acton, Publishing Science Group, 1975, pp. 99-103.

5. Arduino, L.J. and Glucksman, M.A.: Lymph node metastases in early carcinoma of the prostate. J. Urol. 88:91-93, 1962.

6. Attwater, H.L.: Malignant diseases of prostate and bladder. Postgrad. Med. J. 6:6-19, 1930.

7. Bagshaw, M.A. and Kaplan, H.S.: Radical external radiotherapy of localized prostatic carcinoma. Presented at 10th Int. Cong. of Radiol. Montreal, Canada, September 15-18, 1962.

8. Bagshaw, M.A., Pistenma, D.A., Ray, G.R., Freiha, F.S., and Kempson, R.L.: Evaluation of extended field radiotherapy for prostatic neoplasm: 1976 progress report. Cancer Treat. Rep. 61:297-306, 1977.

9. Barringer, B.S.: Radium in the treatment of carcinoma of the bladder and prostate. A review of one year's work. JAMA 68:1227-1230, 1917.

10. Barringer, B.S.: Prostatic carcinoma. J. Urol. 47:306-310, 1942.

11. Bruce, A.W., O'Cleireachain, F., Morales, A., and Awad, S.A.: Carcinoma of the prostate: a critical look at staging. J. Urol. 117:319-322, 1977.

12. Budhraja, S.N. and Anderson, J.C.: An assessment of the value of radiotherapy in the management of carcinoma of the prostate. Brit. J. Urol. 36:535-540, 1964.

13. Byar, D.P. and Mostofi, F.K.: Carcinoma of the prostate: Prognostic evaluation of certain pathologic futures in 208 radical prostatectomies. Examined by the step-section technique. Cancer 30:5-13, 1972.

14. Silverberg, E.: Cancer Statistics. Ca- A Cancer Journal for Clinicians 31: (1):13-28, 1981.

15. Carlton, C.E., Jr., Dawoud, F., Hudgins, P., and Scott, R., Jr.: Irradiation treatment of carcinoma of the prostate. A preliminary report based on 8 years of experience. J. Urol. 108:924-927, 1972.

16. Chu, T.M., Want, M.C., Merrin, C., Valenzuela, L., and Murphy, G.P.: Isoenzymes of human prostate acid phosphatase. Oncology 35:198-200, 1978.

17. Chau, D.T., Veenema, R.J., Muggia, F., and Graff, A.: Acid phosphatase levels in bone marrow: value in detecting early bone metastasis from carcinoma of the prostate. J. Urol. 103:462-466, 1970.

18. Clifton, J.A., Philipp, R.J., Ludovic, E., and Fowler, W.M.: Bone marrow and carcinoma of the prostate. Am. J. Med. Sci. 224:121-130, 1952.

19. Cox, J.D. and Tizerina, A.: Preliminary results of biopsies following irradiation for locally advanced adenocarcinoma of the prostate. Radiology 112: 215-216, 1974.

20. Cox, J.D. and Stoffel, T.J.: The significance of needle biopsy after irradiation for stage C adenocarcinoma of the prostate. Cancer 40:156-160, 1977.

21. Del Regato, J.A.: Cancer of the prostate. JAMA 255:1727-1730, 1976.

22. Deming, C.L.: Results in 100 cases of prostate and seminal vesicles treated with radium. Surg. Gynecol. Obstet. 34:99-118, 1922.

23. Edland, R.W.: Testosterone potentiated radiophosphorus therapy of osseous metastases in prostatic cancer. Am. J. Roentgenol. 120:678-683, 1974.

24. Firusian, N., Mellin, P., and Schmidt, C.G.: Results of 89 strontium therapy in patients with carcinoma of the prostate and incurable pain from bone metastases: A preliminary report. J. Urol. 116:74-768, 1976.

25. Flocks, R.H.: Combination therapy for localized prostatic cancer. J. Urol. 89:889-894, 1963.

26. Flocks, R.H., Culp, D., and Porto, R.: Lymphatics spread from prostatic cancer. J. Urol. 81:194-196, 1959.

27. Flocks, R.H., Derr, H.D., Elkins, H.B., and Culp, D.A.: Treatment of carcinoma of the prostate by interstitial radiation with radioactive gold (198 Au): A preliminary report. J. Urol. 68:510-522, 1952.

28. Fowler, Jr., J.E., Barzell, W., Hilaris, B.S., and Whitmore, Jr., W.F.: Complications of iodine-125 implantation and pelvic lymphadenectomy in the treatment of prostatic cancer. J. Urol. 121:447-451, 1979.

29. Franks, L.M.: The natural history of prostatic cancer. In Progress in Clinical and Biological Research, Prostatic Disease, edited by H. Marberger, H. Maschek, H.K.A. Schirmez, J.A.C. Colston and E. Witkin, New York, Alan R. Liss Inc., 1976, pp. 103-110.

30. Gagnon, J.D., Moss, W.T., and Stevens, K.R.: Pre-estrogen breast irradiation for patients with carcinoma of the prostate: A critical review. J. Urol. 121:182-184, 1979.

31. Gerner-Smidt, M.: Vesicloraphy as a diagnostic aid in cancer and hypertrophy of the prostate. Acta Chir. Scand. 114:387-389, 1957-1958.

32. Gittes, R.F. and Chu, T.M.: Detection and diagnosis of prostatic cancer. Semin. Oncol. 3:123-130, 1976.

33. Golimbu, M., Schinella, R., Morales, P., and Kurusu, S.: Differences in pathological characteristics and prognosis of clinical A2 prostatic cancer from A1 and B disease. J. Urol. 119:618-622, 1978.

34. Grossman, I.: The early lymphatic spread of manifest prostate adenocarcinoma. Am. J. Roentgenol. 120:673-674, 1974.

35. Gursel, E.O., Rezvan, M., Sy, F.A. and Veenema, R.J.: Combination evaluation of bone marrow acid phosphatase and bone scanning in staging of prostatic cancer. J. Urol. 111:53-57, 1974.

36. Gutman, A.: The development of acid phosphatase test for prostatic carcinoma. Bull. N.Y. Acad. Med. 44:63-67, 1968.

37. Gutman, E.B., Sproul, E.E., and Gutman, A.B.: Significance of increased phosphatase activity of bone at the site of osteoblastic metastasis secondary to carcinoma of the prostate gland. Am. J. Cancer 28:485-495, 1936.

38. Henchke, U.K. and Cevc, P.: Dimension averaging: A simple method for dosimetry of interstitial implants. Radiol. Biol. Ther. 9:287-298, 1968.

39. Herr, H.W.: Preservation of sexual potency in prostatic cancer patients after iodine-125 implantations. J. Am. Geriat. Soc. 27:17-19, 1979.

40. Hilaris, B.S., Whitmore, W.F., Batata, M., and Barzell, W.: Behavioral patterns of prostate adenocarcinoma following an iodine-125 implant and pelvic node dissection. J. Radiat. Oncol. Biol. Phys. 2:631-637, 1977.

41. Hilaris, B.S., Whitmore, W.F., Batata, M.A., and Gradstald, H.: Cancer of the prostate. In Hilaris Handbook of Interstitial Brachytherapy, Acton, Publishing Science Group, 1975, pp. 219-234.

42. Hilaris, B.S., Whitmore, W.F., Batata, M.A., Barzell, W., and Tokita, N.: Iodine-125 implantation of the prostate: Dose-response considerations. Front. Radiat. Ther. Onc. 12:82-90, 1978.

43. Watanabe, H., Igari, D., Tanahashi, O., Harada, D., and Saitoh, M.: Transrectal ultrasonotomography of the prostate. J. Urol. 114:734-739, 1975.

44. Huggins, C., Stevens, R.E., and Hodges, C.F.: C.V. studies on prostatic cancer: Effects of castration on advanced carcinoma of the prostate gland. Acta Surg. 43:209-223, 1941.

45. Hulick, P.R.: A review of 147 cases of adenocarcinoma of the prostate treated with radiation therapy at the Wilmington Medical Center, 1967-1974. Delaware Med. J. 50:447-481, 1978.

46. Hultgerg, S.: Results of treatment with radiotherapy in carcinoma of the prostate. Acta Radiol. 27:339-349, 1946.

47. Jewett, H.J., Bridge, R.W., Gray, F.G., and Sheeley, W.M.: The palpable nodule of prostate cancer. Results 15 years after radical excision. JAMA 203:403-406, 1968.

48. Jewett, H.J.: The present status of radical prostatectomy for stages A and B prostatic cancer. Urol. Clin. N. Am. 2:105-124, 1975.

49. Jewett, H.J.: The case for radical perineal prostatectomy. J. Urol. 103: 195-199, 1970.

50. Kabler, R., Farah, R., Greenwald, K., and Cerny, J.C.: Bone marrow acid phosphatase and lymphangiography in the evaluation of patients with carcinoma of the prostate. Read at annual meeting of American Urological Association, Las Vegas, Nevada, May 18, 1976.

51. Kagan, A.R., Gordon, J., Cooper, J.F., Gilbert, H., Nussbaum, H., and Chan, P.: A clinical appraisal of post-irradiation biopsy in prostate cancer. Cancer 39:637-641, 1977.

52. Khan, R., Turner, B., Edson, M., and Dolan, M.: Bone marrow acid phosphatase; another look. J. Urol. 177:79-80, 1977.

53. Kim, J.H. and Hilaris, B.S.: Iodine 125 source in interstitial tumor therapy. Clinical and radiobiologic considerations. Am. J. Roentgenol. 123:163-169, 1975.

54. Lipsett, J.A., Cosgrove, M.D., Green, N., Casagrande, J.T., Melbye, R.W., and George, III, F.W.: Factors influencing prognosis in the radiotherapeutic management of carcinoma of the prostate. Int. J. Radiat. Oncol. Biol. Phys. 1:1049-1058, 1976.

55. Loh, E.S., Brown, H.E., and Beiler, D.D.: Radiotherapy of carcinoma of the prostate: Preliminary report. J. Urol. 106:906-909, 1971.

56. Lytton, B., Collins, J.T., Weiss, R.M., Schiff, Jr., M., McGuire, E.J., and Livolsi, V.: Results of biopsy after early stage prostatic cancer treatment by implantation of iodine-125 seeds. J. Urol. 121:306-309, 1979.

57. Malis, I., Cooper, J., and Wolever, T.H.S.: Breast radiation in patients with carcinoma of the prostate. J. Urol. 102:336-337, 1969.

58. Manual for Staging Cancer, 1977. American Joint Committee for Cancer Staging and End Results Reporting, Chicago, AJCCS, 1977.

59. Maxfield, J.R., Jr., Maxfield, G.S., and Maxfield, W.S.: The use of radioactive phosphorous and testosterone in metastatic bone lesions from breast and prostate. South. Med. J. 51:320-328, 1958.

60. McLaughlin, A.P., Saltzstein, S.L., McCullough, D.L., and Gittes, R.F.: Prostatic carcinoma: Incidence and locations of unsuspected lymphatic metastases. J. Urol. 115:89-94, 1976.

61. McGowan, D.G.: The adverse influence of prior transurethral resection on prognosis in carcinoma of prostate treated by radiation therapy. Int. J. Radiat. Oncol. Biol. Phys. 6:1121-1126, 1980.

62. Mehan, D.J., Brown, G.O., Jr., Hoover, B., and Storey, G.: Bone marrow findings in carcinoma of the prostate. J. Urol. 95:241-244, 1966.

63. Mollenkamp, J.S., Cooper, J.F., and Kagan, A.R.: Clinical experience with supervoltage radiotherapy in carcinoma of the prostate: A preliminary report. J. Urol. 113:374-377, 1975.

64. Mostofi, F.K.: Tumors of the male genital tract. In A Class of Tumor Pathology, edited by F.K. Mostofi and E.B. Price, Jr., Washington, D.C., Armed Forces Institute of Pathology, 1973, pp. 196-252.

65. Nachtsheim, Jr., D.A., McAninch, J.W., Stutzman, R.E., and Goebel, J.L.: Latent residual tumor following external radiotherapy for prostatic adenocarcinoma. J. Urol. 120:312-314, 1978.

66. Neglia, W.J., Hussey, D.H., and Johnson, D.E.: Megavoltage radiation therapy for carcinoma of the prostate. Int. J. Radiat. Oncol. Biol. Phys. 2:873-882, 1977.

67. Nelson, C.M.D., Boatman, D.L., and Flocks, R.H.: Bone marrow examination in carcinoma of the prostate. J. Urol. 109:667-670, 1973.

68. Odell, R.W., Merill, M.D., and Atwood, C.J.: Cobalt-60 teletherapy of localized prostatic carcinoma. A 10-year experience. J. Urol. 105:843-846, 1971.

69. Pasteau, O., and Degrais, P.: The radium treatment of cancer of the prostate. Arch. Roentgen. Ray (London), 19:396-410, 1914.

70. Paulson, D.F. and Uro-Oncology Research Group: The impact of current staging procedures in assessing disease extent of prostatic adenocarcinoma. J. Urol. 121:300-302, 1979.

71. Perez, C.A., Bauer, W., Garza, R., and Royce, R.K.: Radiation therapy in the definitive treatment of localized carcinoma of the prostate. Cancer 40: 1425-1433, 1977.

72. Pontes, J.E., Alcorn, S.W., Thomas, A.J., Jr., and Pierce, J.M., Jr.: Bone marrow acid phosphatase in staging prostatic carcinoma. J. Urol. 114: 422-424, 1975.

73. Pontes, J.E., Choe, B., Rose, N., and Pierce, J.M., Jr.: Indirect immune fluorescence for identification of prostatic acid phosphatase. J. Urol.:117: 459-463, 1977.

74. Pontes, J.E., Choe, B.K., Rose, N.R., and Pierce, J.M., Jr.: Bone marrow acid phosphatase in staging of prostatic carcinoma. How reliable is it? J. Urol. 119:772-776, 1978.

75. Raghavaiah, N.V.: Prostatography. J. Urol. 121:174-177, 1979.

76. Ray, G.: The need for standardized, controlled, perspective trials and less empiricism. Int. J. Radiat. Oncol. Biol. Phys. 2:1041-1044, 1977.

77. Ray, G.R., Piestenma, D.A., Castellino, R.A., Kempson, R.L., Meares, E., and Bagshaw, M.A.: Operative staging of apparently localized adenocarcinoma of the prostate: Results in 50 unselected patients. Cancer 38:73-83, 1976.

78. Ray, G.R. and Bagshaw, M.A.: The role of radiation therapy in the definitive treatment of adenocarcinoma of the prostate. Ann. Rev. Med. 26:567-588, 1975.

79. Reddy, E.K., Mansfield, C.M., and Hartman, G.V.: Prostatic carcinoma results of external radiation therapy (unpublished data).

80. Reif, A., Schlesinger, R., Fish, C., and Robinson, C.: Acid phosphatase isoenzymes in cancer of the prostate. Cancer 31:689-699, 1973.

81. Resnick, M.I., Willar, J.W., and Boyce, W.H.: Recent progress in ultrasonography of the bladder and prostate. J. Urol. 117:444-446, 1977.

82. Reynolds, R.D., Greenberg, B.R., Martin, N.D., Lucas, R.N., Gaffney, C.N., and Hawn, L.: Usefulness of bone marrow serum acid phosphatase in staging carcinoma of the prostate. Cancer 32:181-184, 1973.

83. Rhamy, R.K., Wilson, S.K., and Caldwell, W.L.: Biopsy proved tumor following definite irradiation for resectable carcinoma of the prostate. J. Urol. 107:627-630, 1972.

84. Riehle, R.A., Jr., McCarron, J.P., Jr., Kazam, E., and Muecke, E.C.: Computed tomography in urologic patients: Preliminary assessment. Urology 10:529-535, 1977.

85. Rubenstein, A.B. and Rubnitz, M.E.: Transitional cell carcinoma of the prostate. Cancer 24:543-546, 1969.

86. Smith, S. and Pierson, E.L.: The value of high voltage x-ray therapy in carcinoma of the prostate. J. Urol. 23:331-341, 1930.

87. Sy, F.A., Gursel, E.O., and Veenema, R.J.: Positive random iliac bone biopsy in advanced prostatic cancer. Urology 2:125-128, 1973.

88. Taylor, W.J., Richardson, R.G., and Hafferman, M.D.: Radiation therapy for localized prostatic cancer. Cancer 43:1123-1127, 1979.

89. Thompson, K.R., House, A.J.S., Gothlin, J.H., and Dolan, T.E.: Percutaneous lymph node aspiration biopsy: Experience with a new technique. Clin. Radiol. 28:329-332, 1977.

90. Tong, C.K. Eddy: Parathormone and P 32: Therapy in prostatic cancer with bone metastases. Radiology 98:343-351, 1971.

91. Van der Werf-Messing, B.: Prostatic cancer treated at the Rotterdam Radiotherapy Institute. Strahlentherpie 154:537-541, 1978.

92. Veenema, R.J., Gursel, E.O., Reomas, N., Wechsler, M., and Lattimer, J.K.: Bone marrow acid phosphatase: Prognostic value in patients undergoing radical prostatectomy. J. Urol. 117:81-82, 1977.

93. Wajsman, Z., Chu, M.T., and Rose, N.R.: New diagnostic tests for prostatic cancer? JAMA 238:931-932, 1977.

94. Welsh, J.F. and Mackinney, C.C.: Experience with aspiration biopsies of the bone marrow in the diagnosis and prognosis of carcinoma of the prostate gland. Am. J. Clin. Path. 41:509-512, 1964.

95. Whitmore, W.F.: Hormone therapy in prostate cancer. Am. J. Med. 21: 697-713, 1956.

96. Whitmore, W.F.: The rationale and results of ablative surgery for prostatic cancer. Cancer 16:1119-1132, 1963.

97. Whitmore, W.F.: The natural history of carcinoma of the prostate. Cancer 32:1104-1112, 1964.

98. Whitmore, W.F. Jr., Hilaris, B.S., and Grabstald, H.: Retropubic implantation of iodine-125 in the treatment of prostatic cancer. J. Urol. 108:918-920, 1972.

99. Whitmore, W.F., Jr.: Retropubic implantation of I-125 in the treatment of carcinoma of the prostate. In Progress in Clinical and Biological Research. Prostatic Disease, edited by H. Marberger, H. Haschek, H.R.A. Shermer, I.A.C. Colston, and E. Witkin, New York, Alan R. Liss, Inc., 1976, pp. 222-234.

100. Widmann, B.: Cancer of the prostate. The results of radium and roentgenoray treatment. Radiology 22:153-159, 1934.

101. Wilson, C.S., Dahl, D.S., and Middleton, R.G.: Pelvic lymphadenectomy for the staging of apparently localized prostatic cancer. J. Urol. 117:197-198, 1977.

102. Young, H.H.: The early diagnosis and radical cure of carcinoma of the prostate. Being a study of 40 cases and presentation of radical operation which was carried out in 4 cases. Bull. Johns Hopkins Hosp. 16:315-317, 1905.

103. Zornoza, J., Handel, P., Lukeman, J.M., Jing, B.S., and Wallace, S.: Percutaneous transperitoneal biopsy in urologic malignancies. Urology 9: 395-398, 1977.

chapter 12

COMBINED RADIATION AND CHEMOTHERAPY IN THE TREATMENT OF MALIGNANT DISEASE

Ronald L. Stephens, M.D.

INTRODUCTION

When two modalities, such as radiation and chemotherapy, are introduced simultaneously in the care of a cancer patient, one of three eventualities will of necessity occur. The combined approach may improve the patient's palliation, or increase his or her chance for cure. A second outcome might be neutral without improved palliation, cure, or increased survival. The third eventuality, obviously undesired, could be the interference of palliative effects, or even cure, of one modality by the other.

In all of science, and certainly in oncologic research, there are numerous examples where a combined therapeutic approach initially appeared superior to previous historic experience with either modality alone. On this basis alone the combined approach might even become the standard treatment. Eventually a more time-consuming, prospectively randomized trial would surface, demonstrating not only a lack of superiority for the combined therapy, but possible interference with that therapy which had the greatest chance to cure a given patient. One example might be found in the management of locally advanced head and neck cancer where intensified toxicity (mucositis, myelosuppression, etc.) may well interrupt an important time-dose response for local radiotherapeutic control. Although this is not yet proven, it may one day be acknowledged that the most important immediate post-op care for the recently mastectomized patient with breast cancer is chemotherapy, not the routine use of radiation with the associated delay in referral or even absence of referral to a medical oncologist. Clearly, such issues must await additional observation time and the associated data maturation. However, rather than small, single institutional pilot studies, it will be large randomized, prospective trials which provide convincing guidelines for the combined use of radiation and chemotherapy in any cancer.

In this chapter an effort to review both pilot studies and larger, more meaningful randomized trials will be utilized to establish the current state of the art for several different stages of several different cancers. What will become apparent in this review is how much remains to be done in the systematic evaluation of combined therapy for many of the malignancies.

NON-HODGKIN LYMPHOMAS

No other disease category in oncology, so initially sensitive to either radiation or chemotherapy, is undergoing such a rapid change in therapeutic emphasis as are non-Hodgkin lymphomas (NHL). A safe treatment generalization, based on today's knowledge, is likely to be outmoded by tomorrow's publication.

The importance of histologic subtypes, as well as staging, compound the problem of deciding whether a given patient with NHL will benefit maximally from radiation alone, chemotherapy only, or a combination of the two. Although an important and evolving research tool, the new functional classification of Lukes and Collins does not yet have the decade of clinical correlation associated with the Rappaport morphologic system (57,76). Consequently, therapeutic recommendations for today's patient must depend on this latter system, which broadly divides the NHL into major morphologic groupings of nodular and diffuse. Within each of these two broad categories the prevailing individual cell type, where possible, is further divided into well differentiated, poorly differentiated, and histiocytic. Current treatment attitudes toward these different subtypes range from a wait-and-see policy for the slower-growing, nodular poorly differentiated (NPDL) and diffuse well-differentiated (DWDL) patients to the recognized need for early aggressive treatment for patients with diffuse poorly differentiated (DPDL) and diffuse histiocytic lymphomas (DHL) (73,79). However, the question of which treatment or treatments, for which cell type, and which stage, represents an omnipresent challenge to the oncologist caring for today's patient.

As mentioned, unless there are disease-related symptoms, patients with advanced stage of NPDL and DWDL may do well without treatment, or at most require a single alkylating agent or limited-field radiation. At the other extreme, patients with advanced stages (Ann Arbor III and IV) of aggressive and usually fatal diffuse histiocytic lymphoma (DHL) would now appear to be candidates for primary chemotherapy. Adriamycin and cyclophosphamide in combination with other agents appear to be important drugs for the induction of a sustained complete remission in patients with these stages of DHL (4,5,62,79).

Patients who have undergone reasonably extensive staging and still remain stage I DHL may expect a radiotherapy-only cure in just over one-half the cases (48). Unfortunately, similarly staged patients with stage II DHL fare less well when treated with radiation alone, and available data would suggest that these stage II patients benefit from the addition of chemotherapy (4). Although sufficient follow-up is not available, eventually it may be appropriate for stage II DHL patients to be treated by combination chemotherapy alone.

The other Rappaport cell types and Ann Arbor stages remain confined to the polemics of how much radiation should be used in combination with chemotherapy, or which patients should receive chemotherapy alone. Recently, the National Cancer Institute has retrospectively examined a small number of their patients with the rare histology of nodular histiocytic lymphoma (NHL) (60). Morphologically, the nodular designation would suggest a slower and more benign process, but the histiocytic component portents a potentially aggressive factor. All patients were stage III or IV: and no long-term survivors were found in the five patients treated primarily by radiation; whereas, seven of the eight patients achieving a complete remission with combination chemotherapy were alive and free of disease at a minimum follow-up of 4.5 years. Because of the small numbers of this rare cell type (NHL), one cannot make absolute recommendations for management, but the seeming contribution of combination chemotherapy to survival might suggest an increasing role for chemotherapy in the uncertain area of cell types and stages of NHL which lie between the extremes of local stage I disease and stage IV non-Hodgkin lymphoma.

HODGKIN DISEASE

With the exception of certain childhood malignancies the combination of radiation and chemotherapy has never achieved more in the way of cures than it has in the neoplasm named after Sir Thomas Hodgkin. For well over a century this cancer was considered uniformly fatal. However, during the past three decades a new era of hope has been introduced, due largely to the more aggressive radiotherapeutic posture introduced by Peters (71). At a time when Dr. Peters was revolutionizing the radiotherapeutic attitudes toward Hodgkin disease, favorable reports of active chemotherapeutic agents were beginning to appear (34,68). Although single agents were active in advanced stages of this disease, the responses were usually incomplete, and all too often the duration of remission was measured in weeks. An historic landmark in the drug treatment of advanced Hodgkin disease came with the publication by De Vita and his colleagues at the National Cancer Institute (21). They achieved complete remissions in 35 of 43 patients (81%), utilizing a now classic four-drug combination of nitrogen mustard, vincristine, procarbazine, and prednisone. In a follow-up report, with greatly increased numbers of patients, the complete remission rate was not only sustained, but, it has become apparent that the majority of patients achieving complete remission are free of disease 10 years after six monthly cycles of the above for drug combination (22).

Consequently, it is possible to cure early stages of Hodgkin disease with radiotherapy, and late stages of this same illness with chemotherapy. Conservatively, it is now possible to cure more than two-thirds of the patients with this malignancy, a dramatic improvement for a cancer viewed so pessimistically a bare three decades ago.

Despite this dramatically evolving optimism, therapeutic challenges remain. Radiation and medical oncologists have become increasingly appreciative of the sites where each of their respective modalities fail. Therapeutic success and failure have also bred an increased knowledge of the disease's natural history. Historically this improved understanding resulted from the pioneering use of staging laparotomy by the Stanford group (36). Radiation oncologists now recognize that their failures most often occur in subclinical areas of involvement, outside their radiation ports, or in areas like the mediastinum where port design may attempt to protect normal adjacent structures such as the lungs and heart. This latter problem has only recently become apparent in such publications as the retrospective Harvard experience, where major mediastinal involvement greater than one-third the chest diameter, treated with radiation alone, was associated with excessive local and regional recurrence (59). For some oncologists the x-ray evidence of prominent hilar node involvement, and the massive mediastinal involvement mentioned above, are continued sources of discomfort when radiation alone is utilized to treat bulky disease closely abutting radiosensitive organs and their coverings, such as the lungs and pericardium. Rarely does the thoracic cavity undergo the type of pretreatment staging now commonly performed on the abdominal contents of patients with Hodgkin disease. Hence, the true pathologic extent of active thoracic disease is often unknown. However, the occasional patient who presents with exclusively mediastinal disease, and who undergoes a thoracic diagnosis and staging, serves as a reminder of potential x-ray understaging of the chest cavity. Without pathologic staging it may prove difficult, and often impossible, to differentiate areas of atelectasis from extension into pulmonary parenchyma. One radiotherapeutic approach to this problem encourages the use of 1500 rads over 4 weeks, to one or both lungs, with particular attention to the ipsilateral lung where the most prominent hilar and mediastinal disease resides (49). Interestingly it is this same reference, which describes the use of special subcarinal lead blocks to prevent radiation pericarditis, which fails to deal with this potential site of relapse. Consternation over developing a proper therapeutic philosophy for bulky mediastinal Hodgkin disease has resulted in an additional flurry of recent retrospective analyses (32,60,74). All of these investigators share concern over the high relapse rate in these patients, but differ in their recommendations as to when chemotherapy should be added to radiation. Until larger prospective trials become available many oncologists will continue to recommend additive, or even preradiotherapy chemotherapy, for major intrathoracic involvement, whereas others will advocate withholding chemotherapy until relapse.

Even patients with a favorable surgical stage (II) who also have symptoms (B), are at risk for failure, when treated with radiation alone. These patients, as well as those with splenic involvement (IIIs), continue to perplex physicians faced with deciding which combination of radiation and chemotherapy will optimize a given patient's chance for cure.

This recent concern for massive mediastinal involvement is to some degree an amplification of the earlier recognition by Musshoff of the importance of distinguishing between stage IV "per continuitatem" (local extranodal involvement in continuity with lymph node involvement) and stage IV "per disseminationem" (true distal organ involvement) (65). This revised Ann Arbor staging system gave rise to the E classification, to further delineate a group of patients who might just as well be treated by irradiation alone (i.e., stage IV "per continuitatem" or a revised IIE), and therapy prevent the added morbidity of systemic chemotherapy. Direct extension into adjacent organs or tissues, which will of themselves tolerate the now accepted sterilizing 4000-4500 rad dose, has obvious radiotherapeutic appeal.

In the continuing debate of which modality or combination of modalities to use in a given patient, splenic involvement has created another dilemma. This is particularly true if one accepts the thesis that the spleen, lacking afferent lymphatics, becomes involved by circulation of tumor cells through the splenic artery. If the spleen does indeed become involved by the disease in this fashion it would seem reasonable to accept the need for at least additive systemic therapy in the form of chemotherapy. However, the intellectual debate surrounding splenic involvement has been intensified by those oncologists who believe the spleen may be an exclusive retrograde lymphatic recipient of a cancer which usually has its origin above the diaphragm. For many this issue remains moot, and continues to influence clinicians as they design the initial and often the therapeutic approach to patients with splenic involvement. Relevant to this issue is the recent analysis by the University of Chicago group (20). In their retrospective evaluation of 52 patients with stage III disease, they uncovered a subset of patients whose survival characteristics were greatly influenced by their initial treatment and the anatomic distribution of abdominal involvement. Upper abdominal involvement, including the spleen and/or splenic, celiac, or portal nodes (stage III-1), did not appear to benefit from the addition of chemotherapy to total nodal irradiation. Patients with lower abdominal disease in paraaortic, iliac, or mesenteric nodes (stage III-2) had a significant survival advantage if they received combination chemotherapy in addition to total nodal irradiation. Although they analyzed a smaller number of patients, the Vanderbilt experience was similar, where eight of their nine stage III-2 patients relapsed when treated with irradiation alone (84). Taken together these two studies suggest that splenic involvement per se may not carry the formerly accepted necessity of additive chemotherapy and that the presence of lower abdominal involvement (in stage III disease) may be an important subset of patients to recognize, a be an important subset of patients to recognize, a group whose survival chances will be increased by adding combination chemotherapy to total nodal irradiation. Clearly more data are needed, but any future analyses of patients with stage III Hodgkin disease will of necessity require close attention to disease distribution within the abdominal cavity.

The issue of adding chemotherapy to radiotherapy for intermediate stages of Hodgkin disease (major mediastinal and hilar involvement, splenic involvement, and lower abdominal involvement) would constitute a significant problem, if only to avoid the immediate morbidity and inconvenience of drug treatment. In recent years the long-term follow-up and cure of patients with Hodgkin disease has raised an issue potentially more troublesome than the immediate morbidity of chemotherapy. For many years the development of a second cancer, usually acute myelogenous leukemia, was recognized as either a part of the natural history of Hodgkin disease, or more probably a long-term effect of the primary treatment. Recent analysis of large patient populations and detailed evaluation of the primary treatment, increasingly indict chemotherapy as that treatment modality which significantly increases the risk of a second cancer (15,86). As a consequence the onus of giving enough of one modality, or the right combination of radiation and chemotherapy to optimize the chances of cure in intermediate stages, while minimizing the risk of a second cancer, will continue to be the challenge of future clinical trials in Hodgkin disease.

One can usually find agreement among oncologists regarding which treatment to employ at the extremes of early and late disease. Stages I and IIa Hodgkin disease are clearly best treated with radiation alone, whereas the intermediate stages alluded to above (i.e., IIb, IIIaS, III-2, and major mediastinal disease) will continue to be the subject of ongoing trials. Stages IIIb and IV patients are generally treated with chemotherapy, but at least two pilot studies have been published which add 1500-2000 rads to known disease areas, once a predetermined course of combination chemotherapy is completed (5,25,26,75). Whether the commendable goal of increasing the number of complete remissions by additive radiation will translate to improved cure rates will require longer follow-up, or better designed, truly randomized trials. For the foreseeable future chemotherapy alone will remain the mainstay of treatment in the late stages IIIb and IV Hodgkin disease.

GASTROINTESTINAL TUMORS

For purposes of our discussion the gastrointestinal tract will include published data pertaining to cancers of the esophagus, descending through the intestine and its appendages to the anus. Once again there is a near absence of meaningful randomized trials which seek to establish whether the addition of chemotherapy to radiation will improve tumor response or survival. No doubt the absence of drug activity in late disease, the inability of currently available chemotherapeutic agents to convincingly extend survival in advanced gastrointestinal malignancies, has retarded clinical trials exploring this question. Consequently, current clinical investigation into cancers of the esophagus and rectum often focuses on maximizing local and regional control through various combinations of pre- or postoperative irradiation. Important as these investigations are we will limit our discussion to the very few trials where chemotherapy has been utilized to improve, or to test patient tolerance in the local response and ultimate survival of patients with gastrointestinal malignancies.

An evaluation in the treatment of carcinoma of the esophagus must pay close attention to the level of the esophagus from which the cancer arises, and the histologic particulars of this anatomic structure. Except for those cancers in the distal esophagus, or arising from a Barrett esophagus, the vast majority of cancers in this organ are of the squamous cell type. One Japanese study reported an exhaustive histologic survey of surgical specimens in patients given preoperative irradiation, preoperative bleomycin, or a combination of the two (83). Although significant degenerative changes were seen in the neoplastic cells of all three preoperatively treated groups, no effort, even retrospectively, was made to assess either the effect on resectability or survival by any of the various treatments. Treatment toxicity is inadequately documented, and before a combined approach of irradiation and bleomycin to the mediastinum could be recommended, it would be necessary to conduct a limited feasibility trial. In a well-designed randomized trial, the Eastern Cooperative Oncology Group (ECOG) has failed to demonstrate any advantage for adding bleomycin to radiation in squamous cell carcinoma of the esophagus, and neither symptomatic palliation nor survival were improved in those patients randomized to receive the combination (24). Perhaps other drugs such as cis-platinum or methotrexate, with a lower probability of pulmonary toxicity, would be more suitable for a prospective randomized trial of combined preoperative irradiation and chemotherapy to mediastinal structures. Even more innovative would be the use of chemotherapy before radiation, and before the tumor vessels are altered by radiation therapy.

Published combinations of irradiation and cytotoxic chemotherapy are lacking in distal adenocarcinoma of the esophagus and hepatocellular carcinoma. By way of contrast there are data available for chemotherapy in the more common adenocarcinoma of the pancreas deemed inoperable or unresectable at laparotomy.

Over a decade ago the Mayo Clinic Group published one of the first randomized trials for inoperable pancreatic cancer, comparing radiation alone to radiation plus 5-FU (63). The statistically significant improved mean survival for the combined approach (10.4 months) over the mean survival for radiation alone (6.3 months) should have provided ample impetus for more immediate clinical trials searching for better combined radiation and chemotherapy approaches to inoperable pancreatic cancer. Unfortunately it has taken another decade to bring us to the next significant clinical trial.

One of the most meaningful published trials in pancreatic cancer to date comes from the Gastrointestinal Tumor Study Group (33). A statistically significant survival advantage was apparent for the two study arms, which included chemotherapy, when compared to 6000 rads alone. However, the two arms which included 5-FU, and two different dose regimens of irradiation (6000 rads vs. 4000 rads), failed to demonstrate any survival difference. One may conclude from such a well-designed study, that 5-FU and irradiation are superior to irradiation alone. However, the absence of any cures, and the simple fact that any survival advantage is measured only in months, requires future randomized trials to include improved radiation therapy techniques and/or improved chemotherapeutic regimens.

In patients with unresectable gastric cancer only two randomized trials of radiation and radiation plus chemotherapy have been published. The Mayo Clinic Group has the oldest publication, comparing a total of 3500-4000 rads to the same dose of radiation plus 5-FU (63). The combined approach resulted in a mean survival of 13 months, superior to the mean survival of 5.9 months for radiation alone. More recently Falkson and Van Eden of South Africa have randomly compared radiation plus 5-FU to radiation plus a combination of 5-FU, imidazole carboxamide dimethyl triazeno, vincristine, and bis-chloroethyl nitrosourea (25). Falkson and Van Eden studied 70 patients of which 59 were subject to evaluation. Unlike the Mayo Clinic series, where all patients had limited and locally inoperable disease only, approximately one-fourth of Falkson's patients had distal disease in the liver (nine) or brain (one). Although is is not clear if there was an equal distribution of patients in both arms by anatomical stage of disease and performance status, the overall median survival for all patients receiving the single agent, 5-FU, was 220 days, and for patients receiving the four-drug combination the median survival was 199 days. It would seem that future phase III trials might utilize the 5-FU-radiation combination as a control arm.

The greatest investigative energies in colorectal carcinoma are currently being applied to questions about preoperative irradiation in rectal cancer. Since accurate anatomical staging is so important to randomized trials, the current studies utilizing combinations of chemotherapy and irradiation must of necessity be postoperative in design. Although no data are available, there are currently three cooperative group trials evaluating the relative roles of drug and radiation, alone or in combination, for patients with presumed curative resections, but who have a Duke stage which would increase their chance of recurrence (18). Other cooperative group efforts are underway in patients with known residual, recurrent, or unresectable rectal cancer, but these studies are very early in their inception.

The last gastrointestinal malignancy in which a combined approach has even been anecdotally attempted is that of squamous cell carcinoma of the anus. In the past this uncommon cancer has been approached primarily by surgery, and secondarily by radiation for local surgical failures. In late stages of the disease chemotherapy has been tried, with occasional palliation reported. Bruckner et al. have treated three patients with anal carcinoma who had either failed surgical resection or had subtotal resections utilizing a combination of radiation, and a chemotherapeutic regimen consisting of mitomycin C and continuous 5-FU infusions (8). Follow-up is too short to claim cure, but the substantial toxicity (usually to chemotherapy) was sufficiently tolerable to consider this combined approach in future trials.

GENITOURINARY TUMORS

The concomitant or planned sequential use of radiation and chemotherapy in genitourinary tumors represents one of the most understudied areas in oncology. Carcinoma of the testes has received limited attention with both modalities, but even in this disease most reported investigations utilize a combined approach dictated by individual clinical necessity, rather than a planned prospective assessment of the value of radiation and chemotherapy over radiation alone (10,27). In the Southwest Oncology Group we have attempted to evaluate the relative importance of radiation and chemotherapy in nonseminomatous testes cancer metastatic to the retroperitoneal nodes. Originally this study attempted to examine the role of sandwiching radiation between courses of chemotherapy, vs. sequencing radiation and chemotherapy. It is too early to evaluate the results of this study, but even now it is apparent that there will be insufficient tissue subsets and stages to answer this first objective. However, eventually cure rates of this combined approach will be compared to historical data. Even more interesting will be the results of a planned Northern California Oncology Group study which will take patients with clinically favorable nonseminomatous testicular cancer (at risk with minimal retroperitoneal node involvement) and randomize between retroperitoneal node dissection and radiation. If this study demonstrates equal success for the irradiated patients, and the current claims for the more dramatically successful combination chemotherapy programs are sustained with time, it may well be that certain future patients can be saved the morbidity of surgical node dissection through an aggressive combination of radiation and chemotherapy.

Completed prospective clinical trials which would serve to provide leads in the proper combination of radiation and chemotherapy, vs. either modality alone, are totally lacking in patients with all stages of bladder cancer. In the past few years the introduction of more active compounds such as adriamycin and cis-platinum have provided an impetus for conducting properly designed prospective trials, but such studies are too close to inception to suggest meaningful management generalizations. These drugs with significant activity in late disease have attendant cumulative toxicity or initial nephrotoxicity which necessitates a prospective evaluation to convince oncologists that a combined radiation and a chemotherapeutic approach will actually result in a survival advantage. Only recently have feasibility trials of adding chemotherapy to radiation for locally advanced, nonmetastatic bladder cancer been published (35). In the Yorkshire Urological Cancer Research Group study a combination of adriamycin and 5-FU, limited to four cycles, was given 1-3 months after completing "radical radiotherapy." Although the radical radiotherapy is inadequately defined, the authors claim that toxicity was acceptable and conclude that it is reasonable to conduct prospective trials. One of their 18 patients was considered a fatality from adriamycin cardiomyopathy, emphasizing the need to conduct comparison trials before concluding that any advantage might accrue to patients receiving a combined radiotherapy and chemotherapy approach. Retrospective evaluations such as those of Kenny et al. (50) provide hope that in late disease (Jewett stages C and D) the addition of chemotherpy to radiation may result in a meaningful survival advantage.

For the most part prostatic cancer remains a disease of elderly males for whom palliative hormonal treatment is usually exhausted before chemotherapeutic agents are tried. Historically cancer of this organ has been thought of as a slow-growing malignancy which is often a coincidental finding in surgical specimens removed for benign disease, or an incidental finding in autopsy specimens, where the discovery of carcinomatous foci have no relationship to the patient's death. The discovery, a decade ago, that a 5 mg daily dose of diethylstilbesterol in patients with advanced prostatic cancer contributed to the premature demise of patients from thromboembolic complications has served to perpetuate a conservative attitude to otherwise asymptomatic patients (3). However, more recent assessments of the degree of anaplasia in biopsy specimens and the relationship of anaplasia to survival have suggested that this complacency may be unwarranted in significant numbers of patients with prostatic cancer (70). At a time when attitudes about the natural history of prostatic carcinoma have been evolving away from a potential historic underestimation of the disease's aggressiveness, there has been an enlarging effort to test the efficacy of chemotherapeutic agents. A major source of retardation in quantifying objective response in patients with this disease resides in the propensity of prostatic cancer to spread exclusively as blastic metastases to the bone. In the author's experience only about one-third of patients with advanced prostatic cancer have a disease distribution which allows for accurate tumor measurement on physical exam or x-ray. Despite these limitations, and the inherent conservatism alluded to above, single chemotherapeutic agents showing activity are being discovered. The National Prostatic Cancer Project has established objective responses with the following single agents: 5-FU, cyclophosphamide, estramustine phosphate, and imidazole-4-carboxamide (77). This gradually increasing list of active chemotherapeutic agents comes at a time when radiation oncologists are piloting investigations into radiation as a primary modality for local disease (70). In the study by Perez and his colleagues one finds an excellent argument for primary radiation, but it is also their data which identify a subset of irradiated patients with poorly differentiated prostatic cancer who have a 3-year survival of only 25%. Although there is an absence of published efforts to explore combined radiation and chemotherapy in local disease, it would seem apparent that such an undertaking is justified in patients with poorly differentiated cancer.

Combined radiation and chemotherapy for locally advanced renal cell carcinoma is almost unheard of in the medical literature. To a great degree this paucity of data reflects the absence of meaningful drug activity in advanced kidney cancer, as well as the understandable customary surgical resection on presentation. Exceptional has been the effort of Wiley and associates to combine irradiation and intraarterial actinomycin D in two patients with unresectable disease (93). In one patient without metastatic disease, but disease initially too locally advanced for resection, the combination of irradiation and drug reduced the tumor bulk to one-third of its original size allowing for subsequent resection and a patient free of disease 5 years after the second operation. Admittedly, however, future research into combined radiation and chemotherapy of renal carcinoma will undoubtedly be sluggish until more active drugs are discovered.

GYNECOLOGIC TUMORS

Gestational choriocarcinoma was the first disseminated cancer to be cured by chemotherapy. Unfortunately, of the many cancers which arise in female genitalia, gestational choriocarcinoma is a rare tumor, and because of its dual genetic origin, inadequately reflects the therapeutic challenge presented by cancers arising spontaneously in the genital organs of women. As we examine the spontaneously arising cancers in female genitalia, special attention will be devoted to that organ which frequently gives rise to late diagnosis and from which the largest number of women die.

Equally unfortunate is the tendency for ovarian cancers to arise from epithelial origins, rather than the germ cell origin of the more responsive testicular cancer. Only a few studies in ovarian cancer patients attempt to compare the combination of radiation and chemotherapy to a single modality, and the majority of older published reports were not randomized trials. Radiation methodology varies considerably from one study to the next, and rarely are the drug therapies sufficiently comparable to allow any meaningful comparison between the different studies. Another acknowledged difficulty in evaluating these data in ovarian cancer management centers around problems attendant to the inadequacy of surgical staging. Many patients included in these various trials have had initial surgical incisions which preclude adequate evaluation of those anatomical sites often involved by ovarian cancer. Consequently even those few studies which utilize the now more accepted International Federation of Gynecologists and Obstetrics (FIGO) classification may include significant numbers of patients who are understaged, thereby raising significant doubt as to the accuracy of investigator conclusions. It is important to remember these defects as we examine the published trials which attempt to evaluate which modality, or combination of modalities, is most effective in achieving cure or long-term remission in patients with ovarian cancer. Because of these surgical staging problems, optimal treatment of the earlier stages of ovarian cancer confined to the pelvis (FIGO II or less) must await more properly designed trials which consider accurate surgical and pathological staging. Unfortunately, the bulk of patients with ovarian cancer present with peritoneal spread (FIGO stage III). Even within this category of FIGO stage III patients, problems arise as it becomes increasingly apparent that the patients who can be successfully debulked or have tumor nodules less than 3 cm in size represent individuals with different potentials to respond to radiation. Consequently, studies of individuals with FIGO stage III disease often fail to acknowledge the actual bulk of cancer remaining to be treated.

Cognizant of these deficiencies, one early study in patients with ovarian cancer, with stages comparable to FIGO III, included those who were felt to benefit from melphalan administration, even when subsequent radiation was delivered (78). Selected patients with good responses to melphalan were then given a poorly defined amount of radiation, resulting in a superior survival to patients treated with initial radiation and subsequent melphalan, or to patients treated with melphalan alone. The authors readily acknowledged the selection bias, and make no effort to claim that adding radiation produces a superior survival over patients with this advanced stage treated by melphalan alone. Historically, this study was important because it sanctified the usefulness of chemotherapy in patients with bulky FIGO stage III disease. It left unanswered the question of what the addition of radiation really meant in terms of improved survival in patients having an initial response to chemotherapy. Unfortunately, this question remains unanswered, and there is no present evidence that it is being evaluated in ongoing clinical trials.

Griffiths and his colleagues at the Boston Hospital for Women retrospectively reviewed their experience in different patient groups with ovarian cancer (38). These authors, as have others, properly recognized the importance of evaluating patient survival in terms of the relative success in debulking patients with otherwise similar FIGO stages. Patients with FIGO stage III disease were subdivided into group A, patients who had at least one-half of all gross disease excised and no palpable disease postoperatively. The group B, FIGO stage III, patients had palpable disease after surgery, and significantly shorter median survival times. The addition of postoperative alkylating agent chemotherapy appeared to significantly enhance survival over those patients receiving only irradiation, regardless of whether the patient belonged to group A or group B. Unfortunately, the successfully debulked patients of group A included a large number of patients with FIGO stage II, which served to confound the otherwise encouraging conclusion that chemotherapy was beneficial. The group B patients were all FIGO stage III, and the doubling of median survival in the patients treated with a combined radiation-chemotherapy approach, as opposed to those treated with radiation alone, would suggest the importance of a combined approach in patients with residual bulky disease. However, based on this study alone, the enthusiasm for adding chemotherapy to radiation must be tempered by the realization that this was a retrospective analysis and that the radiotherapy dose and schedule were extremely variable. This last criticism is vital to the extent to which a significant conclusion can be attached to the Griffiths' Boston study results, and serves to remind all oncologists of the necessity to standardize radiation therapy, if firm conclusions are to be reached about the value of additive chemotherapy. This study leaves unanswered what the role of chemotherapy alone might be in patients with bulky FIGO stage III disease. Recently, Haas and her colleagues at the University of Kansas have reported an 80% 2-year disease-free survival in successfully debulked FIGO stage III patients treated with radiation alone, a survival percentage almost twice that of the Griffiths' study mentioned above (39). Continued concern about the need for additive alkylating agent therapy, with its inherent potential for long-term detrimental effect, has been recently enhanced by the preliminary results of the Toronto study (19). This study was a three-armed randomized trial in ovarian cancer, comparing pelvic irradiation alone (4500 rads), pelvic irradiation plus 6 mg/day of chlorambucil for 2 years to pelvic radiation (2250 rads) plus abdominopelvic radiation (2250 rads). Quite properly, patients were stratified by age, stage, histology, and grade, and while all patients had salpingo-oophorectomy and hysterectomy, diaphragmatic visualization was not accomplished. This last circumstance is the only apparent weakness in an otherwise well-conducted clinical trial. Their results reveal a superior actuarial 5-year relapse-free survival for the patient group treated with pelvic and combined abdominopelvic radiation. Ominously, two patients in the chlorambucil group subsequently died from acute leukemia. One other aspect of the Toronto trial deserves special comment, and that relates to the investigators' willingness to deliver abdominal radiation in a port at least 1 cm above the diaphragm, and to avoid liver shielding. This more aggressively designed radiation port would avoid undertreatment of the subdiaphragmatic surfaces, where ovarian cancer so often spreads.

The Eastern Cooperative Oncology Group (ECOG) randomized patients with FIGO stage III ovarian cancer, who were "not completely resectable," to receive radiation only, 8 weeks of chlorambucil, or a combination of the two (61). For a three-armed study, patient numbers were small, and although the overall response rates were not different between the three groups, the radiation-only group had a median survival (94.9 weeks) twice that of the combined treatment group (42.2 weeks), and three times that of the chlorambucil-only group (33.5 weeks). Because of this survival advantage the investigators concluded that radiation therapy alone offered the best chances for long-term survival. This conclusion must be tempered by the realization that there were small numbers of patients in each treatment arm, and that the authors retrospectively acknowledge that 8 weeks of chlorambucil would not be deemed sufficient chemotherapy. Consequently, one can only accept their conclusion with a great deal of reservation. Also of concern is the failure of the ECOG study to quantitate the bulk of tumor left to be treated after surgical resection, a prognosticator already alluded to above and recognized as having significant survival implications in at least two other clinical trials (7,38). In a Gynecologic Oncology Group (GOG) study, similar in design to the ECOG study, the use of sustained prolonged melphalan treatment resulted in survival data not significantly different from radiation alone (7). The GOG study not only incorporated the use of sustained alkylating agent treatment in the chemotherapy-only arm, but recognized the importance of differentiating patients by the relative success of surgical debulking, appreciating the distinction between patients with residual tumor masses greater than 3 cm and those with smaller tumor masses. A Mayo Clinic study comparing cyclophosphamide alone to cyclophosphamide plus radiation failed to demonstrate any survival advantage for the addition of radiation(47). Taken together with the GOG results, one must further question the conclusion of the ECOG study which favored radiation alone.

For the foreseeable future most patients with ovarian cancer will present with advanced FIGO stage III disease, and any solid recommendations for management will await properly designed clinical trials. Despite recognized weaknesses of the just reviewed data, it is these very same studies which have increased our knowledge of the important natural history variables which influence survival, regardless of the treatment. Future trials will need to stratify for degree of anaplasia, histologic subtype, careful quantitation and documentation of surgical debulking, performance status, optimizing chemotherapy agents and treatment duration, and very significantly include radiation ports which treat the abdomen in such a fashion as to include the entire diaphragmatic surfaces.

Unquestionably the decreasing mortality from cervical cancer reflects favorably on the early diagnosis achieved by the now routine use of a Pap smear in gynecologic evaluations. Despite encouraging survival from early diagnosis, and subsequent successful treatment, some patients still present with locally extensive disease. Two initial randomized trials suggested beneficial effects of hydroxyurea when added to radiation in advanced untreated stages of cervical cancer (42,72). Expanding on one of these favorable early trials Hreshchyshyn coordinated a larger GOG study in 104 evaluable patients with FIGO stages III and IV disease (43). All patients were treated with radiation and randomized to receive concomitant hydroxyurea or placebo for 12 weeks. The authors found statistically significant advantages for the hydroxyurea-treated patients in terms of complete tumor regression, progression-free interval, and survival probability. As published, the study appears well conducted, but the evaluation process eliminated roughly 10%, or six patients, treated with hydroxyurea. These six patients were unable to tolerate the combined approach of radiation and a myelosuppressive drug, and were not included in the final analysis which resulted in a significant progression-free interval and survival probability. Despite the encouraging conclusion that hydroxyurea was beneficial in patients treated with radiation, a more convincing argument would have resulted from a statistical analysis which included these six "unevaluable" patients. In summary, future clinical trials, which attempt to assess the value of adding chemotherapy to radiation in advanced cervical cancer will need to follow the careful design of a study like that of GOG, but will need to adopt more rigid criteria in the evaluation process.

HEAD AND NECK

Cytotoxic agents with at least 20% response rates in head and neck cancer include: methotrexate, methotrexate in high dose with leucovorin, bleomycin, cyclophosphamide, hydroxyurea, vinblastine, adriamycin (11), and more recently cis-platinum (85). Those agents most exhaustively studied in combination with radiation include methotrexate, hydroxyurea, 5-FU, and bleomycin. The other compounds with activity, cyclophosphamide, vinblastine, adriamycin, and cis-platinum, have been studied as single agents in only small numbers of patients with head and neck cancer.

In this disease chemotherapy agents have generally been used in conjunction with radiation by either a systemic or intraarterial route. Historically the 1960s was a decade of pilot studies extolling the possible benefits of intraarterial drug administration, either preceding or given conjointly with radiation. Some of the early enthusiasm for the combined treatment, which utilized the intraarterial route of drug administration, was tempered by the significant morbidity attendant to this approach.

The majority of the initial positive reports were nonrandomized, single-institution pilot studies (29,46). Although not a randomized trial, Collin and Johnson evaluated two patient populations, one receiving radiation alone, and the other receiving intraarterial 5-FU prior to radiation (16). While these authors noted good tumor regression in the infusion group, their follow-up ranged from 3-9 years, allowing them to note the absence of any survival advantage or increased cures in the combination approach. Although not randomized, their study groups were reasonably well balanced with regard to age, sex, and TMN staging. The radiation-only group had a lower percentage of T4 lesions with bone involvement (16 vs. 28%), but it is doubtful that this alone would account for the failure of the combined approach to beneficially influence survival. One might argue that 5-FU was a poor drug to select, in view of its inferior activity in this disease. One group of investigators felt their subsequent experience with vinblastine superior to methotrexate, but by the 1970s sufficient experience with intraarterial methotrexate also brought into question whether or not this route provided any real benefit over systemic chemotherapy, plus an enlarged experience was increasingly associated with significant morbidity (81).

Due to the apparent waning interest in the intraarterial route, this approach has little to commend its use, particularly in settings where surgical experience is lacking. The central issue of radiation in head and neck cancer, combined with either systemic vs. intraarterial chemotherapy, is an appropriate question which has never been asked. Until a well-designed, randomized prospective study is conducted in this disease, the exact role of intraarterial drug administration will remain an enigma.

The past two decades have provided us with a rich investigative effort of combining radiation and systemic chemotherapy in patients with head and neck cancer. Perhaps one of the greatest lessons learned from studies in this disease is the necessity to conduct prospective comparative trials. Initial enthusiasm for concomitant radiotherapy and hydroxyurea arose from nonrandomized, noncomparative approaches (44,55,56). The potential problem of hydroxyurea interfering with completion of radiation, due to excessive toxicity of the combination as well as insufficient survival data, would suggest that this combined approach should only be used in a well-designed study. Without a controlled trial with this drug, or any compound capable of intensifying radiation-related mucositis, there is always the hazard that local control and survival may even be impaired by the combined approach.

As with hydroxyurea, the majority of published studies assessing the combination of radiation and a single parenteral or oral chemotherapeutic agent have been nonrandomized pilot studies. The early work of one author, who combined methotrexate and radiation, was appropriately tempered by the caution that larger numbers of patients would need to be studied (17). Other early studies of methotrexate, even when suggestively positive, have suffered from failure to randomize patients, or in instances when randomization was utilized, insufficient patient numbers or survival data to provide convincing data (30,51,52).

One other single agent to receive some study in combination with radiation is bleomycin. Early studies which suggested at least additive effects of radiation and bleomycin in local control of head and neck cancer came from India and Japan (58, 82). Enthusiasm from these positive pilot studies was dampened by the randomized European study, which compared radiation alone to radiation plus bleomycin (13). This randomized trial failed to demonstrate a significant tumor regression or survival advantage for the combined approach. An additional advantage of this European study was its focus on a more limited site of the head and neck cancer, the oropharynx. Recognition that the primary site influences the natural history and survival time in head and neck cancer is often overlooked by investigators evaluating the potential benefits of a combined approach in locally advanced disease. The most recently published pilot study of bleomycin recognizes these limitations and suggests other more restricted investigations prior to proceeding with more costly phase III trials (80).

Only recently have investigators used combinations of cytotoxic chemotherapeutic agents and concurrent radiotherapy in patients with advanced inoperable head and neck cancer. One recent study evaluated cyclophosphamide, vincristine, and bleomycin during the period of radiation, followed by a combination of cyclophosphamide, methotrexate, and bleomycin once the radiation was completed (31). While disease control in the 15 studied patients was excellent, the toxicity was unacceptable, with enhanced radiation mucositis and fatal complications in three patients (20%). In this particular study one might question the inclusion of a drug with minimal activity in this disease, cyclophosphamide. However, an important lesson in toxicity was learned, reinforcing the need for critical evaluation of any proposed combined myelosuppressive approach in this cancer. One other published study of note is the randomized trial of Bezwoda et al. (2), comparing radiation alone to radiation plus a complex seven-drug combination of vincristine, adriamycin, bleomycin, methotrexate, 5-FU hydroxyurea, and 6-mercaptopurine (2). Although the overall response rate for the combination of drugs and radiation was only 10% better than radiation alone (not significant), the twofold increase in survival for the combined approach was significant.

Future combined approaches in inoperable squamous cell carcinoma of the head and neck will undoubtedly explore the possible advantage of administering chemotherapy prior to radiation. The theoretical advantage may well be the improved delivery of drugs to large tumorous masses prior to radiation damage of the tumor vascular bed.

BRAIN TUMORS

In recent years patients with malignant gliomas have been studied in numerous prospective randomized trials, several of which attempt to define the role of combined radiation and chemotherapy. Usually these studies have limited their efforts to patients with proven grades III and IV astrocytomas (glioblastoma multiforme).

Radiation alone has received considerable attention by the Brain Tumor Study Group (BTSG), and the results of their dose-effect relationships have been extensively evaluated in a recent review (89). Patients receiving 4500 rads or less had median survivals which were not statistically different from patients not receiving radiation, although those patients who received 5000, 5500, and 6000 rads had highly significant survival advantages over the patients who had not received radiation. To what degree this survival advantage reflects groups of patients living long enough to receive more radiation over the real benefits of the increased dose is unclear. However, as the authors stress, it is improbable that future investigators will be willing to test this dose-effect relationship in a randomized fashion, nor is such a study necessary. It would appear that future studies of patients with glioblastoma multiforme should include a radiation component which utilizes at least 5000 rads, and preferably 6000 rads.

A pioneering BTSG study which combined radiation and chemotherapy, and compared the combination to each modality alone and an untreated control arm, demonstrated a statistically significant survival advantage of radiation alone over the control group, but an extension of survival was noted when bis-chloroethylnitrosourea (BCNU) was added to radiation (90). The actual median survival times were 17 weeks for the control group, 20 weeks for BCNU alone, 28 weeks for the radiation-only group, and 41 weeks for the combination of BCNU and radiation.

In a later evaluation of this initial (BTSG) study, a different analytic approach resulted in somewhat modified conclusions (91). By redefining the large patient population into "adequately treated" groups, evaluating only those patients who received more than 5000 rads, those who received two or more courses of BCNU (at least 8 weeks), the median survivals in each of the study arms demonstrated modest changes. The best conventional care, or control arm, still had a median survival of 17 weeks, the BCNU-only group now had a medial survival of 25 weeks, radiation alone had an extension to 37.5 weeks, and the median for BCNU and radiotherapy remained constant at 40.5 weeks. By utilizing these altered evaluation criteria, that is, adequately treated patients, the previous additive advantage of BCNU to radiation was less impressive. However, despite the statistically insignificant improvement of combining BCNU and radiation over radiation alone, the combination consistently continued to provide the superior median survival.

Building on this early experience the BTSG systematically evaluated another nitrosourea, methyl-CCNU, comparing this agent as a single therapy to radiation alone, a combination of radiation and methyl-CCNU, and then what appeared to be the best therapeutic combination of their earlier study, BCNU and radiation (92). As in the prior study, radiation was standardized, consisting of 6000 rads, and in this particular trial the radiation-only arm achieved a median survival of 36 weeks. Interestingly, the methyl-CCNU-alone arm and the methyl-CCNU and radiation arm had identical medial survivals of 31 weeks. BCNU and radiation continued to be the superior therapeutic arm, with a median survival of 51 weeks. Although not likely to be significantly different, from a statistical standpoint, it would appear that methyl-CCNU may even detract from the survival achievable by radiation alone. Methyl-CCNU also appears to be an inferior preparation to BCNU when a nitrosourea is used in combination with radiation. This may, in part, relate to the method of administration, that is, oral vs. intravenous.

The Radiotherapy Oncology Group (RTOG) is in the process of completing a trial of radiation alone (6000 rads), radiation plus methyl-CCNU and DTIC, vs. radiation and BCNU in grades III and IV malignant gliomas. Studying this same tumor population the Southwest Oncology Group (SWOG) has been evaluating a three-arm study with radiation and three separate individual chemotherapeutic agents: BCNU, procarbazine, and DTIC. Although both groups continue to evaluate their respective studies, the preliminary results have failed to disclose a chemotherapy agent combined with radiation which is clearly superior to the BTSG's combination of radiation and BCNU.

Future trials in patients with malignant gliomas will necessarily need to include a radiation and BCNU arm, comparing this modest standard approach to new agents, or to BCNU in combination with other drugs which effectively cross the blood-brain barrier. Acceptable approaches might include radiation with BCNU and DTIC, or some combination which includes a drug such as dianhydrogalacticol.

BREAST CANCER

Currently, the most interesting clinical research in breast cancer management is occurring in the area of primary treatment and in the area of additive chemotherapy in surgically treated and staged patients with regional (stage II) spread of their disease. Very little has been done to evaluate the role of combining radiation and chemotherapy for any stage of breast cancer. There is a nonrandomized trial from Italy, where patients with first postmastectomy relapse were treated with a combination of radiation (3500-6000 rads/3-5 weeks) to all sites and chemotherapy (adriamycin, 5-FU, and cyclophosphamide) (66). Duration of freedom from disease was compared with another group of comparable patients treated only with chemotherapy. The authors found that 26% of the combined treatment group was free of disease for 36-48 months, whereas none of the chemotherapy-only group was free of disease. Median survivals were 30 months for patients rendered free of disease by the end of radiation therapy, 24 months for the minority of patients with residual disease when their chemotherapy was started, and only 13 months for the patients who received chemotherapy only. Unfortunately, the nonrandomized nature of this otherwise exceptional trial raises the issue of patient comparability. Although the authors are convinced of the comparability between the two groups, the disclosure of approximately twice as many patients with favorable sites (skin and lymph nodes), and one-half the number of patients with hepatic involvement (unfavorable) being treated by the combined approach, as well as failure to define the number of positive sites in each group, causes concern. Based on the authors' own data it would seem that the conclusion of superiority for the combined approach over chemotherapy may be premature.

In surgically managed patients, where axillary status is known, the presence of breast cancer in lymph nodes should prompt the oncologist to consider a 6-month to 1-year treatment course of chemotherapy. This seems most appropriate in premenopausal patients with stage II breast cancer, where at least three studies have demonstrated the value of chemotherapy as a means of either improving the relapse-free interval or significantly improving survival (6,26,67). Many medical oncologists feel there is a significant advantage to adjuvant chemotherapy even in postmenopausal women with axillary node involvement, although the survival data are not yet available. Consequently, it behooves the radiation oncologist not to forget the importance of axillary node status in dictating the need for additive chemotherapy.

LUNG CANCER

Unlike breast cancer there are numerous published reports evaluating the relative roles of radiation and chemotherapy in patients with carcinoma of the lung. Within the past decade there has been an increasing investigator appreciation for the development of randomized trials by histologic subtypes. The more recent trials correctly separate the small cell (usually oat cell) patients from the other histologies, often referred to as <u>nonoat cell</u> varieties. This separation is justified on the basis of major differences in natural history (37), as well as the in vitro demonstration of heightened growth fractions in the tumors of patients with small cell carcinoma (64). In the future, clinical trials should not allow for this accepted separation of small cell patients, but should further divide the nonoat cell patients into the broad categories of squamous, adeno, and large cell types. It is becoming apparent that detailed histologic review of all cases is important, as mixtures of these cell types may occur in a significant number of patients with lung cancer. For purposes of this review, studies in patients with small cell carcinoma will clearly be separated from other histologies, and where published reports allow, every effort will be made to further subdivide studies with patients having nonoat cell histologies.

For the most part small cell carcinoma ceased to be a surgically treatable form of lung cancer in 1973, when the British published their 10-year follow-up of primary management (28). Long before these published results, which demonstrated the superiority of radiation to surgery as primary management, most oncologists had identified patients with small cell lung cancer as individuals beset by a rapidly growing disease resulting in early death, and which could best be managed by a combination of radiation and chemotherapy. The exact amount and sites of radiation, either to the primary tumor and/or prophylactic whole brain irradiation, and which chemotherapeutic combinations should be administered when, and for how long, remain evolving research questions, the last decade of clinical trials has yielded sufficient data to provide broad guidelines for management of patients with small cell disease. As these trials have evolved, it has become apparent that patients should be staged as <u>limited</u>, disease confined to the thorax and ipsilateral lymph nodes, or all disease that can be included within a single radiation port, and <u>extensive</u>, disease beyond the anatomic distribution of patients with limited disease.

In patients with limited small cell carcinoma, radiotherapy alone may be curative, but 10-year survivals are only in the range of 5% (28). These radiotherapeutic results, based on the data of the Medical Research Council of Britain may actually underestimate the curative potential of radiation in a more modern group of patients with accurately defined limited disease, as the British study was initiated before the importance of staging was fully appreciated. Even so, the low cure rate with radiation alone would indicate that combination chemotherapy should be administered as a part of the treatment for patients with limited disease. However, it would seem premature to rely exclusively on chemotherapy, when at least 5% of such patients may be cured by irradiation. Because most patients with limited disease will die from disseminated disease, it could be argued that these individuals should first receive combination chemotherapy, followed by radiation of the primary, and subsequently returned to chemotherapy for a yet to be defined period of time. While some oncologists would encourage the use of prophylactic whole brain irradiation in patients with limited disease, the single best published study would suggest no advantage for this approach (40). Consequently, the current available data and state of the art would suggest that patients with limited small cell lung cancer are best managed by initial combination chemotherapy, interrupted for radiation of the primary, and a return to combination chemotherapy for a period of 1-2 years.

For patients with extensive small cell carcinoma the primary treatment must of necessity be combination chemotherapy. However, since Hansen first raised the issue of prophylactic brain irradiation (41), at least two prospective studies have attempted to evaluate the role of prophylactic whole-brain irradiation in extensive disease (45,88). Those patients randomized to receive prophylactic brain irradiation had a significant reduction in central nervous system (CNS) metastases, although this did not appear to offer any survival advantage. These findings serve to emphasize the inability of current chemotherapeutic agents to successfully treat subclinical CNS disease and that radiation can prevent the advent of an uncontrollable CNS demise. While one may accept the palliative value of prophylactic brain irradiation in patients with extensive disease, the wisdom of further interrupting systemic chemotherapy to radiate the primary lesion is doubtful. Taken together the combination of radiation to the brain and chest may actually impair the patient's ability to tolerate needed chemotherapy. While occasional patients, under current management standards, may survive longer than 2 years, the majority of responders can only expect a median survival of approximately 9-12 months. Consequently, efforts to improve the chances for cure and increased survival in the immediate future may rest with more aggressive chemotherapy in a protected environment (14) or in the more imaginative setting of autologous bone marrow transplantation.

Over the past decade only a few clinical trials have been published which attempt to evaluate the possible benefits of adding chemotherapy to radiation in patients with nonoat cell varieties of lung cancer. Although randomized, one of the earliest studies to attempt an evaluation of hydroxyurea and radiation vs. radiation alone was clouded by underestimation of the influence of cell types on survival and such small patient numbers as to raise questions about the validity of investigator conclusions (54). Historically speaking, the next major randomized trial attempted to compare radiation alone, chemotherapy alone, and radiation and chemotherapy to a wait-and-see group of patients with lung cancer (23). This Oxford study failed to demonstrate any survival advantage of any of the treatment groups over the wait-and-see patients. Superficially, this data might be utilized to support a "do-nothing" attitude toward patients with the various cell types of lung cancer. Unfortunately, the exclusive dependence on mean survival fails to recognize the occasional patient cured by radiation alone, a problem that might have been minimized by use of median survival rather than mean. Also disconcerting is the then acceptable historical disregard for separating small cell patients from undifferentiated cell types. Adding to this sense of therapeutic frustration in the early 1970s was the Swiss study which suggested a negative effect for the adjunctive use of cyclophosphamide when compared to patients treated with surgery alone (9).

Despite this climate of negativism, more positive reports began to appear. One of the first studies to demonstrate a survival advantage of chemotherapy and radiation, as opposed to radiation alone in patients with nonresectable lung cancer, was the 1972 publication of Bergsagel and his colleagues from Canada (1). Their addition of cyclophosphamide significantly extended survival in patients with oat-cell carcinoma, as well as in patients with other histologies. As patients with adenocarcinoma were excluded from this randomized trial, the other patients would of necessity have been predominantly patients with squamous cell carcinoma. In keeping with this more positive attitude was the pilot study of Tucker and colleagues who assessed the contribution of methotrexate as an additive to radiation in patients with locally inoperable squamous cell lung cancer (87). While the authors were optimistic with reference to the beneficial effects of methotrexate in extending survival, they were appropriately cautious in view of the small numbers of patients actually included in their trial. A positive effect of bleomycin was suggested by Chan and colleagues, who randomized patients with unresectable squamous cell lung cancer to either radiation alone or radiation plus simultaneous drug administration (12). Median survival for the combined approach was more than twice that for radiation alone. Unfortunately, once again, the number of patients in each of the randomized arms was so small as to defy meaningful statistical evaluation, although the concomitant use of bleomycin and radiation did not result in significant pulmonary toxicity. An older randomized study which looked at patients with nonoat cell lung cancer attempted to compare radiation alone to a combination of radiation and hydroxyurea (53). Survival was identical in both groups, suggesting no advantage to radiation and hydroxyurea over radiation alone. Although the number of patients in each arm was 25 or greater, the failure of hydroxyurea to improve survival is clouded by the presence of twice as many patients with adenocarcinoma in the combined treatment arm. Since hydroxyurea is a drug with little activity in adenocarcinoma, the failure of a combined approach may be more reflective of inactivity of the drug in adenocarcinoma than its failure in a combined effort directed at squamous cell lung cancer.

In patients with squamous cell, large cell and adenocarcinoma of the lung, many single agents and combinations have yet to be tested in conjunction with radiation. However, the likelihood of finding an unusually effective combination of radiation and chemotherapy in these otherwise resistant cell types must await the discovery of more active drugs in advanced disease.

REFERENCES

1. Bergsagel, D.E., Jenkin, R.D.T., Pringle, J.F., White, D.M., Fetterly, J.C.M., Klaassen, D.J., and McDermot, R.S.R.: Lung cancer: Clinical trial of radiotherapy alone vs. radiotherapy plus cyclophosphamide. Cancer 30:621-627, 1972.

2. Bezwoda, W.R., deMoor, N.G., and Derman, D.P.: Treatment of advanced head and neck cancer by means of radiation therapy plus chemotherapy - a randomized trial. M.P.O. 6:353-358, 1979.

3. Blackard, C.E., Doe, R.P., Mellinger, G.T., and Byar, D.P.: Incidence of cardiovascular disease and death in patients, receiving diethylstilbesterol for carcinoma of the prostate. Cancer 26:249-256, 1970.

4. Bonadonna, G., Lattuada, A., Monfardini, S., Milani, F., and Banfi, A.: Combined radiotherapy-chemotherapy in localized non-Hodgkin's lymphomas:

5-year results of a randomized study. In Adjuvant Therapy of Cancer II, edited by S.E. Jones and S.E. Salmon, New York, Grune and Stratton, 1979, pp. 145-153.

5. Bonadonna, G., Zucali, R., DeLana, M., and Valagussa, P.: Combined chemotherapy (MOPP or ABVD) - radiotherapy approach in advanced Hodgkin's disease. Cancer Treat. Rep. 61:769-777, 1977.

6. Bonadonna, G., Rossi, A., Tancini, G., Bajetta, E., and Valagussa, P.: CMF adjuvant chemotherapy in operable breast cancer. In Adjuvant Therapy of Cancer II, edited by S.E. Jones and S.E. Salmon, New York, Grune and Stratton, 1979, pp. 227-235.

7. Brady, L.W., Blessing, J.A., Slayton, R.E., Homesley, H.D., and Lewis, G.C.: Radiotherapy (RT), chemotherapy (CT), and combined therapy in stage III epithelial ovarian cancer. Cancer Clin. Trials 2:111-120, 1979.

8. Bruchner, H.W., Spigelman, M.K., Mandel, E., Cohen, C., Deppe, G., Turell, R., and Schiavone, J.: Carcinoma of the anus treated with a combination of radiotherapy and chemotherapy. Cancer Treat. Rep. 63:395-398, 1979.

9. Brummer, K.W., Marthaler, T., and Miller, W.: Effects of long-term adjuvant chemotherapy with cyclophosphamide (NSC-26271) for radically resected bronchogenic carcinoma. Cancer Chemother. Rep. 4:125-132, 1973.

10. Carey, R.W., Weitzman, S.A., Wilkin, E.W., Jr., Chu, A.M. and Prout, G.R., Jr.: Long-term unmaintained remissions after aggressive multidisciplinary treatment of advanced non-seminomatous testicular germ cell tumors. J. Urol. 118:597-600, 1977.

11. Carter, S.: The chemotherapy of head and neck cancer. Semin. Oncol. 4:413-424, 1977.

12. Chan, P.V.M., Byfield, J.E., Kagan, A.R., and Aronstam, E.M.: Unresectable squamous cell carcinoma of the lung and its management by combined bleomycin and radiotherapy. A clinical study of the enhanced results. Cancer 37:2671-2676, 1976.

13. Cochin, Y., Jortay, A., Sancho, H., Eschevege, F., Modelain, M., Desaulty, A., and Gerard, P.: Preliminary results of a randomized E.O.R.T.C. study comparing radiotherapy and concomitant bleomycin, to radiotherapy alone in epidermoid carcinomas of the oropharynx. Eur. J. Cancer 13:1389-1395, 1977.

14. Cohen, M.H., Fossieck, B.E., Gedven, P.J., and Mi-na, J.D.: Intensive chemotherapy of small cell bronchogenic carcinoma. Proc. AACR and ASCO 17:273, 1976.

15. Coleman, C.N., Williams, C.J., Flint, A., Glatstein, E.J., Rosenberg, S.A., and Kaplan, H.S.: Hematologic neoplasia in patients treated for Hodgkin's disease. N. Engl. J. Med. 297:1249-1252, 1977.

16. Collin, F.F. and Johnson, R.O.: Pre-irradiation 5-fluorouracil infusion in advanced head and neck carcinomas. Cancer 27:768-770, 1971.

17. Condit, P.T.: Treatment of carcinoma with radiation therapy and methotrexate. Missouri Med. 65:832-835, 1968.

18. Davis, H.L., Jr., Vontloff, D.D., Rozencweig, W., Handelsnon, H., Soper, W.T., and Mugia, F.M.: Gastrointestinal cancer; esophagus, stomach, small bowel, colorectum, pancreas, liver, gallbladder, and extrahepatic ducts. In Randomized Trials in Cancer: A Critical Reivew by Sikes, edited by M.J. Staquet, New York, Raven Press, 1978, pp. 147-230.

19. Dembro, A.J., Sturgeon, J., Bean, H.A., Beale, F.A.J., Pringle, J.F., Brown, T.C., Gospodarowicz, M., and Bush, R.S.: The effectiveness of adjuvant abdominopelvic irradiation in ovarian cancer. In Adjuvant Therapy of Cancer II, edited by S.E. Jones and S.E. Salmon, New York, Grune and Stratton, 1979, pp. 475-494.

20. Desser, R.K., Golomb, H.M., Ultmann, J.E., Ferguson, D.J., Moran, E.M., Griem, M.L., Vardimanl, J., Miller, B., Oetzel, N., Sweet, D., Lester, E.P., Kinzie, J.J., and Blough, R.: Prognostic classification of Hodgkin's disease in pathologic stage III, based on anatomic considerations. Blood 49:883-893, 1977.

21. DeVita, V.T., Serpick, A.A., and Carbone, P.P.: Combination chemotherapy in the treatment of advanced Hodgkin's disease. Ann. Int. Med. 73:881-895, 1970.

22. DeVita, V., Canellos, G., Hubbard, S., Chabner, B., and Young, R.: Chemotherapy of Hodgkin's disease (HD) with MOP: A 10-year progress report. Proc. AACR and ASCO 17:269, 1976.

23. Durrant, K.R., Ellis, F., Black, J.M., Berry, R.J., Rideholgh, F.R., and Hamilton, W.S.: Comparison of treatment policies in inoperable bronchial carcinoma. Lancet 1:715-719, 1971.

24. Earle, J.D., Gelber, R.D., Moertel, C.G., and Hahn, R.: A controlled evaluation of combined radiation and bleomycin therapy for squamous cell carcinoma of the esophagus. Int. J. Radiat. Oncol. Biol. Phys. 6:821-829, 1980.

25. Falkson, G. and vanEden, E.B.: A controlled clinical trial of fluorouracil plus imidazole carboxamide dimethyl triazeno plus vincristine plus bis-chloroethyl nitrosourea plus radiotherapy in stomach cancer. Med. Pediatr. Oncol. 2:211-217, 1976.

26. Fisher, B., Glass, A., Redmond, C., Fisher, E.R., Barton, B., Duch, G., Carbone, P., Economon, S., Foster, R., Frelick, R., Lermer, H., Levitt, M., Margolese, R., MacFarlane, J., Plotkin, D,, Shibata, H., Volk, H., (and other cooperating investigators). L-phenyl-alanine mustard (L-Pam) in the management of primary breast cancer. An update of earlier findings and a comparison with those utilizing L-Pam plus 5-fluorouracil (5-FU). Cancer 34: 2883-2903, 1977.

27. Folke, E., Per, J., and Britta, W.: Combined therapy with bleomycin against malignant melanomas and testicular tumors. Prog. Biochem. Pharmacol. 11: 219-222, 1976.

28. Fox, W. and Scadding, J.G.: Medical Research Council comparative trial of surgery and radiotherapy for primary treatment of small-celled or oat-celled carcinoma of the bronchus. Lancet 2:63-65, 1973.

29. Friedman, M. and Daly, J.F.: The treatment of squamous cell carcinoma of the head and neck with methotrexate and irradiation. Am. J. Roentgenol. 99: 289-301, 1967.

30. Friedman, M., DeNarvaes, F.N., and Daly, J.F.: Treatment of squamous cell carcinoma of the head and neck with combined methotrexate and irradiation. Cancer 26:711-721, 1970.

31. Fu, K.K., Silverberg, I.J., Phillips, T.L. and Friedman, M.A.: Combined radiotherapy and multidrug chemotherapy for advanced head and neck cancer: Results of a Radiation Therapy Oncology Group pilot study. Cancer Treat. Rep. 63:351-357, 1979.

32. Fuller, L.M., Madoc-Jones, H., Hagemeister, F.B., Rodgers, R.W., North, L.B., Butler, J.J., Martin, R.G., Amble, J.F., and Shullenberger, C.C.: Further follow up of results of treatment in 90 laparotomy-negative stage I and II Hodgkin's disease patients: significance of mediastinal and non-mediastinal presentations. Int. J. Radiat. Oncol. Biol. Phys. 6:799-808, 1980.

33. The Gastrointestinal Tumor Study Group: A multi-institutional comparative trial of radiation therapy alone and in combination with 5-fluorouracil for locally unresectable pancreatic carcinoma. Ann. Surg. 189:205-208, 1979.

34. Gilman, A.: The initial clinical trial of nitrogen mustard. Am. J. Surg. 105-574, 1963.

35. Glashan, R.W., Houghton, A.L., and Robinson, M.R.G.: A toxicity study of the treatment of T3 bladder tumors with a combination of radiotherapy and chemotherapy. Br. J. Urol. 49:669-672, 1977.

36. Glastein, E., Guernsey, J.M., Rosenberg, S.A., and Kaplan, H.S.: The value of laparotomy and splenectomy in the staging of Hodgkin's disease. Cancer 24:709-718, 1969.

37. Green, R.A., Humphrey, E., Close, H., and Patno, M.E.: Alkylating agents in bronchogenic carcinoma. Am. J. Med. 46:416-525, 1969.

38. Griffiths, C.T., Grogan, R.H., and Hall, T.C.: Advanced ovarian cancer: primary treatment with surgery, radiotherapy, and chemotherapy. Cancer 29: 1-7, 1972.

39. Haas, J., Mansfield, C.M., Hartman, G.V., and Reddy, E.K.: Results of the radiation therapy in the treatment of epithelial carcinoma of the ovary. Int. J. Radiat. Oncol. Biol. Phys. 4(2):178, 1978.

40. Hansen, H.H., Dombernowsky, P., Hirsh, F., and Rygar, J.: Intensive combination chemotherapy plus localized or extensive radiotherapy in small cell anaplastic bronchogenic carcinoma (SMAC). Proc. AACR ASCO 18:350, 1977.

41. Hansen, H.H.: Should initial treatment of small cell carcinoma include systemic chemotherapy and brain irradiation? Cancer Chemother. Rep. 4:239-241, 1973.

42. Hreschyshyn, M.M.: Hydroxyurea (NSC-32065) with irradiation for cervical carcinoma - preliminary report. Cancer Chemother. Rep. 52:601-602, 1968.

43. Hreschyshyn, M.M., Aron, B.S., Boronow, R.C., Franklin, E.W., Shingleton, H.M., and Blessing, J.A.: Hydroxyurea or placebo combined with radiation to treat stages III B and IV cervical cancer confined to the pelvis. Int. J. Radiat. Oncol. Biol. Phys. 5:317-322, 1979.

44. Hussey, D.H. and Samuels, M.D.: Combined hydroxyurea and radiotherapy: a new dosage schedule. South. Med. J. 65:137-141, 1972.

45. Jackson, D.V., Cooper, R.F., Ferree, C., Muss, H.B., White, D.R., and Spurr, C.L.: The value of prophylactic cranial irradiation in small cell carcinoma of the lung: A randomized study. Proc. AACR ASCO 18:319, 1977.

46. Jesse, R.H., Geopfert, H., Lindberg, R.D., and Johnson, R.H.: Combined intra-arterial infusion and radiotherapy for the treatment of advanced cancer of the head and neck. Am. J. Roentgenol. 105:20-25, 1969.

47. Johnson, C.E., Decker, D.G., VanHenrik, M., Mussey, E., Malkasian, G.D., and Jorgensen, E.O.: Advanced ovarian cancer: Therapy with radiation and cyclophosphamide in a random series. Am. J. Roentgenol. 114:136-141, 1972.

48. Jones, S.E., Fuks, A., Kaplan, H.S., and Rosenberg, S.A.: Non-Hodgkin's lymphomas: V. Results of radiotherapy. Cancer 32:682-691, 1973.

49. Kaplan, H.S.: Hodgkin's disease. Modern radiotherapy techniques and their results. Ser. Hemat. 6:139-151, 1973.

50. Kenny, G.M., Hardner, G.J., Moore, R.M., and Murphey, G.P.: Current results from treatment of stages C and D bladder tumors at Roswell Park Memorial Institute. J. Urol. 107:56-59, 1972.

51. Kligerman, M.M., Hellman, S., VonEssen, C.F., and Bertino, J.R.: Sequential chemotherapy and radiotherapy. Radiology 86:247-250, 1966.

52. Klimo, J. and Danko, T.: Methotrexate in combination with radiotherapy in the treatment of squamous carcinomas of the head and neck. Neoplasms 21: 451-454, 1974.

53. Landren, R.C., Hussey, D.H., Barkley, H.T., and Samuels, M.L.: Split-course irradiation compared to split-course irradiation plus hydroxyurea in inoperable bronchogenic carcinoma - a randomized study of 53 patients. Cancer 34:1598-1601, 1974.

54. LePar, E., Faust, D.S., Brady, L.W., and Becklof, G.L.: Clinical evaluation of the adjunctive use of hydroxyurea (NSC-32065) in radiation therapy of carcinoma of the lung. Radiol. Clin. Biol. 36:32-40, 1967.

55. Lerner, H.J., Beckloff, G.L., and Goodwin, C.: Concomitant hydroxyurea and radiotherapy in the management of 60 patients with head and neck cancer. Am. J. Surg. 35:525-534, 1969.

56. Lipshutz, H. and Lerner, H.: Three-year observation of combined treatment for far advanced cancer of the head and neck. Am. J. Surg. 118:698-700, 1969.

57. Lukes, R.J. and Collins, R.D.: Lukes-Collins classification and its significance. Cancer Treat. Rep. 61:971-979, 1977.

58. Matsumura, Y., Soda, T., and Motomura, K.: Combined treatment for carcinoma of the paranasal sinuses with irradiation and bleomycin. Eye, Ear, Nose and Throat Monthly 52:25-33, 1973.

59. Mauch, P., Goodman, R., and Hellman, S.: The significance of mediastinal involvement in early stage Hodgkin's disease. Cancer 432:1039-1045, 1978.

60. Mauch, P. and Hellman, S.: Supradiaphragmatic Hodgkin's disease: Is there a role for MOPP chemotherapy in patients with bulky mediastinal disease? Int. J. Radiat. Oncol. Biol. Phys. 6:947-949, 1980.

61. Miller, S.P. and Polock, S.: Comparative evaluation of combined radiation - chlorambucil treatment of ovarian carcinomatosis. Cancer 36:1625-1630, 1975.

62. McKelvey, E.M., Gottlieb, J.A., Wilson, H.E., Haut, A., Talley, R.W., Stephens, R., Lane, M., Gamble, J.F., Jones, S.E., Grozea, P.H., Gutterman, J., Coltman, C., and Moon, T.E.: Hydroxyldaunomycin (Adriamycin) combination chemotherapy in malignant lymphoma. Cancer 38:1484-1493, 1976.

63. Moertel, G.C., Childs, D.S., Jr., Reitemeier, R.J., Colby, M.Y., Jr., and Holbrook, M.A.: Combined 5-fluorouracil and supervoltage radiation therapy of locally unresectable gastrointestinal cancer. Lancet 2:865-867, 1969.

64. Muggia, F.M., Krezoski, S.K., and Hansen, H.H.: Cell kinetic studies in patients with small cell carcinoma of the lung. Cancer 34:1682-1690, 1974.

65. Musshoff, K.: Prognostic and therapeutic implications of staging in extranodal Hodgkin's disease. Cancer Res. 31:1814-1827, 1971.

66. Nervi, C., Arcangeli, G., Concolino, F., and Cortese, M.: Improved survival with combined modality treatment for stage IV breast cancer. Int. J. Radiat. Oncol. Biol. Phys. 5:1317-1321, 1979.

67. Nissen-Meyer, R., Knellren, K., Malmio, K., Mansson, B., and Norin, T.: Surgical adjuvant chemotherapy. Results with one short course with cyclophosphamide after mastectomy for breast cancer. Cancer 41:2088-2098, 1978.

68. Nobel, R., Beer, C.T., and Cutts, J.H.: Role of chance observations in chemotherapy. Vincas rosea. Ann. N.Y. Acad. Sci. 76:882-894, 1958.

69. Osborn, C.K., Norton, L., Young, R.C., Garvin, A.J., Simon, R.M., Berard, C.W., Hubbard, S., and DeVita, V.T.: Nodular histiocytic lymphoma: An aggressive nodular lymphoma with potential for prolonged disease free survival. Blood 56:98-103, 1980.

70. Perez, C.A., Bauer, W., Arza, R., and Royce, R.K.: Radiation therapy in the definitive treatment of localized carcinoma of the prostate. Cancer 40: 1425-1433, 1977.

71. Peters, M.F.: A study of survivals in Hodgkin's disease treated radiologically. Am. J. Roentgenol. 63:299-311, 1950.

72. Piver, M.S., Barlow, J.J., Vongtoma, V., and Webster, J.: Hydroxyurea and radiation therapy in advanced cervical cancer. Am. J. Obstet. Gynecol. 120:969-972, 1974.

73. Portlook, C.S. and Rosenberg, S.A.: No initial therapy for stage III and IV non-Hodgkin's lymphomas of favorable histologic types. Ann. Int. Med. 90: 10-13, 1979.

74. Prosnitz, L.R., Curtis, A.M., Knowlton, A.H., Peters, L.M., and Farber, L.R.: Supradiaphragmatic Hodgkin's disease: Significance of large mediastinal masses. Int. J. Radiat. Oncol. Biol. Phys. 6:809-813, 1980.

75. Prosnitz, L.R., Farber, L.R., Fischer, J.J., and Bertino, J.R.: Low dose radiation therapy and combination chemotherapy in the treatment of advanced Hodgkin's disease. Radiology 107:187-193, 1973.

76. Rappaport, H.: Tumors of the hematopoietic system. In Atlas of Tumor Pathology, Section 3, Fascicle 8, Washington, D.C., Armed Forces Institute of Pathology, 1966, pp. 1-442.

77. Rodriguez, L.H. and Johnson, D.E.: Chemotherapy for metastatic prostatic carcinoma. Cancer Bull. 30:139-141, 1978.

78. Rutledge, F. and Burns, B.C.: Chemotherapy for advanced ovarian cancer. Am. J. Obstet. Gynecol. 96:761-772, 1966.

79. Schein, P.S., DeVita, V.T., Hubbard, S., Chabner, B.A., Cannellos, G.P., Berard, C., and Young, R.C.: Bleomycin, adriamycin, cyclophosphamide, vincristine, and prednisone (BACOP) combination chemotherapy in the treatment of advanced diffuse histiocytic lymphoma. Ann. Int. Med. 85:417-422, 1976.

80. Seagren, S.L., Byfield, J.E., Nahum, A.M., and Bone, R.C.: Treatment of locally advanced squamous cell carcinoma of the head and neck with concurrent bleomycin and external beam radiation therapy. Int. J. Radiat. Oncol. Biol. Phys. 5:1531-1535, 1979.

81. Sealy, R. and Helman, P.: Treatment of head and neck cancer with intra-arterial cytotoxic drugs and radiotherapy. Cancer 30:187-189, 1972.

82. Shanata, V. and Krishnamurthi, S.: The combined therapy of oral cancer. Gann Monogr. 19:159-170, 1976.

83. Soga, J., Fujiniaki, M., Kawaguchi, M.: Bleomycin and irradiation effects on the esophageal carcinoma, a preliminary histological evaluation. Acta Biol. Med. Ger. 19:199-236, 1971.

84. Stein, R.S., Hilborn, R.M., Flexner, J.M., Bolin, M., Stroup, S., Reynolds, V., and Krantz, S.: Anatomical substances of stage III Hodgkin's disease: Implications for staging, therapy and experimental design. Cancer 42: 429-436, 1978.

85. Stephens, R., Coltman, C., Rossof, A., Samson, M., Panettere, F., Al-Surraf, M., Alberts, D., and Bonnet, J.: Cis-dichlorodiammineplatinum (II) in adult patients: Southwest Oncology Group studies. Cancer Treat. Rep. 63: 1609-1610, 1979.

86. Toland, D.M. and Coltman, C.A.: Second malignancies complicating Hodgkin's disease: The Southwest Oncology Group experience. Proc. ACCRASCO 18:351, 1977.

87. Tucker, R.D., Sealy, R., Van Wyk, C., Soskoine, C.L., and LeRoux, R.L.M.: A clinical trial of methotrexate (NSC-740) and radiation therapy for squamous cell carcinoma of the lung. Cancer Chemother. Rep. 4:157-158, 1973.

88. Tulloh, M.E., Maurer, L.H., and Forcier, R.J.: A randomized trial of prophylactic cranial irradiation in small cell carcinoma of the lung. Proc. AACR ASCO 18:268, 1977.

89. Walker, M.D., Strike, T.A., and Sheline, G.E.: An analysis of dose-effect relationship in the radiotherapy of malignant gliomas. Int. J. Radiat. Oncol. Biol. Phys. 5:1725-1731, 1979.

90. Walker, M.D. and Gehan, E.A.: An evaluation of 1-3-bis (2-chloroethyl)-1-nitrosourea (BCNU) and irradiation alone and in combination for the treatment of malignant glioma. Proc. AACR 13:76, 1972.

91. Walker, M.D. and Gehan, E.A.: Clinical studies in malignant gliomas and their treatment with the nitrosoureas. Cancer Treat. Rep. 60:713-716, 1976.

92. Walker, M.D. and Strike, T.A.: An evaluation of methyl-CCNU, BCNU and radiotherapy in the treatment of malignant glioma. Proc. AACR 17:163, 1976.

93. Wiley, A.L., Wirtamen, W., Ansfield, F.J., and Ramirez, G.: Combined intra-arterial actinomycin D and radiation therapy for surgically unresectable hypernephroma. J. Urol. 114:198-201, 1975.

chapter 13

RADIOSENSITIZATION OF HYPOXIC CELLS

Stanley Dische, M.D.

Many attempts have been made to modify radiation response so as to increase the effect in tumors compared with that in normal tissues. The giving of treatment in a number of fractions and the cooling of the skin during irradiation were among methods explored in the early years to improve results. More recently neutrons and pi-mesons, the addition of cytotoxic drugs, and the use of heat have been the subjects of intensive study.

With most of the methods investigated there has been an increased effect both in tumor and in normal tissues, making it difficult to assess the true effect upon the therapeutic ratio. A method of radiosensitization which would be effective in tumor, but not in normal tissues, would obviously be a particularly valuable one as it would be simple to employ and assess.

The importance of the relationship between oxygen tension and radiosensitivity was first established by Gray et al. in 1953 (2). There may be a threefold difference in sensitivity between conditions of good and poor oxygenation of tissue. Thomlinson and Gray (37) suggested that most malignant tumors which were seen in clinical practice contained hypoxic cells which might be protected from radiation injury. As most normal tissues are believed to contain few, if any, hypoxic cells, an effective hypoxic cell sensitizer could be expected to enhance the effect on tumor without altering that in normal tissues.

WAYS OF OVERCOMING THE RADIORESISTANCE OF HYPOXIC CELLS

The early radiation therapists found by clinical observation that the therapeutic ratio was improved by the fractionation of radiotherapy. This was given a biological basis by Thomlinson (36) who showed that there was a progressive reoxygenation of hypoxic cells in tumors during a course of radiotherapy. As tumor cells die and the tumors shrink, the flow and distribution of blood is improved and hypoxic cells become oxygenated. Unfortunately, we have no means to guide us as to the optimum fractionation to employ in any individual patient. The most recent trials have been concerned with treatment being given on two or more occasions within a 24-hr period, but so far no absolute benefit has been demonstrated.

The magnitude of effect decreases when densely ionizing radiation such as neutrons and pi-mesons are employed. Results with considerable promise have been reported and clinical trials are underway. The apparatus remains expensive and does not yet satisfy clinical needs. With neutrons the biological efficiencies in normal structures differ from tissue to tissue as compared with that produced by photons, making it difficult to determine the true alteration in therapeutic radio. Much work remains to be done with the use of neutrons and pi-mesons before their place in radiotherapy can be determined.

The first demonstration in an animal tumor system that hyperbaric oxygen could improve tumor control was by Gray et al. (22). Soon afterward patients were given radiotherapy in a hyperbaric oxygen chamber by Churchill-Davidson and his colleagues (10). In seven of eight patients where half the tumor was treated using hyperbaric oxygen and half under normal conditions, there was evidence histologically of an increased effect when the tumor was biopsied or removed shortly afterward. In the remaining cases there was so much radiation change that no comparison was possible. There followed reports of series of patients with a variety of tumors treated with hyperbaric oxygen who appeared to benefit, and further evaluation has had to wait upon the completion of fully randomized controlled clinical trials.

The results now available vary, particularly according to the site under study. In head and neck cancer the most important work has been that performed at Cardiff (25). In the first trial a dose between 3500-4600 rads was given, depending on the volume to be irradiated, in 10 fractions over 22 days in hyperbaric oxygen or in air. A total of 295 patients was admitted and a highly significant increase in local tumor control was obtained with hyperbaric oxygen, 53% compared with 30% in air ($P = < 0.001$) at the expense of some increase in normal tissue damage in the oxygen. This resulted in a reduced necessity for salvage surgery, but not in any significant improvement in survival. In the second trial, begun in 1971, the identical dose and fractionation was retained for hyperbaric oxygen except where the larynx was in the field of treatment when the dose was reduced by 10%. The control group received a conventional daily fractionation scheme in air. A similar study was conducted at Leeds. When the cases from the two centers were added together it was seen that with hyperbaric oxygen there was a highly significant improvement not only in local control ($P = < 0.001$) but also in survival ($P = < 0.01$) (25, 28). Despite the reduction in dose in the larynx cases, treatment in hyperbaric oxygen remained superior for these cases without any excess of morbidity being shown. Three other randomized trials also report margins in favor of oxygen, but they were concerned with a limited number of cases and statistical significance was not reached (13).

In carcinoma of bladder benefit was shown in one trial performed by Plenk (31), where in 40 patients there was, in survival, a margin in favor of oxygen, also Van den Brenk demonstrated improvement in immediate response in a small group of 16 cases. In the Medical Research Council study, no benefit was seen in a group of 236 cases (Cade et al., 9). There is, at this time, no evidence of long-term benefit being achieved with hyperbaric oxygen in cancer of the bladder.

In carcinoma of the bronchus there have been a series of reported trials by Cade and McEwen (8). With conventional fractionation no benefit has been shown, but using six fractions and a maximum tumor dose of 3600 rads, survival at 2 years after treatment in hyperbaric oxygen was 26% compared with 12.4% in air, and at 4 years 15.9%, compared with 2.5% in air. A total of 123 patients has been included so far. The trend does not reach statistical significance at this time.

In carcinoma of the cervix there is considerable disagreement among the results of randomized studies. In that containing the largest number of cases, the Medical Research Council's study performed at four centers to which 320 cases were added, there was a highly significant increase in local tumor control ($P = < 0.001$) (Table 1). The greatest benefit was seen in stage III where there was also a significant improvement in survival. Some increased morbidity was encountered.

Table 1. Medical Research Council Trial of the Hyperbaric Oxygen Chamber in the Radiotherapy of Advanced Carcinoma of Cervix. Actuarial Local Recurrence-Free Rates According to Center

Center	Treatment Series	Total Patients	Percentages Free of Local Recurrences by Years Since Entry to Trial					Probability of Difference Between Curves Due to Chance
			1	2	3	4	5	
Portsmouth	Oxygen	19	65	58	58	58	58	0.07
	Air	18	46	18	18	18	18	
Oxford	Oxygen	17	45	45	45	45	45	0.11
	Air	17	13	13	13	-	-	
Glasgow	Oxygen	80	89	85	85	85	78	0.03
	Air	82	85	64	61	61	58	
Mount Vernon	Oxygen	45	85	80	70	70	60	0.14
	Air	42	66	55	52	52	49	
All patients	Oxygen	161	80	76	73	73	67	<0.001
	Air	159	68	52	49	49	47	

In a trial concerned with 223 patients in Houston no significant difference was obtained (19). At Leeds in a rather different trial where treatment with a Cathetron was combined with external beam therapy in oxygen or in air, no benefit has been reported (43). A margin in favor of oxygen has been reported by Glassburn et al. (21) and a multicenter study performed by the Radiation Therapy Oncology Group has also shown a margin of benefit in favor of oxygen.

The difference in response seen at different primary sites may be related to the differing patterns of tumor biology. The extent to which hypoxia remains a problem when conventional multifraction therapy is employed is not known. The lack of improvement with hyperbaric oxygen may, on the other hand, be due to the efficiency of conventional multifraction radiotherapy in overcoming the problem of hypoxia without the addition of any other measure or else due to an inefficiency on the part of hyperbaric oxygen to penetrate deeply to hypoxic, though viable, cells. Other factors may be more important than hypoxia in determining radiation failure in some sites. It is possible that in carcinoma of the cervix there are different tumor subtypes which may be differently distributed in the reported series and this may contribute to the contradictory results recorded (13).

There seems no doubt that hyperbaric oxygen does not lead to an increased effect in normal tissues. In the trials showing benefit this seems to outweigh the increase in morbidity, although in these circumstances it is always difficult to give an accurate estimate as to the amount of improvement in the therapeutic ratio which has been obtained. It is important to recognize that increased morbidity in hyperbaric oxygen can be due to two mechanisms. First, the use of hyperbaric oxygen results in a considerable elevation of the oxygen tension in normal tissues. Although the relatively flat portion of the curve relating oxygen tension to radiation sensitivity is reached, it still shows some slope and we must expect some increased radiation effect due to this. The other reason for an elevation in effect is the presence of hypoxic cells in normal tissues. The larynx is the only site where we have certain evidence that this is of significance, but such cells may well exist in other normal structures. The hyperbaric chamber is employed in very few centers at this time. It is a technique that has been with us for over a quarter of a century and one that is very demanding on the patient and the radiotherapy center. During the period of its use many new methods have been introduced into clinical radiotherapy; some are potentially easier to employ and may be used in a wider range of cases. The future for hyperbaric oxygen remains uncertain and much depends on the results of clinical trials of these other methods now in progress.

Chemical Hypoxic Cell Sensitizers

Oxygen is the best known and the most effective radiosensitizer of hypoxic cells. It is, however, metabolized in the cells through which it diffuses and so may not reach the cells distant to the capillaries. The rationale for the use of sensitizing drugs is that although they may be less active than oxygen they are, for practical purposes, not metabolized in the cells through which they diffuse and are, therefore, able to reach the distant hypoxic cells in high concentration.

In 1963, Adams and Dewey (1) suggested, on the basis of the few radiosensitizing compounds then available and their effects upon hypoxic bacteria, that the electron affinity of these compounds and their ability to sensitize was directly related. Subsequent work has fully supported this and the principle has been most valuable in the search for more active sensitizers. Progress towards a clinical application was slow until the discovery that metronidazole (Flagyl), a drug familiar in medicine as a trichomonacide, was an active sensitizer (4). The relatively low toxicity of this compound enabled a dramatic sensitization of animal tumors known to contain hypoxic cells. In 1973, metronidazole was first given to patients in doses likely to achieve sensitization, however, in order to do so doses of the order of 10-12 g were required, and this single dose can be compared with 200-400 mg three times daily given in the treatment of trichomonas or anaerobic infections (12, 40).

On theoretical grounds, based on electron affinity, it was predicted that the 2-nitroimidazoles would be more efficient than the 5-nitroimidazole, metronidazole. A Roche experimental compound, RO-07-0582 now called misonidazole, was found to be a more active radiosensitizer. The drug has been tested in many different animal tumor systems and a highly significant improvement in results obtained (20) This improvement, shown in single-dose work, has now been confirmed using multiple fractions up to a total of 20 fractions in animal studies (35).

Clinical Experience with Metronidazole

When the work with metronidazole began in 1973 there were considerable problems due to nausea and vomiting on administration of a large amount of the drug. Urtasun et al. established a regime for use in glioblastoma when metronidazole was given on three occasions in the week for a period of 3 weeks (40). He performed a randomized, controlled clinical trial giving 3000 rads as total dose in nine fractions in an overall time of 18 days. A statistically significant difference in survival was demonstrated. Although the control group fared less well than patients treated by other schemes of radiotherapy, the improvement in survival of those given metronidazole suggests that there was increased cell kill, giving evidence for an enhanced response using a chemical sensitizing agent. The introduction of misonidazole and the evidence that it was a more effective sensitizing agent has resulted in the diversion of interest away from metronidazole. The results of giving metronidazole to consecutive series of patients have been recorded and some randomized studies are underway. At this time, apart from the work by Urtasun, there are no hard data on which to make an assessment of the value of metronidazole.

Clinical Experience with Misonidazole

Misonidazole was a drug virtually unknown in medicine at the time of its introduction as an effective hypoxic cell sensitizer in 1974. The initial administration to patients was performed at Mount Vernon Hospital in November 1974 (23). In a series of eight patients given single doses of between 4-10 g, serum concentrations were achieved similar to those obtained in animals where radiosensitization had been truly demonstrated. There were some gastrointestinal disturbances, particularly in the patients given high doses, but otherwise in the single-dose study, tolerance was good. Promising results were obtained from studies of skin reaction in hypoxic skin and in the response of tumor in patients where multiple nodules were irradiated with and without the sensitizer (15,38).

In 1975 patients were given multiple doses of the drug and neurological problems were encountered with the drug for the first time. Despite this there has been wide interest and the work has now been taken up by centers for radiotherapy all over the world.

The Administration of Misonidazole to Man

Misonidazole is readily absorbed in the stomach and a peak level in the plasma is achieved normally between 1-2 hr after administration. After the peak there is a period of slow fall which extends for about 5 hr, and this has been called the plateau period (Fig. 1). All misonidazole levels given are actually estimates of total nitroimidazoles. The subsequent decline in concentration tends to be logarithmic with a mean half-life of 12.8 hr (S.D. 3.0 hr). The mean plateau concentration achieved per gram of misonidazole given is 23.4 μg/ml (17). The variance is reduced by correcting for body weight and still further by correcting for surface area. This confirms the general use of surface area when calculating the dose for any one patient. The mean plateau concentration achieved per gram of misonidzole is lower in men (21.2 μg/ml) than in women (25.9 μg/ml). On the other hand the half-life of the drug in women is 11.9 hr compared with 13.4 hr in men. These differences remain after correction for body size. There is a linear relationship between dose given and the plasma concentration in the plateau period. The half-life of the drug in plasma seems largely independent of the amount given, but with small doses may be associated with a slightly shortened half-life (17).

A large number of studies of the concentration of drug in normal and tumor tissue have been made. Most values have been in the range of 60-100% of the plasma concentration at the time of estimate (32). The inclusion of a small amount of normal fat in the specimen may considerably lower the result because the partition coefficient of water/fat for misonidazole is about 2:1 (3). The concentration in tumor and normal tissues rises and falls with that in the plasma with, in some cases, only a slight delay. Recent studies at Mount Vernon have shown an inverse relationship between the degree of necrosis seen histologically in tumor samples and the concentration of misonidazole (32). This may account for some low values found in some biopsy samples of tumor. It seems most probable that in most cases such necrotic tissue contains no viable cells and low values of misonidazole are of no clinical significance. There seems little doubt that misonidazole is a freely diffusing compound which reaches hypoxic cells, but data as to distribution in human tissues or on a cellular basis remain to be gathered.

Although the drug diffuses deeply into tumor tissue, the dose limit, due to toxicity, has encouraged efforts to achieve high local doses by direct diffusion. Awaad et al. (5) reported their findings from the introduction of misonidazole into the bladder 2 hr before cystectomy for carcinoma secondary to schistosomiasis. In five of seven cases concentrations of the order of 400 μg/g were detected in tumor, but not in normal bladder tissues. We have repeated this work obtaining a rather more varied range of tumor concentrations. Further work is proceeding.

Tolerance and Toxicity of Misonidazole in Man

Gastrointestinal Disturbances

Using current dose regimes giving between 6-30 doses of the drug we are encountering no gastrointestinal disturbances. These do occur with high single doses as was found in our original work and have also been reported by other workers.

Neurotoxicity

Convulsions have now been reported in three patients: In the two which occurred at Mount Vernon, doses considerably above our present maximum recommended level were employed, and in one the patient showed an unusually high

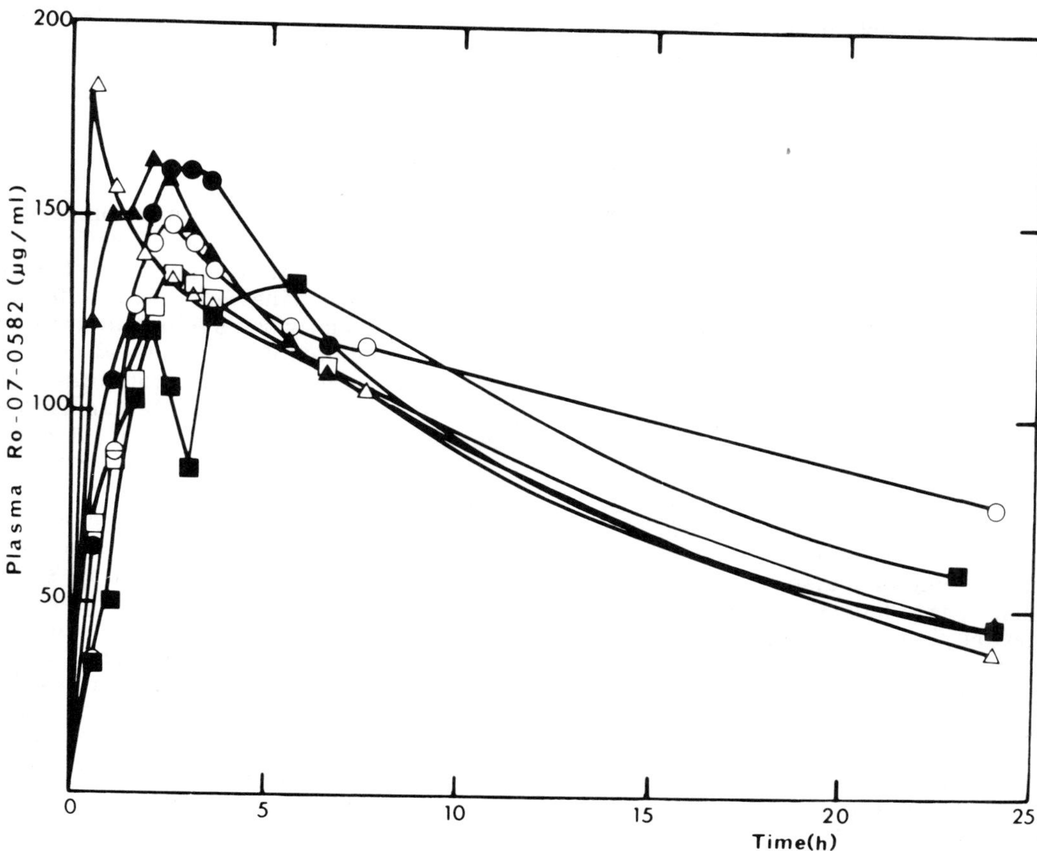

Figure 1. Plasma total nitroimidazole concentration obtained in one patient after each of six doses of 5 g of misonidazole (2.5 g per square meter of surface area). This is one of the patients treated early in the studies before the dose measurement of 12 g per square meter of surface area was established.

plasma concentration in relation to the actual dose given. In both, convulsions commenced 20 hr after administration of the last dose of misonidazole. These were easily controlled with Valium (diazepam), but there was considerable impairment of brain function which showed only a partial improvement before each of the patients died due to advanced malignant disease. With dose restriction and monitoring, the conditions leading to these episodes should not recur.

In an initial series of 14 patients given multiple doses of misonidazole and where the total dose was approximately 15-16 g/m^2 of surface area, 11 suffered a peripheral neuropathy. It took the form of numbness and paresthesia in the hands and feet with the most troublesome symptoms persistent in the feet. Some suffered cramplike pains which extended up into the calves. Usually the symptoms subsided after a period of several weeks, but in some they persisted until death and two patients are troubled still at 2 years. No motor loss has been demonstrated in our patients, but minor changes have been reported by other workers. Electromyelography has shown in our patients a sensory peripheral neuropathy with a mild motor component.

With the reduction of dose to 12 g/m^2 of surface area given over a period of at least 17 days, the incidence of peripheral neuropathy was reduced to 30%. Now with monitoring of the serum concentrations and appropriate reduction of dose in some cases, this has been halved and in most cases any neuropathy observed is of mild severity and of no great importance. There is an occasional patient with more troublesome and persistent symptoms, but these account for no more than 2 or 3% of all patients given the drug. It may be that a larger total dose can be given either when the period of treatment exceeds 4 weeks or when the drug is given in a single weekly dose. Further work is required to show whether this is truly so, and a collaborative effort involving five centers where work with misonidazole is proceeding may, by pooling of data, lead to an early answer to this and other questions of concentration with tolerance (16).

Transient peripheral neuropathy appearing about 12 hr after administration of the drug may follow large doses. We observed this to settle in 24 hr and not to be associated with a later established neuropathy. Transient confusional states may occur. In one patient after four doses each of 4 g we observed transient changes in the plantar responses and deep reflexes in the legs during a period of confusion. The episode occurred following a fall in the hemoglobin concentration to 9 g. With withdrawal of the drug, recovery was complete. Urtasun (41) reported a convulsion occurring after a confusional episode in a man of 85 who received eight doses of 2 g of misonidazole over a period of 19 days. Postmortem showed evidence of drug-induced toxic effect in the brain. Other confusional episodes have been reported, but in these cases recovery was complete after withdrawal of the drug. Confusional disturbances are not uncommon in elderly patients with large neoplasms, and in such patients who are given misonidazole it may be difficult to tell if the drug is contributing. It is possible that elderly patients who are suffering some degree of cerebral anoxemia due to impairment of vascular supply, together with anemia, may suffer a neurotoxic effect given doses well within the range considered safe and where the plasma concentrations of drug reach normal levels. It is best not to administer the drug to such patients, or if such patients are given the drug, to monitor carefully, suspending treatment at the first suspicion of a confusional episode.

Skin Rash

Hypersensitivity skin rashes have now been recorded in seven cases. The incidence is from 1-2% of all cases administered the drug. Usually a maculopapular rash on the hands, legs, and feet appears during the course of drug therapy and quickly settles when the drug is discontinued (29, 34).

Auditory Symptoms

Deafness has been reported where patients have been given large doses on a weekly basis. It seems transitory and full recovery occurs (27, 30).

Plasma Concentration Measurements and Misonidazole Toxicity in Man

Using the maximum safe dose, 12 g/m^2 of surface area, given in no less than six treatments over a period of 17-18 days, neurotoxicity occurs in less than 30% of patients. In a series of 45 patients given identical misonidazole therapy (six doses over 17-18 days to a maximum of 12 g/m^2 of surface area), those who suffered peripheral neuropathy showed significantly higher plateau values in plasma and tissue exposure as indicated by the product of the plateau concentration and the half-life (17). Therefore, it is important to monitor the plasma concentrations, not only to pick up those few patients who show unusually high values and who are especially at risk for development of misonidazole toxicity, but also to pick out those who show values in the upper part of the normal range when a small reduction of misonidazole dose may appreciably reduce the risk of peripheral neuropathy. Because in any one patient fairly consistent readings are obtained throughout the course of treatment, only a limited number of plasma concentration estimations are necessary, perhaps at the time of the first three treatments.

Evidence as to the Ability of Misonidazole to Sensitive Hypoxic Cells in Man

In our original study of the administration of the drug to man, an attempt was made to determine whether the drug could sensitize hypoxic cells in man using a technique where normal and artificially hypoxic skin was irradiated (14, 15). With a radiostrontium plaque, doses ranging from 800-1100 rads were given to areas of skin 15 mm square with the limb surrounded by a bag of oxygen. Although the erythema that followed was poorly related to dose, the subsequent pigmentation, usually at 6-8 weeks, was in most cases closely related. For irradiation under hypoxia an Esmarch bandage, a sphygmomanometer cuff at 200 mm of mercury, and the replacement of the oxygen in the bag by nitrogen were employed. Under these hypoxic conditions, approximately 1600 rads were required to produce the pigmentation which follows a dose of 800 rads given under oxic conditions. The drug greatly increased the radiation response of skin made temporarily hypoxic but did not significantly alter the response in oxic skin. The relative sensitizing efficiency is a measure expressing as a percentage the restoration of the sensitivity of the hypoxic cells to that of those under oxic conditions. In six patients given misonidazole in a range of doses, the efficiencies extended from 27-71%. These values can be compared with 11-14% in the three patients given metronidazole (15).

The Enhancement of Tumor Response in Man

A further study was made to determine whether any differences could be detected in the response of tumors in patients with multiple, observable, or measurable metastases (38). Seven patients took part in the study. The main method employed was the measurement of subcutaneous nodules treated under different conditions. Observations were made in the period of regression after treatment and if the patient survived long enough when regrowth occurred. The most satisfactory situation for study occurred in a young woman with multiple subcutaneous metastases from carcinoma of the cervix. Measurement of two groups each of seven nodules with a mean diameter of 12.6 mm showed a significant difference (P = 0.05) of the time of regrowth after single doses of 960 and 1120 rads, thus giving a measure of the ability of the system to discriminate. Regrowth seen in the third group of seven nodules treated with a lower radiation dose of 800 rads, combined with a dose of misonidazole, was similar to that seen after 960 rads alone, indicating a dose enhancement factor of 1:2.

In a second patient with a metastases in lung from a primary carcinoma of breast, no enhancement was detected. In a third case there was fairly clear evidence of enhancement, though this did not reach significance in the period of survival of the patient; while in the fourth with diffuse infiltration of tumor in wide areas of skin there was delay of regrowth when misonidazole was added to the standard dose. In the other cases it was not possible to make any estimate of effect.

Further work in patients with multiple deposits of tumor has been reported by Dawes et al. (11) and Ash (3). In both series a majority of cases studied gave evidence for increased response when misonidazole was given with radiotherapy. In one of the cases reported by Ash, radiotherapy was given in 10 fractions using less than 200 rad dose increments and increased delay in tumor regrowth was demonstrated.

These studies demonstrate that misonidazole can lead to increased kill of hypoxic cells in man, as in animals. They give great encouragement towards the use of the drug in man, but only randomized, controlled clinical trials can show whether a significant improvement in cure can result.

Effect Upon Normal Tissues in Man

In a few experiments in animals some enhancement of normal tissue effects has been observed, but only when high doses of radiation and misonidazole have been combined and the tissue irradiated was known to contain a concentration of hypoxic cells.

It must be recognized that there is an essential difference between the effects to be expected with hyperbaric oxygen and with a chemical sensitizing agent. The radiation response of tissues which are normally well oxygenated will be enhanced in hyperbaric oxygen by perhaps the equivalent of a 3% elevation in dose because of the continued gradual elevation of the line linking radiation response and oxygen tension through high concentrations of oxygen (13). The addition of misonidazole in the concentrations which are to be used clinically in well-oxygenated tissue may be expected to result in virtually no increment of effect (2).

There is, however, the possibility of an enhancement of effect in normal tissues containing a concentration of hypoxic cells. It remains to be seen if such an enhancement will be significant in the fractionated courses of radiotherapy to be employed. So far, in all tissues, immediate radiation reactions have been observed which have been similar to those expected with the dose and fractionation regime employed. It is too early to make any observations as to long-term effects.

The larynx presents a special problem because it contains a considerable concentration of hypoxic cells. Using misonidazole in the current restricted dosage in fractionated radiotherapy, it is unlikely that increased normal tissue effects will be observed, but careful observation is required.

A problem of interpretation of results with regard to normal tissue effects may be present in clinical trials using misonidazole combined with an unusual fractionation regime and this is discussed below.

Regimes of Administration of Misonidazole in Man

The neurotoxicity of misonidazole in man limits the dose which can be given. We must, therefore, consider carefully how best to use this drug in clinical radiotherapy. Among the possibilities are that it may be given:

1. With every treatment in a multifraction course given over a number of weeks.

2. With each of a reduced number of fractions so that a higher radiation dose is combined with a high dose of sensitizer.

3. With some of the treatments in a multifraction course of radiotherapy, the remaining treatments being given without administration of the drug.

4. Combined with multiple radiation treatments in 1 day taking advantage of the relatively long half-life of the drug in man.

If using the last three schemes we may give six doses, then we can hope to achieve 50-60 μg/g in the tumor at the time of radiotherapy (Fig. 2) when an enhancement ratio of 1. 6 or greater can be achieved, which is similar to that with neutrons.

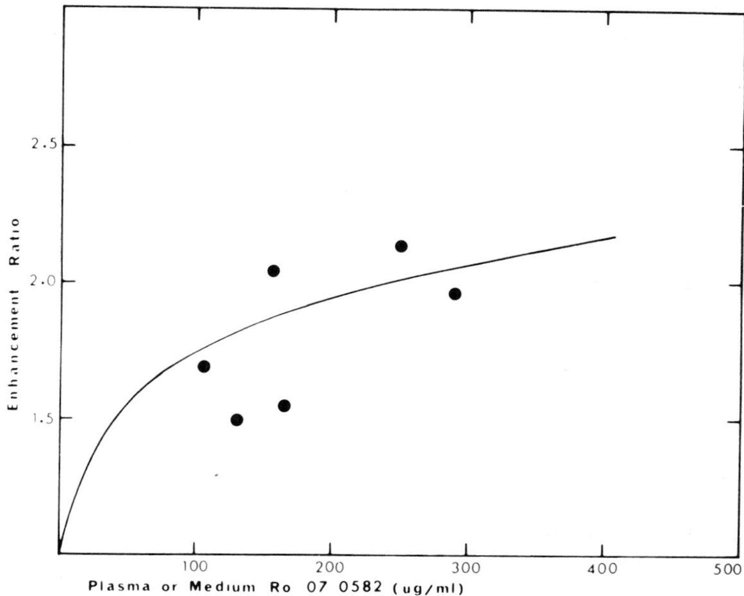

Figure 2. The sensitizing efficiency of Ro 07-0582. Continuous line: Data for sensitization of hypoxic Chinese hamster V79 cells cultured and irradiated in vitro. (Ref. 2) •: Data for sensitization of hypoxic human skin. (Adapted from Ref. 15.)

If we give misonidazole daily in a multifraction course over 4 or 6 weeks, we may be dividing our dose into 20 or 30 fractions. Tumor concentrations of around 24 and 20 μg/g may be achieved, giving us enhancement ratios of about 1:25 and 1:3. Because of the shape of the curve linking enhancement ratio with dose and the steep rise in enhancement at low doses, we have only just over half the degree of radiosensitization by dividing the dose for daily fractionation (Fig. 2).

On the other hand, biological evidence suggests that the reverse is true with radiation dose because of the shape of the survival curves for oxic and hypoxic cells. Particularly when doses start falling below 400 rads, the amount of sensitization of hypoxic cells may also fall steeply. Below 200 rads the curves are often drawn so close together that there may not be a theoretical advantage in altering cells from the hypoxic to the oxic state. However, the conditions applying at this dose level are difficult to exactly simulate in the laboratory and the subject remains one of discussion.

In the Medical Research trial of hyperbaric oxygen in the treatment of carcinoma of cervix, two centers (Mount Vernon and Glasgow) used multiple fractions of radiotherapy (27 and 20 fractions)(Table 1). There was a highly significant improvement in local tumor control ($P =< 0.001$). This dose suggests that there is an oxygen effect at the 200 rad dose level and so the addition of an hypoxic cell sensitizer may give benefit in a conventional course of radiotherapy.

There is also the independent cytotoxic effect of the nitroimidazoles (24). We still do not know whether at the level of dose possible in man this effect is going to be an important one with misonidazole. We know, however, that it is the duration of exposure rather than its height which is most important in producing the greatest cytotoxicity so daily administration rather than biweekly or weekly is more likely to be effective. There is further work to be done before we can take this into consideration.

When misonidazole is given with only some of the treatments in a course of radiotherapy, it is usually combined with a greater radiation dose than that used in fractions given without it. As a result a number of unorthodox regimes of radiotherapy are being employed. The regime itself without sensitizer needs to be tested, as well as conventional therapy. This leads to three-limbed trials and ethical problems with use of the unorthodox regime without sensitizer.

It is unfortunately true that there are many different pathways of use of the hypoxic cell sensitizers which are open to exploration. If too many are explored, then questions will take many years to be answered. Collaboration in clinical trials at national and international levels is important.

Dose Regimes

Misonidazole is presently supplied by the Roche Company in capsules containing 500 mg and 100 mg. Schemes for administration of misonidazole have been devised based on the total allowed dose of 12 g/m^2 surface area and the strength of these preparations.

Currently Used Dose Regimes

Using single doses per week and fractionation over long periods, a higher dose, perhaps 15 g/m^2, may prove safe but more data is needed.

We often employ a six dose regime given twice weekly for 3 weeks. We divide the permitted dose (12 g/m^2 of surface area) by 6 and if the dose falls between half-gram levels give the lower dose using 500 mg capsules. If the plasma concentration permits, we can later elevate the dose to the higher dose level. The plateau and 24 hr concentrations are determined after the first dose and the half-life calculated. If initial readings are above the line in Fig. 3 we make appropriate reductions in dose (33). Subsequently, we take plateau levels only at the second, fourth, and sixth dose to monitor the course.

Because of the relatively long half-life of the drug some 10-30% of the plateau concentration remains at 24 hr. This means that in daily administration the dose on the second day will result in a higher level. When the drug is continued on every day the concentration on the second and subsequent days tends to remain constant. In an effort to obtain uniform concentration at every treatment the dose on the first day can be increased.

Although the adjustment of dose does give a more even concentration at time of treatment, the variations are relatively small and sometimes may not be easily discernible among the variations which must be expected from day to day. We have concluded that the complications which may result from varying the dose due to confusion on the part of the patient do not make this variable dosage worthwhile and recommend a uniform dose throughout treatment. Table 2 is employed for calculation of dose for patients.

The plasma concentration is monitored the first 3 days during the plateau period and percentage reductions made in the dose if the concentration of plasma is greater than 30 μg/ml when 20 doses are administered, 28 μg/ml when 24 are given and 25 μg/ml when 30 doses are given. Subsequently, we tend to monitor the

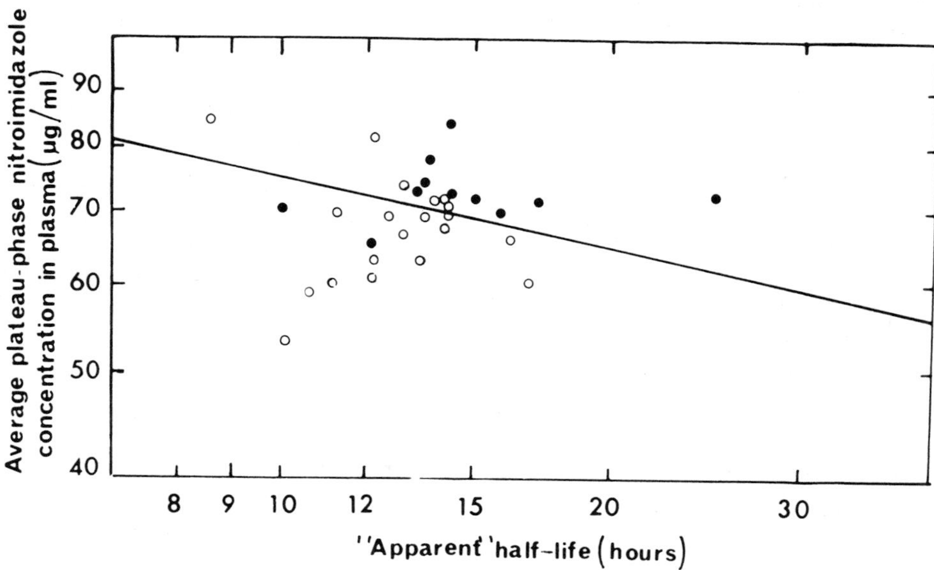

Figure 3. Chart employed for adjustment of dose when patient given six doses based on a total of 12 g per square meter of surface area. The • indicates a patient who developed neuropathy and ○ a patient who did not, using the same regime.

plasma concentration once a week just to make sure there is no accumulation of drug, but in our experience this is extremely rare. It is important to emphasize that if there is evidence or suspicion of neurotoxicity administration of the drug should be suspended. If neurotoxicity is not confirmed the drug can always be restarted.

An interesting recent development is the observation that patients who have been receiving steroids and diphenylhydantoin have a low incidence of neurotoxicity compared with other patients given similar doses of misonidazole (6,44). A halving of the half-life of the drug in serum has been shown, but the results of a full investigation are now awaited. This may lead to new techniques for administration of misonidazole as a radiosensitizer.

Clinical Trials

At this time misonidazole is under clinical trial in radiotherapy centers all over the world. These range in scale from single department projects to international cooperative ventures. The sites of tumor commonly under study are squamous carcinoma in the head and neck region, glioblastomas, and carcinoma of cervix. However, tumors at many other sites are also included. Many different regimes are being employed.

Some interim observations have been recorded but none of the trials have reached the stage of full assessment. Bleehen et al. (6) with glioblastomas has used single weekly doses of misonidazole combined with radiotherapy in a 4-week course of treatment when smaller doses of radiotherapy are also given without the drug. These patients are compared with one control group given similar radiation without the drug and another given conventional radiotherapy. So far no significant difference in survival has emerged with 56 cases in the study. We have performed randomized trials in carcinoma of bronchus using six fractions of radiation plus misonidazole (44 cases); carcinoma of bladder, 20 fractions of radiotherapy plus misonidazole (26 cases); carcinoma of breast, 25 fractions of radiotherapy plus misonidazole (12 cases); and results are as yet similar in those given misonidazole and in the controls (18).

In carcinoma of the uterine cervix we have now treated 10 cases with misonidazole using 24-30 doses of the drug. All have shown apparent complete regression at the time of radium application, and only one in follow-up has shown recurrence in the treated volume. Bulk regression has been shown to correlate closely with subsequent result (18), and this gives encouragement that misonidazole may offer benefit in carcinoma of the cervix.

Table 2. Calculation of Dose for Patients

	Number of doses			Daily dose
	20	24	30	mg
Surface Area	2.0			1200
	1.8			1100
	1.7	2.0		1000
	1.5	1.8		900
Square Metres	1.3	1.6	2.0	800
	1.2	1.4	1.8	700
	-	1.2	1.5	600
			1.3	500

CONCLUSIONS

Despite all the efforts to improve methods of treatment, a large number of patients with malignant disease fail to be cured of tumor at the primary site of disease. To improve this situation, the exploration of methods to increase the radiosensitivity of the hypoxic tumor cell is among the most promising undergoing present evaluation. The great attraction lies in the possibility of an increase in effect in tumor with little or no effect in normal tissues. The promising results shown in some trials of neutron therapy and hyperbaric oxygen gave support to the view that the oxygen effect is important in the radiotherapy of human malignant disease. The extent of the problem, however, remains to be demonstrated and only a totally effective hypoxic cell sensitizer will show this. There is, nevertheless, great encouragement for work in this field. To achieve this purpose the chemical agents which specifically sensitize hypoxic cells to radiation are attractive and give the possibility of use in every patient in every radiotherapy center, without the addition of costly, complex, or expensive apparatus or techniques.

Misonidazole is the first hypoxic cell sensitizer to reach the stage of full clinical testing. The dose which may be given, however, is limited because of neurotoxicity, and it remains to be seen how effective it will be when employed in clinical radiotherapy. Preliminary observations suggest that it might prove of value in squamous carcinomas arising in the head and neck region and in the uterine cervix, but it may not prove beneficial in the radiotherapy of tumors at other sites (18). A large effort is currently being made to produce new chemical sensitizing agents which will be more effective and give greater benefit to patients with malignant disease.*

* I wish to thank Dr. M.I. Saunders and past and present research staff for all their work and support. My colleagues in radiobiology have given me much advice and encouragement, in particular Professor G. E. Adams, Professor J. F. Fowler, and Dr. O.C.A. Scott. Mrs. Eileen Davis has kindly prepared the manuscript.

The support of the Medical Research Council is gratefully acknowledged.

REFERENCES

1. Adams, G.E. and Dewey, D.L.: Hydrated electrons and radiobiological sensitization. Biochem. Biophys. Res. Comm. 12:473-477, 1963.

2. Adams, G.E. and Dische, S.: Care with radiosensitizers. Br. J. Radiol. 52: 920-921, 1979.

3. Ash, D., Smith, M.R., and Bugden, R.D.: The distribution of misonidazole in human tumors and normal tissues. Br. J. Cancer 39:503-509, 1979.

4. Asquith, J.C., Foster, J.L., Willson, R.L., Ings, R., and McFadzean, J.A.: Metronidazole ('Flagyl'). A radiosensitizer of hypoxic cells. Br. J. Radiol. 47:474-481, 1974.

5. Awaad, H. K., El-Merzabani, M. M., and Burgers, M. V.: Penetration of misonidazole after intravesical administration in cases of carcinoma of the bilharzial bladder. Br. J. Cancer 37:Suppl. III:297-298, 1978.

6. Bleehen, N.M., Wiltshire, C.R., and Workman, P.: Clinical and experimental studies with misonidazole, with special reference to factors which may affect its biological half life. In Proceedings of 6th International Congress of Radiation Research, Tokyo, May 13-19, 1979.

7. Brady, L.W., Plenk, H.P., Hanley, J.A., Glassburn, J.R., Kramer, S., and Parker, R.G.: Hyperbaric oxygen therapy for carcinoma of the cervix. Stage IIB, IIIA, IIIB, and IVA: Results of a randomized study by the Radiation Therapy Oncology Group. Int. J. Rad. Oncol. Biol. Phys. 7:991-998, 1981.

8. Cade, I.S. and McEwen, J.B.: Clinical trials of radiotherapy in hyperbaric oxygen at Portsmouth (1964-1976). Clin. Radiol. 29:333-338, 1978.

9. Cade, I.S., McEwen, J.B., Dische, S., Saunders, M.I., Watson, E.R., Halnan, K.E., Wiernik, G., Perrins, D.J.D., and Sutherland, I.: Hyperbaric oxygen and radiotherapy: A Medical Research Council trial in carcinoma of the bladder. Br. J. Radiol. 51:876-878, 1978.

10. Churchill-Davidson, I., Sanger, C. and Thompson, R.H.: High pressure oxygen and radiotherapy. Lancet 1:1091-1095, 1955.

11. Dawes, P.J.D.K., Peckham, M.J., and Steel, G.G.: The response of human tumors metastases to radiation and misonidazole. Br. J. Cancer 37:Suppl III: 290-296, 1978.

12. Deutsch, G., Foster, J.L., McFadzean, J., and Parnell, M.: Human studies with high dose metronidazole: A non-toxic radiosensitizer of hypoxic cells. Br. J. Cancer 31:75-80, 1975.

13. Dische, S.: Hyperbaric oxygen. The Medical Research Council trials and their clinical significance. Br. J. Radiol. 51:888-894, 1978.

14. Dische, S. and Zanelli, G.D.: Skin-reaction - a quantitative system for measurement of radiosensitization in man. Clin. Radiol. 27:145-149, 1976.

15. Dische, S., Gray, A.J., and Zanelli, G.D.: Clinical testing of the radiosensitizer Ro 07-0582. II. Radiosensitization of normal and hypoxic skin. Clin. Radiol. 27:159-166, 1976.

16. Dische, S., Saunders, M.I., Anderson, P., Urtasun, R.C., Kärcher, K.H., Kogelnik, H.D., Bleehen, N., Phillips, T.L., and Wasserman, T.H.: The neurotoxicity of misonidazole. The pooling of data from five centers. Br. J. Radiol. 51:1023-1024, 1978.

17. Dische, S., Saunders, M.I., Flockhart, I.R., Lee, M.E., and Anderson, P.: Misonidazole. A drug for trial in radiotherapy and oncology. Int. J. Radiat. Oncol. Biol. Phys. 5:851-860, 1979.

18. Dische, S., Saunders, M.I., and Anderson, P.: Misonidazole in the clinic at Mount Vernon. Cancer Clin. Trials 3:175-178, 1980.

19. Fletcher, G.L., Lindberg, R.D., Caderao, J.B., and Taylor Wharton, J.: Hyperbaric oxygen as a radiotherapeutic adjuvant in advanced carcinoma of the uterine cervix. Preliminary results of a randomized trial. Cancer 39:617-623, 1977.

20. Fowler, J.F., Adams, G.E., and Denekamp, J.: Radiosensitizers of hypoxic cells in solid tumors. Cancer Treat. Rev. 3:227-256, 1976.

21. Glassburn, J.R., Damsker, J.I., Brady, L.W., Faust, D.S., Antoiniades, J., Prasvinchai, S., Lewis, G.C. Jr., Torpie, R.J., and Asbell, S.A.: Hyperbaric oxygen and radiation in the treatment for advanced cervical carcinoma. In Fifth International Hyperbaric Congress Proceedings, II, Philadelphia, Simon Fraser University, 1974, pp. 813-819.

22. Gray, L.H., Conger, A.O., Ebert, M., Hornsey, S., and Scott, O.C.A.: The concentration of oxygen dissolved in tissues at the time of irradiation as a factor in radiotherapy. Br. J. Radiol. 26:638-648, 1953.

23. Gray, A.J., Dische, S., Adams, G.E., Flockhart, I.R., and Foster, J.L.: Clinical testing of the radiosensitizer Ro 07-0582. I. Dose tolerance, serum and tumor concentration. Clin. Radiol. 27:151-157, 1976.

24. Hall, E.J. and Biaglow, J.: Ro 07-0582 as a radiosensitizer and cytoxic agent. Int. J. Radiat. Oncol. Biol. Phys. 2:521-530, 1977.

25. Henk, J.M. and Smith, C.W.: Radiotherapy and hyperbaric oxygen in head and neck cancer. Interim report of 2nd clinical trial. Lancet 2:104-105, 1977.

26. Henk, J.M., Kunkler, P.B., and Smith, C.W.: Radiotherapy and hyperbaric oxygen in head and neck cancer. Lancet 2:101-103, 1977.

27. Kogelnik, H.D., Meyer, H.J., Jentzsch, K., Szepesi, T., Karcher, K.H., Maida, E., Mamoli, B., Wessely, P., and Zaunbauer, F.: Further clinical experience of a phase I study with the hypoxic cell radiosensitizer misonidazole. Br. J. Cancer 37:Suppl. III:281-285, 1978.

28. Medical Research Council: A report of the Medical Research Council's Working Party on Radiotherapy and Hyperbaric Oxygen. Lancet 2:881-884, 1978.

29. Partington, J., Koziel, D., Chapman, D., Rabin, H., and Urtasun, R.C.: A new side effect of the hypoxic cell sensitizer misonidazole. Cancer Treat. Rep. 63:123-125, 1979.

30. Phillips, T.L., Wasserman, T.H., Johnson, R.J., and Rubin, D.J.: The hypoxic cell sensitizer programme in the United States. Br. J. Cancer 37:Suppl. III:276-280, 1978.

31. Plenk, H.P.: Hyperbaric radiation therapy. Preliminary results of a randomized study of cancer of the urinary bladder and review of the 'oxygen experience.' Am. J. Roentgenol. 114:152-157, 1972.

32. Rich, T.A., Dische, S., Saunders, M.I., Stratford, M., and Minchinton, A.: The influence of necrosis on the concentration of misonidazole in human tumors. In: Proceedings of Conference on Combined Modality Cancer Treatment: Radiation Sensitizers and Protectors, Key Biscayne, Florida, October 3-6. Int. J. Radiat. Oncol. Biol. Phys., 1979.

33. Saunders, M.I., Dische, S., Anderson, P., and Flockhart, I.R.: The neurotoxicity of misonidazole and its relationship to dose, half-life and concentration in the serum. Br. J. Cancer 37:Suppl. III:268-270, 1978.

34. Saunders, M.I., Dische, S., Kogelnik, H.D., Sealy, R., and Lenox-Smith, I.: Skin reashes associated with the administration of the 2-nitro-imidazole-misonidazole. Cancer Treat. Rep. 64:263-268, 1980.

35. Sheldon, P.W. and Fowler, J.F.: Radiosensitization by misonidazole (Ro 07-0582) of fractionated x-rays in a murine tumor. Br. J. Cancer 37:Suppl. III: 242-245, 1978.

36. Thomlinson, R.H.: Proceedings of Carmel Conference on time and dose relationship in radiation biology as applied to radiotherapy. Brookhaven National Lab. Report No. 50203, Carmel, California, 1969, p. 242.

37. Thomlinson, R.H. and Gray, L.H.: The histological structure of some human lung cancers and the possible implications for radiotherapy. Br. J. Cancer 9: 539-549, 1955.

38. Thomlinson, R.H., Dische, S., Gray, A.J., and Errington, L.M.: Clinical testing of the radiosensitizer Ro 07-0582. III. Regression and re-growth of tumor. Clin. Radiol. 27:167-174, 1976.

39. Urtasun, R.C., Sturmwind, J., Rabin, H., Band, J.R., and Chapman, J.D.: "High-dose" metronidazole: A preliminary pharmacological study prior to its investigational use in clinical radiotherapy trials. Br. J. Radiol. 47:297-299, 1974.

40. Urtasun, R.C., Band, P., Chapman, J.D., Feldstein, M.L., Mielke, B., and Fryer, C.: Radiation and high dose metronidazole in supratentorial glioblastomas. N. Engl. J. Med. 294:1364-1367, 1976.

41. Urtasun, R.C.: Personal communication, 1978.

42. Van den Brenk, H.A.S.: Hyperbaric oxygen in radiation therapy. An investigation of dose-effect relationships in tumor response and tissue damage. Am. J. Roentgenol. Rad. Ther. Nucl. Med. 102:8-26, 1968.

43. Ward, A.J., Dixon, B., and Stubbs, B.: A clinical appraisal of hyperbaric oxygen in cervix cancer (Abstract). Br. J. Radiol. 51:150-151, 1978.

44. Wasserman, T.H., Phillips, T.L., Van Raalte, G., Urtasun, R.C., Partington, J., Koziel, D., Schwade, J.G., Gangji, D., and Strong, J.M.: The neurotoxicity of misonidazole: Potential modifying role of Phenytoin Sodium and Dexamethasone. Br. J. Radiol. 53:172-173, 1980.

chapter 14

PARTICLE RADIATION THERAPY

Morton M. Kligerman, M.D.
Edward A. Knapp, Ph. D.

The use of ionizing radiation in treatment of cancer began almost immediately after the discovery of x-rays by Roentgen in 1896. Modern radiotherapy is dated from the early 1930s when Coutard responding to the investigations of his colleagues Regaud and Ferroux (26) began to treat squamous cell cancers of the tonsils, hypopharynx, and larynx (8) with fractionated and protracted radiotherapy. The voltage and output of these early x-ray therapy machines were low. However, dose quantitation had progressed from the use of milliampere seconds and erythema dose to the roentgen (R) as the measurement of dose. Except for isolated high voltage units - the 600 kV unit at the Foundation Curie and the 1 million volt unit developed at the Columbia-Presbyterian Medical Center - the available x-ray generators in the 1930s and 1940s were predominately those generating between 150 and 250 kV. A major improvement at the end of this period was the design of a constant potential 180 kV unit, to be followed in the early 1940s by a 250 kV constant potential unit.

Radiotherapy entered the supervoltage era in a practical way when radioactive cobalt was produced easily and cheaply by the atomic reactor. However, in the early 1940s two forms of electron accelerators were developed in the United States. One of these was the betatron invented by Kerst (17) and the other was the linear accelerator, developed by Ginzton (11). Both of these accelerators produced supervoltage x-rays by having a stream of high-energy electrons strike a metal target. The betatron, a circular accelerator, was the generator used initially for therapeutic applications because it produced high energy at relatively low cost. However, the intensities were low. Furthermore, because of the massive weight and size of the magnets, early clinical betatrons were cumbersome. Technically, therefore, the development of the isocentric mount by Howard-Flanders (16), and its adaptation to cobalt units and linear accelerators accentuated the ability to apply accurate, multiportal, beam-directed external radiation therapy. The higher-intensity capabilities of flexible linear accelerator units have allowed these systems largely to displace the betatron for cancer therapy.

The linear accelerator itself has evolved in the course of the last 35 years. The first linear accelerators were of the traveling wave type, pioneered in physics research at Stanford University, and first adapted to medical use by The Varian Associates. The invention of the side-coupled cavity electron linac (23) at the Los Alamos Scientific Laboratory provided a major simplification of electron linear accelerator systems pioneered again in medical applications by The Varian Associates. The introduction of these units reduced the cost of linac facilities by a factor of two and increased reliability appreciably. Side-coupled cavity electron linear accelerator units are extensively employed in hospitals where they provide a compact, reliable, and relatively low-cost radiation source, well adapted to isocentric mounting. Presently, units based on this principle dominate the medical radiation source market.

RADIOBIOLOGICAL BACKGROUND TO PARTICLE THERAPY

The biological principle of Regaud, mentioned earlier, pointed the way to the use of fractionated radiotherapy. Until the early 1950s, interpretation of results observed in curative cancer treatment with ionizing radiations was based on the concept that young tissues (including neoplasms) were more sensitive to all chemical and physical agents than older (normal) tissues. Puck and Marcus discovered the method of cloning tumor cells and observed their quantitative responses to x-ray (25) Elkind and Sutton, using this technique (9), showed that the initial low-dose portion of the single-dose survival curve was characterized by a shoulder, which represented the ability of a particular type of cell to repair radiation sublethal damage. Beyond the shoulder, increasing dose results in cell killing directly proportional to the dose (Fig. 1). A cell line with a broad shoulder can withstand larger daily fractions of radiation and recover as compared to a cell line with a smaller shoulder. One of the important factors in the ability to cure patients with radiation therapy is this differential repair capability favoring normal tissue survival over that of the tumor cells which arise within the specific normal tissue.

Gray and his group (13) showed the relationship between radiosensitivity and the presence or absence of oxygen. Specifically, hypoxic cells are up to three times as resistant to conventional x-rays or gamma rays as oxygenated cells. The implication for the survival of some tumor cells, which can be found to be hypoxic in almost any tumor, was apparent. Furthermore, Teresima and Tolmach (32) revealed that cells varied in their sensitivity to conventional radiations while in different phases of the cell cycle. The observation that cells in a tumor could be resistant to ionizing radiation because of hypoxia or because of their stage in the cell cycle was recognized as a cause for the survival of some tumor cells, which, after apparent complete regression of a tumor, provided the nidus for regrowth.

In an attempt to overcome the protection that some tumor cells enjoy because of hypoxia, Churchill-Davidson et al. (7) placed patients in hyperbaric chambers and raised the pressure to three and four atmospheres before applying external radiation. The method has not gained wide acceptance, principally because it is cumbersome and not tolerated by claustrophobic patients. Additionally, however, increased effects on the normal tissues were observed (31). Only one study, using an unconventional fractionation scheme (15), demonstrated statistically that ionizing radiation treatments under the hyperbaric state were superior to treatments in atmospheric air.

Small daily fractions, less than 200 rads/fraction, are advantageous for treatment of solid tumors. If the dose is small enough so that it would be within the shoulder (repair portion) of the normal tissue single cell survival curve, while at the same time being large enough to fall on the exponential portion of the tumor cell curve, a favorable situation exists for the possibility of eliminating all of the tumor cells by multiple fractions while permitting recovery of the normal tissue. This is illustrated in Fig. 1 by the dotted line representing such a daily fraction size cutting the curves B, representing a tumor cell line, and C, representing normal tissue cells.

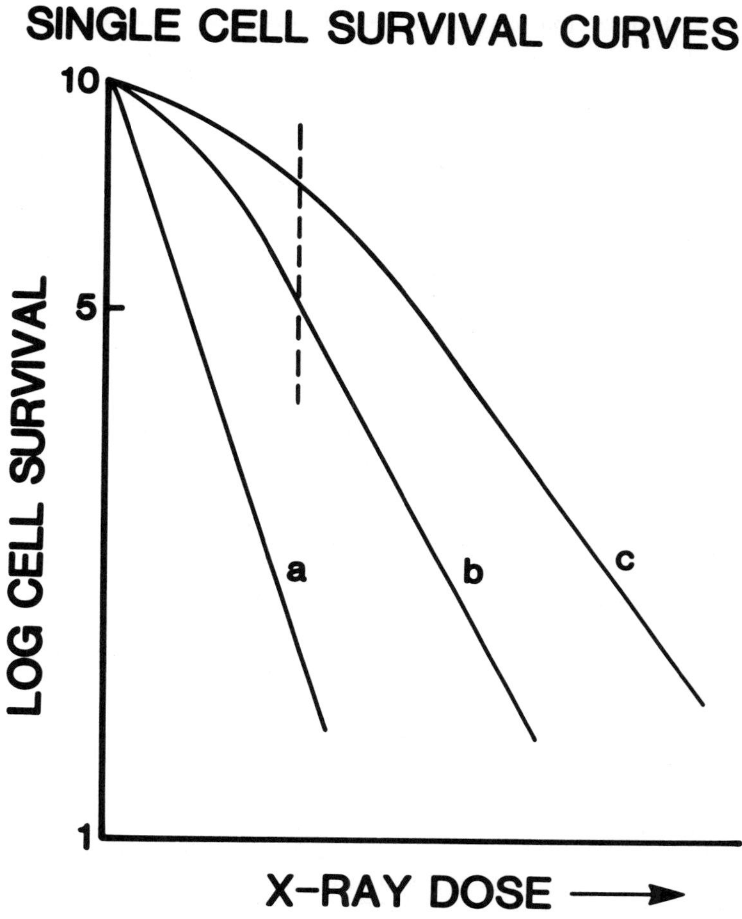

Figure 1. Representational comparison of single cell survival curves. Curves b and c represent response of tumor cell and normal tissue cells, respectively. The shoulder (curving portion at the top) is a measure of the cell repair capacity. The wider the shoulder, the greater the ability to repair sublethal damage. The straight line portion, exponential portion, represents the sensitivity of the cell. Note that the sensitivity of both the tumor cell and the normal cell is essentially the same, but the normal tissue has greater repair capacity than the tumor cell which is a principal reason why tumors can be cured by radiation therapy. Curve a represents cell survival after treatment by a high LET beam, e.g., neutrons. Note that the repair capacity (shoulder) is eliminated and the sensitivity (slope of the exponential portion) increased. High LET beams are, therefore, more effective in destroying cells than low LET beams.

When fractionated radiation is undertaken, two other factors must be considered. First, redistribution of the number of cells in each of the phases of the cell cycle occurs. This is due to mitotic delay caused by the radiation followed by partial synchronization of the cells as they escape from this delay. Not all cell lines are most sensitive in the same phase of the cell cycle, though usually the sensitive phases are in the early portion of the DNA synthesis phase and in the mitotic phase. Bullen et al. (3) attempted to determine when breast tumors were in the synthetic phase by giving patients ^{32}P and, with a suitable probe, recording when the activity in the tumor showed a significant increase. Assuming that this was the synthetic phase, he irradiated the patients at that moment. Whether the majority of tumor cells would remain continually in a particular sensitive phase with continued fractions is unknown. Perhaps the study of multicellular tumor spheroids (35) grown from a patient's tumor, using multiple fractions of radiation at different times following one or two priming doses, might provide a guide to the clinical treatment of that patient.

In addition to the significance of repair and redistribution in fractionated radiation, two other factors, reoxygenation and repopulation, are important. The importance of hypoxia in clinical tumor resistance to radiotherapy has been mentioned earlier. Small daily fractions destroy the well-oxygenated and, therefore, sensitive cells near the capillary supply, permitting oxygen to diffuse farther out into the tumor, reaching cells which had previously been hypoxic. As cells are eliminated, other cells that had been too far from the capillary to be oxygenated are brought physically closer to the capillary. With reoxygenation, sensitivity is reestablished. This is the mechanism by which protracted fractionated radiation overcomes the disadvantage of hypoxia in many tumors (34).

Repopulation is a factor in radiotherapy delivered in small daily fractions. The degree of repopulation is dependent upon the combination of the sensitivity of the cell and the cell cycle time. If the daily dose of radiation is such that a substantial number of actively dividing cells, the clonogenic fraction, remain, and if the division time is relatively short, there could be a net gain of tumor cells within the ensuing 24 hr. This occurs in the tumor that continues to grow under radiotherapy. One approach to this problem is increasing the daily fraction size, but this must not be so large as to totally interfere with the repair capacity of the normal tissue cells. If such is the case, giving two or more fractions of radiation each day, the superfractionation scheme, should be considered (29).

To further improve the results of radiotherapy, methods must be developed by either physical or chemical means to increase the differential effect of ionizing radiation on the tumor, which would result in increased killing of tumor cells, as compared to cells of normal tissues. This chapter explores the future possibilities of radiotherapy through alteration of biological effects to improve cancer control. The discussion will center around the possible contribution of new machines.

PARTICLE RADIATION THERAPY

One of the greatest interests in radiotherapy today is the prospect for the treatment of tumors with particle irradiation. Protons, neutrons, heavy ions, and negative pi-mesons (pions) have some or all of the following characteristics: (1) the ability to heavily damage the DNA molecule with breaks in both strands, so that repair of damage to this critical module is severely impaired; (2) a high degree of localization of the energy in the region of the tumor with sparing of the surrounding normal tissues; (3) the ability to overcome the relative radioresistance of hypoxic tumor cells to conventional radiation; and (4) a reduction of the variation in sensitivity which cells exhibit with respect to conventional radiation in the several stages of the cell division cycle. Only pions possess all four of these qualities.

For any form of ionizing radiation to be effective, an ionizing event must take place within the molecule. The transfer of energy causes a disruption in the molecule. For the purpose of this discussion, radiation may be divided into two types, those which produce low linear energy transfer (LET) as opposed to those which produce high linear energy transfer. Figure 2 is a diagrammatic representation of these two different types of radiation. Low LET beams include x-rays and gamma rays, and electrons, protons, and pions in flight through the tissues. One can see that low LET radiation has a relatively low density of ionizing events per unit distance as the beam passes through tissue. The number of ionizing events in relation to a critical molecule is relatively small. Furthermore, in the case of DNA, if an event takes place on a single strand, this is rapidly repaired by appropriate enzymes using the corresponding DNA strand as a template.

In contrast, high LET beams characterized by neutrons, heavy ions, and stopped pions are densely ionizing as illustrated. Not only is a relatively wide segment of the molecule disrupted, but both strands are involved so that repair is difficult (see Fig. 1, curve a) or, if it takes place, frequently results in an inappropriate hookup of the fragments. Linear energy transfer can be quantified according

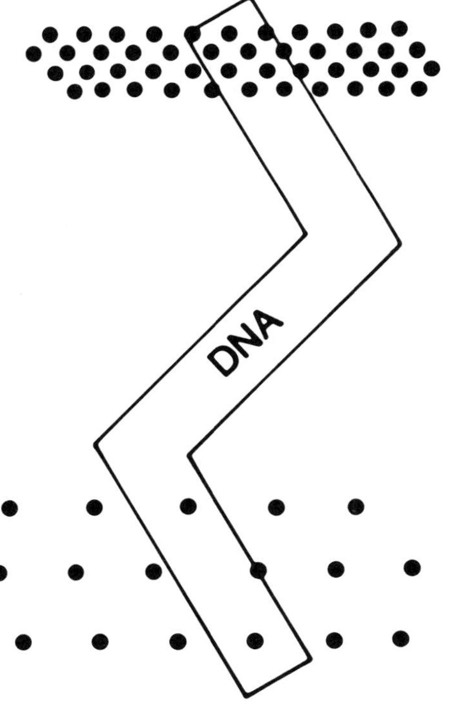

Figure 2. An ionizing event must take place within a critical molecule to create an injury which could result in cell death. The density of ionizing events, black dots, is relatively sparse in low linear energy transfer (LET) radiations. Single strand injuries in DNA can be rapidly repaired. High LET radiations create large double-stranded injuries which the cell has difficulty repairing. This accounts for the difference in biological response between low and high LET radiations.

to the kilovolts deposited within the radius of a micron surrounding the point of ionization. Though there is some disagreement as to the number of kilovolts per micron which would designate a beam as high LET or not, the values frequently mentioned are between 50 and 100 kV/μ or greater. Low LET radiations, therefore, are those beams which deposit less than 50 kV/μ.

Three of four particles - protons, heavy ions, and pions - are charged particles. The neutrons, as the same suggests, is without charge. Charged particles have a finite range in tissue with the maximum depth dependent on the amount of energy with which they are propelled. Furthermore, the amount of energy deposited as they traverse the tissue is characterized by an initial portion where the dose deposited is essentially equal (Fig. 3). This segment is descriptively called the plateau. As the particle proceeds through the tissues, it loses energy and begins to move slower. Therefore, more ionizing events take place. This causes a peak of increased ionization at the end of the particle's range. This is the stopping region of the particle's tragectory or Bragg peak. Because of the increased ionization at the end of a finite range, a high dose can be shaped to that of the tumor. For therapeutic purposes, the peak region of the charged particle beams must be

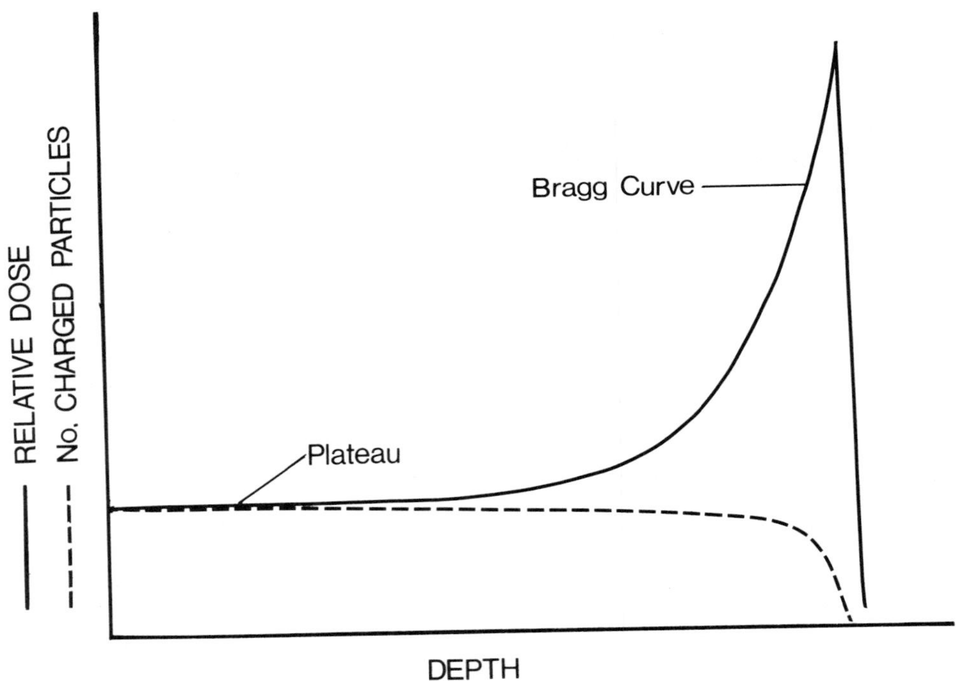

Figure 3. Charged particle beams have a finite range in tissue. The depth of the stopping region or Bragg peak is proportional to the energy with which the particle is propelled. Different from noncharged beams, particles deposit essentially the same amount of energy as it traverses tissue, the plateau, at the beginning of its course since it has high energy and, therefore, great speed. As the particles interact with matter, they lose energy, and, therefore, they slow down. When the particles slow down, more ionizing events take place because the particle spends more time in this region. The increased ionization creates the high peak of dose. The lower curve documents the number of particles remaining in the beam.

spread, or widened, to a diameter that would be clinically useful to cover the size of tumor volumes to be treated. The process of widening the peak region is called modulation. In the case of the pion beam where the peak region is a combination of high- and low-energy transfer radiation, modulation also involves changing the proportion of these two different kinds of radiation at different points in the peak region.

Figure 4 is a diagrammatic representation of the depth dose characteristics of two charged particle beams, proton and pions, as well a cobalt 60 generated gamma beam and a neutron beam. Note the plateau and modulated peak regions of the charged particle beam. The vertical striped regions in the pion beam and neutron beam are an indication of the high LET fraction. The neutron beam is 100% high LET. The depth dose characteristics of the gamma rays of cobalt and a mildly energetic neutron beam are the same. The difference is that the cobalt beam is 100% low LET radiation, and the neutron beam, 100% high LET radiation.

NEUTRON SOURCES

If neutron therapy is to become a standard treatment for cancer, reliable, low-cost neutron sources must be developed for use in the standard medical environment.

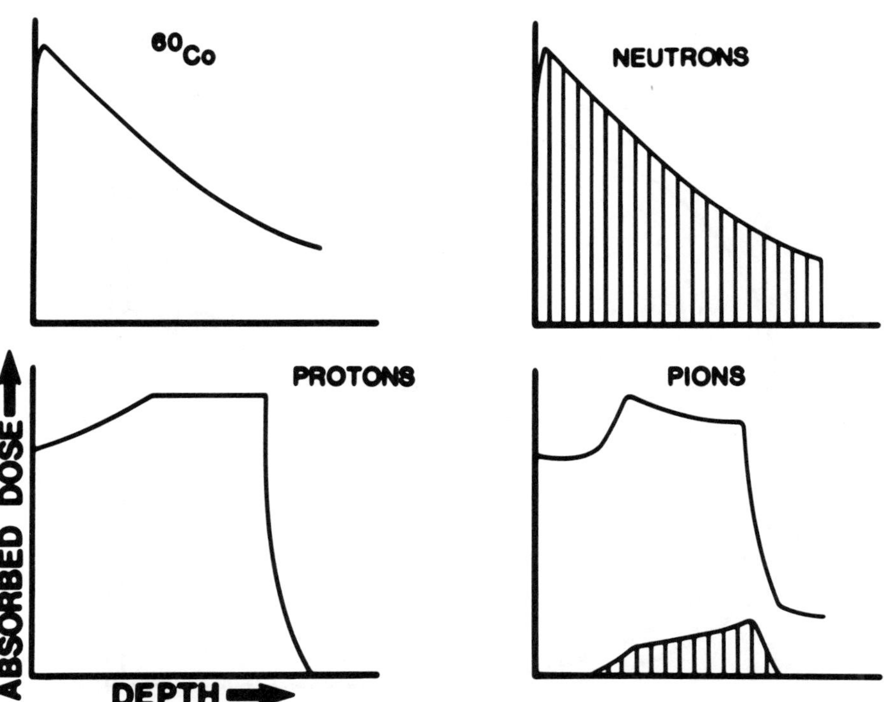

Figure 4. Comparison of low and high LET depth dose curves and neutron and charged beams of ionizing radiation. Note the similarity of ^{60}Co and neutron depth dose distributions; but neutrons are approximately three times as effective in cell killing as ^{60}Co beams because neutrons interfere with cellular repair. Note that both proton and pion beams have peaks (spread for therapeutic use) of energy distribution of finite range. However, in the pion peak, there is a mixture of high and low LET radiation which gives a biologic response different from either a pure high or pure low LET beam (see text).

Four sources have been discussed that might be able to fulfill this requirement: (1) the D-T generator, (2) the cyclotron, (3) the ion linear accelerator, or (4) the synchroton.

In the D-T generator, a relatively low-energy (a few hundred kilovolt) deuterium beam strikes a tritium target producing 14 MeV neutrons via the exothermic reaction $D + T \longrightarrow n + He^4$ Past experience with this generator indicates that it suffers serious difficulties in providing an adequate dose rate for cancer therapy at reasonable source distances. Furthermore, source lifetimes tend to be short, with associated high maintenance costs. However, a new neutron generator has been developed by the Cyclotron Corporation of America in conjunction with the University of Pennsylvania and will be installed in the department of radiation therapy in the spring of 1981. The target structure differs in that a relatively thick (300-400 μg) layer of chromium is used to surface the copper base of the target, replacing the usual rare earth surface. This target can withstand 450 mA and is expected to last in the neighborhood of 1000 hr or better. The reason for the limitation of 1000 hr will not be the target, but rather the amount of tritium which will be available in the sealed tube. This tube will be mounted in an isocentric head. The dose rate which has been measured at 125 cm is 22 rads/min (2). The addition of small amounts of oxygen in the sealed tube which is evacuated to 10^{-7} mmHg appears to increase neutron production (2).

The cyclotron (see Fig. 5) is the most thoroughly tested approach to providing a neutron therapy source at the present time. Typically, neutrons are produced by

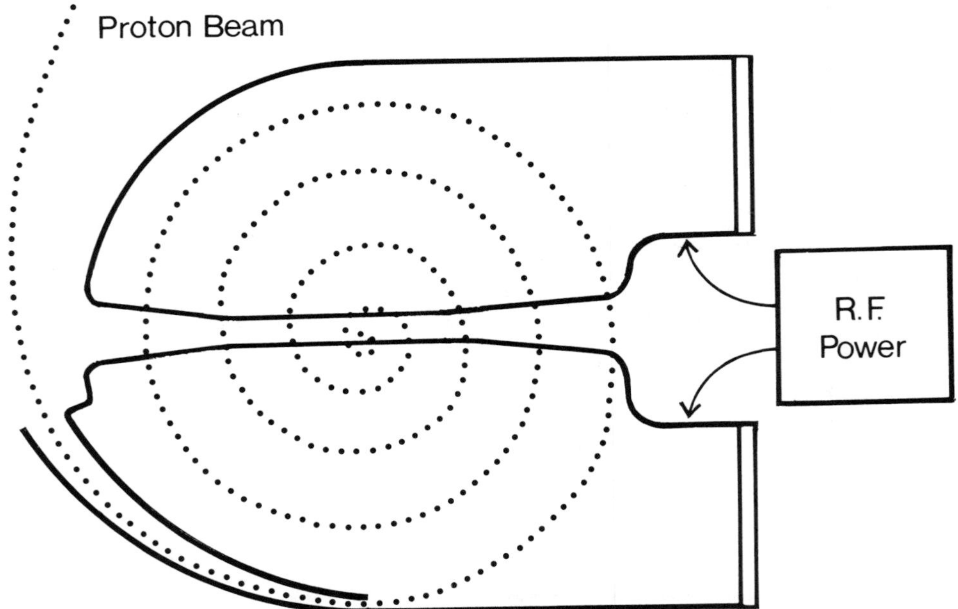

Figure 5. A cyclotron operates by cyclically adding voltage to particles as they circulate in larger and larger orbits in a constant magnetic field. Illustrated is a typical orbit of a particle from injection at the center of the device to extraction from the outer edge of the device. The particle gains its voltage as it crosses between two "Dee's" which sustain a radiofrequency (R. F.) oscillation powered by a high-frequency transmitter. As in the case of the drift tube linac, the particle is shielded within the Dee structure during voltage reversal.

a high-energy proton deuteron beam (30-40 MeV energy) striking a beryllium metal target. Cyclotrons tend to be quite large and complex, but do provide a high-intensity neutron beam of good quality. Isocentric dose delivery is possible with a magnetic channel to transport the primary proton or deuteron beam to a suitably located target which can be rotated to the desired therapy location. A typical cyclotron-based neutron generator, as produced by an industrial firm for medical applications, will cost $2 to $4 million, not including the building in which it is to be used.

For neutron generation, a proton or deuteron linear accelerator (see Fig. 6) is also capable of producing a suitable proton or deuteron beam of 30-40 MeV energy with excellent beam properties. The development of this neutron source is now in progress at Los Alamos and promises to be very compact, cost-efficient, and reliable for hospital installation. Isocentric capabilities should be even easier to address with the ion linear accelerator than with the cyclotron.

PROTON SOURCES

A source of protons suitable for providing therapeutic quality beams should have an energy of about 200 MeV and a current of about 1 μamp. Either a proton synchrotron (see Fig. 7) or a proton linear accelerator would be suitable for providing these particles. However, for the very low intensity required, a synchrotron probably would be most economical.

HEAVY ION SOURCES

The only economically viable radiation source for heavy ion therapy is the synchrotron, long used as a source of high-energy ions for physics research. A synchrotron is a relatively complex circular particle accelerator, in which a ring of magnets guides the accelerated particles in closed orbits. As the magnetic field is raised in the guide field, a radiofrequency cavity adds energy to the ions to keep them synchronous in their constant radius orbits. Generally, an ion linear accelerator is used as an injector into a synchrotron.

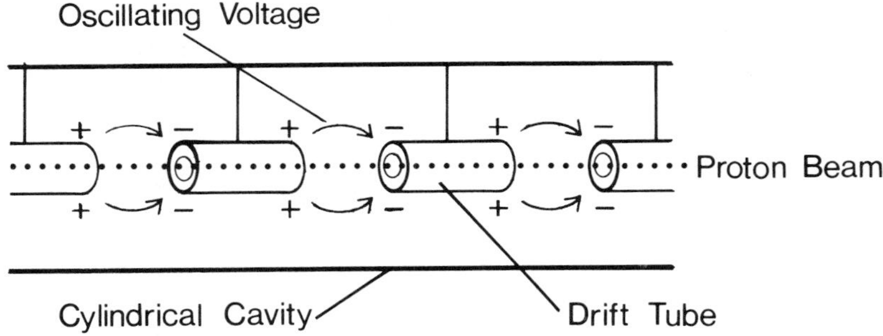

Figure 6. An ion linear accelerator, such as the drift tube linac, adds energy to nuclear particles by a series of voltage impulses generated in radiofrequency-powered resonant cavities, all arranged in a straight line. The drift tubes are suspended in a hollow cylindrical cavity. The voltage oscillates at a radiofrequency rate on the ends of the drift tube; the length of the tube is cut so the particle is hidden within the drift tube during voltage reversal, and is accelerated by the voltage when it is of the correct sign. Particle confinement along the bore axis is accomplished with focusing magnets within the drift tubes.

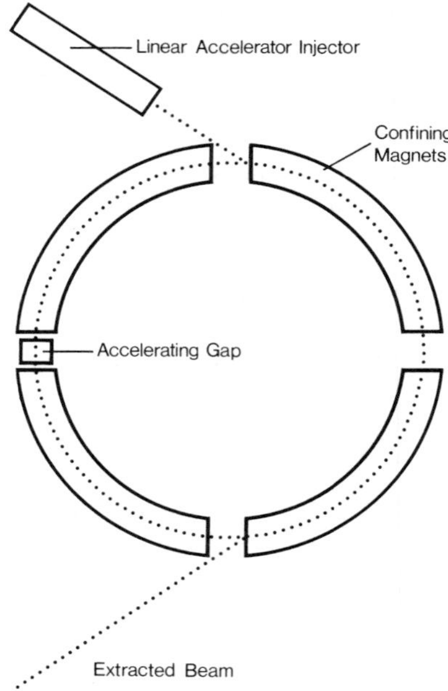

Figure 7. A synchrotron (top view illustrated) operates somewhat like the cyclotron in that the particles are confined to circular orbits with a magnetic field and the voltage is added each circulation by a radiofrequency voltage on an accelerating gap. However, the synchrotron uses a ring of magnets. As the energy is raised, the magnetic field is raised simultaneously to maintain a constant radius orbit. The synchrotron is suitable for much higher energies than the cyclotron, but generally operates at much lower intensity levels. It usually requires a linear accelerator for injection to avoid very low magnetic field values at initial injection.

In heavy ion cancer therapy, the primary accelerated beam is used for therapy, in distinction to the secondary beams used in neutron, pion, or x-ray therapy, and thus the intensity of the accelerated beam can be quite low. Accurate beam distribution can be accomplished by using a magnetic beam scanning technique and variable thickness absorbers to vary the depth at which the ions come to rest.

Generally, the radius or curvature of heavy ions suitable for cancer therapy in a magnetic channel is so large that an isocentric delivery system would be quite awkward, although not impossible. The clinical tests of heavy ion therapy being undertaken at the Lawrence Berkeley Laboratory in Berkeley, California, using the Bevelac synchrotron, utilize a fixed horizontal beam for treatment. Accelerators with multiple treatment capability (several treatment rooms and shared beam facilities) may make heavy ion therapy cost-effective, even though the installation is very expensive relative to conventional x-ray therapy or neutron therapy units.

PION SOURCES

Negative pi-mesons or pions are secondary particles produced by collision of protons or electrons with nuclei at very high energy. The probability of production in any given collision is quite low, requiring a high accelerated beam power to produce sufficient pions for therapeutic dose levels. Electrons are approximately 30 times less efficient than protons per unit beam power in producing pions. Both electron-accelerator and proton-accelerator-based pion therapy systems have been proposed, with extremely efficient pion collectors being required in the electron linac case. With the proposed PIGMI proton linac pion therapy system being studied at the Los Alamos National Laboratory, a 650 MeV, 30 μ amp proton beam is required to produce sufficient pions for adequate treatment times. It uses a highly efficient pion collector to produce a large-diameter, single-port pion beam. A fixed horizontal or vertical mount is required for this design. Researchers at Stanford University have devised an extremely clever superconducting orange peel spectrometer pion collector, which has 60 channels all focusing their pions in the center of the spectrometer. This may be efficient enough to be used with an electron-linac-based pion source. However, based on this design a spectrometer is now in operation at SIN in Switzerland using protons as the bombarding particle.

In either the proton or electron-based source design, a linear accelerator system is required to deliver the beam power necessary to produce adequate pions for therapy. Significant advances in linear accelerator science over the past few years make reliable accelerators quite achievable for this application. Proposed systems typically have lengths of 50-100 m, adequately short to be situated under the parking lot of most modern urban hospitals. Location in a well-shielded tunnel is a requirement, due to possible radiation produced by misguided beams. Again, as in the case of the heavy ion therapy systems, costs are high. However, multiple use of the primary beam to separate treatment rooms and efficient pion collectors can increase the cost/benefit ratio.

NEUTRONS

The first clinical application of neutrons in cancer therapy was reported by Stone and coworkers (23, 28) in 1940 and 1942. Though tumor control was observed in patients with gastric and other radioresistent tumors, the experiment was terminated because of severe late normal tissue damage resulting in death for some patients. Recognizing that an understanding of the biological effects of neutrons, lacking in the late 1930s, could make neutron cancer therapy possible, Fowler and coworkers (10) explored the biological and physical parameters of the neutron beam. They demonstrated that neutrons were less dependent than x-rays on the presence of oxygen for cell killing to be effected. This and other differences in the biological effect of neutrons have been discussed earlier. Following the biological experiments, clinical trials were instituted at Hammersmith Hospital, London. Using 7.5 MeV neutrons and a dose schedule of 1560 rads/12 treatments/26 elapsed days, Catterall (5) reported complete regressions and a low recurrence rate for squamous cell cancers and adenocarcinoma, as well as soft tissue sarcomas. Prospectively, comparing neutron therapy with photon treatment in advanced cancers of all sites, Catterall found "persisting control" in 54 of 71 patients treated with neutrons as compared with 12 patients out of 63 with "persisting control" who were treated with photons.

From the Netherlands Cancer Institute, Battermann and Bruer (1) report an 80% control rate in head and neck tumors. Of the 43 evaluable patients, they found that recurrence was most likely in very large primary tumors of the tongue with bilateral neck nodes. There was some laryngeal edema in all patients when this structure was in the field. Also, subcutaneous fibrosis was such that a dose reduction of 5% has been instituted if portals are larger than 80 cm^2. These investigators point to an interesting local result in the treatment of 11 cases of parotid tumors. Four are alive between 2 and 20 months. Two deaths were due to complications in patients who were treated with neutrons for recurrences after curative doses of supervoltage photons. No tumor was seen at autopsy, however. Of the 28 deaths in the evaluable head and neck patients, 7 died of metastases without local recurrence and 12 died of intercurrent disease.

There was 72% local control rate in advanced urinary bladder, rectum, and female genital cancer; however, 15% of these patients developed severe intestinal complications. As a result, the total dose was reduced to 1620 rads in subsequent patients. The authors believe their local control rate is "much higher" with neutrons than they believe can be obtained with conventional treatment. Control clinical trials were started in May, 1978.

Many believed that malignant gliomas would be a tumor ideal for high LET treatment. At the University of Washington using a 21 MeV cyclotron, 37 patients with grades III and IV lesions have been treated (14). The mean survival time was 10.8 and 7.5 months in histological grades III and grade IV lesions, respectively. These results are not as good as historical controls treated with photons at the University of Washington, and the neutron-treated group did not show the same degree of functional improvement as compared to the photon-treated patients. However, of the 15 patients who were autopsied, viable tumor cells were seen in only one patient. The tumor had been replaced by necrotic material and reactive astrocytes. Also, deterioration of the white matter distant from the tumor site occurred and may have been the actual cause of death in these patients.

A pilot study of fast neutron therapy was begun in 1972 by the radiotherapy department of the M. D. Anderson Hospital using the Texas A & M University cyclotron (TAMVEC) (24). At first the neutrons were those produced by 16 MeV deuterons on beryllium (d→Be neutrons). When 50 MeV d→Be neutrons became available in 1973, locally advanced gynecological tumors were added to the study. In January, 1977, a prospective clinical trial was begun comparing photon treatment with a mixture of neutrons (2 days/week) and photons (3 days/week). In 91 patients subjected to the pilot study ending December, 1976, 17 were treated with neutrons only, 20 received a neutron boost after whole pelvis photon irradiation, 34 were treated with mixed beam, and 20 were treated with photons only. The results and complications reported are seen in Table 1. In viewing the complications, Hussey points out that by chance the neutron-only group collected the greatest number of patients with the most advanced disease and that these were mainly treated early in the study before dose-time schedules for neutrons were well worked out. The mixed-beam technique was selected for the randomized trial because in the pilot study it developed the best therapeutic ratio, e.g., almost the highest local control rate with a complication rate equal to the lower rate seen with neutrons and not significantly different from the photon control complication rate. Seventy-five patients with advanced cervical cancer were randomized between photons and the mixed neutron-photon schedule. Analyzed 9 months after the last patient admitted to the trial, the data showed no significant difference in local control, frequency of complications, and patient survival.

In her report to the third meeting on fundamental and practical aspects of the application of fast neutrons and other high LET particles in clinical radiotherapy, Mary Catterall stated that "fast neutrons, in the treatment regimen used at Hammersmith Hospital, promise a significant advance in the treatment of some tumors." However, when this writer takes all the information available on neutron trials from Great Britain, Europe, Japan, and the United States, the data do not look too promising. When neutron generators designed for and dedicated to clinical use are available for randomized trials, perhaps a clear superiority of neutrons will be found.

Table 1. Pilot Study Results for Locally Advanced Gynecological Cancer (April 1973-December 1976); Unlimited Follow-up, Analysis August 1978)

	Neutrons Only	Neutron Boost	Mixed Beam	Photons
Local control	5/17 (29%)	11/20 (55%)	18/34 (53%)	8/20 (40%)
IIB CA Cx	-	1/2	1/1	1/2
IIIA CA Cx	0/2	3/6	8/14	5/9
IIIB CA Cx	1/7	5/8	6/13	1/7
IV CA Cx	1/2	1/1	0/1	1/1
Other sites	3/6	1/3	3/5	0/1
Survival	1/17 (10%)	9/20 (45%)	13/34 (38%)	6/20 (30%)
IIB CA Cx	-	1/2	1/1	1/2
IIIA CA Cx	0/2	2/6	5/14	2/9
IIIB CA Cx	0/7	3/8	6/13	2/7
IV CA Cx	0/2	1/1	0/1	1/1
Other sites	1/6	2/3	1/5	0/1
Complications	2/17[a] (12%)	4/20[b] (20%)	4/34[c] (12%)	2/20[d] (10%)

Note: Results from the M.D. Anderson-TAMVEC Program of Neutron Therapy Testing. The mixed photon and neutron beam program was selected for randomization with photon treatment since it gave essentially the same local control rate as the neutron boost, but with a reduced complication rate.

a - 1 sigmoiditis, 1 small bowel obstruction.
b - 1 proctitis, 2 small bowel obstructions, 1 small bowel necrosis.
c - 1 proctitis, 2 small bowel obstructions, 1 small bowel necrosis.
d - 1 vault necrosis, 1 small bowel obstruction.

HEAVY IONS

Phase I and II trials of heavy ion radiotherapy are nearing completion at the Lawrence Berkeley Laboratory at the University of California. Helium ions are accelerated in the 184 inch Synchrocyclotron. Carbon, neon, and argon ions are accelerated by the Bevalac. Castro and coworkers (4) point out the reduction in the oxygen enhancement ratio (OER) - the smaller the ratio, the smaller the dependence on the presence of oxygen to accomplish cell killing - afforded by all heavy ions. This radiation is a modest advantage in the case of helium compared to low LET radiations, but the advantage is marked with carbon, neon, and argon. However, all heavy ions can be planned to deposit their energy in a manner that limits the high-dose area to the tumor-bearing volume. This sparing of the normal tissues is the major advantage of helium ions, a property shared with proton beams. The Bragg peak of heavy ions is less than 1 cm in width. To make the peak region available for clinical use, a family of filters made of brass, ridge filters, spread the peak to widths between 4 and 14 cm.

One-hundred and ninety-four patients treated with helium ions and forty-nine patients treated with other heavy ions were reported by Berkley (4). The major sites treated were head and neck, intracranial tumors, thoracic tumors, abdomen/retroperitoneal, and pelvic tumors. In addition, 22 ocular melanomas have been treated by helium ions alone. Twenty of these were stable or regressing. The largest experience has been with pancreatic carcinoma. After 52 patients had been treated, a randomized trial comparing helium ion therapy with photon treatment was begun. Only 23 patients have been entered so far. As yet, no difference in survival of either group of pancreatic tumors is evident.

Little improvement has been found by Castro in treating esophageal carcinomas with helium ions. Experience with helium ions in brain and stomach irradiation is limited, but is encoraging enough that these sites will be the object of trials with heavier ions so that the benefit of the increased biological effect can be added to the benefit of locaization. However, the Berkeley group wish to treat an additional 50 patients with carbon, neon, and argon before embarking on phase III trials with heavy ions. At that time, the sites with the highest priority for trial will be glioblastoma, advanced head and neck tumors, localized cancer of the pancreas, and bone and soft tissue sarcomas.

PROTONS

As with helium ions, the advantage of proton therapy is the ability to localize the high dose in the treatment volume with relative sparing of the normal tissues. In certain sites, Suit and coworkers (30) believe that though biological advantages are lacking, the dose distribution of protons is superior to that which can be obtained with photons. Since 1973, 140 patients have been treated using the Harvard cyclotron and conventional fractionation schemes. Because the proton is a charged particle, its range can be limited in tissue with rapid decrease in dose at the end of the range. The beam also exhibits rapid fall off laterally. This characteristic of rapid fall off on all margins of the peak make this an excellent beam for high-dose localized radiotherapy. Limitation of the high-dose region compared to photon treatment, and elimination of critical structures from the high dose volume should permit higher doses. The increase in dose is expected to result in increased tumor control.

Suit does not believe the RBE of the Harvard proton beam exceeds 1.10. Treatment is given four times a week with 191 rads/fraction. Great care is taken to ensure in the daily setup, which can require multiple portal filming during a single treatment session. In most instances (choroidal melanomas being the major exception), the proton treatment is limited to a boost at the end of photon therapy. In 44 patients with cancer of the prostate treated in this manner the greater portion of the rectal wall is spared, resulting in marked reduction in proctitis. The photon boost raises the usual photon dose by 6-9%. It is delivered through a peritoneal portal. The urethra in the center of the prostate now becomes the dose-limiting tissue. To date there has been only one recurrence in the 44 patients treated. Sarcoma of bone adjacent to the central nervous system is a candidate for proton beam treatment. Five such patients have been managed without evidence of CNS damage.

Thirty-six patients with choroidal melanomas have been treated by pure photon beam. Though the optimum total dose is still being determined by treating at two dose levels, treatment is given in five fractions over 7-9 days. Patients have been observed as long as 48 months. There have been no local failures. Complications have been few. Three patients developed partial cataracts, and three have developed mild glaucoma which is controlled medically.

In summary, higher doses in smaller treatment volumes have been achieved using protons with tolerable normal tissue reaction. The investigators are enthusiastic about continuing the evaluation of proton therapy.

NEGATIVE PI-MESONS

As stated earlier negative pi-mesons (pions) are charge particles which act as a low LET radiation as they transverse tissue in the plateau region, and combine low and high LET radiation in the peak region. The pion beam, therefore, combines the shaping capabilities of other charge particles and the advantage of high LET radiation in the region of the tumor. It should be pointed out, however, that the combination of high and low LET radiation in the peak region alters the biologic response to one which interferes with repair of the cell, but not the sensitivity of the cell. Because of this biology, different than that seen with low LET or a pure high LET beam, the potential for therapeutic gain was hypothesized (18) for pion therapy. It is believed that the biological difference could be as important as the highly localized disposition of radiation of which all particle beams are capable. The first patient to be tested with pion therapy occurred on October 21, 1974 at the Clinton P. Anderson Meson Physic's Facility in Los Alamos, New Mexico, by a team of scientists from the Cancer Research and Treatment Center of the University of New Mexico and from the Los Alamos Scientific Laboratory (19). At the present time, two additional facilities have begun testing pion beams using skin nodule experiments. They are the Tri-University Meson Facility (TRIUMF) in Vancouver, Canada (12), and The Swiss Institute for Nuclear Research (SIN) (33). The ability to follow a patient with multiple metastatic tumor nodules in the skin, which had been treated with several doses of x-rays or pions as part of the determination of the RBE for skin, gave the opportunity to assess, in a preliminary way, whether therapeutic gain did exist. Though the data are not large (20), all 16 of the nodules had disappeared after treatment, permitting observation of the time required for regrowth of the lesions. A therapeutic gain of 37.5% favoring pions was estimated.

Observations on the pion patients treated in phase I and II studies are summarized below (19, 20, 23). At the initiation of the New Mexico program, many sites were examined for the response of the normal tissue as well as the tumor within it. Sites that appeared of greatest interest were the brain, head and neck, rectum, urinary bladder, prostate, and the pancreas. No patient had complete regression of the tumor unless a minimum of 2700 peak pion rads were given. As each new site was treated, low doses were first given. These were esclated as long as acute reactions of the normal tissues remained minimal. Since the experience with neutrons showed a lack of correlation between the acute response of a normal tissue and late effects - the latter could have a higher RBE - the maximum dose delivered in the pion peak was kept at certain levels until sufficient time could elapse for the repair of acute reactions and the appearance of any late reactions. It was the impression that in at least some of the tumors, notably prostatic cancers, the lesions disappeared more rapdily than one would expect with conventional radiation. Furthermore, if the daily dose rate was kept between 110-125 rads the normal tissue reactions appeared less than what one would expect for the concomitant tumor regression. The rectal and bladder mucosa appeared to tolerate pion radiation, given with this size of fraction better than the normal tissues of the head and neck, although no serious difficulty was experienced in treating patients with tumors in the latter region.

Prior to May, 1980, 140 patients were treated with pion radiotherapy at the Los Alamos Meson Physic's Facility. Ninety-seven tumors in ninety-six patients received therapy with curative intent. They were analyzed with regard to local control, survival, and the relationship between acute and chronic reactions. Sixty-eight patients were treated by pions alone. Nineteen patients had the addition of conventional radiation and ten patients were treated with pions followed by surgery. The reason for the addition of conventional radiation on the one hand and surgery on the other was mainly due to the low doses which were given early in the program. A cautious approach was taken to the escalation of pion doses since there was concern that an unexpected untoward effect might occur in a particular tissue. Therefore, early, a large safety factor dictated an underdosage in advanced lesions which often resulted in persistence not unexpected. It was soon learned that even when doses of 3000 and 3500 rads were given tumors did not always disappear. At the same time, the mucosal reaction was minimal or nonexistent, indicating that considerable normal tissue tolerance remained. In order to ensure that each patient had the best opportunity for complete regression of his lesion, appropriate conventional therapy of some type was added. Surgical procedures were used when normal tissue reactions were moderate and a small persistent mass remained.

A working tolerance dose-fractionation overall time schedule has been established which is being used in conjunction with randomized phase III trials of pion radiotherapy. This working tolerance dose is 4500 maximum peak pion rads in 36 fractions/50 days. It is these authors' impression that for small volumes a daily maximum peak pion dose of 125 rads is tolerated. However, for large volumes such as required for many of the pelvic cases, the daily fraction size is better tolerated by the normal tissues if the dose is reduced by 5-7%. The working RBE is, therefore, between 1.5 and 1.6.

The majority of patients in the analysis leading to the working tolerance dose were advanced neoplasms of the head and neck, 36 patients, and high-grade gliomata, 23 patients. There were also 15 patients with T3 and T4 adenocarcinoma of the prostate. Last, patients with locally advanced unresectable adenocarcinoma of the pancreas were treated. There were also some patients with carcinoma of esophagus, lung, stomach, skin, uterus, cervix, urinary bladder, and rectum. This occurred early in the administration of pion radiotherapy when a search was being made for sites which might respond in an unusually salutory way. All of these sites were used in assessing the toxicity of the several normal tissues.

Table 2 shows local control in those 68 patients treated with pions only. Note the improvement in overall survival in spite of a zero result for all pancreatic cases as the dose was increased to the 4000-5000 maximum peak pion rad range. However, it should be noted that when tumors persisted at 5000 rads, additional pion treatment did not effect tumor response. These latter were truly pion-resistant tumors.

When the initial decisions were made as to what type of patients would be assessed for the trials of pion radiotherapy, it was decided that patients would be accepted whose disease site or advanced stage rendered them relatively incurable by conventional means. Patients with tumors with an expected survival over 20% were excluded. At that time it was believed that locally advanced prostatic carcinoma fell into this group. Prostate cancers showed a 100% response to pion treatment. Subsequently, it has been demonstrated that conventional radiation gives a follow-up of approximately 50% in T3 and T4 lesions which are confined to the pelvis. Therefore, after the accession of 25 patients with prostatic carcinoma, the study

Table 2. Local Control, Pion Only, By Site and Dose

Site	Dose (π^- Rad Maximum)				
	2700-3999	4000-4999	5000	Local	Control
Head and neck	1/4	4/9	0/3	5/16	(31%)
Brain	1/10	2/6	0/0	3/16	(19%)
Prostate	4/4	11/11	0/0	15/15	(100%)
Pancreas	0/5	0/5	0/0	0/10	(0%)
Other	3/6	1/4	0/1	4/11	(36%)
Total	9/29	18/35	0/4	27/68	(40%)

Note: Of the 68 tumors treated with pions only, there is a suggestion of a dose-response curve in that better control occurs in the 4000-5000 rad group. Note also that control was not improved if tumors required more than 5000 rads. This was also true when pion treatment was augmented by additional amounts of radiation therapy or surgery once a high dose of pions was given.

was closed so that the pion patients could be observed over a 3-5 year period. If there is any indication that control in this group of 25 is improved significantly over that seen with conventional treatment, then a randomized study will be undertaken comparing pion therapy with conventional radiation. The reverse was true in the case of the pancreas. Results have been dismal. In fact, many patients developed metastasis to the liver or lung while they were being worked up for pion therapy or developed metastases during treatment even though all tests were negative for distant metastases before pion therapy began. A new program has been started which includes treatment of the prostate and its regional nodes plus conventional irradiation to the entire liver. At the rate of 150 rads/day, 2500 rads are given to the liver prophylactically. The patients being selected must show negative CT and radionuclide scans as well as a negative liver biopsy before they are accepted for this program.

Another group of tumors which deserve mention are the malignant gliomas. When all 23 patients which have been treated are taken into account, there is a suggestion that survival of both grade III and grade IV lesions is improved over conventional treatment.

Tables 3 and 4 show the acute and chronic reactions of normal tissues to pion irradiation. A dose response is noted. More importantly, however, the data available indicate that the acute reactions are predictive of the chronic reactions. The latter is at a lower degree of severity than the acute reaction at each level. This is different from what had been seen with neutron therapy where chronic reactions of the normal tissues were often more severe than the relatively mild to moderate acute reactions.

Summarizing pion radiotherapy, it may be said that phase I and phase II trials have been completed with the development of a working tolerance dose. Phase III trials are underway.

Table 3. Acute Reactions to Pion Irradiation Alone

(π - R Maximum)	Severity	No. Patients	Av. Severity
2700-3999	0	2	
	1	9	1.7
	2	13	
	3	4	
4000-4999	0	0	
	1	11	
	2	12	2.0
	3	12	
5000	0	0	
	1	0	
	2	1	2.8
	3	3	

Note: A dose-response curve for acute reactions is seen. Severity I are mild symptoms such as injection only in the mucous membranes of the mouth. Severity II would be a patchy pseudodiphtheric membrane in the mucosa of the mouth, while severity III would be a confluent mucositis.

Table 4. Chronic Reactions Related to Pions

(π - R Maximum)	Severity	No. Patients	Av. Severity
2700-3999	0	9	
	1	10	1.0
	2	9	
	3	0	
4000-4999	0	9	
	1	16	
	2	8	1.1
	3	2	
5000	0	0	
	1	2	
	2	2	1.5
	3	0	

Note: The chronic responses are symptomatically less than the acute reactions. If this persists with the addition of more patients, it would represent a distinct advantage over neutron therapy where frequently there is an increased chronic reaction as compared to the acute reaction. Note that in the range of dose selected as the working dose fractionation schedule, namely between 4000 and 5000 rads, the late reactions are clearly acceptable.

CONCLUSIONS

Phase I and II trials have been completed or nearing completion for all of the four types of particle beams. Phase III trials are underway. At the present time, it is still unclear as to whether particle radiotherapy will be advantageous in a reasonable percentage of patients to make it worth general community support. The outcome of the present trials should yield this answer over the next 3-5 years.

REFERENCES

1. Battermann, J.J. and Bruer, K.: Results of fast neutron radiotherapy at Amsterdam. In High LET Radiations in Clinical Radiotherapy, edited by G.W. Barendsen, J. Broerse, and K. Bruer, London, Pergamon Press, 1979.

2. Bloch, P.: Personal communication, 1981.

3. Bullen, M.A., Freundlich, H.F., Hale, B.T., Marshall, D.H., and Tudway, R.C.: The activity of malignant tumors and response to therapeutic agents, studied by continuous records of radioactive phosphorus uptake. Postgrad. Med. J. 39:265-277, 1963.

4. Castro, J.D., Quivey, J.M., Saunders, W.M., Woodroff, K.H., Chen, G.T.Y., Lyman, J.T., Pitluck, S., Tobias, C.A., Walton, R.E., and Peters, T.C.: Clinical results in heavy particle therapy. In Lawrence Berkeley Laboratory Publication #11220, Berkeley, Calif., December 1980, pp. 305-318.

5. Catterall, M., Sutherland, I., and Bewley, D.K.: Second report on results of a randomized clinical trial of fast neutrons compared with x- or gamma rays in treatment of advanced tumors of head and neck. Br. J. Radiol. 1:16-42, 1977.

6. Catterall, M.: Observation on reactions of normal and malignant tissue to a standard dose of neutrons. In High LET Radiation in Clinical Radiotherapy. Ed. by G.W. Barendsen, J. Broerse, K. Bruer, Pergamon Press, London, 1979, pp. 11-15.

7. Churchill-Davidson, I., Sanger, C., and Thomlinson, R.H.: Oxygenation in radiotherapy. II. Clinical application. Br. J. Radiol. 30:406-422, 1957.

8. Coutard, H.: Roentgen therapy of epitheliomas of the tonsil hypopharynx and larynx. Am. J. Roentgenol. 28:313-331, 1932.

9. Elkind, M.N. and Sutton, H.: Radiation response of mammalian cells grown in culture. I. Repair of x-ray damage in surviving Chinese hamster cells. Radiat. Res. 13:556-593, 1960.

10. Fowler, J.F., Morgan, R.L., and Wood, C.A.P.: Pre-therapeutic experiments with fast neutron beam from the Medical Research Council Cyclotron (MRCC)1. The biological and physical advantages and problems of neutron therapy. Br. J. Radiol. 36:77-80, 1963.

11. Ginzton, E.D., Hansen, W.W., Kennedy, W.R.: A linear electron accelerator. Rev. Sci. Inst. 19:89-108, 1948.

12. Goodman, G.: Personal communication, 1981.

13. Gray, L.H., Conger, A.D., Ebert, N., Hornsey, S., and Scott, O.C.A.: The concentration of oxygen dissolved in tissues at the time of irradiation as a factor in radiotherapy. Br. J. Radiol. 26:638-648, 1953.

14. Griffin, T., Blasko, J., and Laramore, G.: Results of fast neutron beam radiotherapy pilot studies at the University of Washington. In High LET Radiation and Clinical Radiotherapy, edited by G.W. Barendsen, J. Broerse, and K. Bruer, London, Pergamon Press, 1979, pp. 23-29.

15. Henk, J.M., Kunkler, P.B., Shah, N.K., Smith, C.W., Sutherland, W.H., and Wassiff, S.B.: Hyperbaric oxygen in radiotherapy of head and neck carcinoma. Clin. Radiol. 21:223-231, 1970.

16. Howard-Flanders, P.: The development of the linear accelerator as clinical instrument. Acta Radiologica 116:649-655, 1943.

17. Kerst, D.W.: The betatron. Radiology 40:115, 1943.

18. Kligerman, M.M.: Potential for therapeutic gain similar to pions by daily combination of neutrons and low LET radiation. Med. Hypotheses 5:257-264, 1979.

19. Kligerman, M.M., West, G., Dicello, J.F., Sternhagen, C.J., Barnes, J.E., Loeffler, R.K., Dobrowolski, F., Davis, H.T., Bradbury, J.N., Lane, T.F., Petersen, D.F., and Knapp, E.A.: Initial comparative response to peak pions and x-rays of normal skin and underlying tissue surrounding superficial metastatic nodules. Am. J. Roentgenol. 126:261-267, 1976.

20. Kligerman, M.M., Sala, J.M., Wilson, S., and Yuhas, J.M.: Investigation of pion treated human skin nodules for therapeutic gain. Int. J. Radiat. Oncol. Biol. Phys. 4:263-265, 1978.

21. Kligerman, M.M., Sala, J.M., Smith, A.R., Knapp, E.A., Tsujii, H., Bagshaw, M.A., and Wilson, S.: Tissue reaction and tumor response with negative pi mesons. J. Can. Assoc. Radiol. 31:13-18, 1980.

22. Kligerman, M.M., Bush, S., Kondo, M., Wilson, S., and Smith, A.R.: Results of phase I-II trials of pion radiotherapy. Proceedings of the Second Rome International Symposium on Biological Bases and Clinical Implications of Tumor Radioresistance (in press).

23. Knapp, E.A.: Resonantly coupled wave accelerator structure for electron and proton linac applications. IEEE Transactions Nuclear Science, NS-16:329, 1969.

24. Morales, P., Hussey, D.H., Maor, M., Fletcher, G.F., and Wharton, T.: Report of the M.D. Anderson study of neutron therapy for locally advanced gynecological tumors (in manuscript).

25. Puck, T.T. and Marcus, P.E.I.: Action of x-rays on the mammalian cell. Gen. Exp. Med. 103:653-656, 1956.

26. Regaud, C. and Ferroux, R.: Est il possible de sterilise le testicle du lapin adults par une dose massive de rayons X scans produire de lesion grave de la peau? C.R. Soc. Biol. (Paris) 97:330-333, 1927.

27. Stone, R.S., Lawrence, J.H., and Aebersold, P.C.: Preliminary report on use of fast neutron in treatment of malignant disease. Radiology 35:322-327, 1940.

28. Stone, R.S. and Larkin, Jr., J.C.: Treatment of cancer with fast neutrons. Radiology 39:608-620, 1942.

29. Suit, H.D.: Superfractionation. Int. J. Radiat. Oncol. Biol. Phys. 2:591-592, 1977.

30. Suit, H.D., Goitein, M., Munzenrider, J.E., Verhey, L., Gragoudas, E., Koehler, A.M., Urano, M., Shipley, W.U., Linggood, R.M., Friedberg, C., and Wagner, M.: Clinical experience with proton beam radiation therapy. J. Can. Assoc. Radiol. 31:35-39, 1980.

31. Tapley, N. du V.: Personal communication, 1960.

32. Teresima, T. and Tolmach, L.J.: Variation in several responses in HeLa cells to x-radiation during the division cycle. Biophys. J. 3:11-33, 1963.

33. von Essen, C.F.: Personal communication, 1979.

34. Withers, H.R.: Biological basis for high-LET radiotherapy. Radiology 108: 131-137, 1973.

35. Yuhas, J., Li, A., Martinez, A., Ladman, A.: A simplified method of production and growth of multicellular tumor spheroids. Cancer Res. 37:3639-3643, 1977.

chapter 15

PRIVATE PRACTICE OF RADIATION THERAPY AND THE LAW OF MEDICAL MALPRACTICE

Walter G. Gunn, M.D., J.D.

"I suggest that the key to a wholeness of life in medicine is the intensity of the experience itself, and that our great gift is to be able to live at the point of intensity, where our spirits might grow" (23).

SECTION I. THE PRIVATE PRACTICE OF RADIATION THERAPY

This chapter will attempt to address neither the detailed economics of private practice in the United States nor consideration of departmental layout and planning. Rather extensive information on these topics is available both from the American College of Radiology and from sequences of articles appearing in Medical Economics and other parascientific publications (6,22,30). The reader is urged to consult these excellent sources when considering setting up a new department or renovating an existing one, either in a hospital or freestanding center. Decisions on the organization of a group radiotherapy practice, the incorporation of professionals and paraprofessionals, and office management and patient flow techniques are made easier by the topics considered in these resumes and handbooks.

In Section I we will concern ourselves with practical advice to the newly graduated radiotherapists. We will analyze the various types of private practice and some of the administrative and ethical standards by which physicians are governed in 1982. We will touch upon practice in hospitals and in freestanding centers, consider those persons and consultants whose work intersects with our own, and conclude with a forecast of where we may be headed. Along the way we will dispense some recommendations on the relationship of the radiotherapist to his patients, to his colleagues, to the town, and to the gown.

DEFINITIONS AND DIRECTIONS

By private practice we mean the situation where a doctor interacts with a patient and bills him for his services. The fact that the billing may be done by the hospital or a clinic group is irrelevant to this definition. In a sense a contract for a specific exchange of medical care for an agreed payment is <u>implied-in-fact</u>, and this is generally what the medical profession designates as fee for services. Inherently it excludes physician-on-salary arrangements such as those provided by medical schools or governmental organizations. With radiotherapists the variations on this contractual theme are but two: (1) There is ordinarily a hospital or technical component to the patient's bill, similar to that of the diagnostic radiologist, and intended to compensate the billing agent for various unusual direct and indirect expenses such as the cost and maintenance of linear accelerators. (2) Radiotherapy is, almost exclusively, a referral practice, i.e., the radiotherapist may hang out a shingle but does not just accept anyone walking in off the street. Customarily patients are sent to him by other physicians.

Radiotherapists in private practice may work alone or with other therapists in a hospital or office, or be associated with diagnostic radiologists as part of a general practice of radiology, or be one of a number of physicians working in a multidiscipline clinic or group. Another working place is the freestanding facility by which is generally meant a building standing separate from and independent of a hospital but serving certain functions formerly performed by a subsection of the hospital, e.g., outpatient surgery, radiation therapy, etc. Such an entity is a logical outgrowth of attempts to curb rising hospital costs coupled with the desire for independence from the hospital by physicians who cater primarily to outpatients, for example, radiation therapists, plastic surgeons, etc. We are concerned here with those workers in radiotherapy at private hospitals, clinic groups and offices, and freestanding centers.

To this author, it seems best for the radiotherapist to practice as part of a group, and preferably with a group of other radiotherapists, either as a separate team, or as part of a larger entity, such as a multidiscipline clinic. I believe that the opportunity to discuss clinical problems each day with one's peers is a powerful antidote to what Osler (20) called "the corroding effect of routine" and a stimulus to keep current regarding developments in one's field. It is, of course, also of benefit if referring physicians and related specialists such as medical oncologists, surgeons, pathologists, and radiologists are close at hand or just down the corridor. To me this is the outstanding advantage of the multidiscpline clinic. The hospital combines this advantage with having inpatients nearby, though it may have some not-so-desirable administrative constraints. The freestanding facility offers the most freedom but does not conveniently provide referring clinicians or inpatients in person.

The solo radiotherapist will have difficulty obtaining suitable coverage for meetings and vacations. Even the well-trained general radiologist who has had 1 or 2 years of radiotherapy and remains interested in the field will be an inadequate substitute, particularly for the patients who have become used to and dependent upon "their" doctor, the radiotherapist. Such doctor-patient relationships can be among the most intimate and meaningful in all of medicine. No other clinician, except possibly the psychiatrist, sees patients daily for many weeks and pays such attention to their minor symptoms, granting that these are often clues to treatment side effects or manifestations of their disease. To have a stranger, even an associate, come in to direct the daily care of the cancer patient during treatment is unsettling to the patient. This is difficult enough for the substitute radiotherapist who has seen the patient occasionally; for the diagnostician not primarily interested in therapy it is, in my view, an impossible task.

Michael Radetsky (23) has eloquently stated the need of physicians to maintain the capacity for wonder, for human sharing and growth of the spirit. The solo practitioner, preoccupied with his daily round and bereft of frequent interchange of ideas with his peers, may begin imperceptibly to experience, in Radetsky's words "the impoverishment of our own capacities for responsiveness and growth . . ."

If possible, therefore, the preferred mode of private practice is as part of a group of radiotherapists. Failing this, an association with interested and concerned radiodiagnosticians may work out. Least satisfactory is true solo practice.

I have seen radiotherapy practiced in conjunction with medical oncology both as full partnership and as close membership in a group. At best, short-term coverage is all that is possible between these allied specialists. Although they may share many of the same patients, the demands of the two specialties are diverse enough that one should not ask for or rely on coverage by the other.

DEGREES OF FREEDOM

The choice of private practice as against salaried employment in an academic center or governmental organization for reasons of greater freedom of practice is becoming illusory. On the one hand most salaried therapists must follow the rules set forth by their employer, and these, while usually administrative and not hampering of professional decision making, can be irksome enough. At the same time the private practitioner of radiotherapy works under a host of superimposed constraints as well, and these externals to his practice markedly narrow his freedom of work. Hospitals, for example, can no longer ignore the concern of consumer groups and governmental bodies in the acquisition of expensive hardware such as supervoltage equipment, though enough loopholes still exist so that clever and determined individuals can maneuver past state guidelines. The federal health service agencies, in concert with state issuance of certificates of need, constitute a lead-in to national health control of medical care delivery. Professional standards review organizations are another federal concept, and though designed for quality control of medical care, they have containment notions in the background. Thus, while participation in peer review criteria for quality of care seems laudable, the physician must understand that he is undergoing this self-regulation with guided prodding from the federal government. Third, there is no question but that such devices for patient billing as a "relative value scale" of services are regarded as price-fixing by the Federal Trade Commission, the protests of the American College of Radiology notwithstanding.

Organized medicine and physicians' unions, of course, rail at these administrative encroachments. There can be little doubt, however, that their efforts, though meaningful in the short term, will serve at best as no more than delaying tactics to full government takeover of physician and hospital care at least for the chronic diseases. If this assessment seems unduly pessimistic I would only proffer two points: (1) In the early 1970s provisions for renal dialysis coverage via Medicare for patients of any age were attached to and passed by the Congress as an innocuous-appearing provision on another bill. So in that limited sense, there is already national health insurance in place and functioning. Some would say that the high cost of renal dialysis ought to be covered. I am inclined to agree, which leads to the next point: (2) If chronic renal disease, why not cancer? Is one a worse catastrophe than the other? And perhaps it is time that such long-term, debilitating, and financially disastrous diseases were placed under some sort of catastrophe insurance for hospital and physician care.

THE FREESTANDING RADIATION CENTER

While the freestanding center might seem ideally suited as a form of private practice relatively free from administrative strictures, there are several considerations that suggest such an approach will play but a minor part in American radiation therapy practice. Of perhaps most significance is the image of a hospital as the focus of a cancer treatment center both to the public and to governmental grant-giving agencies alike. Currently a major push is underway by many medical schools to become the site of regional cancer centers and so qualify for federal grants to develop their own programs as well as become clearing houses for smaller grants to be disbursed in their regions. It seems not unreasonable to envision the community hospitals becoming satellites of the major cancer centers in this effort. Such is not to say that this development may not be for the best in the nationwide effort at cancer control, but only to imply that regional centers may determine treatment programs of their choosing and require conformity before loosening the purse strings. I suggest only that one's freedom of practice may be lessened by several degrees if this development continues. It would appear that interdisciplinary team approach is a catch phrase in this effort and the freestanding center devoted solely to radiation therapy may find itself on the outside looking in. In addition, the local tax structure is set against the private practice of radiation therapy outside hospitals in that the private therapists must pay business and property taxes on his equipment and buildings. The business property (read linear accelerator, computer, simulator) may be taxed at 2-3% annually, based on the original purchase price, and real property taxes may constitute an additional 2-3% of the value determined by the tax assessor. Most hospitals, being not-for-profit institutions, will be free of these taxes. Thus, the radiotherapist at a freestanding center will face certain inherent economic disadvantages, particularly if his case load is limited. Add to this the professional problem of being physically separate from the inpatient population and daily hospital give and take of joint clinics, and it is not hard to see a limited future for such centers.

A partial solution might be to organize the freestanding center under a nonprofit or cancer foundation umbrella, thereby avoiding onerous taxes. A portion of such services must then be available for charity cases as well. Ideally the open staff arrangement is best, so that any qualified radiation therapist in the community can treat his patients at the center. The few centers in the United States organized on this basis seem to work well. The referring doctor has his choice of radiotherapist and the patient does not suffer from any limitation of equipment. After treatment is complete, the patient can be followed by the therapist either at the open facility or at his own separate nonmachine-equipped office.

I submit that the nub of this problem is that hospitals, and radiation therapists, want to have the best of both worlds. Therapists want to work at well-equipped and staffed centers, but feel insecure when bound to relatively short-term contracts, so often want outside offices and other security, such as minimum guarantees. Hospitals want "their" man, knowing he will be always available; they fear giving a long-term contract lest his performance not always measure up, and realize that as time passes the therapist will become locked-in since advancing age will make him less desirable elsewhere. Time is thus on the hospital's side. Neither side is secure enough to create the logical solution. In my view the open staff concept in or out of hospital is the best for all parties, including the hospital, the therapist, and particularly the patient. It may be that federal pressures for national health insurance and cost containment will push the parties further in the direction of open staff. Certificate of need requirement would indicate that continued duplication of underused expensive radiation facilities is not the answer.

RIGHTS AND DUTIES

The American College of Radiology has enunciated in considerable detail (1) the responsibilities of the radiologist. In a hospital he should have "definite and adequate hours of attendance" and "have the privilege of admitting patients." The chief of radiology should have the right to select radiologic personnel as well.

Inasmuch as the therapeutic radiologist may function as a member of the radiology department, he should play proportionately the same role.

The College emphasizes the importance of periodic reports to the medical staff on the diagnostic and therapeutic services rendered, as well as the need for indexing all therapy records on a suitable pathological basis (2). In addition both the College and AMA advise separate billing by radiologists for professional services. While not yet nearly universally accepted by hospitals (15),* this precept seems to have found easier acceptance since federal sources responsible for cost containment have wondered aloud as to whether or not such practices as percentages of gross contract do not amount to fee splitting between hospital and radiologist, particularly where the radiologist is not named. Both the American Medical Association and the Joint Commission on Accreditation of Hospitals, an organization supported by the American Hospital Association, have also raised this question. Hospital leaders have more generally become aware of this potential problem as well.

Ideally it would seem sensible for the radiotherapist in private practice in a hospital to bill patients for his professional services on his own billhead while the hospital bills each patient separately for the cost incurred in its service. The latter may include direct costs for personnel (including support persons in physics, nursing, treatment, dosimetry, etc., if such are hospital employees), fixed overhead such as building costs and utilities, plus amounts to be set aside for equipment repair and eventual replacement. The hospital may also bill for indirect costs, e.g., the radiotherapy department's contributions to the overall hospital functioning including total plant maintenance, salaries for administrative personnel, etc. The indirect costs should probably be distinctly less than the direct costs unless the radiotherapy department occupies a significant proportion of the overall hospital square footage. It is not unknown for hospitals to claim that the radiotherapy department is losing money in an effort to persuade the physician to accept a change in his contract. In such circumstances the therapist will be well advised to inspect the cost figures referred to above.

The radiotherapist in a clinic group practice should have the same responsibilities and prerogatives as those of his colleagues, and his income should be based upon the value of his professional medical services and his other services and contributions to the group (3).

THE NEW MAN IN TOWN

The new radiotherapist in town should visit established therapists since, though they may be friendly competitors, they may also provide useful background information on local medical and hospital policies. One of the best ways to find out information is to go directly to them, preferably in advance of accepting a job, and ask questions. Most will be friendly and eager to help; some will be grateful that a colleague is arriving to take on some of the patient load; rarely, and then only in radiotherapist-impacted areas, will one be threatened by the new man. It is important to arrange for state medical licensing, narcotic registration, and compliance with state laws regarding equipment registration well before starting the new job. Hospital staff privileges may take a matter of months, so it is wise to initiate those applications long before appearing on the scene.

---

* A survey conducted by the College in early 1975 revealed that 64% of the membership of the College was billing separately from hospitals.

The follow-up of patients by the radiotherapist can be a touchy subject. It may seem self-evident that cancer patients in general and radiotherapy patients in particular should be followed by those administering treatment (17). It strikes this author that a radiotherapist who does not follow patients whom he has treated may fairly be considered as somewhat negligent. The American College of Radiology emphasizes that careful follow-up in all treatment cases is essential both as material for staff conferences and for clinical research purposes. A cancer registry, if available, is one way to accomplish this. Where a patient is treated only for palliation and where two or more physicians interested and competent in cancer are on the case, by agreement the therapist could relinquish follow-ups to the others provided he keeps himself informed regarding the case. To relinquish this role where a patient has been treated for cure or via radical irradiation would be unwise. Many nononcologists do not understand the importance of such close follow-up, and the new radiation therapist would do well to explain this to his potential pool of referring physicians at the outset. One way to do this is as part of a general talk on cancer care to the hospital medical staff early in the therapist's career.

LIAISON WITH THE UNIVERSITY

It is important for the private practitioner to maintain some teaching or research relationship with a nearby medical school. Whether in solo or private group practice, the therapist needs, more than most, interaction with those in training programs and research because the pace of clinical work in cancer seems to take a quantum leap about every 5 years. Conversely, the private practitioner has much practical information to impart to the resident in training as regards the practicalities of work outside the teaching center. Such mutual exchange permits the private therapist to keep up, share a feeling of being at the forefront of the action, and even help the goals of the larger research group by bringing in his own cases. I would suggest a half day per month as a minimum for this effort, and more where the center is not geographically distant. If a clinical faculty appointment is offered, it represents an extension of status and privilege to the practitioner and should only be accepted if one can deliver teaching time on a regular basis.

PHYSICS AND SUPPORTING PERSONNEL

The radiotherapist in private practice will need the services of a physicist, even if only part time. Increasing governmental emphasis on quality control plus the probing interest of courts and plaintiff's attorneys into the precise details of each treatment given, force the therapist to evaluate every facet of technical details of therapy. The physicist is uniquely qualified to perform this task, and his imprimatur on treatment records, calibrations, and machine output carries much weight in official and courtroom deliberations. A favorite query directed to the radiotherapist in a malpractice case these days is "When did you have your machine last calibrated prior to the incident in question, doctor?" The radiotherapist had better be ready for that one. His indispensable aide will be the physicist. Particularly important are repeat output calibrations after electrical or wiring work is done involving a machine or treatment room.

Funds to support a salary for full-time physics and computer-dosimetry services will flow easily enough in a busy department where the radiotherapist can show to hospital administrators the need for sophisticated treatment planning, beam shaping, and calibrations. For the smaller department which may not need such ancillary help more than 1 or 2 days/week, a billing maneuver known as the <u>head tax</u> may make it possible to hire a consulting physicist and his supporting services on a part-time basis. Essentially each patient is billed one time, at nominal fee, for the expense of quality control for that individual case. This will include checking calculations on the treatment chart, calibrating machines, evaluating department standards, and such other duties as may arise. Computer or dosimetrist-calculated plans can be charged for separately, and form another cash-flow mechanism by which the independent physicist can amortize his expensive equipment.

My personal preference is to have such part-time supporting persons work a full day when they are in attendance, rather than to share them with other facilities on half-day or hourly arrangements. Traveling between various offices or hospitals is time consuming and inefficient at best, and at worst one facility may be waiting several hours while the physicist is delayed doing an urgent treatment plan at another place. At the outset it is important to spell out precisely on paper what is expected. Often working situations may change, new personnel be employed, and the original smooth-running relationship is set aside or disappears for reasons no one is exactly sure of. At such times it helps to go back to a job description or employment agreement to clarify how things were set up at the start.

THE REFERRING PHYSICIAN

The relationship of the radiation therapist with his referral base of private physicians is all important; and rapport with clinicians, particularly surgical subspecialists and medical oncologists, determines not only better overall patient management but also efficiency of practice in that those patients who should be followed by the appropriate specialist are followed.

Working closely with the medical oncologist does not mean yielding one's ability to make decisions or consultative opinions simply in favor of harmony at all costs. The radiotherapist is unique in that he is, in effect, a general practitioner of cancer care. His skills are devoted to specific treatment and consultation in any organ system where cancer is found. To abdicate his primacy as a cancer consultant is foolish. Particularly gullible is he where he subserves his skills to a department of oncology for administrative convenience. Perhaps one could not do better than to echo the words of Moss (19): "How long does it take the therapist to learn that one loses freedom of clinical management with every loss of administrative responsibility. . . . Looking to others to solve one's administrative problems leads to decisions modifying budget, personnel, patient referral, space, equipment, staff salaries. . . ." In another sense the same is true as regards treatment in the private facility vis-à-vis various bureaucratic entities.

The referring physician must be kept informed of developments on his patient. When the patient first visits the therapist the case should be evaluated, then discussed with the referring physician and all other physicians involved. This is time consuming but vitally important so that all concerned may know what to expect. Often patients and relatives will tell these physicians of symptoms or ask questions to which they may not know the answers. My practice has been to send copies of the initial radiotherapy consultation to all doctors concerned, letters of completion at the close of radiotherapy, and during treatment to give them verbal progress reports from time to time. Needless to say, copies of all significant x-ray and laboratory reports should also be sent along as these are obtained.

The patient must be kept aware of the important role of his other physicians. Often close attachments will form between the cancer patient and radiotherapist, so much so that at times the patient will stop going back to his family doctor or referring physician. This must absolutely not be allowed to happen for many reasons, not the least of which is that the radiotherapist is usually ill equipped to handle either the host of other diseases that may affect the patient or the righteous wrath of the referring physician.

SOME PRACTICAL POINTERS

A miscellany of do's and don't's may ease the passage of the new radiotherapist into private practice:

1. Do look over a new position on the scene before accepting it. If possible, work on a short-term or locum basis before making the commitment. The most responsible job offers are from those who spell out their disadvantages along with their advantages. The therapist, in turn, should indicate what he has to offer as well as what he wants.

2. Do maintain your equanimity no matter how provoked by circumstances, e.g., a peevish patient, a belligerent relative, an impatient physician. Losing one's composure, no matter how provoked, never helps a situation.

3. Do spend plenty of time with the patient, particularly at the first visit, including a detailed history and physical since this is the best way to get to know him. Work through the nature of his tumor with him and his spouse. Be frank but realistically encouraging. Take plenty of time with the consent form.

4. Do emphasize to the patient the importance of his other physicians and their necessary role in helping restore him to health.

5. Do maintain a sense of humor. Don't be afraid to put an arm around the patient, to rejoice with him at small triumphs, to listen to family troubles (which often explains symptoms ascribed to radiations).

6. Don't neglect the importance of relating to voluntary agencies such as the American Cancer Society. Often their volunteer drivers are the ones responsible for getting your patients to you. The Visiting Nurses Association and similar groups can play an important role in maintaining good nursing care in the home where patients need this type of support or where there are severe reactions to treatment. When they call upon you to serve on committees or give talks to lay groups, be sure to accept. It can only help your practice. Be happy to give tours of your office and equipment.

7. Don't take a hospital percentage of the net contract or a salary, unless you are in a teaching situation.

8. Do carry adequate malpractice insurance; at least $1-3 million in these times.

9. Do join your County Medical Society. Simultaneously join the Union of American Physicians.

10. Do play a role in the internal affairs of your hospital medical staff. Volunteer for a committee or two and serve seriously and faithfully.

11. Don't be afraid to talk to the respected physicians of integrity on your staff and to ask for advice in critical political situations. Obviously this is best done in advance of trouble, if possible.

12. Do keep precise and legible treatment records and notes, preferably typed and initialed. Give an annual or biennial report to the medical staff on the statistics of cases treated and consultations. Discuss at that time in detail some especially interesting cases.

PATHS AHEAD

Several writers have addressed the task of ensuring that the patient receives the best treatment and yet remains within the setting of the community hospital or office management. Certainly a heavy proportion of cancer patients in this country will find it, at the least, inconvenient to be transported long distances to major cancer treatment centers. One alternative is hospitalization, now prohibitively expensive, at such centers during a course of therapy. Funding agencies are not in the temper to permit that approach, and ordinarily being an inpatient during radiation therapy is both unnecessary and psychologically unsound. The concept of a domiciliary facility adjacent to major hospitals has not caught on in the United States, but is effective in smaller countries such as Great Britain. It has the advantage that low-cost temporary housing with kitchen facilities could be provided for patient and spouse. The closest American version of this approach is the motel, though costs remain high for the family and eating all meals out neither ensures good nourishment nor eases the financial drain.

We are left then with the community hospital-private office concept of radiotherapy to care for many cancer patients. Actually, it may be a uniquely American solution that the cancer patient can get personalized service with quality of care equal to if not better than that provided by major cancer centers (21) if certain conditions are met: adequately trained physicians and personnel, supervoltage facilities, and supporting services such as physics and dosimetry on a regular and quality-controlled basis. A logical extension of this is to tie in such community facilities with a major teaching center. Several years ago Dr. Charles Stetson (28), then president of the American Radium Society, spelled out the problem and pointed toward a solution: ◦ . . The development of specialized cancer facilities must be a cooperative venture among groups of hospitals . . . One man centers treating fewer patients cannot be justified any longer." Now in the late 1970s and early 1980s some efforts (13) are being made, with signal success, in this direction. It may be that the joint center with its major cooperating hospitals and centralized resources will become the pattern. Such centers provide a horizontal department of radiotherapy in that the therapists work primarily at their community facilities and maintain frequent contact with referring physicians, yet are simultaneously the staff or faculty members of the central major center. Select patients can be treated at the central facility, e.g., with electron or high LET irradiation or where major professional backup is required such as elaborate treatment preparation involving anesthesia, high-energy photons, etc. Yet the follow-up can be done in the community facility or hospital of origin by the radiotherapist involved initially. With such a system the patient has the best chance for optimum treatment; there is a better opportunity for keeping the referring physician content since he is well informed at all steps; and the radiotherapist has the advantage of being welcomed at patient conferences and ward rounds at the major center and of playing a vital role therein.

SECTION II. THE LAW OF MEDICAL MALPRACTICE: ITS CONTACT POINTS WITH RADIATION THERAPY

OVERVIEW

The legal system in the United States touches upon more than just crimes and lawsuits. It includes an increasing array of regulations by administrative agencies at federal, state, and local levels. As shown in Section I, radiation rules and regulations set out by the various federal and state agencies concerned with radiation protection have established the norms for individual exposure, safety requirements, and equipment control and licensing. In this section, however, we will focus on the troublesome issue of medical malpractice and how it impinges on the radiotherapist.

Civil actions ordinarily involve one person or entity suing another, unlike criminal actions where the state (or society) is the plaintiff. A judgment in a civil action means that someone will have to pay in damages, and customarily does not imply a jail term or guilt. An example of civil action at the federal level is an antitrust suit against a major corporation doing business in more than one state, while in state courts a common civil action is a tort.

Legal scholars have wrestled with the definition of a tort over the years. Basically it consists of a civil wrong committed by one person against another (excluding breach of contract), for which the law gives the remedy of an action for damages. There are many types of torts, some intentional, some not. Battery is one type of intentional tort, involving a harmful or offensive touching without consent. Thus body contact in a football game is not battery because the players have given their consent, either formally or by implication. Similarly a person standing in line to receive a vaccination, even though not speaking English, impliedly gives consent when she holds her arm out to receive the abrasions. In recent years with medical cases the requirement that the consent be informed has emerged, and lawyers and defendants in this country wrestle daily with the definition of just how much information informed consent requires. The surgeon operating for a ruptured appendix with a specific consent form signed by the patient may find that more pathology is present in the abdomen than just the appendix. If he has to remove part of the colon and a complication develops from this deliberate act, he may be liable for battery if the patient chooses to bring an action against him.

Some states have defined lack of informed consent as a separate tort entirely, when it involves medical procedures. Where an untoward outcome results but no intentional harmful touching and no negligence occurred, a suit just for lack of informed consent may yield an award for the plaintiff.

Another cause of action, not in tort but in contract, is the breach of warranty. Much as in the warranty for a manufactured product, when a physician guarantees or warrants the results of his procedure, he may be liable for any less than perfect result. This should be distinguished from words of reassurance. Statements like "You'll look just as good as new after your nose-bobbing operation" or "You won't be able to tell where the cancer was after we finish irradiating your nose" are the type of things that lead to such suits (29).* Particularly where the outcome is unexpected but negligence cannot be shown, this is a potential cause of action.

---

* One case held in dictum that there were qualitative differences between physicians' contracts and others' since the doctor's therapeutic reassurance that his patient will be all right must not be converted into a binding promise by the disappointed or quarrelsome.

Far and away, however, the most common cause of action in a medical misadventure is negligence. Here no intention is required. The action stems from a relationship between two persons wherein one has a duty of care toward the other. Thus, the person who buys a rail ticket for a journey can assume that the carrier will provide her with a safe journey, and if an accident occurs to which the passenger has not contributed, the carrier will usually be liable in damages for injuries sustained. In like manner the relationship between doctor and patient implies that the doctor has a duty of care toward that patient, and the standard of his conduct is judged by that of the reasonable physician acting in his situation. If he is a specialist, the standard is that of the equivalent specialist in the same situation. In former years the standard differed depending on whether the physician worked in a rural area or in the large city where it was assumed he was more in touch with medical advances. With the coming of the jet and electronic age, however, this locality rule has largely withered except in a few jurisdictions.

In negligence, after showing what the standard of care is, the plaintiff must prove, usually by the testimony of expert witnesses, that the defendant doctor (or hospital or physicist, etc.) violated that standard. This ordinarily requires testimony by physicians in the same field as the defendant, because of the medical complexity of most cases. No expert would be needed for the jury to infer negligence where a scissors is left in the abdomen by a surgeon, but most cases are not so straightforward. The defendant may also employ his own experts, and it is left to the jury to decide to whom to give greater credence, considering the facts of the case and attendant circumstances.

There are other elements for the plaintiff to prove, however. He must show that the doctor's dereliction from duty was not only the actual cause of the injury claimed but that it was close enough in time to the injury to be the source of the damage, and that there was no foreseeable intervening injury that could have interrupted the chain of causation. Thus, for example, where a radiotherapist delivers doses of the order of 6000-7000 rads into the pelvis for prostate carcinoma there is a significant chance of late radiation injury to small bowel and bladder and other organs within the beams. If the patient later brings an action in negligence, he will have to show that the radiation injury to the bowel was the proximate cause of the subsequent perforation and fistula. And where the therapist can point to a later attempt at radical prostatectomy (in which he was not involved) the radiotherapy will not be considered to be the proximate cause of the plaintiff's injuries. Of course, such a case of doctors accusing each other practically ensures a result for the plaintiff, if the surgeon is also named in the suit.

Two other requirements in negligence are that an injury must have resulted and that the plaintiff has not contributed to the injury. Thus, if I drive an auto 75 mph down a crowded avenue past a school in session, that is certainly negligent behavior. But if I do not hit anything (or frighten any parents into having a heart attack) there is no basis for an action in negligence. There has to be an actual injury for a case to stand. In medicine this does not imply that there has to be a good outcome. Some cases receiving irradiation may not be benefited in the least. If, however, what we do harms them, then we may be liable.

The plaintiff must not have contributed to her own injury. For example, the patient postmastectomy and postirradiation develops a swollen arm. She sues the surgeon and radiotherapist in negligence. But at trial it comes out that she is a professional bowler and bowls for several hours 3 nights a week with that arm. Certainly she has contributed to her own injury and defendant may escape liability on that basis. An enterprising plaintiff's attorney, however, will also have filed a cause of action in lack of informed consent alleging that the doctors should have informed the patient that extensive use and pressure on the lymphatics of that arm would not be prudent. A much closer case. Some states follow the doctrine of contributory negligence by the patient on an all or none basis, i.e., if the patient has herself been even minimally at fault, negligence by the defendant is not sufficient for damages. Other states follow, and the trend is toward comparative negligence, i.e., the degree of fault on a percentage basis is estimated and this subtracted from the damages.

INFORMED CONSENT

The physician who treats patients with cancer needs some guidelines as to how "informed" informed consent must be. On the one hand we have an instinctive feeling that the patient should know what she is in for; on the other hand, we do not want to so frighten her in naming all remotely possible consequences of treatment or no treatment as to ruin the doctor-patient relationship. The seminal case of Cobbs v. Grant (8) indicated many of the specific details that should be spelled out in an informed consent, while at the same time stating that a minicourse in medical science was not required. That case held that where a given procedure inherently involved a known risk of death or serious bodily harm, the doctor had certain duties of disclosure, viz., the explanation in lay terms of any complications that might possibly occur. The scope of the physician's duty to the patient must be measured by the patient's need, and that need is whatever is material to his decision.

How can we translate this into a vehicle for conveying information to the cancer patient without terrorizing him? The physician (not a nurse or technician) should explain: (1) the procedure, (2) its purpose, (3) risks, (4) likely consequences with and without treatment, (5) alternatives available, and (6) advantages and disadvantages of one course of treatment over another. Once this has been done, he should be certain the patient understands, repeating the explanation to a relative if necessary, and then memorialize the discussion in two steps: (1) by writing or dictating a note in his records indicating the substance of the conversation, identifying the patient's responses and (2) by having the patient sign a specific customized consent form containing the essential points of the conversation. Fig. 1 is an example of a thorough specific consent form for a patient scheduled for surgery following a radiation complication. Frustrating as it may seem, this is still not enough to ensure that the patient has received truly informed consent, as will be indicated in the next section. It will go much further, however, to evidence an intent to inform than many of the consent forms now used. As a record made in the ordinary course of business, it is entitled to great weight in the event of subsequent litigation. There is no duty to make disclosure of risks when the patient decides of his own free will that he does not wish to be so informed. This too must be evidenced in the chart. The obligation to inform exists even if the patient tells the therapist to do whatever he thinks is right.

Increasingly frequent causes of action for medical malpractice based on negligence are linked with allegations of lack of informed consent, particularly where the outcome is untoward but it cannot be shown that the physician was other than conscientious. As in all questions of medical negligence, if due care is used, the physician is not liable for unfortunate results (12), though he is liable for negligent departure from customary and accepted standards used in exposing patients to x-rays (24).

General
Plastic
Vascular
Thoracic Surgery
Endoscopy

4528 W. Cermak Rd.
Chicago, Illinois 60625
Telephone: (312) 384-2000

Date: January 12, 1975 - 10:30 a.m.

Dr. Goodman has explained to me the full extent of the surgical procedure designed to bring tissue with good blood supply to the posterior vagina and eliminate the painful irradiated tissue.

This may take months to heal properly. The entrance to the vagina will be full of pubic hair. This hair may be removed by electrolysis later, if desired.

I realize that adequate sexual function cannot be guaranteed. Some numbness may be expected for a time, but eventual full sensation is hoped for. An additional procedure to enlarge the opening of the vagina may be necessary at some time, months later, but every attempt to avoid this will be made.

Possible complications include wound disruption, infection, hematosis or excessive bleeding, rectovaginal fistula, urinary infection, and slough of the flaps.

Signed______________________

Witness:

____

Figure 1. John L. Goodman, M.D., P.C.

A patient at a VA Hospital was given preoperative irradiation for rectal cancer with a dosage far in excess of normal. Resulting reactions led to permanent injury. Defendant doctors justified their departure from standard treatment on the basis of a research paper delivered at a recent conference. The radiologists admitted that the patient was not told the procedure was experimental, and the court held that damages could be based not only on negligence but on failure to obtain informed consent (4,14).

Where a patient is a minor, parental consent must be obtained before treatment is begun. With an incompetent or senile patient the guardian or near relative should sign the consent form. Emergency situations, though rare in radiation therapy, are instances where consent need not be obtained before starting treatment where the standard of practice is to treat such conditions. Actually, most urgent treatment situations are accompanied by a cooperative patient.

Another variant on informed consent is the situation when a patient leaves the hospital against medical advice, or terminates treatment unilaterally despite your best efforts. Here again you are presented with the task of informing him, and a relative if available, about risks of stopping treatment. He must be aware of what he can expect with tumor spread. Put the substance of the conversation in your notes, write him a letter about it with a copy for the file, and call the referring physician to help in reasoning with him. If he hints at or wants consultation, be happy to arrange it. Forget the ego problem. If your opinion is wrong, you should be happy to have it corrected; if right, it will be pleasant to have it reinforced.

There are many cases where an unexpected outcome is the sole basis of the suit. In effect the patient says "If I had known this would have happened to me, I never would have consented to the treatment," and the doctor must show that indeed the patient was informed that such an outcome was possible, not always an easy thing to do. Even the best of consent forms do not cover every eventuality, and a resourceful plaintiff's attorney can show that a signed consent form, even though naming specifically the possible injury, does not constitute informed consent. His basis for this will be the contention that the relation between doctor and patient is inherently unequal, that the patient is relatively helpless in such a situation and is coerced into signing whatever form the doctor presents, particularly with a disease like cancer where the patient has little choice but to accept the recommended treatment, fearing disease and death as the alternative. It is one thing to explain the details of treatment, but quite another to spell out potential consequences. In cancer practice many of us leave the patient with but little choice of acceptance of treatment or not. The relationship is inherently unequal, and to balance that fact we must take exquisite care to see that patients and their relatives know what to expect, no matter how remote, if such complications can be profound.

In a perceptive essay relating to the rights of patients undergoing experimental treatment, John Fletcher (10) probes the factors impinging on the patient to limit his autonomy. Foremost is the threat of serious illness. Second, arrangements at august medical institutions tend to diminish the patient's willingness to complain or question. This is particularly true where treatment is free and the disease is life threatening. Third, the investigator's expectations for the patient are a strong force which may operate to limit the subject's freedom. The patient is eager not to disappoint. In greater or lesser degrees those factors operate in clinical situations at all levels, from the Clinical Center at the National Institutes of Health to the smallest community hospital. We may realistically ask: "How informed can a consent be? Does the patient ever have absolute freedom of decision?"

It is human nature to reflect ruefully on the outcome of a course of action where it turns out unfortunately, and to blame someone else for the mishap. How is the physician to protect himself from the disgruntled patient who insists she would not have consented if she had been adequately informed? Courts in the various states are provided with model jury instructions which attorneys can request the judge to make just before the jury retires to consider its decisions. One from California (7) may serve as an example of how to deal with the human nature question posed above: " . . . Even though the patient has consented to a proposed treatment . . . the failure of the physician . . . to inform the patient . . . before obtaining such consent is negligence and renders the physician . . . subject to liability for any injury (proximately) resulting from the treatment if a reasonably prudent person in the patient's position would not have consented to the treatment if he had been adequately informed of all the significant perils." It is perhaps particularly true in cancer work that an inherent coercion of the patient exists, and we recognize this when we go through the ritual of having the patient sign a consent form before beginning treatment. The ritual is important, nonetheless, not just to protect ourselves from potential liability for lack of informed consent, but also as a form of protection to the dignity of the patient as we work through the form of the ritualistic words with compassion and understanding. Both actors in this scene know that the patient does not have much of a choice. Once the therapist and referring physician have reasoned through to their decisions, the patient is truly in a dependent and unequal position with them. This may be the moment in the entire history of the case calling for the utmost tact and gentleness. The patient's decision, unless irrational, will be to go along with that of her doctors. That very inequality of discussions is all the more reason for painstaking care in working through the case once again with the patient.

DIAGNOSTIC PROBLEMS

Surgeons and pathologists are occasionally sued for failure to perform a biopsy or for misinterpretation of results. Where the reasonably careful physician would determine that a biopsy is indicated before treatment, failure to advise or perform the procedure may constitute negligence.

The physician or gynecologist who watches an ovarian mass or cyst slowly enlarge over several months may find himself the target of a malpractice suit if the jury believes an expert who testifies that 1 or 2 months at most is the longest one should wait on such a case. Even if the subsequent surgery for ovarian carcinoma is successful in eradicating the cancer, or even if the tumor would have been incurable in any case, juries and courts may hold that such delay evidenced a lack of due care and either that treatment would have been easier (9) on the one hand or that it would have made for a more comfortable and pleasant existence on the other.

While an incorrect diagnosis of cancer often leads to unnecessary surgery and presumably considerable mental suffering, the reverse is more serious. Where there is failure to diagnose cancer (false negative), the result can lead to the death of the patient and extremely high jury awards are likely to ensue. Formerly expiration of the statute of limitations was the usual good defense, but recent changes in the law whereby the statute does not begin to run until the negligence is discovered have altered that. Thus, in a New York case (18) the physician concluded that the patient had Hodgkin disease and treated the patient for 10 years before checking on the tests. The original diagnosis was incorrect but the court held that the statute of limitations was a good defense. Such a verdict would probably now go for the patient, since courts in recent years have used the discovery doctrine to expand the time limit within which suits must be brought.

What lessons can radiotherapists learn from these cases? Although delay in diagnosis of malignancy does not usually lie at the therapist's doorstep initially, it is worth noting that where the therapist practices radiation oncology and follows up previously treated patients, he may, in theory, be liable should there be any undue delay in diagnosis of further manifestations of cancer. There are no cases on this point as yet. The cancer patient is not the type of person who ordinarily is prone to bring suit, particularly where her original treatment was carefully and conscientiously given. But it must be said that one of the primary purposes of follow-up is to detect signs of recurrence, metastasis, or new disease, and where that diagnosis is fumbled or unaccountably delayed, the radiotherapist may find himself at the receiving end of a malpractice action based on negligence.

More likely is the fact that treatment not based on histological confirmation is fraught with hazard. In my opinion the radiotherapist should review with the hospital pathologist personally any cases which could be considered at all equivocal. The surgeon, after all, takes extreme care to be sure of the histologic diagnosis before performing a mastectomy. Should the radiotherapist do less merely because his weapon is an invisible ray? The therapist should insist upon having the microscopic slides sent where any outside cases are referred for consultation or treatment and should review this material with his pathologist. The long-term radiation effects and potential liability are both too profound to do anything less.

We are led next to the question: "When will you treat in the absence of a histologic diagnosis?" My answer is almost never. Certainly there are instances where biopsy is realistically not attainable, e.g., in some expanding lesions of the brain stem, for reasons of excessive morbidity or mortality from the biopsy procedure itself. There also are cases where the clinical and roentgenographic appearance is so characteristic, and the attempt at biopsy sufficiently morbid, to make it acceptable to proceed to treatment without histologic confirmation. Thus, an adult with acromegaly and an expansile lesion of the pituitary can be treated with the diagnosis of eosinophilic adenoma without resort to biopsy. But be careful, for example, of treating superior vena caval obstruction in haste because the chest film may show an upper mediastinal widening. And before placing beams on a man with medically inoperable presumed bronchus carcinoma, at least try to have a positive sputum cytology or mediastinal tomograms showing carina splaying or tracheal compression.

One of the reasons given for the rising cost of medical care is the increasing practice of defensive medicine by physicians, largely due to the threat of being sued for overlooking a diagnosis. In 1975 insurance companies seemed to quadruple their rates while simultaneously staging a mass exodus from the field of underwriting medical liability insurance. Numbers of claims and jury verdicts rose geometrically. Most of the increased premium costs were passed on to patients. National hospital expenditures totaled $46.6 billions in 1975, and if even 5% of all hospital costs were in fact for defensive practices, the total national cost of defensive medicine in hospitals alone is of the order of $2 billion per year. In a 1978 report (11) Gerg et al. attribute 8% of all laboratory charges and 15% of diagnostic x-ray charges to defensive medical practices. Radiotherapists are not especially vulnerable to the charge of practicing defensive medicine, since most lab studies are indeed indicated during and following treatment. Reflex ordering of expensive scans, films, and laboratory tests, however, is not sound radiotherapy practice.

Failure to diagnose properly is responsible for roughly 14% of claims, while improper treatment accounts for 86% overall. Forty percent of claims result in eventual payment, and although the median payment has been small ($2000), three percent of claims will exceed $100,000 (25). About 18-20% of the premium dollar is returned to the patient, suggesting that the current restitution system leaves something to be desired both in efficiency and fairness. No figures are available for the typical radiotherapeutic misadventure, but it is probably safe to assume that claims will probably be for rather profound and chronic side effects for the most part and will be for substantial sums. On the other hand, the cancer patient is ordinarily in the geriatric group, grateful for care, and not prone to sue for the untoward outcome, unless there has been gross negligence or she has been totally misinformed.

MALPRACTICE INSURANCE

The rising cost of insurance premiums has prompted many physicians to "go bare" in the states where this is allowed. Their reasoning includes a reluctance to pass along these increased fees to the patient as well as a general outrage at outlandish jury awards of recent years. It seems to me that being uninsured is shortsighted, primarily because the physician has become the middleman in a redistribution of resources when the patient suffers a catastrophe. While granting that cases of medical negligence do occur and are compensable, I submit that there are many instances in which an unfortunate outcome in the absence of negligence results in a medical and financial catastrophe for the patient, and that juries determine such events should be compensable. Casting about for a rationale upon which to base a claim, they may seize upon or believe that lack of informed consent is as good a basis as any upon which to base an award. After all, the physician is, or ought to be, heavily insured, and the depth of that insurance pocket may be the currently most acceptable way for society to restore balance in the interest of the injured patient. Unfortunately for the physician such an award carries with it a stigma concerning his competence, deserved or not. If he is uninsured, it may also carry a back-breaking liability of future payment obligations or wreck his medical practice. Some potential solutions include: (1) basing malpractice awards on an unfortunate outcome basis, thus compensating patients on a no-fault system (26), similar to auto insurance liability statutes now operative in several states; (2) setting up scales of compensation for patients similar to those in various workers' compensation schemes for industrial injury, where again no permanent stigma attaches to the author of the injury; and (3) requiring "catastrophic" insurance on every person, either supplied by the employer or by government with or without the individual's contribution for medical costs above a certain amount, e.g., $25,000.

In 1978 in California, a state court decision (5) may have made "going bare" an unacceptable risk for physicians for another reason. In that case involving several defendants it was determined that the percentage of liability of each would be assessed according to his percentage of fault, as determined by the jury. Heretofore, the uninsured defendant would often not be named by the plaintiff since he would often be judgment proof, at least as to significant amounts. Where there were several defendants, the plaintiff would go only after those sure to be susceptible of goodly financial remuneration, such as hospitals or insured physicians. This case, however, makes it far more likely that uninsured defendants will be brought in, if not by plaintiffs then almost surely by their codefendants (and their insurers), so that they will have their percentages of fault determined and thereby reduce the relative amounts of liability incurred by those insured.

Most forms of medical liability insurance written up to 1975 were of the occurrence type, i.e., the physician was insured for any actionable act or omission that occurred during the time when the insurance was in force, regardless of when the claim was made. Where a physician carried insurance in 1970, for example, and during that year irradiated a child with a plantar wart, if 20 years later (long after the physician had retired and ceased carrying insurance) the patient developed cancer in the irradiated area and sued the physician for malpractice, the doctor would be covered by his insurance policy written in 1970. It is quite another question, of course, whether the limits of his 1970 liability policy would be sufficient to compensate the patient in the eyes of a jury which had lived with inflation for the ensuing 20 years.

The occurrence-type policy, therefore, served well during a period such as that up to about 1970 when awards were fairly modest and inflation had not become rampant. As awards and incidence of claims began to rise steeply during the 1970s, however, two things became obvious: (1) Insurers jumped their annual premiums drastically and began to leave the underwriting market as the medical liability business became less profitable and (2) it became increasingly difficult for physicians not only to pay the higher premiums required but to predict what kind of coverage they would need for an award that might not be decided until many years later.

A partial solution to this problem has been the claims-made medical liability insurance policy (16). Such coverage insures the physician for any claims that are filed during the period that the policy is in effect. It can also insure him for any claims filed during that period arising from any acts, errors, or omissions prior to coverage except those he knew might result in a claim, and those otherwise insured by an occurrence-type policy. Where the individual retires or moves to another area, many companies provide for coverage by the doctor purchasing, at a percentage of the previous annual premium, "tail" coverage for the incurred but as yet unreported claims. Such policies provide the doctor with a much more accurate idea of costs, despite inflationary trends, and where such companies or self-insured trusts are sound physician-managed organizations, a significant savings in premium dollars can result. Radiotherapists will find themselves about halfway up the scale in premium dollars required, somewhere above internists and pediatricians and significantly below such high-risk occupations as obstetrics, orthopedics, plastic surgery, and anesthesiology.

RECORDS

Should a patient have access to his medical record? In all states such records can be subpoenaed where there is a legal action and many states require the physician or hospital to provide access for an authorized patient representative, and several directly to the patient in some circumstances. Four (31) require open access to the patient on request, and the statutes of Wisconsin and California even include sanctions for refusal to disclose requested records. It would appear that although ownership of records may remain with doctor or hospital, the trend is toward permitting open access to the patient or his representative.

Patient-carried records are a recent innovation and have much to commend them. Certainly in our modern consumer-oriented and sophisticated society there is little need to hide anything from the patient apart from psychiatric notes and where the patient would be disturbed by reading gloomy prognostic details. The American Society of Internal Medicine has endorsed a two-tiered system, delivering to the patient the permanent or official record on his request and maintaining coownership of that portion. The active working portion of the record is kept by the physician (still reachable by subpoena) and contains material of subjective nature, working hypotheses, speculations, etc. My own practice is to hand over all records and notes to our patients for their perusal any time they wish, not, however, to be taken from the department. Such records can be subpoenaed, of course, and we copy and mail (or better, give to the patient to hand carry) to any physician to which follow-up care is to be transferred.

The actual record of radiation therapy daily treatments or data sheet is written in ink once the daily treatments have been given. We do not make erasures, but if a mistake is made, a simple stroke through the incorrect numerals with the correct figure placed alongside is much more satisfactory. Attempted erasures are never perfect, and they always raise the query "Have these records been altered?" in the mind of the reviewer (27). And altered records, no matter how well intended, mean a lost case if doses of radiation are in question.

A RADIOTHERAPIST'S PHILOSOPHY

I am not especially sanguine that an early or simple solution of the malpractice problem can be achieved. Perhaps uniquely among professionals, the physician is puzzled when he is charged with malpractice and may become defensively stubborn. This attitude works against his best interests. Part of the problem may be that as physicians we are unaccustomed to being accused of negligent behavior, let alone admitting that we have made mistakes. It would serve us better, I submit, to look at malpractice in much the same light as we look at liability for misfunction of an automobile. I do not imply that the consequences are not far more serious, but only that no one is perfect, least of all the physician. The human body has enough variations in physiology, in reactions to drugs, and in responses to treatment that it is only surprising that untoward outcomes do not occur more often that they do. Perhaps among those who deal with cancer in particular might it be said that we skate perpetually on thin ice. Daily we deal with an inexorable disease, with patients often old and frail, and with therapeutic agents powerful and potentially lethal. The surprise is that there are not more claims against radiotherapists for "therapeutic misadvantures." The reasons would include the very fact that not much is expected with a patient doomed to die without treatment. Not much of what we do is really elective.

How often do we hear a physician admit a mistake? And yet that may be the one best preventive for an action in negligence. The doctor who sees that a misdiagnosis occurred or an untoward result of therapy happened, is well-advised to say to the patient or relative: "I'm sorry, we tried our best but overlooked this approach" or "Mrs. Jones, I miscalculated on your treatment dose. We'll watch your reaction very carefully for the next several weeks. Please call me if you have any symptoms in between visits." Patients do not want to sue doctors. What they cannot stand, however, is being condescended to, being talked down to, and covering up. Do these things and you are asking for a suit.

I am sure that there are many unconscious reasons why the physician has a particular horror of suit. The physician is hurt because he is accused of negligence, whereas the lawyer or other professional would not have the same emotional reaction were he in a similar position. We cannot understand why patients should be so ungrateful when we have only tried to help them. It may be that as physicians we are accustomed to the image of being looked up to by the patient; and the expression "Doctors who play God" may have more than a grain of truth in it. I think we unconsciously start believing that what we are doing for the patient must be right (otherwise why would we be doing it?) and we find it particularly ego-shattering to be challenged on that ground.

STRATEGY WHEN SUED

But what if we are beyond prophylaxis, and you have been served with a complaint, what then?

1. As indicated before, carry adequate malpractice insurance. Do not try to go bare. The risks and consequences are not worth it.

2. Do not deal with opposing lawyers directly. Notify your insurance carrier.

3. Tell your lawyer all the facts. Conceal nothing. The lawyer-client privilege will prevent others from probing these disclosures to him. Any questionable things should be related to him. When concealed, they may turn into unpleasant courtroom surprises.

4. Do not try to change your records to clarify your case. Changes are easily detected, and if brought to the attention of a jury, regardless of the merits of your case, you have lost.

5. Misplaced records are also hard to explain. Therefore, when you become aware that an action is brewing, put them in a safe place. Keep a second file containing correspondence on the case and your notes on it separate

from the patient's chart, since it will not be protected by the attorney-client privilege if the chart is subpoenaed and your notes are handed over along with the chart.

6. Research the details in the case. Keep lists of local and national experts on potential points you think may be inquired into in the case. These can help your defense attorney.

7. Keep another list of leading articles and texts helpful to him in his research.

8. Do not discuss the case with your colleagues and friends. Such information has a peculiar way of getting back to the opposition and may give them useful points to probe.

9. Try to relax. Being sued puts you in an elite group. Many very illustrious physicians have been named in complaints. There will be some unaccustomed stress ahead, but you have faced and overcome tougher problems, like getting into medical school, for instance.

CONCLUSIONS

Large awards are becoming a societal mechanism whereby injured patients are compensated for grievous financial loss. Juries intuitively understand that such a loss must be compensated by damages, at least until some fairer coverage of catastrophe can be devised. The physician may be the person caught in the middle of this dilemma, being the unintentional victim of a social injustice in that he is considered as having the pocket deep enough, via insurance, to compensate the patient for an untoward result and financial catastrophe. Part of this, but only a part, stems from rights and entitlements of the patient in the late twentieth century. Unfortunate side effects for the physician are damage to his reputation, regardless of any fault, and being called to account by various state medical boards. He may suffer loss of referrals and certainly will experience an unaccustomed form of stress.

Major overhaul of the tort system is not the answer, though some steps in that direction may help. An injury caused by a negligent act deserves fair compensation, and minor adjustments in the laws, e.g., limiting attorney contingent fees and requiring screening panels before lawsuits are filed, may restore some balance and reason to awards as well as discouraging nuisance suits. It remains unfortunately true that the major cause of medical malpractice awards is medical malpractice.

Pending a longer-term resolution of the medical liability problem, the physician would be well advised to carry adequate malpractice insurance, preferably on a <u>claims-made</u> basis and using a physician-sponsored insurance company with a good track record. The physicist should likewise carry such a policy, if he is an independent contractor.

Given the fact that the traditional doctor-patient relationship (authority figure vs. dependent figure) is deteriorating, whether or not spurred by the malpractice crisis, this may not be altogether unfortunate, since it may lead to a greater willingness by the patient to assume more responsibility for his own health.

The radiation therapist is well advised to give particular attention to the details of securing informed consent for the treatment of his patients. He should be at least as meticulous about this as he is about the details of treatment itself. He should carefully explain the patient's diagnosis and the treatment planned. He must outline short and long-term side effects. He must indicate alternatives to treatment. This should be documented on a suitable consent form and a note summarizing the discussion placed in the patient's chart. If this means spending an extra half-hour or so again with the patient and her relatives, spend it.

Informed consent is important so that patients know what to expect and what the alternatives are, but may not be much of a legal hazard for radiotherapists because of the notion that the reasonably prudent patient would not refuse treatment where the alternative is an inexorable downhill course.

Prophylaxes against malpractice suits for radiotherapist and physicist: Work together on quality control in details of daily treatment and planning. Double-check calculations. Run a beam output check each day. Repeat calibrations whenever any electrical or equipment change is made in a treatment room or whenever any work is done by outside manufacturers, e.g., beam-alignment lasers installed, beam modifiers constructed, changes in x-ray tubes or wave guides, etc. Do not treat cancer, with the exceptions noted, without a histological diagnosis.

REFERENCES

1. A Guide for Radiologists, American College of Radiology, Chicago, 1977.
2. A Guide for Radiologists, American College of Radiology, Chicago, 1977, p. 5.
3. A Guide for Radiologists, American College of Radiology, Chicago, 1977, p. 9.
4. Ahern, v.: Veterans' Administration, 537 F 2d, 1098, CCA 10, 1976.
5. American Motorcycle Assn. v. Superior Court, 20 Cal. 3d 578 P. 2d, 899, 146 Cal. Rptr. 182 (1978).
6. Buck, M.L.: How to Build a More Rewarding Medical Practice, Executive Reports Corp., Engelwood Cliffs, N.J., 1970.
7. Calif. BAJI 6.11 (1977 rev.) Reality of Consent - (emphasis supplied).
8. Cobbs v. Grant, 104 Cal. Rptr. 505, 502, P. 2d 1, 8 Cal. 3d 229.
9. Cullum v. Seifer, 81 Cal. Rptr. 381, Cal. 1969.
10. Fletcher, J.: Realities of patient consent to medical research. In Biomedical Ethics and the Law, edited by J. Humber and R. Almeder, New York, Plenum Press, 1976.
11. Gerg, M.L., Glieve, W.A., and Elkhatib, M.B.: The extent of defensive medicine: Some empirical evidence. Legal Aspects of Medical Practice 6:25, 1978.
12. Gore v. Brockman, 119 S.W. 1082, Mo. 1909.
13. Hellman, S.: The joint center for radiation therapy. In Frontiers in Radiation Therapy and Oncology, Vol. 8, Baltimore, Karger, 1973, pp. 76-80.
14. Holder, A.R.: Medical Malpractice Law, 2nd edition, New York, Wiley, 1978, p. 150.

15. Independent Practice: A Guide from the ACR, 1977, American College of Radiology, Chicago.

16. Kroll, S.: The professional liability policy "claims made." Forum 13: 842, 1978.

17. Lynch, P.: Radiation therapy in a small community. In Progress in Radiation Therapy, Vol. II, edited by F. Buschke, New York, Grune and Stratton, 1962.

18. McQuinn v. St. Lawrence County Laboratory, 283 NYS ed. 747, N.Y., 1967.

19. Moss, W.: Opinion: Out of the frying pan into the fire. Radiology 118:741, 1976.

20. Osler, Sir W.: Nurse and Patient in Aequanimitas, 3nd edition, Philadelphia, Blakiston's, 1932, p. 159.

21. Phillips, R.: Current work and future plans of the Russell A. Firestone Radiation Treatment Center. Cancer 22:697, 1968.

22. Planning Guide for Radiologic Installations - Fascicle I: Radiation Therapy Installations. Committee on Department Planning, American College of Radiology, Chicago, 1976.

23. Radetsky, M.: Sounding board: Recapturing the spirit in medicine. N. Engl. J. Med. 298:1142, 1978.

24. Simonaites, J.E.: Radiation therapy. JAMA 220:1807, 1972.

25. Rudov, M.H., Myers, T.I., and Mirabella, A.: Medical malpractice insurance claims files closed in 1970. In Report of the Secretary's Commission on Medical Malpractice, U.S. Department of Health, Education and Welfare, Washington, D.C., 1973.

26. Shapiro, E.: The history of medical malpractice in the United States. In The Influence of Litigation on Medical Practice, edited by C. Wood, New York, Grune and Stratton, 1977.

27. Shindell, S.: Medicolegal aspects of pelvic surgery. In Te Linde's Operative Gynecology, 5th edition, edited by R. Mattingly, Philadelphia, Lippincott, 1977, pp. 13-23.

28. Stetson, C.: Cancer management and radiotherapy centers. Am. J. Roentgenol. 91:3, 1965.

29. Stewart v. Rudner. (Mich. 1957) 349 Mich. 459, 84 N.W. 2d 816.

30. The Whys and Wherefores of Corporate Practice, Medical Economics Book Division, Oradell, N.J., 1970.

31. Tucker, G.: Patient access to medical records. Legal Aspects of Medical Practice 6:45, 1978.

INDEX